Management of Severe Traumatic Brain Injury

Terje Sundstrøm • Per-Olof Grände
Niels Juul • Carsten Kock-Jensen
Bertil Romner • Knut Wester
Editors

Management of Severe Traumatic Brain Injury

Evidence, Tricks and Pitfalls

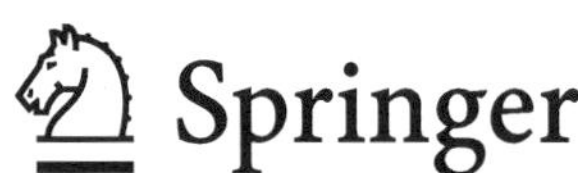

Editors
Terje Sundstrøm, M.D.
Department of Neurosurgery
Haukeland University Hospital
Bergen
Norway

Department of Surgical Sciences
and Department of Biomedicine
University of Bergen
Bergen
Norway

Per-Olof Grände, M.D., Ph.D.
Department of Anaesthesia
and Intensive Care
Lund University and Lund University
Hospital
Lund
Sweden

Niels Juul, M.D.
Department of Anaesthesia
Aarhus University Hospital
Aarhus C
Denmark

Carsten Kock-Jensen, M.D.
Department of Neurosurgery
Aarhus University Hospital
Aarhus C
Denmark

Bertil Romner, M.D., Ph.D.
Department of Neurosurgery
Copenhagen University Hospital
Copenhagen
Denmark

Knut Wester, M.D., Ph.D.
Department of Surgical Sciences
University of Bergen
Bergen
Norway

Department of Neurosurgery
Haukeland University Hospital
Bergen
Norway

ISBN 978-3-642-28125-9 ISBN 978-3-642-28126-6 (eBook)
DOI 10.1007/978-3-642-28126-6
Springer Heidelberg New York Dordrecht London

Library of Congress Control Number: 2012936153

Printed on acid-free paper

Springer is part of Springer Science+Business Media (www.springer.com)

Foreword I

The Scandinavian Neurotrauma Committee (SNC) with its President Carsten Kock-Jensen has done a real service for those who care for severe traumatic brain injury (TBI) patients. These comprehensive TBI management recommendations allow the practitioner easy access to triage decisions and all possible diagnostics and therapeutics from injury site through rehabilitation with supporting evidence. While it is based on local expertise, it is heavily supported by current literature – a combination that hopefully makes implementation that much easier.

The first step to improving TBI outcomes is to assess the literature. The next, more difficult step is implementation. Changing TBI practice is a mandate since it is proven to dramatically reduce morbidity and mortality. Application of the Brain Trauma Foundation Guidelines (www.braintrauma.org) has been proven to improve patient outcomes and significantly reduce costs due to better patient outcomes (Faul et al., *Journal of Trauma*, 2007):

1. Patients are twice as likely to survive if BTF guidelines are followed.
2. Proportion of patients with "good" outcomes rose from 35% to 66%.
3. Proportion of patients with "poor" outcomes fell from 34% to 19%.
4. Potential savings – $3.8 billion (US national).

Similarly, a 50% reduction in deaths, even adjusted for confounding factors such as age, GCS, pupils, hypotension, and CT characteristics, has been achieved in New York State over the last 10 years (BTF article in submission) with an active TBI quality assurance program supported by an Internet database (TBI-Trac) and a free guidelines assessment tool at www.tbiclickandlearn.com. The reduction in deaths was accompanied by an increase in intracranial pressure monitoring in those patients that were recommended to have monitoring as described in the BTF Guidelines.

Taking these Scandinavian TBI Guidelines and developing courses and tracking tools for compliance will ensure that the authors' hard work will not be in vain, and more importantly, many TBI patient lives will be saved and the quality of life improved.

Jamshid Gahjar, President,
The Brain Trauma Foundation

Foreword II

It is with great pleasure and with tremendous respect for the dedication and hard work performed by the Scandinavian Neurotrauma Committee (SNC), that I have witnessed the creation of the Scandinavian "Practical guide to the management of severe traumatic brain injury." The SNC, which was initiated by the Scandinavian Neurosurgical Society, has since its foundation been dedicated to updating the Scandinavian neurosurgeons, neurointensivists, and neuroanaesthesiologists on the optimal treatment of patients with traumatic brain injury (TBI). This is the third major publication by the SNC. The first publication in 2000 covered guidelines for the management of minimal, mild, and moderate head injuries, and this was followed in 2008 by guidelines for the prehospital management of severe TBI. Even though we consider Scandinavia as being one of the safest places on planet Earth, head injuries are still a major cause of morbidity and mortality, health-care costs, and catastrophic emotional turmoil for the victims and their families.

This book covers the subject of TBI from A to Z in a very systematic and evidence-based fashion, formulated in such a way that it presents smooth and easy reading. The recurring paragraphs of *Tips, tricks, and pitfalls* are an ingenious way of highlighting the essentials. This book is relevant, both for the trainees in all specialties involved in the management and treatment of patients with TBI, but also a well-written update for the seasoned physician – trauma treatment has improved. However, we should not only focus on what we can do for the head injured patients, i.e., preventing secondary brain injury, we should also get far more involved in preventing the primary brain injury. This means getting more involved in the political agenda and promoting trauma prevention initiatives.

I am very proud of the work performed by the SNC, and I am sure that you will enjoy reading this book as much as I did. It should be found in any and all units dealing with trauma patients.

Jannick Brennum, President,
The Scandinavian Neurosurgical Society

Acknowledgements

The SNC would especially like to acknowledge the following institutions, all the contributing authors and the sponsors of committee meetings. Without you, this book project would not have been possible. Thank you!

Institutions

The Brain Trauma Foundation
New York, USA

Department of Neurosurgery
Aarhus University Hospital
Aarhus, Denmark

Department of Anaesthesia and Intensive care
Aarhus University Hospital
Aarhus, Denmark

Department of Neurosurgery
Copenhagen University Hospital (Rigshospitalet)
Copenhagen, Denmark

Clinic for Neurosurgery
University Hospital of Oulu
Oulu, Finland

Department of Neurosurgery
Reykjavik University Hospital
Reykjavik, Iceland

Department of Neurosurgery
University Hospital of North Norway
Tromsø, Norway

Department of Neurosurgery
Haukeland University Hospital
Bergen, Norway

Department of Neurosurgery
Karolinska University Hospital
Stockholm, Sweden

Department of Anaesthesia and Intensive Care
University Hospital of Lund
Lund, Sweden

Department of Anaesthesia and Intensive Care
Halmstad Regional Hospital
Halmstad, Sweden

Department of Neurosurgery
Umeå University Hospital
Umeå, Sweden

Authors
Bellander, Bo-Michael
Bloomfeld, Eric
Brennum, Jannick
Dahl, Bent Lob
de Hoog, Bram
Enblad, Per
Engström, Martin
Eskesen, Vagn
Feldt-Rasmussen, Ulla
Fink-Jensen, Vibeke
Gahjar, Jamshid
Grände, Per-Olof
Guttormsen, Anne Berit
Hermansson, Ann
Hernæs, Jennie
Hillered, Lars
Howells, Tim
Ingebrigtsen, Tor
Johnsen, Birger
Juul, Niels
Frennström, Jan
Kauppinen, Mikko
Klose, Marianne
Kock-Jensen, Carsten
Koefoed-Nielsen, Jacob
Kølsen-Petersen, Jens-Aage
Koskinen, Lars-Owe D.
Kvåle, Reidar
Langhorn, Leanne Enggaard
Marklund, Niklas
Møller, Jens Kjølseth
Naredi, Silvana
Nielsen, Rasmus Philip
Nielsen, Troels Halfeld
Nordström, Carl-Henrik
Olivecrona, Magnus
Rasmussen, Mads
Reinstrup, Peter
Riis, Jens Jakob
Romner, Bertil

Ronne-Engström, Elisabeth
Rønning, Pål André
Rosenlund, Christina
Skandsen, Toril
Skrede, Steinar
Sollid, Snorre
Sørensen, Leif Hovgaard
Springborg, Jacob Bertram
Steiness, Morten Zebitz
Sundstrøm, Terje
Tietze, Anna
Ulvik, Atle
Undén, Johan
Vik, Anne
Wang, Mikala
Welling, Karen Lise
Wester, Knut
Wulf-Eskildsen, Helle
Åstrand, Ramona

Sponsors
Meda Denmark
Codman Johnson & Johnson
Roche Diagnostics
Storz

Contents

Part VI Peroperative Anaesthesia

Part VII Monitoring in Neurointensive Care

Introduction

Terje Sundstrøm, Carsten Kock-Jensen, Niels Juul, Bertil Romner, and Knut Wester

TBI is a major cause of morbidity and mortality in the Nordic countries. About 200 per 100,000 inhabitants are each year admitted to hospital with a head injury (Ingebrigtsen et al. 2000a). The TBI mortality rate varies from around 10 per 100,000 in Denmark, Norway and Sweden, to approximately 20 per 100,000 in Finland (Sundstrøm et al. 2007). The management of TBI constitutes a tremendous organizational challenge to health-care professionals and health-care organizers. During the last two decades, physicians and health-care planners have increasingly understood the need to have organized and integrated systems of trauma care, reflecting the increased appreciation of quality assurance in modern health-care services.

Evidence-based guidelines for the practice of clinical medicine provide recommendations based on the best scientific evidence available. The Brain Trauma Foundation (BTF) published their first evidence-based guidelines for the management of severe TBI in 1995 (www.braintrauma.org). The second revised edition was published in 2000, and the latest edition in 2007. Several other TBI guidelines have also been developed, all aiming to improve the quality of care in and between prehospital services, primary hospitals, neurosurgical departments, neurointensive care units and rehabilitation facilities.

The Scandinavian Neurotrauma Committee (SNC) was founded after an initiative from the Scandinavian Neurosurgical Society in 1998 (www.neurotrauma.nu). The major objective of the SNC is to improve the management of neurotrauma patients in the Nordic countries. The committee is comprised of dedicated neurosurgeons, neurointensivists and neuroanaesthesiologists from Denmark, Finland, Iceland, Norway and Sweden (population 25 million, 21 neurosurgical centres). The SNC published guidelines for the management of minimal, mild and moderate head injuries in 2000 (Ingebrigtsen et al. 2000a, b; Romner et al. 2000a, b). These guidelines are implemented throughout most of the Nordic region. In 2008, guidelines for the prehospital management of severe traumatic head injury were published in collaboration with the Brain Trauma Foundation (BTF) in the USA (Bellander et al. 2008; Juul et al. 2008; Sollid et al. 2008).

The SNC decided in 2007, in cooperation with the BTF, to work for a comprehensive manual of TBI management throughout the entire chain of care. A major goal was to create a template for good TBI care for our neurosurgical centres. In this perspective, it was of significant importance to recruit recognized professionals from most centres in Scandinavia, and from most of the involved specialities in neurotrauma care. Another important objective was to develop a practical and basic manual for young neurosurgeons and neuroanaesthesiologists dealing with severe TBI.

The authors performed literature searches, not only with reference to the BTF guidelines from 1995 and later revisions but also within other areas of the medical field, which is reflected in the index of this book. The evidence was classified into three levels according to quality and reliability (based on the United States Preventive Services Taskforce, the National Health Services (UK) Centre for Reviews and Dissemination, and the Cochrane Collaboration). The classifications were refined through an independent review process and consensus discussion in the SNC.

- *Level I evidence*: Properly designed (prospective) randomized controlled trial (the gold standard of clinical practice).
- *Level II evidence*: Prospectively collected data or retrospective analyses based on clearly reliable data on well-defined populations. This level includes prospective trials that did not meet the strict criteria for Level I evidence, as well as non-randomized studies, observational studies, cohort studies, and so forth.
- *Level III evidence*: Descriptive studies and expert opinions.

There are only a few areas in this book that have Level I evidence. Most of the recommendations that are given are based on Level II or Level III evidence. As a whole, the scientific foundation for management of severe TBI is extensive, but rarely grounded on high quality evidence.

Each chapter has been given a standardized set-up, unless it has been clearly not practicable. The reader is given initial *Recommendations* based on levels of evidence. An *Overview* gives a short theoretical run through the relevant literature with emphasis on the newest and the most important older articles. A section with *Tips, tricks, and pitfalls* provides some general rules, practical advice and expert views. The *Background* gives a thorough look on the relevant literature, and a final section deals with *Specific paediatric concerns*.

The members of SNC hope that these guidelines will prove useful for those confronted with the clinical and scientific problems of severely brain-injured patients, and that they might help to establish a systematic and sustainable health-care system from injury through rehabilitation, and finally to the survivors' re-entry in society.

References

Bellander BM, Sollid S, Kock-Jensen C, Juul N, Eskesen V, Sundstrøm T, Wester K, Romner B (2008) Prehospital management of patients with severe head injuries. Scandinavian guidelines according to Brain Trauma Foundation. Lakartidningen 105:1834–1838

Ingebrigtsen T, Rise IR, Wester K, Romner B, Kock-Jensen C (2000a) Scandinavian guidelines for management of minimal, mild and moderate head injuries. Tidsskr Nor Laegeforen 120:1985–1990

Ingebrigtsen T, Romner B, Kock-Jensen C (2000b) Scandinavian guidelines for initial management of minimal, mild, and moderate head injuries. J Trauma 48:760–766

Juul N, Sollid S, Sundstrøm T, Kock-Jensen C, Eskesen V, Bellander BM, Wester K, Romner B (2008) Scandinavian guidelines on the pre-hospital management of traumatic brain injury. Ugeskr Laeger 170:2337–2341

Romner B, Ingebrigtsen T, Kock-Jensen C (2000a) Scandinavian guidelines for management of head injuries. Evidence-based management of minimal, mild and moderate head injuries. Ugeskr Laeger 162:3839–3845

Romner B, Ingebrigtsen T, Kock-Jensen C (2000b) Scandinavian guidelines for management of head injuries. Evidence-based management of minimal, mild and moderate head injuries. Lakartidningen 97:3186–3192

Sollid S, Sundstrøm T, Kock-Jensen C, Juul N, Eskesen V, Bellander BM, Wester K, Romner B (2008) Scandinavian guidelines for prehospital management of severe traumatic brain injury. Tidsskr Nor Laegeforen 128:1524–1527

Sundstrøm T, Sollid S, Wentzel-Larsen T, Wester K (2007) Head injury mortality in the Nordic countries. J Neurotrauma 24:147–153

Members of the Scandinavian Neurotrauma Committee

Denmark

Dahl, Bent Lob
Juul, Niels
Kock-Jensen, Carsten (President)
Romner, Bertil
Rosenlund, Christina
Springborg, Jacob Bertram

Finland

Mikko Kauppinen

Iceland

Ingvar Olafsson

Norway

Sollid, Snorre
Sundstrøm, Terje (Secretary)
Wester, Knut

Sweden

Bellander. Bo-Michael
Grände, Per-Olof
Koskinen, Lars-Owe D.
Reinstrup, Peter
Undén, Johan

Editorial Board

Sundstrøm, Terje (Chief executive editor)
Grände, Per-Olof (Anaesthesia and intensive care editor)
Juul, Niels (Anaesthesia and intensive care editor)
Kock-Jensen, Carsten (Chairman of the board)
Romner, Bertil (Neurosurgical editor)
Wester, Knut (Assistant executive editor)

Review Committee

Dahl, Bent Lob
Grände, Per-Olof
Juul, Niels
Kock-Jensen, Carsten
Romner, Bertil
Rosenlund, Christina
Sundstrøm, Terje (Co-chairman)
Wester, Knut (Co-chairman)

Part I

Epidemiology

1 Epidemiology

Snorre Sollid and Tor Ingebrigtsen

Take-Home Messages

- Trauma is among the leading causes of death in the world. The problem is increasing.
- In the population below 44 years, trauma is the leading cause of death in the western world.
- The majority of deaths happen within the first hour after injury.
- Head injury as the cause of death among trauma victims consists of up to 50%.
- Traffic accidents are the number one cause in fatal injuries, and falls are the number one among nonfatal injuries.
- Seventy to eighty percent of all head injuries are minor, 10% are moderate, and 10% are severe.
- A positive trend towards a decrease in accidents and mortality rates is documented in North Europe, mostly due to prevention of accidents.

S. Sollid
Department of Neurosurgery,
University Hospital of North Norway,
9038 Tromsø, Norway
e-mail: snorre.sollid@unn.no

T. Ingebrigtsen
University Hospital of North Norway,
9038 Tromsø, Norway
e-mail: tor.ingebrigtsen@unn.no

1.1 Trauma Epidemiology

Individual treatment of injured persons is the basis of our trauma and health-care systems. Epidemiological research analyses the impact of injury to the health and mortality of the general population. To prevent and effectively treat patients exposed to trauma, we need knowledge of the epidemiology. Basic health indicators are as crucial for understanding the health situation as are the Glasgow Coma Scale score (GCS) and pupil reaction of a brain-injured patient. A health indicator is a variable describing a single numeric measurement of an aspect of health within a population for a specific period of time, normally a year. Basically, two types of health indicators are used. The first type describes survival or mortality. The second type measures the burden of a specific disease or risk factors. By combining the years of life lost (YLL) and the loss of healthy years, the health impact of a disease can be presented as the disability-adjusted life years (DALY). Table 1.1 shows the most used parameters to describe trauma epidemiology.

1.2 Global Perspectives

Trauma as a general health problem was previously remarkably neglected. During the last two decades, the impact of trauma on the global health has been understood. This fact has been greatly influenced by the pioneering work of Christopher

T. Sundstrøm et al. (eds.), *Management of Severe Traumatic Brain Injury*,
DOI 10.1007/978-3-642-28126-6_1, © Springer-Verlag Berlin Heidelberg 2012

Table 1.1 Health indicators most used in trauma epidemiology

Measure	How to calculate	What it expresses
Incidence rate	The number of new cases in a given time period divided by the total population from which they are drawn	A measure of the risk of developing some new condition within a specific period of time
Prevalence rate	The total number of persons with the observed condition (old and new cases) divided by the total population from which they are drawn	A measure of how common a condition is within a population at a certain time
Mortality rate	The number of persons dying from the condition per unit time (e.g. year) divided by the total population from which they are drawn	A measure of the number of deaths in a population, scaled to the size of the population within a specific period of time
Case fatality rate	The number of persons dying from the condition per unit time (e.g. year) divided by the total number of persons in the population with the same condition	A measure of the ratio of deaths within a designated population of people with a particular condition over a certain period of time
Years of life lost (YLL)	Reference age (life expectancy in the population) minus age of death = years of life lost	A measure of potential years of life lost. The reference age corresponds to the life expectancy of the population, commonly set at age 75
Years lived with disability (YLD)	Reference age minus age of onset of condition/disease = YLD	A measure of the years lived with the impact of disability
Disability-adjusted life year (DALY)	YLL + YLD = DALY	A measure of overall disease burden, expressed as the number of years lost due to ill health, disability or early death
Quality-adjusted life years (QALY)	(Reference age minus age of onset of condition) multiplied by 'weight' value	A measure of disease burden, including both the quality and the quantity of life lived

Murray and Allan Lopez (Murray and Lopez 1997). Under the direction of the World Health Organization (WHO), regular publications describing the global burden of all major diseases in all countries of the world have been published. The last update was published in 2004 (WHO 2004). These studies indicate that injury represents about one-tenth of the global public health problem. Injury causes about 12% of the global burden of disease and 9% of all deaths in the world. For specific regions and age groups, trauma is an even more common cause of death and disability. Trauma is the leading cause of death in the ages between 1 and 44 years in the western world (MacKenzie 2000). If both intentional and unintentional injuries are put together, they account for more years of life lost than cancer, heart disease or HIV. While death only represents the tip of the iceberg, it is estimated that for every injury death, there are 18 hospital discharges and 250 injury-related visits to the emergency departments. Due to the increasing number of motor vehicles in densely populated regions, it is estimated that trauma will become the fourth most common cause of death within 2020 (Murray and Lopez 1997).

Because of this, trauma is a major health problem, which emphasises the importance of both prevention and treatment. Prevention has the highest impact on trauma death. Studies have shown that as many as 75% of the trauma deaths occur during the first hour after the accident (Wisborg et al. 2003). Most of them are not treatable due to the severity of the traumatic lesions. Reaching the trauma scene within this limited time is a practical problem.

1.3 Causes

Studies of the relative importance on a global basis of each type of injury show that road traffic accidents (RTA) are the number one type of injury causing death in the world, followed by falls, violence and suicide. This pattern varies significantly between regions and age groups. When it comes to nonfatal injury, falls are the leading cause followed by RTA (MacKenzie 2000). There is a difference in the cause of injury between the ages. Falls are the major aetiology in the younger and older age groups, while traffic accidents are the most usual cause in the intermediate age groups.

Alcohol as an important risk factor for injuries is well known. As many as one-third of all trauma deaths involve alcohol, and more than one-half of all traffic fatalities among young persons are alcohol-related.

1.4 Traumatic Brain Injury Epidemiology

It is difficult to obtain the real incidence of head injury due to the lack of a definitive classification of the term and the lack of reliable data. Most published rates include both hospitalised patients and prehospital deaths. Some publications also include persons treated only in an emergency department. Comparison of such studies should therefore be done with these differences in mind. The same problem comes into consideration when it comes to the prevalence of traumatic brain injury (TBI). The global burden of disease reports does not specify which organ trauma causes death. It is known from other studies that brain injury is a major factor causing 30–50% of all trauma deaths (Jennett 1996). The mortality rate due to head injury is easily obtained in most western countries, where national death registries are common. The data quality in such databases is moderate (Sundstrøm et al. 2007). In-hospital studies describing the case fatality rate and fractions of the different severities are not a good source for understanding head injury as a public health problem. Most patients dying from trauma do so within the first hour (Wisborg et al. 2003). Despite these limitations, there are some data available to describe the most important trends in TBI epidemiology.

1.4.1 Incidence

Most published incidences of TBI include hospitalised and/or prehospital patients plus deaths identified from local authorities (Tagliaferri et al. 2006). Most incidence rates are in the range 150–300 per 100,000 population per year for European countries, with an average of 235 per 100,000 population per year. These rates include all severities. Within Europe, the incidence ranges from as high as 546 per 100,000 to as low as 91 per 100,000 population per year. Comparisons in other regions also show large variation in incidence rates. Aggregated data show incidence rates of 103, 226, 344 and 160 per 100,000 per year in the USA, Australia, Asia and India, respectively. These differences are largely explained by the differences in data collection, but it is reasonable to assume actual differences in the occurrence of trauma and head injury as well. During the last two decades, a decreasing number of TBI admissions have been reported (Colantonio et al. 2009). First of all, there is a decline in the number of minor TBI admitted to hospital. This is most likely due to a change in the referral policy, with routines for handling these patients on an outpatient or emergency room (ER) basis (Muller et al. 2003). This development may have contributed to an increasing proportion of hospitalised patients being classified as moderate or severely injured.

1.4.2 Severity

Severity classification of TBI could be based on several different classification systems. The severity could be classified according to the level of consciousness (Glasgow Coma Scale – GCS), the anatomic damage to the brain (Abbreviated Injury Scale – AIS), the total load of anatomic damage to the body (Injury Severity Score – ISS) or the length of post-traumatic amnesia. The GCS has become the standard for assessing initial TBI severity. The severities are described as minor, moderate or severe. According to the Head Injury Severity Scale (HISS), GCS, length of post-traumatic amnesia and neurological deficits are factors affecting severity. The severity expresses the risk of death or the probability of developing an intracranial lesion in need of neurosurgical treatment. In most published studies, the distribution between the severities is approximately 70–80%, minor; 10%, moderate; and 10%, severe (Tagliaferri et al. 2006).

1.4.3 Mortality and Case Fatality Rates

In addition to the severity description mentioned above, two other severity measures of TBI are used to describe the TBI epidemiology. The mortality rate describes the number of TBI-associated deaths in the general population. It is usually expressed per 100,000 population per year. The case fatality rate expresses the outcome among those exposed to TBI. The reported rates in the literature show large differences. During the last 150 years, the mortality rates in patients with severe TBI have decreased by almost 50% (Stein et al. 2010). This decline varied through this period. From the late 1800s to 1930, the decline in mortality was approximately 3% per decade. An even higher decline was observed in the period from 1970 to 1990. Between these periods, and after 1990, the rates are steady. These figures do not describe the variations between different geographic regions and health-care systems.

The lack of precise death diagnosis in trauma cases could both under- and overestimate the number of deaths due to TBI. The case fatality rate is largely affected by the total number of TBI included, by the frequency of severe TBI and by the number of patients with co-morbidity or injury. Most studies only describe the in-hospital case fatality rate. An overall case fatality rate also includes those patients who die prehospital. Comparison of such rates between different populations and institutions, and between periods of time, should therefore be done with caution. Due to the proportional shift in the severity grade among TBI patients admitted to hospital, mortality rate is a better parameter than case fatality rate to monitor fatal outcomes after TBI.

1.4.4 Prevalence and Outcome

Prevalence is the measure of the total amount of TBI at one point in time or in one period in a population. It includes all those with a TBI sequela such as impairment, disability, handicap or complaint plus all newly diagnosed cases at the defined time or time interval. Prevalence describes the burden of TBI to the health-care system and the society, but not the real outcome of TBI. To capture all consequences of TBI influencing daily living in such a way that it defends the term "sequela" is difficult and demanding. Thus, it is not surprising that so few studies have attempted to ascertain the prevalence level of TBI in a community or nation.

Population-based or case studies examining outcome following the acute hospitalisation phase usually describe outcome by the Glasgow Outcome Scale (GOS) (Jennett and Bond 1975). It is difficult to perform comparisons between studies due to variation in inclusion criteria and the time of scoring. Some large studies with reasonable follow-up periods provide useful data. European Brain Injury Consortium (EBIC) published a European survey in 1999 (Murray et al. 1999). The study group contained 796 severely or moderately head-injured patients with a 6-month follow-up. Thirty-one percent died, 3% had a permanent vegetable state, 16% were severely disabled, 20% moderately disabled, and 31% had a good recovery.

The GOS does not describe the nature of the persistent disabilities or impairments following TBI. Studies focusing on this are inconsistent when it comes to the parameters described. All reports show that TBI consequences are persistent for a long period of time, for some patients life-long. Changes in employment, physical complaints and problems with memory, disabilities and neuropsychological difficulties appear to be common. These complaints are described after all severities of TBI. However, such complaints may not be found in all TBI victims, and studies are needed to map which factors affect outcome.

Another way to explain the burden of TBI to the society is to calculate the economical costs such injuries cause. The costs include both direct and indirect costs. Direct costs are the monetary value of real goods and services that are provided for health care. Indirect costs are the monetary loss imposed on the society because of interruption of productivity by the injured person. Such calculations are complex and can only give an impression of the magnitude of the problem.

1.5 Prevention

Prevention is always better than cure and much less expensive. To prevent injuries, we need to reveal their causes. Behind the RTAs, falls and other causes of trauma, there are factors susceptible to influence. Trauma is not only bad luck, but an endpoint of explainable events that are possible to prevent. We need to reduce the burden of preventable accidents.

Injury prevention strategies cover a variety of approaches: education, engineering modification, law enforcement/enactment, evaluation, economic incentives and empowerment. Prevention can be targeted at both population and individual scale, encompassing numerous strategies, techniques or programs designed to eliminate or reduce its occurrence. As an example, traffic and automobile safety can be increased by numerous different actions:

- *Engineering*: create a safe driving environment, such as seat belts, airbags, child seat, safer roads with physical dividers
- *Education*: promote seat belt use, promote child safety seats
- *Enforcement and enactment*: primary seat belt laws, speed limits, impaired driving enforcement, motor- and bicycle helmet laws
- *Economic incentives*: reduce taxes on safety equipment

Despite the documented need for prevention of injuries, there is a disappointing lack of scientific focus upon this problem. Only a small but increasing number of evidence-based injury control interventions have been published (Stelfox and Goverman 2008). Despite this, several studies have shown positive effects on the incidence of injury, morbidity and mortality of community-based injury prevention (Tellnes et al. 2006; Timpka et al. 1999).

In recent years, studies covering Scandinavia have shown a positive trend towards a significant decline in head injury mortality (Sundstrøm et al. 2007). This progress has also been experienced in Great Britain (Patel et al. 2005). The most probable explanation for this achievement is the systematic preventive work accomplished in these countries, not the medical treatment delivered.

Neurosurgeons, trauma surgeons, anaesthesiologist and other health-care workers rarely engage in epidemiological research and injury prevention. This is disappointing. It is our responsibility to provide society in general and politicians and other decision makers in special with the information they need to prevent the trauma epidemic. We and especially our leaders must bear the burden of promoting unpopular but necessary preventive measures, such as reduced speed limits. This responsibility lies just as clearly on us as the responsibility for prevention of infectious disease does to specialists in that field.

References

Colantonio A, Croxford R, Farooq S, Laporte A, Coyte PC (2009) Trends in hospitalization associated with traumatic brain injury in a publicly insured population, 1992–2002. J Trauma 66:179–183

Jennett B (1996) Epidemiology of head injury. J Neurol Neurosurg Psychiatry 60:362–369

Jennett B, Bond M (1975) Assessment of outcome after severe brain damage. Lancet 1:480–484

Mackenzie EJ (2000) Epidemiology of injuries: current trends and future challenges. Epidemiol Rev 22:112–119

Muller K, Waterloo K, Romner B, Wester K, Ingebrigtsen T (2003) Mild head injuries: impact of a national strategy for implementation of management guidelines. J Trauma 55:1029–1034

Murray CJ, Lopez AD (1997) Alternative projections of mortality and disability by cause 1990–2020: Global Burden of Disease Study. Lancet 349:1498–1504

Murray GD, Teasdale GM, Braakman R et al (1999) The European Brain Injury Consortium survey of head injuries. Acta Neurochir (Wien) 141:223–236

Patel HC, Bouamra O, Woodford M, King AT, Yates DW, Lecky FE (2005) Trends in head injury outcome from 1989 to 2003 and the effect of neurosurgical care: an observational study. Lancet 366(9496):1538–1544

Stein SC, Georgoff P, Meghan S, Mizra K, Sonnad SS (2010) 150 years of treating severe traumatic brain injury: a systematic review of progress in mortality. J Neurotrauma 27:1343–1353

Stelfox HT, Goverman J (2008) The number, content, and quality of randomized controlled trials in the prevention and care of injuries. J Trauma 65:1488–1493

Sundstrøm T, Sollid S, Wentzel-Larsen T, Wester K (2007) Head injury mortality in the Nordic countries. J Neurotrauma 24:147–153

Tagliaferri F, Compagnone C, Korsic M, Servadei F, Kraus J (2006) A systematic review of brain injury epidemiology in Europe. Acta Neurochir (Wien) 148: 255–268

Tellnes G, Lund J, Sandvik L, Klouman E, Ytterstad B (2006) Long-term effects of community-based injury prevention on the island of Vaeroy in Norway: a 20-year follow up. Scand J Public Health 34:312–319

Timpka T, Lindqvist K, Schelp L, Ahlgren M (1999) Community-based injury prevention: effects on health care utilization. Int J Epidemiol 28:502–508

WHO (2004) The global burden of disease: 2004 update. http://www.who.int/healthinfo/global_burden_disease/2004_report_update/en/index.html. WHO Library Cataloguing-in-Publication Data

Wisborg T, Hoylo T, Siem G (2003) Death after injury in rural Norway: high rate of mortality and prehospital death. Acta Anaesthesiol Scand 47:153–156

Part II

Classification and Assessment

2 Classification of Head Injury

Ramona Åstrand and Bertil Romner

Recommendations

Level I

There is insufficient data to support a Level I recommendation for this topic.

Level II

There is insufficient data to support a Level II recommendation for this topic.

Level III

The Glasgow Coma Scale (GCS) is the most frequently used scoring system for assessment and classification of traumatic brain injury.

2.1 Overview

Head injuries can be categorized in several ways: by mechanism of injury (closed or penetrating injury), morphology (fractures, focal intracranial injury, diffuse intracranial injury), or severity of injury (mild to severe).

Immediate triage and assessment of the severity and probable survival of the traumatized patient should be made whenever possible already at the scene of injury. Of useful help are the various trauma scores that have been developed to triage the patients for proper care and evaluate the severity of injury. The scores are based on physiological and/or anatomical features, as well as patient responses. Physiological scores are exemplified by Glasgow Coma scale (GCS) (Teasdale and Jennett 1974), the Revised Trauma Score (RTS) (Champion et al. 1989), and the Pediatric Trauma Score (PTS) (Tepas et al. 1987). The Injury Severity Score (ISS) is an anatomical score based on the Abbreviated Injury Scale (AIS) that provides an overall score of the patient (Baker et al. 1974).

The GCS has been the most valuable and frequently used scoring system for assessing the severity of a head trauma.

To estimate severity of brain injury after head trauma, various classification systems of head injury have been proposed and modified throughout the years. Most of them are based on the patients' level of consciousness according to the GCS, as e.g. the Head Injury Severity Scale (HISS) (Stein and Spettell 1995). The Swedish Reaction Level Scale 85 (RLS) is a somewhat

> **Tips, Tricks, and Pitfalls**
>
> - Severe head injury is defined as a patient with conscious level of GCS 3–8 (RLS 4–8) after head injury.

R. Åstrand • B. Romner (✉)
Department of Neurosurgery, 2092,
Rigshospitalet, 2011 Copenhagen, Denmark
e-mail: ramona.aastrand@rh.regionh.dk;
bertil.romner@rh.regionh.dk

T. Sundstrøm et al. (eds.), *Management of Severe Traumatic Brain Injury*,
DOI 10.1007/978-3-642-28126-6_2, © Springer-Verlag Berlin Heidelberg 2012

- Traumatic brain injury is defined as primary or secondary injury to the brain after trauma.
- The definition of a paediatric patient varies in Scandinavian hospitals, with an upper age limit either below 16 or 18 years.
- Neurologic assessment, including GCS and pupil response, should be assessed as soon as possible either prehospital or at admission, preferably before sedation and intubation, for a more correct classification of the severity.
- Intoxicated patients are challenging to classify and should be treated with higher awareness. The GCS score may be decreased by 2–3 points due to heavy alcohol intoxication or drug use; a problematic confounding factor when assessing the level of consciousness in a head-injured patient.

simpler scale than the GCS, though less frequently used outside of Sweden (Starmark et al. 1988a).

2.2 Background

In the 1960s, there was a common belief amongst neurosurgeons that, aside from evacuating occasional hematomas or elevating depressed fractures, little could be done to influence outcome after head injury. However, with improvement of intensive care and resuscitation, the challenge for neurosurgeons was to assist in reducing mortality and morbidity for these severely head-injured patients. Pathological studies in Glasgow showed that by avoiding potentially preventable secondary brain damage, one could limit the degree of disabilities in survivors (Reilly et al. 1975).

Complications, such as the development of intracranial haematomas or increased intracranial pressure, were difficult to recognize; hence treatment was delayed. These concerns lead to the development of the Glasgow Coma Scale by Jennett and Teasdale in 1974 (Teasdale and Jennett 1974). The scale was initially designed as a research tool for assessment of the comatose patient, but is now one of the most frequently used scales in triage of head injuries and in daily assessment of severe head injury. The drawback of using the GCS is the confounding effect of alcohol or other drugs, especially during the first few hours after injury. Heavy alcohol intoxication has been associated with a reduction of 2–3 points in GCS in assaulted patients (Brickley and Shepherd 1995).

2.2.1 Classification Systems

In 1981, Rimel and colleagues defined minor head injury as a head trauma with patient's GCS score of 13–15 at admission, loss of consciousness (LOC) less than 20 min, and a duration of hospital admission less than 48 h (Rimel et al. 1981). About a decade later, Stein and Spettell introduced a modified classification system, the Head Injury Severity Scale (HISS), a five-interval severity scale (minimal through critical) based primarily on initial GCS score. The HISS scale also includes the aspects of retrograde amnesia, loss of consciousness, and focal neurological deficits for each severity intervals (Stein and Spettell 1995).

In 2000, the Scandinavian Neurotrauma Committee (SNC) presented guidelines of management of adult head injury (Ingebrigtsen et al. 2000), using a modified version of the HISS classification, by classifying head injuries into minimal, mild, moderate, and severe (Table 2.1):

- Minimal head injury is presented by a patient with GCS 15 at admission and with no LOC or focal neurological deficits.
- Mild head injury is defined as initial GCS of 14–15, brief LOC (<5 min) and no focal neurological deficits.
- Moderate head injury defines a patient with initial GCS of 9–13 and/or focal neurological deficits or LOC ≥5 min after head trauma.
- Severe head injury includes all patients with an initial GCS score of 8 or below, hence, unconscious patients.

The definitions of mild and moderate head injury vary in the literature, especially with regard

Table 2.1 Classification of head injuries according to SNC in 2000 (Ingebrigtsen et al. 2000)

HISS category	Clinical characteristics
Minimal	GCS = 15, no loss of consciousness
Mild	GCS = 14 or 15, brief (<5 min) loss of consciousness or amnesia, or impaired alertness or memory
Moderate	GCS = 9–13, or loss of consciousness ≥5 min, or focal neurologic deficit
Severe	GCS = 3–8

to the importance of a GCS score of 13 and the duration of loss of consciousness.

Commotio cerebri is a clinical definition of an awake patient with posttraumatic amnesia possibly due to brief LOC after head trauma, but without any apparent brain injury. Amnesia is most often retrograde, but in some cases even antegrade amnesia is present, i.e. the inability to recall new memories after the head injury event.

2.2.2 Primary and Secondary Brain Injury

Primary brain injury refers to the immediate brain damage caused upon impact. This includes cerebral contusions, shearing lesions (diffuse axonal injuries – DAI), lacerations from a foreign body, and acute subdural or epidural hematomas. Secondary brain injury refers to progressive cerebral oedema, which is more commonly seen in children, ischemia, and the expansion of cerebral contusions and the surrounding focal oedema, which causes an increase in intracranial pressure (ICP) within the confined skull and can eventually lead to cerebral herniation and death.

2.2.3 Assessment Scales

The GCS has been the most valuable and frequently used scoring system for assessing severity of neurologic injury after head trauma. The scale is divided in three parts: eye response, verbal response, and motor response, adding to a total score of 3–15 points. The GCS scale has, however, been considered difficult to apply on especially preverbal children (Yager et al. 1990) since their ability to express themselves verbally or nonverbally in a consistent manner is limited. The response from an infant is also clearly different from an adult. Reilly et al. were the first to design the paediatric version of the GCS, where verbal responses were reported as appropriate words, social smiles, cries, irritability, and agitation (Reilly et al. 1988; Simpson and Reilly 1982). Some modifications of the scale have later also been made to suite even the youngest children and infants (Table 2.2). The paediatric GCS scale has proved to be accurate in evaluating preverbal children with head trauma with regard to the need for acute intervention (Holmes et al. 2005).

In Sweden, the most practiced scale for assessment of the level of consciousness is the Swedish Reaction Level Scale 85 (RLS) (Johnstone et al. 1993; Starmark et al. 1988a, b). This scale evaluates the consciousness in an inverted manner to the GCS, with a scoring range from 1 (best) to 8 (worst), and without specific focus on the verbal response (Table 2.3). This has made the score more practical to use, particularly on neurologically traumatized patients (who also may suffer from aphasia) and children, as well as more easily remembered in acute situations.

The Revised Trauma Score (RTS) is a numeric grading system for estimating the severity of injury. It is composed of the GCS, systolic blood pressure, and respiratory rate, each giving rise to a score between 0 and 4. The severity of injury is estimated by the total sum of the three parameters, where the highest score is 12, hence, the least severe injury (Table 2.4).

The Injury Severity Score (ISS) is an anatomical score that provides an overall score of the patient with multiple injuries after severe trauma (Table 2.5). It is based on the AIS score, which

Table 2.2 The Glasgow Coma Scale

Glasgow Coma Scale			
	Standard	*Paediatric version*	
		1–4 years	<1 year
Eye opening			
4	Spontaneous	Open	
3	To speech	To voice	
2	To pain	To pain	
1	None	No response	
Verbal response			
5	Orientated	Oriented, speaks, interacts	Coos, babbles
4	Confused conversation	Confused speech, consolable	Irritable cry, consolable
3	Words (inappropriate)	Inappropriate words, inconsolable	Persistent cry, inconsolable
2	Sounds (incomprehensible)	Incomprehensible, agitated	Moans to pain
1	None	No response	No response
Best motor response			
6	Obey commands	Normal spontaneous movement	
5	Localizes pain	Localizes pain	
4	Flexion, withdraws to pain	Withdraws to pain	
3	Flexion, abnormal to pain	Decorticate flexion	
2	Extension (to pain)	Decerebrate extension	
1	No response	No response	
3–15	*Total score*		

Table 2.3 The Swedish Reaction Level Scale

Reaction Level Scale (RLS 85)	Score
Fully awake. Oriented	1
Lethargic. Confused. Contact after mild stimuli	2
Stupor. Confused. Contact after rough stimuli or pain	3
Unconscious. Localizes to pain	4
Unconscious. Withdraws to pain	5
Unconscious. Abnormal flexion to pain	6
Unconscious. Abnormal extension to pain	7
No response to painful central stimuli	8

determines six body regions (head, face, chest, abdomen, extremities and pelvis, and external). The three most severely injured regions are squared and added to produce the ISS. The ISS correlates to mortality, morbidity, hospital stay, and other measures of severity, but is not considered a good tool for triage (Baker and O'Neill 1976; Baker et al. 1974).

2.3 Specific Paediatric Concerns

The head injury classification systems mainly apply to adults, although in clinical practice the SNC classification is also used on children and adolescents. This is mainly due to the lack of specific head injury classification systems for children. In some hospitals, the level of consciousness is more properly evaluated with use of the paediatric GCS score (Reilly et al. 1988). The Pediatric Trauma Score (PTS) has been developed as an assessment score for trauma severity in children (Table 2.6), but its use in Scandinavia has so far been limited.

Definitions of mild to moderate head injury in children vary even more extensively in the literature than for adults, especially with regards to the duration of LOC (AAP 1999; Schutzman et al. 2001). Other clinical factors, such as scalp haematoma, low age (<2 years), history of excessive vomiting, and suspected skull fracture and post-traumatic seizures, have in former studies and proposed guidelines been considered as risk factors for developing an intracranial complication (Dunning et al. 2006; Holmes et al. 2004;

Table 2.4 The Revised Trauma Score scale

Revised Trauma Score (RTS)			
GCS score	Systolic blood pressure (mmHg)	Respiratory rate (breaths/min)	Coded value*
13–15	>89	10–29	**4**
9–12	76–89	>29	**3**
6–8	50–75	6–9	**2**
4–5	1–49	1–5	**1**
3	0	0	**0**

RTS score <11 indicates a more severe trauma and need for immediate treatment
*Total RTS score = the sum of the coded values for every category (GCS, systolic blood pressure and respiratory rate)

Table 2.5 The Injury Severity Scale

Injury Severity Scale (ISS)			
Region	Injury description (examples)	AIS	Square top three
Head and neck	No injury	0	
Face	Minor injury	1	
Thorax	Moderate injury	2	
Abdomen and viscera	Serious injury	3	*
Bony pelvis and extremities	Severe injury	4	*
External structures	Critical injury	5	*
Injury Severity Score = sum:			*0–75*

Lethal injury (incompatible with life) = Abbreviated injury scale (AIS) 6 = ISS 75
*The three most severe injuries are squared and added, to produce the final ISS score

Table 2.6 The Pediatric Trauma Score scale

Pediatric Trauma Score (PTS)			
	Category		
Component	+2	+1	−1
Size (kg)	≥20	10–20	<10
Airway	Normal	Maintainable	Unmaintainable
Systolic BP (mmHg)	≤90	90–50	<50
CNS	Awake	Obtunded/LOC	Coma/decerebrate
Open wound	None	Minor	Major/penetrating
Skeletal	None	Closed fracture	Open/multiple fractures

Sum total points: −6 to +12. Score < 9 = potentially significant trauma

Schutzman et al. 2001), requiring hospitalisation or further radiological investigation (Schutzman and Greenes 2001).

The definition of severe head injury in children still include all with GCS 3–8 (Adelson et al. 2003).

References

Adelson PD, Bratton SL, Carney NA, Chesnut RM, du Coudray HE, Goldstein B, Kochanek PM, Miller HC, Partington MD, Selden NR, Warden CR, Wright DW (2003) Guidelines for the acute medical management of severe traumatic brain injury in infants, children, and adolescents. Chapter 1: Introduction. Pediatr Crit Care Med 4:S2–S4

Baker SP, O'Neill B (1976) The injury severity score: an update. J Trauma 16:882–885

Baker SP, O'Neill B, Haddon W Jr, Long WB (1974) The injury severity score: a method for describing patients with multiple injuries and evaluating emergency care. J Trauma 14:187–196

Brickley MR, Shepherd JP (1995) The relationship between alcohol intoxication, injury severity and Glasgow Coma Score in assault patients. Injury 26:311–314

Champion HR, Sacco WJ, Copes WS, Gann DS, Gennarelli TA, Flanagan ME (1989) A revision of the Trauma Score. J Trauma 29:623–629

Committee on Quality Improvement, American Academy of Pediatrics and Commission on Clinical Policies and Research, American Academy of Family Physicians (1999) The management of minor closed head injury in children. Pediatrics 104:1407–1415

Dunning J, Daly JP, Lomas JP, Lecky F, Batchelor J, Mackway-Jones K (2006) Derivation of the children's head injury algorithm for the prediction of important clinical events decision rule for head injury in children. Arch Dis Child 91:885–891

Holmes JF, Palchak MJ, Conklin MJ, Kuppermann N (2004) Do children require hospitalization after immediate posttraumatic seizures? Ann Emerg Med 43: 706–710

Holmes JF, Palchak MJ, MacFarlane T, Kuppermann N (2005) Performance of the pediatric glasgow coma scale in children with blunt head trauma. Acad Emerg Med 12:814–819

Ingebrigtsen T, Romner B, Kock-Jensen C (2000) Scandinavian guidelines for initial management of minimal, mild, and moderate head injuries.The Scandinavian Neurotrauma Committee. J Trauma 48: 760–766

Johnstone AJ, Lohlun JC, Miller JD, McIntosh CA, Gregori A, Brown R, Jones PA, Anderson SI, Tocher JL (1993) A comparison of the Glasgow Coma Scale and the Swedish Reaction Level Scale. Brain Inj 7: 501–506

Reilly PL, Graham DI, Adams JH, Jennett B (1975) Patients with head injury who talk and die. Lancet 2: 375–377

Reilly PL, Simpson DA, Sprod R, Thomas L (1988) Assessing the conscious level in infants and young children: a paediatric version of the Glasgow Coma Scale. Childs Nerv Syst 4:30–33

Rimel RW, Giordani B, Barth JT, Boll TJ, Jane JA (1981) Disability caused by minor head injury. Neurosurgery 9:221–228

Schutzman SA, Barnes P, Duhaime AC, Greenes D, Homer C, Jaffe D, Lewis RJ, Luerssen TG, Schunk J (2001) Evaluation and management of children younger than two years old with apparently minor head trauma: proposed guidelines. Pediatrics 107: 983–993

Schutzman SA, Greenes DS (2001) Pediatric minor head trauma. Ann Emerg Med 37:65–74

Simpson D, Reilly P (1982) Pediatric coma scale. Lancet 2:450

Starmark JE, Stalhammar D, Holmgren E (1988a) The Reaction Level Scale (RLS85). Manual and guidelines. Acta Neurochir (Wien) 91:12–20

Starmark JE, Stalhammar D, Holmgren E, Rosander B (1988b) A comparison of the Glasgow Coma Scale and the Reaction Level Scale (RLS85). J Neurosurg 69:699–706

Stein SC, Spettell C (1995) The Head Injury Severity Scale (HISS): a practical classification of closed-head injury. Brain Inj 9:437–444

Teasdale G, Jennett B (1974) Assessment of coma and impaired consciousness. A practical scale. Lancet 2:81–84

Tepas JJ 3rd, Mollitt DL, Talbert JL, Bryant M (1987) The pediatric trauma score as a predictor of injury severity in the injured child. J Pediatr Surg 22:14–18

Yager JY, Johnston B, Seshia SS (1990) Coma scales in pediatric practice. Am J Dis Child 144:1088–1091

Primary Clinical Assessment

3

Jacob Bertram Springborg and Vagn Eskesen

Recommendations

Level I

Data are insufficient to support Level I recommendations for this subject.

Level II

The Glasgow Coma Scale score (GCS) is a reliable indicator of the severity of TBI; the Injury Severity Score (ISS) can be used to predict severity in patients with multitrauma.

Level III

When pupil fixation or dilation is observed, cerebral herniation should be suspected and appropriate interventions initiated. However, like other patients, patients with TBI may demonstrate iridoplegia, which is not due to herniation.

3.1 Overview

As part of the primary care of patients with TBI, some form of assessment of the severity of the injury is needed. Outside the hospital and in the primary care facility, this assessment is currently mostly based on a clinical examination. Different scoring systems have been designed to assess the level of consciousness and such scoring should together with pupil examination be used repetitively to recognise improvement or deterioration over time. Furthermore, the primary clinical evaluation of the patient can be used as a predictor of long-term outcome.

J.B. Springborg (✉) • V. Eskesen
University Clinic of Neurosurgery,
Copenhagen University Hospital, Blegdamsvej 9,
2100 Copenhagen, Denmark
e-mail: jacob.springborg@rh.regionh.dk;
vagn.eskesen@rh.regionh.dk

Tips, Tricks, and Pitfalls

- Do not use simultaneous verbal and tactile stimuli when evaluating the GCS. Start with verbal commands and proceed only to painful stimuli if the patient does not follow commands. Also, remember to start with a near midline painful stimulus to appreciate if the patient localises.
- Remember that not all 'fixed and blown' pupils are caused by ipsilateral cerebral herniation. Most neurosurgeons know of patients who have been operated on the wrong side because of a false localising sign and because a CT scan was not done for time reasons.
- Pupillary abnormalities in a patient that is conscious are almost never a sign of cerebral herniation.

T. Sundstrøm et al. (eds.), *Management of Severe Traumatic Brain Injury*,
DOI 10.1007/978-3-642-28126-6_3, © Springer-Verlag Berlin Heidelberg 2012

Table 3.1 Glasgow coma scale

Adult GCS		Paediatric GCS	
Eye opening		*Eye opening*	
Spontaneous	4	Spontaneous	4
To speech	3	To speech	3
To pain	2	To pain	2
None	1	None	1
Verbal response		*Verbal response*	
Oriented	5	Coos, babbles	5
Confused	4	Irritable cries	4
Inappropriate words	3	Cries to pain	3
Sounds	2	Moans to pain	2
None	1	None	1
Motor response		*Motor response*	
Obey commands	6	Normal spontaneous movements	6
Localises to pain	5	Withdraws to touch	5
Withdraws to pain	4	Withdraws to pain	4
Abnormal flexion	3	Abnormal flexion	3
Abnormal extension	2	Abnormal extension	2
None	1	None	1

3.2 Background

3.2.1 Measures of Consciousness

In 1974, Teasdale and Jennett introduced the GCS as an objective measure of the level of consciousness 6 h after TBI (Teasdale and Jennett 1974), and in 1976 the scale was adjusted to its current form (Teasdale and Jennett 1976) (Table 3.1). It has since become the most widely used early clinical measure of the severity of TBI. The GCS allows repetitive and relatively reliably recordings of the level of consciousness and a standardised method of reporting the findings (Braakman et al. 1977; Menegazzi et al. 1993; Matis and Birbilis 2008). The GCS evaluates three independent responses to stimuli: eye opening, verbal response, and best motor response. In patients unable to follow commands, a painful blunt stimulus is applied, first near the midline, e.g. to the supraorbital nerve, to see if the patient localises, and if not so, peripherally, e.g. to the nail bed, to see if the patient withdraws. The motor score is based on the extremity with the best response and the eye opening score on the eye with the best response.

Other scales have been designed to evaluate the level of consciousness, such as the Swedish Reaction Level Scale (Starmark et al. 1988), which has eight values and resembles an enhanced GCS motor score, and the Full Outline of UnResponsiveness (FOUR) Score, which besides eye and motor function includes brain stem and respiratory function (Wijdicks et al. 2005). Most of the other scales are reliable and valid, but none have gained the same general acceptance and use as the GCS, which should therefore be considered gold standard. However, one should keep in mind that the use of the scale has expanded beyond the original intension and the limitations of the scale should be acknowledged (Matis and Birbilis 2008).

In intubated patients or in patients with lesions causing aphasia or cervical medullary dysfunction, the use of the GCS is problematic as the verbal or motor scores of these patients may be difficult to interpret. Likewise, patients may have additional injuries to the extremities complicating the assessment of the best motor score. Furthermore, the GCS score can be affected by a number of pre- and posttraumatic systemic factors that may impair the neurological response, e.g. alcohol, drugs, hypoglycaemia, hypotension, hypoxia, or sedation. Therefore, these conditions should be corrected prior to the evaluation of the GCS, or if not possible, the GCS should be recorded as a modified GCS. Finally, ocular or facial trauma can hinder the evaluation of the eye or verbal response, and pre-existing factors such as hearing impairment, dementia, or psychiatric diseases may affect the evaluation of especially the verbal response. To overcome the problem with the evaluation of the verbal score of intubated patients, different models have been proposed to predict the verbal score from the eye and motor score (Rutledge et al. 1996; Meredith et al. 1998). However, these attempts have been questioned (Chesnut 1997).

Several studies have confirmed the predictive value of the GCS in estimating outcome after TBI (Narayan et al. 1981; Rocca et al. 1989; Fearnside et al. 1993; Alvarez et al. 1998). However, as the CGS is a combined score of 120 different possible eye-verbal-motor combinations summing up to just 13 different scores (3–15), it is not surprising that different patients with the same initial GCS score may have different outcomes, which has in fact been demonstrated in the general trauma population (Healey et al. 2003). In addition, these authors have demonstrated that most of the predictive power of the GCS resides in the motor score and that a mathematical transformation of the motor score gives an almost perfectly calibrated line between predicted and actual mortality (Healey et al. 2003). However, the design of that study leaves some unanswered questions about the reliability of the collected GCS values and the external validity of the study, which as mentioned included general trauma patients (National Trauma Data Bank). Nevertheless, others have confirmed that in patients with TBI, the motor score is the single most precise predictor of mortality (Kung et al. 2010). However, the National Trauma Data Bank end point 'survival to discharge' and mortality are poor indices of outcome for the head injury population, completely neglecting the quality of life in survivors.

3.2.2 Clinical Examination of the Pupils

This is an important aspect of neurological assessment and is not included in the GCS score. Pupil assessment is defined as each pupil's size and response to light stimulation. Pupil asymmetry is defined as more than 1 mm difference between the two pupils, and an absent light response ('fixed pupil') is defined as less than 1 mm constriction on bright light. The light reflex depends on a normally functioning lens, retina, optic nerve, brain stem, and oculomotor nerve. The parasympathetic pupillary constrictory nerve fibres run from the Edinger-Westphal nucleus in the high midbrain with the oculomotor nerve to the ciliary ganglion and from that with the short ciliary nerves to the pupillary constrictory muscles. The direct light response assesses the ipsilateral optic and oculomotor nerve and the consensual light response assesses the ipsilateral optic and contralateral oculomotor nerve. The examination is generally easy and quick.

Increased intracranial pressure causing cerebral uncal herniation may compress the oculomotor nerve resulting in a reduction of parasympathetic tone in the pupillary constrictory muscles and thereby ipsilateral pupil dilation and an absent light reflex. Bilateral fixed and dilated pupils are consistent with direct brain stem injury or marked elevation of ICP with central herniation. Metabolic or circulatory disturbances including hypoxia, hypotension, or hypothermia may, however, also be associated with pupil asymmetry or abnormal light reactivity (Meyer et al. 1993). Therefore, resuscitation and stabilisation should be initiated before evaluation of the pupils.

Direct trauma to the eye or oculomotor nerve, e.g. from skull fracture through the sphenoid bone, may cause pupil dilation and thereby mimic severe intracranial injury or herniation. Moreover, traumatic carotid dissection may cause Horner's syndrome with ipsilateral pupil constriction from decreased sympathetic tone making the contralateral pupil appear dilated (Fujisawa et al. 2001). However, in Horner's syndrome, there is ptosis associated with the miotic eye, and the contralateral pupil appearing dilated will have a normal reaction to light. This assessment may be tricky in the acute setting. Finally, in patients with severe swelling of the orbital regions, the evaluation of the pupils can be challenging.

In summary, pupillary function can be an indicator of brain injury after trauma, but is neither a specific indicator of severity or involved anatomy. Nonetheless, studies support the assessment of pupils after severe TBI as both a guide to decision making and for prognostic reasons (Braakman et al. 1977; Chesnut et al. 1994; Halley et al. 2004).

3.2.3 Systems Designed to Grade Patients with Multiple Injuries

The most commonly used is the ISS (Baker et al. 1974), which is based on the Abbreviated Injury Scale (AIS). The AIS is an anatomical scoring system first introduced in 1969 (MacKenzie et al. 1985). The system describes single injuries, and injury severity is ranked on an ordinal scale of 1–6 with 1 being minor, 3 serious, 5 severe, and 6 an unsurvivable injury. The ISS provides an overall score for patients with multiple injuries. Each injury is assigned an AIS score and is allocated to one of six body regions (head, face, chest, abdomen, extremities including pelvis, and external). Only the highest AIS score in each body region is used. The three most severely injured body regions have their scores squared and added to produce the ISS score. The ISS score takes values from 0 to 75. If an injury is assigned an AIS score of 6 (unsurvivable injury), the ISS score is automatically assigned to 75. The ISS score correlates linearly with mortality, morbidity, hospital stay, and other measures of severity. Its weaknesses are that any error in AIS scoring increases the ISS error, many different injury patterns can give the same ISS score, and injuries to different body regions are not weighted. Also, as a full description of patient injuries is not known prior to a full clinical investigation and potential surgery, the ISS, along with other anatomical scoring system, is not useful as a triage tool. As multiple injuries within the same body region are only assigned a single score, a modification of the ISS, the "New Injury Severity Score" (NISS), has been proposed (Osler et al. 1997). This is calculated as the sum of the squares of the top three AIS scores regardless of body region. The NISS has been found to statistically outperform the traditional ISS score and is possibly a more accurate predictor of mortality in TBI (Lavoie et al. 2004).

3.3 Specific Paediatric Concerns

Standard GCS scoring of non-verbal children is inapplicable. The responses of children change with development, so the GCS requires modification for paediatric use (Table 3.1) (Matis and Birbilis 2008). In children with severe TBI, the GCS is an independent predictor of mortality, as in adults (White et al. 2001; Holmes et al. 2005; Tude Melo et al. 2010). However, in children, pupil examination seems to be of less value (Halley et al. 2004; Chan et al. 2005).

References

Alvarez M, Nava JM, Rué M, Quintana S (1998) Mortality prediction in head trauma patients: performance of Glasgow Coma Score and general severity systems. Crit Care Med 26:142–148

Baker SP, O'Neill B, Haddon W, Long WB (1974) The injury severity score: a method for describing patients with multiple injuries and evaluating emergency care. J Trauma 14:187–196

Braakman R, Avezaat CJ, Maas AI, Roel M, Schouten HJ (1977) Inter observer agreement in the assessment of the motor response of the Glasgow "coma" scale. Clin Neurol Neurosurg 80:100–106

Chan HC, Adnan WAW, Jaalam K, Abdullah MR, Abdullah J (2005) Which mild head injured patients should have follow-up after discharge from an accident and emergency ward? A study in a university hospital setting in Kelantan, Malaysia. Southeast Asian J Trop Med Public Health 36:982–993

Chesnut RM (1997) Appropriate use of the Glasgow Coma Scale in intubated patients: a linear regression prediction of the Glasgow verbal score from the Glasgow eye and motor scores. J Trauma 42:345

Chesnut RM, Gautille T, Blunt BA, Klauber MR, Marshall LE (1994) The localizing value of asymmetry in pupillary size in severe head injury: relation to lesion type and location. Neurosurgery 34:840–845

Fearnside MR, Cook RJ, McDougall P, McNeil RJ (1993) The Westmead Head Injury Project outcome in severe head injury. A comparative analysis of pre-hospital, clinical and CT variables. Br J Neurosurg 7:67–279

Fujisawa H, Marukawa K, Kida S, Hasegawa M, Yamashita J, Matsui O (2001) Abducens nerve palsy and ipsilateral Horner syndrome: a predicting sign of intracranial carotid injury in a head trauma patient. J Trauma 50:554–556

Halley MK, Silva PD, Foley J, Rodarte A (2004) Loss of consciousness: when to perform computed tomography? Pediatr Crit Care Med 5:230–233

Healey C, Osler TM, Rogers FB, Healey MA, Glance LG, Kilgo PD, Shackford SR, Meredith JW (2003) Improving the Glasgow Coma Scale score: motor score alone is a better predictor. J Trauma 54: 671–678

Holmes JF, Palchak MJ, MacFarlane T, Kuppermann N (2005) Performance of the pediatric glasgow coma scale in children with blunt head trauma. Acad Emerg Med 12:814–819

Kung W-M, Tsai S-H, Chiu W-T, Hung K-S, Wang S-P, Lin J-W, Lin M-S (2010) Correlation between Glasgow coma score components and survival in patients with traumatic brain injury. Injury 49:940–944

Lavoie A, Moore L, LeSage N, Liberman M, Sampalis JS (2004) The New Injury Severity Score: a more accurate predictor of in-hospital mortality than the Injury Severity Score. J Trauma 56:1312–1320

MacKenzie EJ, Shapiro S, Eastham JN (1985) The Abbreviated Injury Scale and Injury Severity Score. Levels of inter- and intrarater reliability. Med Care 23:823–835

Matis G, Birbilis T (2008) The Glasgow Coma Scale – a brief review. Past, present, future. Acta Neurol Belg 108:75–89

Menegazzi JJ, Davis EA, Sucov AN, Paris PM (1993) Reliability of the Glasgow Coma Scale when used by emergency physicians and paramedics. J Trauma 34:46–48

Meredith W, Rutledge R, Fakhry SM, Emery S, Kromhout-Schiro S (1998) The conundrum of the Glasgow Coma Scale in intubated patients: a linear regression prediction of the Glasgow verbal score from the Glasgow eye and motor scores. J Trauma 44:839–844

Meyer S, Gibb T, Jurkovich GJ (1993) Evaluation and significance of the pupillary light reflex in trauma patients. Ann Emerg Med 22:1052–1057

Narayan RK, Greenberg RP, Miller JD, Enas GG, Choi SC, Kishore PR, Selhorst JB, Lutz HA, Becker DP (1981) Improved confidence of outcome prediction in severe head injury. A comparative analysis of the clinical examination, multimodality evoked potentials, CT scanning, and intracranial pressure. J Neurosurg 54:751–762

Osler T, Baker SP, Long W (1997) A modification of the injury severity score that both improves accuracy and simplifies scoring. J Trauma 43:922–925

Rocca B, Martin C, Viviand X, Bidet PF, Saint-Gilles HL, Chevalier A (1989) Comparison of four severity scores in patients with head trauma. J Trauma 29:299–305

Rutledge R, Lentz CW, Fakhry S, Hunt J (1996) Appropriate use of the Glasgow Coma Scale in intubated patients: a linear regression prediction of the Glasgow verbal score from the Glasgow eye and motor scores. J Trauma 41:514–522

Starmark JE, Stålhammar D, Holmgren E (1988) The Reaction Level Scale (RLS85). Manual and guidelines. Acta Neurochir (Wien) 91:12–20

Teasdale G, Jennett B (1974) Assessment of coma and impaired consciousness. A practical scale. Lancet 2:81–84

Teasdale G, Jennett B (1976) Assessment and prognosis of coma after head injury. Acta Neurochir (Wien) 34:45–55

Tude Melo JR, Di Rocco F, Blanot S, Oliveira-Filho J, Roujeau T, Sainte-Rose C, Duracher C, Vecchione A, Meyer P, Zerah M (2010) Mortality in children with severe head trauma: predictive factors and proposal for a new predictive scale. Neurosurgery 67:1542–1547

White JR, Farukhi Z, Bull C, Christensen J, Gordon T, Paidas C, Nichols DG (2001) Predictors of outcome in severely head-injured children. Crit Care Med 29:534–540

Wijdicks EFM, Bamlet WR, Maramattom BV, Manno EM, McClelland RL (2005) Validation of a new coma scale: the FOUR score. Ann Neurol 58:585–593

Part III

Prehospital Management

Prehospital Management of Severe Traumatic Brain Injury (TBI)

4

Snorre Sollid

Recommendations

Level I

There are insufficient data to support a Level I recommendation for this topic.

Level II

There are insufficient data to support a Level II recommendation for this topic.

Level III

Trauma Systems

All regions should have an organised trauma care system.

It is not recommended to perform craniotomy on head injury patients at hospitals without neurosurgical expertise.

Protocols are recommended to direct Emergency Medical Service (EMS) personnel for patients with severe traumatic brain injury (TBI).

Patients with severe TBI should be transported directly to a facility with immediately available CT scanning, prompt neurosurgical care, and the ability to monitor intracranial pressure (ICP) and treat intracranial hypertension.

The mode of transport should be selected so as to minimise total prehospital time for the patient with TBI.

Prehospital Treatment

Avoid hypoxemia (arterial haemoglobin oxygen saturation [SaO_2] <90%) and correct immediately when identified.

An airway should be established in patients who have severe TBI (GCS<9), the inability to maintain an adequate airway, or hypoxemia not corrected by supplemental oxygen by the most appropriate means available.

When endotracheal intubation is used to establish an airway, confirmation of placement of the tube in the trachea should include lung auscultation and end-tidal CO_2 ($ETCO_2$) determination.

Patients should be maintained with normal breathing rates ($ETCO_2$ 35–40 mmHg), and hyperventilation ($ETCO_2$ <35 mmHg) should be avoided unless the patient shows signs of cerebral herniation.

Hypotensive patients should be treated with isotonic fluids.

Hypertonic resuscitation is a treatment option for TBI patients with a Glasgow Coma Scale Score (GCS) <9.

Paediatric Considerations

In the paediatric population, there is no prehospital evidence that directly associates oxygenation and blood pressure to patient outcome. In-hospital data in children indicate that hypotension is linked to poor outcome.

S. Sollid
Department of Neurosurgery,
University Hospital of North Norway,
9038 Tromsø, Norway
e-mail: snorre.sollid@unn.no

T. Sundstrøm et al. (eds.), *Management of Severe Traumatic Brain Injury*,
DOI 10.1007/978-3-642-28126-6_4, © Springer-Verlag Berlin Heidelberg 2012

No data exist regarding the relationship between prehospital assessment of the GCS and outcome in paediatric patients. Hospital data from the emergency department, paediatric critical care, and neurosurgical services indicate that the GCS and the paediatric GCS (PGCS) are reliable indicators of the severity of TBI in children.

4.1 Overview

Traumatic injury is the leading cause of early death and lifelong disability. If the trauma victim suffers from a head injury, the mortality rate is as high as 30% compared to 1% without TBI. Half of those who die from TBI do so within the first 2 h of injury. It is known that not all neurological injuries after the trauma are caused by the primary injury. Secondary injury evolves over the ensuing minutes, hours, and days. This secondary injury can result in increased mortality and disability. Consequently, the early and appropriate management of TBI is critical to the survival of these patients.

To deliver optimal treatment, management, and transport in the early phase after TBI, adequate assessment of the patients is essential.

Emergency Medical Services (EMS) providers are often the first health-care providers for patients with TBI. Treatment often begins in the field by EMS providers who have varied skills, backgrounds, and qualifications. They continue this care during transport to the hospital. Thus, prehospital assessment and treatment is the first critical link in providing appropriate care for individuals with severe head injury.

In this chapter, we will describe the basic assessment methods for TBI patients and the treatment and transport options for the severely head injured patients.

Tips, Tricks, and Pitfalls

- For BP monitoring in children, use an appropriately sized paediatric cuff. When a blood pressure is difficult to obtain because of the child's age or body habitués, documentation of mental status, quality of peripheral pulses, and capillary-refill time can be used as surrogate measures.
- Patients suffering from TBI should be monitored for hypoxemia and hypotension. The percentage of blood oxygen saturation should be measured continuously with a pulse oximeter. Both systolic and diastolic blood pressure should be measured as often as possible, continuously if possible.
- GCS should be measured repeatedly in the prehospital management of TBI patients.
- GCS/PGCS should be determined after assessment and stabilisation of airways and circulation and prior to administration of sedatives or paralytic drugs.
- The GCS is a clinical test demanding appropriate training in interaction with the patient. Beware that strength of voice and pain stimulation may differ between testers. Thus, only one tester should evaluate the patient in the prehospital phase, if possible.
- When evaluating the pupils, remember that a direct blow to the orbit may give a dilated pupil!
- Prehospital endotracheal intubation performed by untrained personnel could be harmful to the patient.
- For the paediatric TBI patient, hypotension should be treated with isotonic solutions.

4.2 Background

4.2.1 Prehospital Assessments

4.2.1.1 Assessment of Oxygenation and Blood Pressure

Hypoxemia (<90% arterial haemoglobin oxygen saturation) or hypotension (<90 mmHg systolic blood pressure [SBP]) in the prehospital setting are significant parameters associated with a poor outcome in adult patients with severe TBI.

In severe TBI, secondary insults occur frequently and exert a profound negative influence on outcome. This influence appears to differ markedly from that of hypoxemic or hypotensive episodes of similar magnitude occurring in trauma patients without neurological involvement. Hypoxia and hypotension were among the five most powerful predictors of bad outcome in the Traumatic Coma Data Bank study (Chesnut et al. 1993). Hypotension was defined as a single observation of Systolic Blood Pressure (SBP) < 90 mmHg and hypoxia as PaO_2 < 60 mmHg by arterial blood gas analysis. Similar results were found in a study from Italy (Stocchetti et al. 1996). Among 50 patients with TBI, 55% had oxygen saturation <90% measured at the scene prior to intubation. The outcome was strongly influenced by the hypoxia and hypotension. The same deleterious effect of hypotension and hypoxia is also seen in children (Pigula et al. 1993).

The value of 90-mmHg threshold for SBP must be regarded as rather arbitrary. It is advocated to aim at a blood pressure higher than this threshold. In the calculation of the Cerebral Perfusion Pressure (CPP) = (MAP) − (ICP), a higher blood pressure is necessary to achieve an optimal perfusion of the brain if the ICP is elevated.

4.2.1.2 Assessment of Consciousness: Glasgow Coma Scale Score

For more details on this topic, see Chap. 3.

Prehospital measurement of the Glasgow Coma Scale score (GCS) is a significant and reliable indicator of the severity of the TBI, particularly in association with repeated scoring and improvement or deterioration of the patient over time.

The GCS has become the most used repeatable neurological test for measurement of the level of consciousness after TBI. The test was developed in 1974 by (Teasdale and Jennet 1974). The GCS permits a repetitive and moderately reliable standardised method of reporting and recording ongoing neurological evaluation even when performed by a variety of health-care providers.

The GCS evaluates three independent responses: eye, motor response, and verbal response. For patients not able to follow command, the best motor and eye response is scored after a standardised stimulus. The stimulus should preferably be applied to an area innervated by a cranial nerve. Painful areas are the mastoid or the eyebrow.

The GCS score can be affected by several pre- and post-traumatic factors. Treatable causes to low GCS such as hypoglycaemia and alcohol/narcotic overdose should be determined and treated. Other important factors, such as hypotension and hypoxia, also lower GCS. Airway control and fluid resuscitation should therefore be performed prior to GCS assessment.

The predictive value of a low prehospital GCS has been shown in several studies, both for adults and children (Servadei et al. 1998; White et al. 2001). The change in GCS from the scene of the accident to the Emergency Department is a stronger prognostic factor for survival and outcome. Those patients with an improvement of the GCS score of more than 2 points had a favourable outcome compared with those who deteriorated or had no improvement. Servadei et al. showed that the need for acute decompressive surgery for ASDH was more likely among deteriorating patients (Servadei et al. 1998).

4.2.1.3 Assessment of the Pupils

No data specific to pupillary assessment in the prehospital setting support its diagnostic and prognostic value for TBI patients. In-hospital data show that the pupillary exam is important for diagnosis, treatment, and prognosis. Therefore, despite the absence of prehospital data, it is recommended that pupils are assessed in the field.

Protocol for measuring pupils:

1. Evidence of orbital trauma should be noted.
2. Pupils should be measured after the patient has been resuscitated and stabilised.
3. Note left and right pupillary finding.
   - Unilateral or bilateral dilated pupil(s)
   - Fixed and dilated pupil(s)

Definitions:

Asymmetry is defined as >1-mm difference in diameter.

A fixed pupil is defined as <1-mm response to bright light.

Pupillary asymmetry of less than 1 mm has no pathological significance (Meyer 1947).

To assess the pupil size, symmetry and reaction to light are essential components of the post-traumatic neurological exam. The light reflex depends on an intact afferent system, an intact brainstem, and an intact efferent system. The direct and indirect (consensual) light reflex test could identify a life-threatening herniation syndrome or ischemia of the brain stem.

Unilateral pressure or destruction to the III cranial nerve produces a dilated pupil on the same side. A direct trauma to the orbit may do the same. Bilateral dilated and fixed pupils are caused by direct or indirect affection of the brain stem.

A lot of other conditions are associated with dilated pupils and abnormal reactivity. Metabolic or cardiovascular disturbances including hypoxemia, hypotension, and hypothermia may give abnormal pupils and reaction. It is therefore important to resuscitate and stabilise the patient before assessing pupillary function (Meyer et al. 1993).

Even though pupil size and reactivity is an important indicator of brain trauma and prognoses of the head injury, it is an unspecific indicator of injury severity or involved anatomy. Data from 608 patients with severe TBI were assessed for the reliability of pupillary asymmetry in predicting the presence and location of intracranial mass lesions (Chesnut et al. 1994). Pupillary asymmetry had a positive predictive value of 30%. Of the affected patients 80% had a contralateral lesion to the pupil finding. Anisocoria had a sensitivity of 40% and a specificity of 67%; even when the pupils were different by more than 3 mm, there was a 43% positive predictive value.

4.2.2 Prehospital Treatment

4.2.2.1 Treatment: Airway, Ventilation, and Oxygenation

In ground-transported patients in urban environment, it is not recommended to use paralytics routinely to assist endotracheal intubation in patients who are spontaneously breathing and maintaining a SpO_2 above 90% on supplemental oxygen.

Hypoxemia is a strong predictor of outcome in the TBI patient (Chesnut et al. 1993). Data from the Traumatic Coma Databank showed a significant increased risk of death among TBI patients with hypoxemia (PaO_2 < 60 mmHg). Simultaneous hypotension further increased the risk. Optimal oxygenation and assessing the airways are therefore the primary goal in the early treatment. Hypoxemia could be corrected using supplemental oxygen administrated through a bag/mask for patients with adequate respiration or to perform endotracheal intubation for administration of oxygen.

Several studies have shown that prehospital endotracheal intubation performed by untrained personnel could be harmful to the patient (Davis et al. 2003). In urban areas with short prehospital transport times, it is therefore warranted not to intubate. Induced hypoxemia due to long or failed intubation and involuntary hyperventilation are the main causes for this recommendation. Such acts could induce cerebral ischemia. In trauma systems staffed with trained personnel regularly performing the procedure and the opportunity to monitor both the tube position and adequate ventilation, intubation could be performed without unwarrantable risks (Helm et al. 2006). One small retrospective study reported no statistically significant difference in survival in children with TBI who were intubated in the field compared with those ventilated with bag mask ventilation, which is a safe alternative (Gausche et al. 2000).

The use of ETCO2 monitoring reduces the risk of hyperventilation and misplacement of the endotracheal tube (Silvestri et al. 2005) and should be used if intubation is performed.

4.2.2.2 Fluid Resuscitation

Haemorrhage following trauma is the major cause of hypovolaemia and hypotension. This reduces the peripheral and cerebral oxygen delivery and could cause secondary injury to the brain. This is especially dangerous to the TBI patients with a post-traumatic decreased cerebral perfusion in the first hand. In adults, hypotension is defined as a systolic blood pressure (SBP) of <90 mmHg. In children, hypotension is defined as SBP less than the 5th percentile for age or by clinical signs of shock. For more exact values, see Sect. 4.3.

The deleterious effect of hypotension on outcome after TBI is well documented (Chesnut et al. 1993). Despite this fact, there is much less evidence that reducing or preventing this secondary insult improves outcome.

The goal of prehospital fluid resuscitation is to support oxygen delivery and optimise cerebral haemodynamics.

Isotonic crystalloid solution is the fluid most often used in the prehospital setting. However, little data have been published to support its use. Wade et al. showed a beneficial effect of hypertonic solutions (Wade et al. 1997). The total load of evidence is so far not convincing enough to recommend one treatment over the other. The most recent randomised controlled study by Cooper et al. did not show any significant difference in outcome between patients with TBI and hypotension treated with hypertonic saline compared with isotonic crystalloid (Cooper et al. 2004).

4.2.2.3 Treatment in Case of Cerebral Herniation

Mild or prophylactic hyperventilation ($ETCO_2$ < 35 mmHg) should be avoided. Hyperventilation therapy titrated to clinical effect may be necessary for brief periods in cases of cerebral herniation or acute neurological deterioration.

Patients should be assessed frequently for clinical signs of cerebral herniation. The clinical signs of cerebral herniation include dilated and uncreative pupils, asymmetric pupils, a motor exam that identifies either extensor posturing or no response, or progressive neurologic deterioration (decrease in the GCS Score of more than 2 points from the patient's prior best score in patients with an initial GCS < 9).

In patients who are normoventilated, well oxygenated, and normotensive – and still have signs of cerebral herniation – hyperventilation should be used as a temporary measure and discontinued when clinical signs of herniation resolve.

Hyperventilation is administrated as:

- 20 breaths per minute in an adult
- 25 breaths per minute in a child
- 30 breaths per minute in an infant less than 1 year old

The goal of hyperventilation is $ETCO_2$ of 30–35 mmHg. Capnography is the preferred method for monitoring ventilation.

There is solid evidence for the reducible effect of hyperventilation upon ICP (Lundberg et al. 1959). Vasoconstriction with a subsequent reduction in cerebral blood flow could however induce cerebral ischemia. Prophylactic hyperventilation worsens outcome in TBI patients (Muizelaar et al. 1991). The use of hyperventilation should be restricted to selected patients showing signs of cerebral herniation and finished when the patient improves. It appears that in some patients with progressive cerebral oedema, hyperventilation can temporarily stop herniation. In patients who have objective evidence of herniation, the benefits of hyperventilation in delaying the process outweigh the potential detrimental effects.

Osmotherapy, first of all Mannitol, has long been accepted as an effective tool for reducing intracranial pressure, even though no positive prognostic effect has been proven (Smith et al. 1986). So far, no good evidence supports the use of Mannitol in the prehospital setting. Hypertonic saline offers an attractive alternative to Mannitol as a brain targeted hyper-osmotic therapy. Its ability to reduce ICP has been demonstrated to be as effective as Mannitol (de Vivo et al. 2001).

Despite this knowledge, hyper-osmotic therapy could be considered in the prehospital setting in situations where the transport facilities, monitoring, and personnel equals that of an intensive care setting (advanced air ambulances) and long prehospital transport times.

4.2.3 Decision Making Within the Emergency Medical Service EMS System: Dispatch, Scene, Transportation, and Destination

Prehospital recognition of TBI, the decisions made, and responses performed are important elements in the prehospital setting which need structural systems. Good prehospital trauma systems are based on:

(a) Information gathered by EMS call-takers and dispatchers to determine if a patient potentially has a significant brain injury.

(b) Dispatcher decisions about the type of personnel to be dispatched, resources to be deployed, and the priority for the response.
(c) Prehospital care provider assessment of the overall neurological situation through evaluation of the mechanism of the injury (i.e., vehicular deformation, windshield violation, the use or non-use of seat belts, or other safety devices), the scene, and the patient examination.
(d) Based on the overall assessment, prehospital interventions are initiated to prevent or correct hypotension or hypoxemia and to address other potential threats to life or limb. At this step, the decision regarding the level of responder dispatched to the scene impacts patient care.
(e) Prehospital care providers select a transport mode (e.g., ground ambulance, helicopter, plane – red lights and siren versus neither).
(f) Prehospital care providers select the appropriate destination facility.

All trauma patients benefits from treatment at a level I trauma centre (Guss et al. 1989). Direct transport to a Level I trauma centre improves survival and outcome in TBI patients (Hartl et al. 2006). Prehospital trauma systems may differ, due to large geographical differences concerning hospital structure, transport systems and distances, and personnel qualifications. It is warranted to make systems to secure optimal assessment, treatment, and fast transport to a hospital with sufficient neurotrauma care. It is not recommended to perform head injury surgery at local or central hospitals without neurosurgical expertise (Wester 1999; Wester et al. 1999).

4.3 Specific Paediatric Concerns

In children, hypotension is defined as SBP less than the 5th percentile for age or by clinical signs of shock. Usual values are:

Age	SBP
0–28 days	<60 mmHg
1–12 months	<70
1–10 years	<70 + 2× age in years
>10 years	<90

For preverbal children (under the age of 2 years), a modified GCS for children should be used (Paediatric GCS – PGCS). As for adults, the GCS/PGCS should be determined after assessment and stabilisation of airways and circulation and prior to administration of sedatives or paralytic drugs.

For the paediatric TBI patient, hypotension should be treated with isotonic solutions.

As for adults, the GCS/PGCS should be determined after assessment and stabilisation of airways and circulation and prior to administration of sedatives or paralytic drugs.

In a metropolitan area, paediatric patients with severe TBI should be transported directly to a paediatric trauma centre if available.

Paediatric patients with severe TBI should be treated in a paediatric trauma centre or in an adult trauma centre with added qualifications to treat children in preference to a Level I or II adult trauma centre without added qualifications for paediatric treatment.

References

Chesnut RM, Marshall LF, Klauber MR et al (1993) The role of secondary brain injury in determining outcome from severe head injury. J Trauma 34:216–222
Chesnut RM, Gautille T, Blunt BA, Klauber MR, Marshall LE (1994) The localizing value of asymmetry in pupillary size in severe head injury: relation to lesion type and location. Neurosurgery 34:840–845
Cooper DJ, Myles PS, McDermott FT et al (2004) Prehospital hypertonic saline resuscitation of patients with hypotension and severe traumatic brain injury: a randomized controlled trial. JAMA 291:1350–1357
Davis DP, Hoyt DB, Ochs M et al (2003) The effect of paramedic rapid sequence intubation on outcome in patients with severe traumatic brain injury. J Trauma 54:444–453
De Vivo P, Del Gaudio A, Ciritella P, Puopolo M, Chiarotti F, Mastronardi E (2001) Hypertonic saline solution: a safe alternative to mannitol 18% in neurosurgery. Minerva Anestesiol 67:603–611
Gausche M, Lewis RJ, Stratton SJ et al (2000) Effect of out-of-hospital pediatric endotracheal intubation on survival and neurological outcome: a controlled clinical trial. JAMA 283:783–790
Guss DA, Meyer FT, Neuman TS et al (1989) The impact of a regionalized trauma system on trauma care in San Diego County. Ann Emerg Med 18:1141–1145
Hartl R, Gerber LM, Iacono L, Ni Q, Lyons K, Ghajar J (2006) Direct transport within an organized state trauma

system reduces mortality in patients with severe traumatic brain injury. J Trauma 60(6):1250–1256

Helm M, Hossfeld B, Schafer S, Hoitz J, Lampl L (2006) Factors influencing emergency intubation in the prehospital setting – a multicentre study in the German Helicopter Emergency Medical Service. Br J Anaesth 96:67–71

Lundberg N, Kjallquist A, Bien C (1959) Reduction of increased intracranial pressure by hyperventilation. A therapeutic aid in neurological surgery. Acta Psychiatr Scand Suppl 34:1–64

Meyer BC (1947) Incidence of anisocoria and difference in size of palpebral fissures in five hundred normal subjects. Arch Neurol Psychiatry 57:464–468

Meyer S, Gibb T, Jurkovich GJ (1993) Evaluation and significance of the pupillary light reflex in trauma patients. Ann Emerg Med 22:1052–1057

Muizelaar JP, Marmarou A, Ward JD et al (1991) Adverse effects of prolonged hyperventilation in patients with severe head injury: a randomized clinical trial. J Neurosurg 75:731–739

Pigula FA, Wald SL, Shackford SR, Vane DW (1993) The effect of hypotension and hypoxia on children with severe head injuries. J Pediatr Surg 28:310–314

Servadei F, Nasi MT, Cremonini AM, Giuliani G, Cenni P, Nanni A (1998) Importance of a reliable admission Glasgow Coma Scale score for determining the need for evacuation of posttraumatic subdural hematomas: a prospective study of 65 patients. J Trauma 44:868–873

Silvestri S, Ralls GA, Krauss B et al (2005) The effectiveness of out-of-hospital use of continuous end-tidal carbon dioxide monitoring on the rate of unrecognized misplaced intubation within a regional emergency medical services system. Ann Emerg Med 45:497–503

Smith HP, Kelly DL Jr, McWhorter JM et al (1986) Comparison of mannitol regimens in patients with severe head injury undergoing intracranial monitoring. J Neurosurg 65:820–824

Stocchetti N, Furlan A, Volta F (1996) Hypoxemia and arterial hypotension at the accident scene in head injury. J Trauma 40:764–767

Teasdale G, Jennett B (1974) Assessment of coma and impaired consciousness. A practical scale. Lancet 2:81–84

Wade CE, Grady JJ, Kramer GC, Younes RN, Gehlsen K, Holcroft JW (1997) Individual patient cohort analysis of the efficacy of hypertonic saline/dextran in patients with traumatic brain injury and hypotension. J Trauma 42:S61–S65

Wester K (1999) Decompressive surgery for "pure" epidural hematomas: does neurosurgical expertise improve the outcome? Neurosurgery 44:495–500

Wester T, Fevang LT, Wester K (1999) Decompressive surgery in acute head injuries: where should it be performed? J Trauma 46:914–919

White JR, Farukhi Z, Bull C et al (2001) Predictors of outcome in severely head-injured children. Crit Care Med 29:534–540

5 What the Neurosurgeon Wants to Know: What, Who, When, and Where?

Knut Wester

The recommendations in this chapter are purely based on common sense and practical knowledge.

During the first-emergency contact between the referring hospital/the prehospital unit and the neurosurgical department, the following information should be given by the referring partner or asked for by the neurosurgical unit. Our recommendation is that this information is given and collected/filed in a systematic, standardised fashion, e.g. by using and filling in an information sheet as shown at the end of this chapter. This sheet may be copied and/or modified and should be spread and available in the neurosurgical unit.

NB! Remember to notify the anaesthesiology personnel and the CT/MR laboratories about the patient immediately!

K. Wester
Department of Surgical Sciences,
University of Bergen,
Jonas Lies Vei 65, 5021 Bergen, Norway

Department of Neurosurgery,
Haukeland University Hospital,
Jonas Lies Vei 65, 5021 Bergen, Norway
e-mail: knut.gustav.wester@helse-bergen.no

5.1 What?

Current Consciousness Level and Neurological Status

GCS score (total and each category)?

- Any signs of herniation?
  - Pupillary dilatation (uni- or bilateral)?
  - Extension spasms?
- Any other coarse neurological deficit (hemi-para, or tetraparesis)?

Injury Mechanism

- High velocity (yes/no)?
- Traffic accident?
  - Car collision? Speed? Driver? Passenger?
  - MC? Speed? Other vehicles involved?
  - Bicycle? Other vehicles involved?
  - Pedestrian! Hit by what and at which speed?
- Fall?
  - From which height?
- Violence?
  - Blunt blow? By what?
  - Penetrating injuries?
- Multitrauma (yes/no)?
  - External/internal blood loss?
  - Indications of fractures (extremities, pelvic, spine)?
  - Adequate ventilation?

T. Sundstrøm et al. (eds.), *Management of Severe Traumatic Brain Injury*,
DOI 10.1007/978-3-642-28126-6_5, © Springer-Verlag Berlin Heidelberg 2012

- Any indication of a neck injury?
  - Para- or tetraparalyses?
  - Localised neck pain?
  - Is the neck stabilised before the transport?
- Is the patient otherwise stable for transport?
  - If not, what needs to be done and where?

Radiological Examinations

- Radiological examinations performed and findings

5.2 Who?

Name

Age

Gender

Any previous medical conditions?

- Anticoagulant medication (yes/no)?
- Hydrocephalus with CSF shunt (yes/no)?
- Other?

5.3 When?

Approximate time of accident

Time of contact with the neurosurgical unit

5.4 Where?

Site of accident.

Present location of the patient and transport to the neurosurgical unit?

- In hospital or in ambulance?
- How far from the neurosurgical unit?
- How soon can the patient be in the neurosurgical unit?
- Who accompanies the patient?
  - Anaesthesiology personnel?
  - Other?

Present location of the patient and transport to the neurosurgical unit

- Is the patient in a hospital
- Or in an ambulance?
- How soon can the patient be in the neurosurgical unit?
- Who accompanies the patient?
  - Anaesthesiology personnel?
  - Other?

Neurotrauma emergency sheet – notify anaesthesiology and radiology!

Message received by: .... (**signature**)	
Name:	**Gender**: **M/F**
D.O.B.:	**Date and time of first contact**:
Approximate time of accident:	**Site of accident**:

The patient's condition:

GCS score (total and each category):	Total:	Eyes:	Motor:	Verbal:
Herniation?				
Unilateral pupillary dilatation:	Yes/no			
Bilateral pupillary dilatation:	Yes/no			
Extension spasms:	Yes/no			
Any other coarse neurological deficit: If yes: what?	**Yes/no**			

Radiological examinations performed and findings:	
Multitrauma:	**Yes/no**
External/internal blood loss?	
Fractures?	
Adequate ventilation?	
Any indication of a neck injury?	**Yes/no**
Is the neck stabilised?	Yes/no
Any previous medical conditions?	
Anticoagulant medication?	Yes/no
Hydrocephalus with CSF shunt?	Yes/no
Other?	Yes/no
Injury mechanism.	
High velocity?	Yes/no
Traffic accident?	
Vehicle?	
Fall? From which height?	
Violence?	

6 Transportation: Choice of Anaesthetic Drugs

Niels Juul

Recommendations

Level I

There are insufficient data to support a Level I recommendation for this topic.

Level II

There are insufficient data to support a Level II recommendation for this topic.

Level III

None of the intravenous anaesthetic or analgesic drugs used in daily practice has any significant advantages over others, and they can all be used en route to hospital. Side effects of the different drugs must be taken into consideration when the choice of anaesthetic drug is taken.

6.1 Overview

Ischemic neuronal injury is characterised by early death mediated by excitotoxicity and by apoptosis. Current evidence indicates that volatile anaesthetic agents, apart from nitrous oxide, barbiturates, and propofol, can protect neurones against ischemic injury caused by excitotoxicity. In the case of volatile agents and propofol, neuroprotection may be sustained if the ischemic insult is relatively mild; however, with moderate to severe insults, this neuronal protection is not sustained after a prolonged recovery period. This suggests that these agents do not protect from delayed neuronal death caused by apoptosis. The long-term effects of any anaesthetic drug on ischemic cerebral injury are not yet defined.

Any opioid can be used, but the influence on ventilation must be taken into consideration. Careful titration must be utilised in the spontaneously breathing patient. Opioids have been shown to reduce the neuroendocrine stress response after traumatic head injury and are consequently of paramount importance in the treatment of TBI victims.

Ketamine has been in bad standing in the neurosurgical community for many years due to the alleged intracranial hypertension after use. New investigations indicate that ketamine is safe and the previous showed rise in ICP probably was caused by increased $PaCO_2$.

Tips, Tricks, and Pitfalls

- Use the drug you are most familiar with.
- It is better to use an anaesthetic drug you are familiar with, and therefore know the influence of on the circulation, instead of choosing a drug with a theoretical better cerebral profile that is unfamiliar to you. A drop in blood pressure or an unexpected

N. Juul
Department of anaesthesia,
Aarhus University Hospital, Noerrebrogade 44,
8000 Aarhus C, Denmark
e-mail: nieljuul@rm.dk

T. Sundstrøm et al. (eds.), *Management of Severe Traumatic Brain Injury*,
DOI 10.1007/978-3-642-28126-6_6, © Springer-Verlag Berlin Heidelberg 2012

high or low CO_2 may create more havoc in the injured brain than use of a suboptimal anaesthetic drug since the differences between the drugs detected in clinical trials are minor.

- Titrate your drugs. It is even more important en route to hospital to avoid hypotension. Give 50–75% of the expected drug dose and wait for the result before adding more. Remember: many of the severely head injured patients have additional injuries and are prone to be hypovolaemic and will require smaller doses of drugs.
- Muscle relaxants should be avoided when possible. The neurosurgeon needs to obtain a full GCS when the patient arrives at the neurosurgical department.

6.2 Background

Considering the patient with TBI, there are minor differences between different anaesthetic regimes. With the focus on avoidance of hypotension and hypoxia, it is important that the treatment team sticks to the drugs best known to them.

For obvious reasons total intravenous anaesthesia is recommended for transport of TBI patients. Thiopentone is by tradition the drug of choice in neuroanaesthesia, and numerous experimental and clinical studies have been carried out proving the benefit in patients with head injury (Shapiro 1985). From experimental and clinical studies, it is clear that propofol produces a dose related decrease in ICP, EEG activity, cerebral blood flow, and cerebral metabolism. When used cautiously, the negative effect on blood pressure is shown to be mild (Weinstabl et al. 1990). Midazolam has been shown to have the same effect on the cerebral circulation as thiopentone.

Opioids are strong respiratory depressants; therefore, they should be used carefully in the spontaneously breathing patient where intracranial pathology is suspected. On the other hand, opioids reduce the neuroendocrine stress response in the trauma patient, and they are indispensable in the treatment of TBI victims. All currently used opioids have been tested in head-injured patients, and the effect on ICP was found to be minor; however, the effect seen on blood pressure is significant. In a study on patients undergoing craniotomy, remifentanil, alfentanil, and fentanyl were compared; no difference in the effect on blood pressure or heart rate was seen (Coles et al. 2000). During the period between intubation and skin incision, remifentanil anaesthetised patients have been found more prone to hypotension, indicating that remifentanil should be omitted as the opioid of choice in the emergency room (Warner 1999).

Muscle relaxants should be used to facilitate tracheal intubation. It is important to create the best working conditions when you perform tracheal intubation in a patient with a stiff neck collar. Succinylcholine or a nondepolarising muscle relaxants can be used. The relative high risk of aspiration should be balanced against the minor risk of increased ICP, when succinylcholine is being used. Use of muscle relaxants during neurointensive care treatment do not diminish ICP or result in a better outcome (Juul et al. 2000).

Ketamine has been studied intensively in the 1970s and afterwards abandoned in neuroanaesthesia due to the cerebral vasodilatation, even though it has intrinsic neuroprotective qualities. However, recently it has been argued that in many of the older studies ketamine was administrated to patients during spontaneous ventilation where an increase in $PaCO_2$ might have been responsible for the observed cerebral vasodilatation and increase in ICP. A study of intracranial hypertension in pigs showed a decrease in ICP when ketamine was administered in normoventilated animals, indicating that ketamine can be used safely in intubated and CO_2-monitored TBI patients (Schmidt et al. 2008).

Considering the patient with TBI, there are minor differences between different anaesthetic regimes. With the focus on avoidance of hypotension and hypoxia, it is important that the treatment team uses the drugs best known to them.

6.3 Specific Paediatric Concerns

Propofol is not recommended for use in children <1 month old. Propofol should be used with caution in paediatric practice.

A data sheet with calculated doses of all relevant drugs should be printed before transport of all paediatric patients.

References

Coles JP, Leary TS, Monteiro JN, Brazier P, Summors A, Doyle P et al (2000) Propofol anesthesia for craniotomy: a double-blind comparison of remifentanil, alfentanil and fentanyl. J Neurosurg Anesthesiol 12:15–20

Juul N, Morris GF, Marshall SB, Marshall LF (2000) Neuromuscular blocking agents in neurointensive care. Acta Neurochir Suppl 76:467–470

Schmidt A, Øye I, Akeson J (2008) Racemic, S(+)- and R(−)-ketamine do not increase elevated intracranial pressure. Acta Anesthesiol Scand 52:1124–1130

Shapiro HM (1985) Barbiturates in brain ischaemia. Br J Anaesth 57:82–95

Warner DS (1999) Experience with remifentanil in neurosurgical patients. Anesth Analg 89:533–539

Weinstabl C, Mayer N, Hammerle AF, Spiss CK (1990) The effect of bolus propofol administration on the intracranial pressure in craniocerebral trauma. Anaesthesist 39:521–524

Part IV

Admission, Diagnostics and Planning

Trauma Team Alert

7

Christina Rosenlund

Recommendations

Level I

There are insufficient data to support a Level I recommendation.

Level II

Patient outcome is directly related to the time elapsed between trauma and properly delivered definite care.

Trauma outcome is improved if critically injured patients are cared for in trauma centres.

Level III

Level and timing of communication between the prehospital system and the primary receiving hospital influences timeliness in patient treatment and transfer to definite care.

7.1 Overview

Before the transfer is effectuated:

1. Ensure that the patient's ABCDEs are appropriately managed (see Sect. 9.2).
2. Do not wait for test results other than those necessary to ensure hemodynamic and respiratory stability.
3. Ensure that the level of care does not deteriorate, including the care delivered during transport to definite care.
4. Ensure that the proper written information is following the patient.
5. Contact the trauma team leader when transfer is initiated.

Information provided directly to the trauma team leader at the receiving hospital should include:

1. Patient identification.
2. Brief history of the incident, including pertinent prehospital data.
3. Initial findings in the primary hospital.
4. Patient's response to the therapy administered.

7.2 Background

The primary injury during trauma is inevitable. The secondary injury, however, is developing in the minutes and hours following trauma and the timing, and prioritising of treatment is of crucial importance to the patient outcome. It is the responsibility of the prehospital personnel and their medical director to ensure that appropriate patients arrive at appropriate hospitals and to alert the receiving hospital as early as possible. It is essential that doctors assess their own capabilities and limitations, as well as those of their institution, to allow for early recognition of

C. Rosenlund
Department of Neurosurgery,
Odense University Hospital,
Sdr. Boulevard 29, 5000 Odense, DK
e-mail: chrisstenrose@gmail.com

T. Sundstrøm et al. (eds.), *Management of Severe Traumatic Brain Injury*,
DOI 10.1007/978-3-642-28126-6_7, © Springer-Verlag Berlin Heidelberg 2012

patients who may be safely cared for in the local hospital and those who require transfer for definite care. Once the need for transfer is recognised, arrangements should be expedited and not be delayed for diagnostic procedures that do not change the immediate plan of care. Transfer agreements must be established as early as possible to provide for the consistent and efficient movement of patients between institutions. The patient must be as respiratory and circulatory stabile as possible and should be transferred with personnel capable of monitoring and giving treatment to the trauma patient. The information accompanying the patient should include a written record of the problem, clinical findings, treatment given, and patient's status at the time of transfer in addition to demographic and historical information pertinent to the patient's injury (Mullins et al. 1994; Schoettker et al. 2003; Sharar et al. 1988).

7.3 Specific Paediatric Concerns

The recommendation regarding paediatric trauma patients follows the adult protocol.

References

Mullins PJ et al (1994) Outcome of hospitalized injured patients after institution of a trauma system in an urban area. JAMA 271:1919–1924

Schoettker P et al (2003) Reduction of time to definite care in trauma patients: effectiveness of a new checklist system. Injury 34:187–190

Sharar SR et al (1988) Air transport following surgical stabilization: an extension of regionalized trauma care. J Trauma 28:794–798

The Trauma Team

8

Christina Rosenlund

Recommendations

Level I

There are insufficient data to support a Level I recommendation.

Level II

Implementation of standardised trauma evaluation, trauma centres, and better pre-hospital care has shortened the time from the trauma scene to definite care.

Level III

Implementation of trauma teams has reduced the time spent at primary trauma care and the frequency of overseen injuries.

C. Rosenlund
Department of Neurosurgery,
Odense University Hospital,
Sdr. Boulevard 29, 5000 Odense, DK
e-mail: chrisstenrose@gmail.com

Tips, Tricks, and Pitfalls

- The team leader should not participate in the practical management of the patient but should concentrate on keeping track of the process.
- Speak out loud whenever you take an assignment. Teamwork is essential.
- Step away from the scene whenever you are without an assignment.

8.1 Overview

Receiving and treating severely injured patients involve many different groups of personnel and medical specialties which constitute the trauma team. The trauma team is typically formed by a surgeon, an anaesthesiologist, emergency department nurses, anaesthesiology nurses, and a radiologist. It is important that the trauma team and the trauma team settings are well organised and of high quality since the acute diagnostics and treatment can be very challenging. Systematic and strict procedures should be outlined in a trauma manual. The trauma team should have a team leader (often the surgeon) who is responsible for coordinating the process, gathering information, and making the final decisions for further treatment. Airway resuscitation equipment should be checked and easily assessable. Warmed intravenous crystalloid solutions should be available. Appropriate monitoring capabilities should be present.

T. Sundstrøm et al. (eds.), *Management of Severe Traumatic Brain Injury*,
DOI 10.1007/978-3-642-28126-6_8, © Springer-Verlag Berlin Heidelberg 2012

8.2 Background

Death due to injury occurs in one of three periods, first described in 1982, the first period being within seconds to minutes after the injury. The second period is within minutes to several hours following injury. The third peak occurs within hours to days or weeks following trauma and is due to sepsis or multiple organ failure. The development of standardised trauma training, better pre-hospital care, development of trauma centres, and protocols for intensive care of injured patients has improved the prognosis and altered the picture. The golden hour of care after injury is characterised by rapid assessment and resuscitation, which are the fundamental principles of Advanced Trauma Life Support – the ATLS program. Forty-seven countries are now providing this program to their doctors. Studies have shown significant effect on morbidity and mortality following implementation (Ali et al. 1993; Anderson et al. 1997; van Olden et al. 2004; Williams et al. 1997). The principles are founded on the fact that the injuries causing the deaths within the second period are intracranial haematomas (epi- and subdural), thoracic injuries causing problems with the airways, breathing, or circulation, and abdominal or extremity injuries causing massive bleeding; for the ABCDE principle, see Chap. 9.

8.3 Specific Paediatric Concerns

The recommendation regarding paediatric patients follows the adult protocol.

References

Ali J et al (1993) Trauma outcome improves following the Advanced Trauma Life Support program in a developing country. J Trauma 34:890–899

Anderson ID et al (1997) Advanced Trauma Life Support in the UK: 8 years on. Br J Hosp Med 57:272–273

van Olden GDJ et al (2004) Clinical impact of advanced trauma life support. Am J Emerg Med 22:522–525

Williams MJ et al (1997) Improved trauma management with Advanced Trauma Life Support (ATLS) training. J Accid Emerg Med 14:81–83

Trauma Protocol (ABCDE) 9

Christina Rosenlund

Recommendations

Level I

There are insufficient data to support a Level I recommendation.

Level II

There are insufficient data to support a Level II recommendation.

Level III

Implementation of systematic trauma protocols has shortened the time interval to definitive care and reduced the frequency of overseen injuries.

9.1 Overview

Systematic evaluation and re-evaluation of the patient following the ABCDE principles will diminish the risk of overlooking injuries in the patient. Primary focus in the first 5 min is to discover the most critical injuries. The secondary survey is more thorough and will reveal the injuries causing problems later (Enderson et al. 2001; Esposito et al. 2005).

C. Rosenlund
Department of Neurosurgery,
Odense University Hospital,
Sdr. Boulevard 29, 5000 Odense, DK
e-mail: chrisstenrose@gmail.com

Tips, Tricks, and Pitfalls

- (**A**irway) Nasopharyngeal airway is NOT an option in patients with skull base fractures.
- (**A**) The presence of gastric contents (vomiting) in the oropharynx represents a significant risk of aspiration. Suction and rotation (log roll) are indicated.
- (**A**) Abusive and belligerent patients may in fact have hypoxia and should not be presumed intoxicated.
- (**A**) Performing a needle cricothyroidotomy with jet insufflation can provide the time necessary to establish a definite airway when all other options have failed, and hypoxia and patient deterioration are a threat.
- (**B**reathing) Patients with a penetrating thoracic trauma are presumed to have a pneumothorax until proven otherwise.
- (**B**) Both tension pneumothorax and massive haemothorax are associated with decreased breath sounds. Hyperresonance in percussion confirms a pneumothorax, dullness a haemothorax. Definite diagnosis, however, is made by x-ray (noise in the trauma settings can make the differentiation impossible!).
- (**B**/**C**irculation) Pressure pneumothorax and cardiac tamponade can cause shock. Pneumothorax is much more frequent than tamponade.

T. Sundstrøm et al. (eds.), *Management of Severe Traumatic Brain Injury*,
DOI 10.1007/978-3-642-28126-6_9, © Springer-Verlag Berlin Heidelberg 2012

- **(C)** Until proven otherwise, bleeding is the reason for shock in a trauma patient!
- **(D**isability) Intracranial haemorrhage is almost never the reason for shock – at least not because of bleeding! Important exception: infants!
- **(ABCDE)** Initial monitoring and tests:
  - Pulse oximetry
  - Capnography (intubated patients)
  - Invasive blood pressure
  - Continuous ECG
  - Temperature
  - Urinary catheter
  - Plain X-ray (thorax, pelvis)
  - FAST (abdomen)

9.2 Background

The initial 5 min:

Airway:

- Assess airway patency simultaneously with securing the cervical spine. Bleeding, facial fractures, direct trauma against head/neck, or unconsciousness can cause problems handling the airway.
- GCS < 9 indicates intubation.
- See (alertness, colour, breathing movements, lesions/obstructions).
- Listen (breathing sounds/noise, speech).
- Feel (trachea in midline).

Endotracheal intubation includes sedation. Four-person procedure: a skilled intubator, a person fixating head and cervical spine, a person providing cricoid pressure, and a person giving medication and providing suction and tube whenever necessary.

If a definite airway is not obtainable through endotracheal intubation, a surgical airway is necessary. This is done through the cricothyroid membraneeitherasaneedleorsurgicalcricothyroidotomy, in which the latter is to consider as a definite airway with insertion of a small endotracheal or a tracheostomy tube through the membrane.

Temporary options to a definite airway includes chin lift, jaw thrust, oropharyngeal airway, nasopharyngeal airway (see Tips, Tricks, and Pitfalls), laryngeal mask airway, multilumen oesophageal airway, laryngeal tube airway, and of course oxygen provided either directly through the established airway, through a nasal catheter, or a mask (American College Committee on Trauma 2008).

Breathing:

- See (movement of the thorax, lesions).
- Listen (percussion, stethoscope).
- Feel (fractures of ribs/sternum, subcutaneous emphysema).
- Measure respiratory frequency, pulse oximetry (and end-tidal CO_2).
- Signs of tension pneumothorax, haemothorax, unstable thorax (at least two fractured adjacent ribs, flail chest), and cardiac tamponade.

Open pneumothorax can be immediately handled by placing a closed bandage on the lesion, fastening it to the skin on three sides and with the fourth open as a one-way valve. This gives a closed pneumothorax/simple pneumothorax. A tension pneumothorax is managed by placing a large-calibre needle into the second intercostal space in the midclavicular line of the affected hemithorax.

Massive haemothorax is treated by placing one or more chest tubes into the pleural cavity.

Treatment of an unstable thorax is primarily intubation and ventilation.

Cardiac tamponade is diagnosed using ultrasound and treated initially by pericardiocentesis under ECG monitoring (American College Committee on Trauma 2008).

Circulation:

- Shock is defined as insufficient perfusion of the organs and is presented by a clinical picture with symptoms and objective findings from all the organ-related systems.
- Stop apparent bleeding by compression.
- Introduce two large-calibre intravenous catheters. Other peripheral lines, cutdowns, intraosseous, and central venous lines should be used when necessary in accordance with the shock level of the patient and the skill level of the doctor.
- Draw blood samples for blood type, cross-match, haemoglobin, electrolytes, arterial blood gases, toxicology studies, and, if indicated, pregnancy test.

- Administer warmed crystalloids (lactated Ringer's or normal saline). Initial bolus of 20 ml/kg, which can be repeated.
- If continued need for volume, administer synthetic colloids and blood products (SAG-M, plasma, blood platelets).
- Evaluate response. Circulatory parameters have to normalise, not just stabilise!
- The goal of resuscitation is a systolic blood pressure >100 mmHg (if an aortic aneurism/aortic rupture = 100 mmHg, to reduce risk of rupture and further bleeding). Head trauma patients should have a systolic blood pressure >120 mmHg to ensure sufficient cerebral blood flow.
- Seek the source of bleeding!
- Reasons for shock: bleeding, bleeding, bleeding, tension pneumothorax, neurogenic (medullary compression), cardiac tamponade (American College Committee on Trauma 2008).

Disability:

- Glasgow coma scale score.
- Pupil reaction, size, and form.
- Movement of the extremities.
- Indication for intubation at GCS < 9 (American College Committee on Trauma 2008).

Exposure:

- Undress the patient in order to make a complete and thorough examination/inspection including the back, but at the same time, avoid hypothermia which can cause complications, especially coagulopathies.
- Use warmed fluids.
- Use blankets to cover the patient.
- High room temperature in the resuscitation area.

Reassess ABCDE throughout the initial treatment period. Make sure that the intervention actually provides the response expected (American College Committee on Trauma 2008).

9.3 Specific Paediatric Concerns

The recommendations regarding paediatric patients follow the adult protocol, apart from the different reference values in children and the alertness regarding the shorter interval between seemingly normal values during monitoring and the sudden deterioration leading to a shorter period for resuscitation, if alertness is not appropriate.

NB! Intracranial bleeding may on rare occasions cause hypovolaemic shock before neurological deterioration in small infants!

References

American College Committee on Trauma (2008) Advanced trauma life support for doctors, 8th edn. American College of Surgeons, Chicago, pp 1–244

Enderson BL et al (2001) The tertiary trauma survey: a prospective study on missed injury. J Trauma 50:367–383

Esposito TJ et al (2005) General surgeons and the Advanced Trauma Life Support course: is it time to refocus? J Trauma 59(6):1314–1319

Multi-trauma Triage

10

Christina Rosenlund

Recommendations

Level I

There are insufficient data to support a Level I recommendation.

Level II

There are insufficient data to support a Level II recommendation.

Level III

Use the ABCDE principles to prioritise and make triage decisions.

Tips, Tricks, and Pitfalls

- Keep disaster plans simple. Complex and detailed plans are destined to fail.
- All available information including vital signs should be used to make each triage decision.
- Treat the most injured patients first in case of multiple casualty incidents; save the greatest number of lives in case of mass casualty events.
- Ensure fully interoperable communication systems and redundant with capability for both vertical and horizontal communications.
- Security must be ensured for providers, patients, supplies, and systems needed for disaster care, such as transport and communications.

10.1 Overview

Triage is the process of prioritising patient treatment during mass casualty events. The principles are following the devise: do the most good for the most patients using available resources. The principles of triage are applied when the number of casualties exceeds the medical capabilities that are immediately available to provide usual and customary care. Time is of essence.

10.2 Background

Disaster is derived from the Latin words for evil and star. Falling stars are seldom seen and when they are, they vanish from view almost immediately and do not re-enter the collective consciousness until the next star falls. Preparation

C. Rosenlund
Department of Neurosurgery,
Odense University Hospital,
Sdr. Boulevard 29, 5000 Odense, DK
e-mail: chrisstenrose@gmail.com

T. Sundstrøm et al. (eds.), *Management of Severe Traumatic Brain Injury*,
DOI 10.1007/978-3-642-28126-6_10, © Springer-Verlag Berlin Heidelberg 2012

for a future disaster is essential for managing it when it suddenly is there.

Multiple casualty incidents in which the patient care resources are overextended but not overwhelmed can stress local resources such that triage focuses on identifying the patients with the most life-threatening injuries. *Mass* casualty events are disasters in which patient care is overwhelmed and can exhaust local resources such that triage focuses on identifying those patients with the greatest possibility of survival. Each hospital must determine its own thresholds, recognising that the hospital disaster plan must address both *multiple* casualty incidents and *mass* casualty events. Simple disaster plans, education and implementation of the plans, as well as disaster drills and exercises should be effectuated and evaluated frequently in order to be prepared if the disaster should appear (Roccaforte et al. 2002).

Triage is not a one-time, one-place event or decision. It first occurs at the scene of the event when deciding which patients should be transported to the hospital facilities, then outside the hospital when deciding which patients to enter the preoperative room and later in the preoperative area, deciding which patients should be entering the operating room or the intensive care unit. Triage schemes in mass casualty events should adopt an approach that separates patients with minor injuries from those with more serious injuries, before proceeding with evaluation and sustentative treatment of patients with major injuries. Unsalvageable patients receive terminal or comfort care only after other patients have been treated (Sever et al. 2006). The ABCDE principles as well as the principles of transportation should be followed as in single casualty incidents, but alternative thinking can be necessary. Safety and security is, however, of extreme importance no matter how many casualties there are. Volunteers are priceless if they are able to join in without being instructed and hence are trained prior to the disaster; otherwise they can be of more harm than help to the process.

10.3 Specific Paediatric Concerns

The recommendations regarding paediatric patients follow the adult protocol.

References

Roccaforte JD et al (2002) Disaster preparation and management for the intensive care unit. Curr Opin Crit Care 8(6):607–615

Sever MS et al (2006) Management of crush-related injuries after disasters. N Eng J Med 354(10):1052–1063

Cervical Spine Injury

11

Christina Rosenlund

Recommendations

Level I

The complication rate is significantly increased following high-dosage steroid infusion.

The mortality is increased, and the outcome is poorer for spinal injury patients with head trauma that have received high-dosage steroid infusion.

There is no significant effect of standardised steroid infusion in patients with spinal cord injury.

Level II

There are insufficient data to support a Level II recommendation.

Level III

One can attempt to prevent secondary injury following spinal trauma by immobilisation on a spine board, using a cervical collar and careful transport.

11.1 Overview

Vertebral column injury must always be considered in patients with traumatic injuries. The patient should therefore be immobilised on scene. Attend to life-threatening injuries first, minimising the movement of the patient until vertebral fractures or spinal cord injuries have been excluded. Obtain as much information as possible from the patient history and physical examination and as soon as possible in order to establish a baseline in the patient's neurological status. The examination of awake, alert, sober, neurologically normal and painless patients can be limited to a physical examination only, if there are no positive findings. All other patients should have performed a radiological examination as well; preferably CT imaging of the spine, but if that is not an option, then an AP and lateral view of the cervical spine and first thoracic vertebra, an open-mouth view of the odontoid process and if indicated, also an AP and lateral view of the thoracic and lumbar spine. If the plain x-ray does not rule out the possibility of a spinal injury, transportation to a centre with further examination facilities should be effectuated. Physical examination of the spine includes palpation of the vertebral column (log-rolling the patient), looking for visible lesions, neurological evaluation (motor and sensory deficits including reflexes) and rectal exploration.

Tips, Tricks, and Pitfalls

- Immobilisation on the spine board should be of as short duration as possible (less than 2 h) in order to prevent decubitus ulcers.
- Cervical spine fractures are in 10% of incidences associated with a second vertebral column fracture.

C. Rosenlund
Department of Neurosurgery, Odense University Hospital, Sdr. Boulevard 29, 5000 Odense, DK
e-mail: chrisstenrose@gmail.com

T. Sundstrøm et al. (eds.), *Management of Severe Traumatic Brain Injury*,
DOI 10.1007/978-3-642-28126-6_11, © Springer-Verlag Berlin Heidelberg 2012

- CT scans are the radiologic examination of choice, but you should be aware that disc and ligament fractures/lesions are difficult and in some cases impossible to see on CT imaging.
- Spinal shock is a reversible condition and defined by the flaccidity and loss of reflexes seen after spinal cord injury whereas neurogenic shock refers to impairment of the sympathetic pathways in the cervical or upper thoracic spinal cord. Both conditions, however, indicate spinal cord injury.
- Neurogenic shock includes loss of vasomotor tone and in sympathetic innervations to the heart, causing vasodilatation, pooling of blood and, consequently, hypotension and failure of the heart to respond to hypovolaemia with tachycardia. The blood pressure may not be restored by fluid resuscitation alone, and vasopressors may be necessary as well as atropine in counteracting hemodynamically significant bradycardia.
- The ASIA (American Spinal Injury Association) score can very well be used to classify the spinal cord injury.
- Injuries located at C6 or higher can result in partial or total loss of respiratory function.

11.2 Background

Approximately 5% of patients with brain injury have an associated spinal injury, and 25% of patients with spinal cord injury have at least a mild traumatic brain injury. Approximately 55% of spinal injuries occur in the cervical region, 15% in the thoracic region, 15% at the thoracolumbar junction and 15% in the lumbosacral area. Approximately 10% of patients with a cervical spine fracture have a second vertebral column fracture. The mortality following cervical spine injury is between 4.4% and 16.7% according to the available literature (Enderson et al. 2001). Five percent of the patients are in a process of deterioration at arrival or during their stay in the hospital. This is usually due to ischemia or progression of spinal cord oedema, but it may also be the result of failure to handle the patients correctly by providing adequate immobilisation. Early decompression (<8 h) of the spinal cord in case of a mechanical compression (vertebral column fracture, disc rupture, ligament lesion, haematoma) has essential impact on the final outcome in case of incomplete para- or quadriplegia (American College Committee on Trauma 2008).

The Nascis II and III study together with the Cochrane meta-analysis performed by Bracken reveals that routine steroid infusion in case of spinal cord injury is not related to a better outcome regarding the spinal cord lesions and that the risk of complications to this treatment (pneumonia, sepsis) as well as the risk of deterioration in case of a simultaneous brain injury is significantly increased. It is therefore not recommended to use steroid routinely (Bracken et al. 1990; 1998).

11.3 Specific Paediatric Concerns

The recommendations regarding paediatric patients follow the adult protocol.

References

American College Committee on Trauma (2008) Advanced trauma life support for doctors, 8th edn. American College of Surgeons, Chicago, pp 1–244

Bracken MB et al (1990) A randomized controlled trial of methylprednisolone or naloxone in the treatment of spinal cord injury: results of the second National Spinal Cord Injury Study. N Engl J Med 322: 1405–1411

Bracken MB et al (1998) Methylprednisolone or tirilazad mesylate administration after acute spinal cord injury: 1-year follow up: results of the third National Spinal Cord Injury Study. N Engl J Med 89:699–706

Enderson BL et al (2001) The tertiary trauma survey: a prospective study on missed injury. J Trauma 50: 367–383

12 Radiological Evaluation of Head Traumas

Helle Wulf Eskildsen, Anna Tietze, and Vibeke Fink-Jensen

Recommendations

Level I

Data are insufficient to support Level I recommendations for this subject.

Level II

A CT scan of the head is recommended as first line examinations for a patient with head injury.

Evaluation of vascular injuries requires specific angiography series with contrast (CT, MRI, DSA).

Level III

MRI within the first days after trauma should be reserved for patients where the CT does not sufficiently explain the clinical state of the patient.

V. Fink-Jensen • A. Tietze • H.W. Eskildsen (✉)
Department of Neuroradiology,
Aarhus University Hospital,
Noerrebrogade, 8000 Aarhus C, Denmark
e-mail: vibefink@rm.dk; antz@cfin.dk; helleski@rm.dk

12.1 Overview

CT imaging is the examination of choice in the acute setting because it is readily available, fast, offers full body investigation with detailed imaging including imaging of bones with reconstruction in all planes and allows close observation of the patient.

CT of the head is in most places performed with helical technique, as multidetector CT scanners are readily available in most trauma centres. This will allow reconstruction in all planes and evaluation of both soft tissues and bones from one scan series. It is recommended to include the facial skeleton from the hard palate in cranial direction including the mandible if there is clinical evidence of that region being involved. Some centres perform one scan series that cover the cervical spine, facial skeleton, brain and skull in one. In most, if not all centres, a radiologist will be on call to evaluate these examinations.

Haematomas will appear white (hyperdense) in the right window setting, whereas ongoing bleeding will appear darker (hypodense), and older haematomas will be similar to grey matter (isodense).

Contusions of the brain parenchyma appear as focally darker areas around punctate haemorrhages, often more apparent on later scans.

Diffuse cerebral oedema is seen as a diminished differentiation of grey-white matter boundaries, sulcal obliteration, narrowing of the basal cisterns, and often also the ventricular system.

T. Sundstrøm et al. (eds.), *Management of Severe Traumatic Brain Injury*,
DOI 10.1007/978-3-642-28126-6_12, © Springer-Verlag Berlin Heidelberg 2012

Also the falx and tentorium will appear whiter than normally against the brain parenchyma. Focal oedema is seen darker against the surrounding more normal parenchyma, but also with the above-mentioned signs.

Diffuse axonal injury (DAI) is often underestimated or not seen on CT. MRI is the examination of choice for DAI, where lesions will appear as small black spots on T2-weighted gradient echo series, but MRI is not as readily available as CT and is far more complex to perform with traumatised patients. MRI should therefore be reserved for those patients where CT within the first days after trauma does not sufficiently explain the clinical state of the patient.

One should always evaluate:

- Scalp lesions – lacerations, foreign bodies, oedema and/or subgaleal haematomas
- Skull fractures – including the facial bones
- Extra-axial lesions – epidural haemorrhage, subdural haemorrhage, subarachnoid haemorrhage and/or intraventricular haemorrhage
- Intra-axial lesions – intraparenchymal haematomas, contusions, oedema with or without herniation and/or DAI

The possibility of vascular injuries should also be considered. Cranial CT is usually performed as a non-contrast study and more specific angiography series (CT, MRI or angiography) with contrast may be necessary.

Tips, Tricks, and Pitfalls: CT Imaging of the Head

To avoid overlooking critical injuries in the immediate setting, perform a systematic evaluation using three different window settings:

- Brain parenchyma window (Level 30–40 Hounsfield Units (HU), Window: 65–120 HU)
  - Is the ventricular system of normal size, symmetrical and in the midline?
  - Is there any blood extra- or intra-axial?
  - Is the grey-white matter differentiation normal? Are there any focal lesions?
  - Are the cortical sulci discernible and symmetrical, or are they narrowed or even obliterated?
  - Are the basal cisterns of normal size and symmetrical?
  - Are there any scalp lesions?
- Subdural window (L: 70–100 HU, W: 150–300 HU):
  - To avoid overlooking smaller subdural haematomas due to the density of bone and artefacts at the interface between bone and soft intracranial tissue, use a subdural window. This will allow you to detect a thin layer of sub- or epidural blood.
- Bone window (L: 500 HU, W: 2000–4000 HU):
  - Are there any fractures involving the skull base or the calvarium? If so, are there dislocations and/or fragments?
  - Is the optical canal intact?
  - Is the carotid canal intact?
  - Are there any indirect signs of fracture, i.e. opacification of the nasal sinuses and/or mastoid cells or intracranial air bubbles?
  - Are there fractures of the facial bones?
  - Are there any foreign bodies extra- or intra-cranially?

Especially regarding fractures, make good use of the possibility of three dimensional reconstructing.

12.2 Background

Intracranial lesions can be subdivided into extra- and intra-axial lesions.

12.2.1 Extra-axial Lesions

Epidural Haematomas (Fig. 12.1)

- Located between tabula interna and dura.
- Ninety percent of cases occur in association with

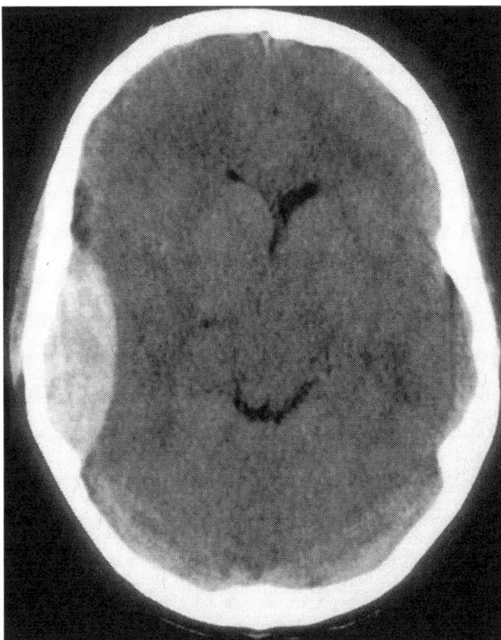

Fig. 12.1 Epidural haematoma

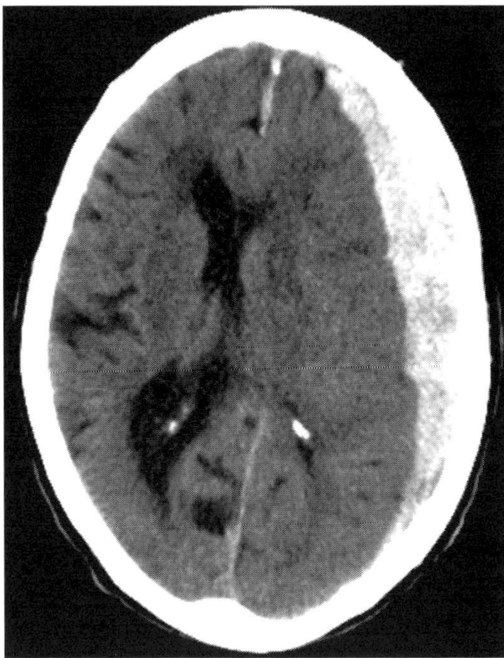

Fig. 12.2 Acute subdural haematoma

skull fractures involving the middle meningeal artery or less common one of the venous sinuses.

- Rarely crosses sutures but can cross the midline.
- Usually a biconvex appearance.

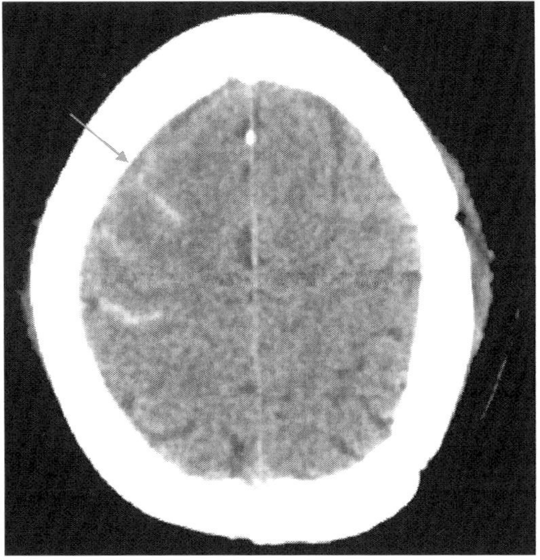

Fig. 12.3 Acute traumatic subarachnoid haemorrhage

Subdural Haematomas (Fig. 12.2)

- Located between dura and arachnoid.
- Venous bleeding from superficial bridging cortical veins.
- Cross sutures but not midline.
- Often located along falx cerebri or tentorium cerebelli.
- Concave appearance toward brain surface.
- Chronic subdural haematomas appear dark, fresh bleeding in a chronic subdural haematoma will appear as white areas, often in compartments.
- After 2 days to 2 weeks, subdural haematomas can become isodense and very difficult to discern from the brain. Look for shift of midline or difference of right and left hemisphere sulci.

Traumatic Subarachnoid Haemorrhage (Fig. 12.3)

- Fresh blood found focally in most cases in a few sulci over the convexities or in the basal cisterns often the interpeduncular.
- It may look as though the sulci are effaced, when in fact it is blood replacing the CSF.
- If there is abundant and diffuse spread of SAH, one should always consider rupture of an aneurism. Perhaps that was the cause for the traumatic incident to happen.

Intraventricular Haemorrhage

- Seen as fresh blood (white on CT) in the ventricular system.

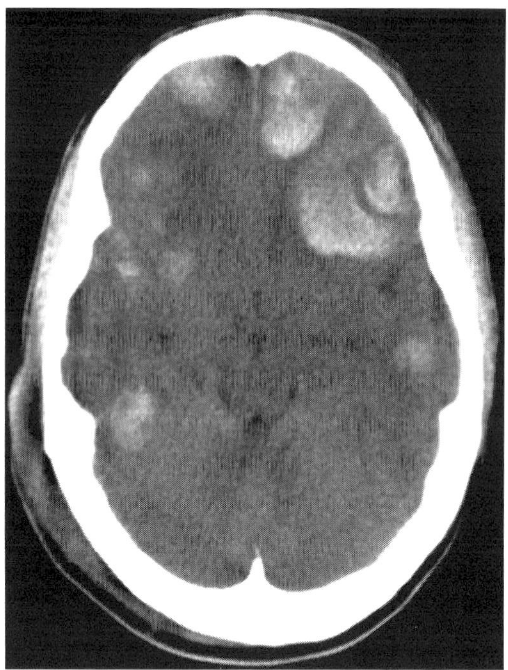

Fig. 12.4 Multiple brain contusions

- Can be caused from direct trauma with tearing of subependymal veins, breakthrough from parenchymal hematoma or reflux from SAH.
- Often, the intraventricular bleeding is seen as blood at the back of the occipital horns with a blood-CSF level. Even very small amounts of blood can be detected here (Parizel et al. 2005).

12.2.2 Intra-axial Lesions

Cerebral Contusions (Fig. 12.4)

- The most common injury of the parenchyma.
- Are seen as punctate haemorrhages that after a few days are surrounded by oedema, often multiple, located near the brain surface supratentorially.
- Are caused as the brain hits the skull base or the falx/tentorium and are therefore often located inferiorly and anteriorly in the frontal and temporal lobes.

Intracerebral Haematomas.

- Larger than contusions.
- Located deeper within the brain parenchyma.
- Frequently progress during the first few posttraumatic days, especially if a surgical

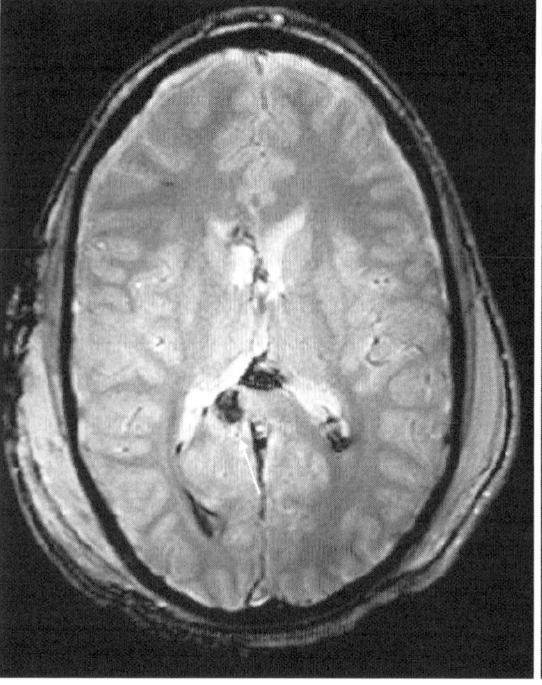

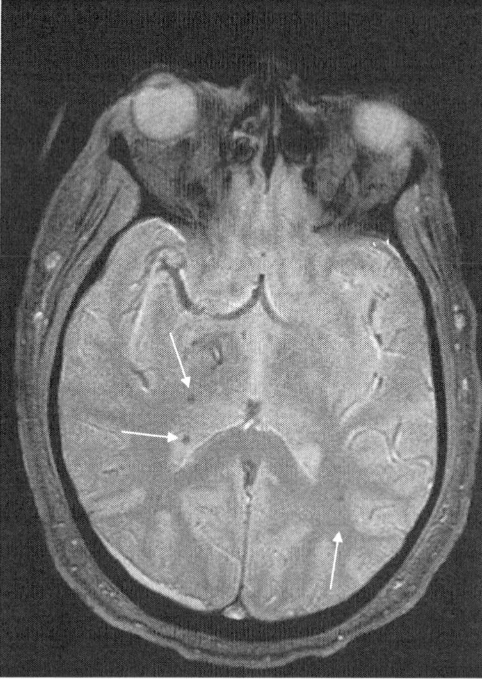

Fig. 12.5 Diffuse axonal injury, DAI and intraventricular haemorrhage

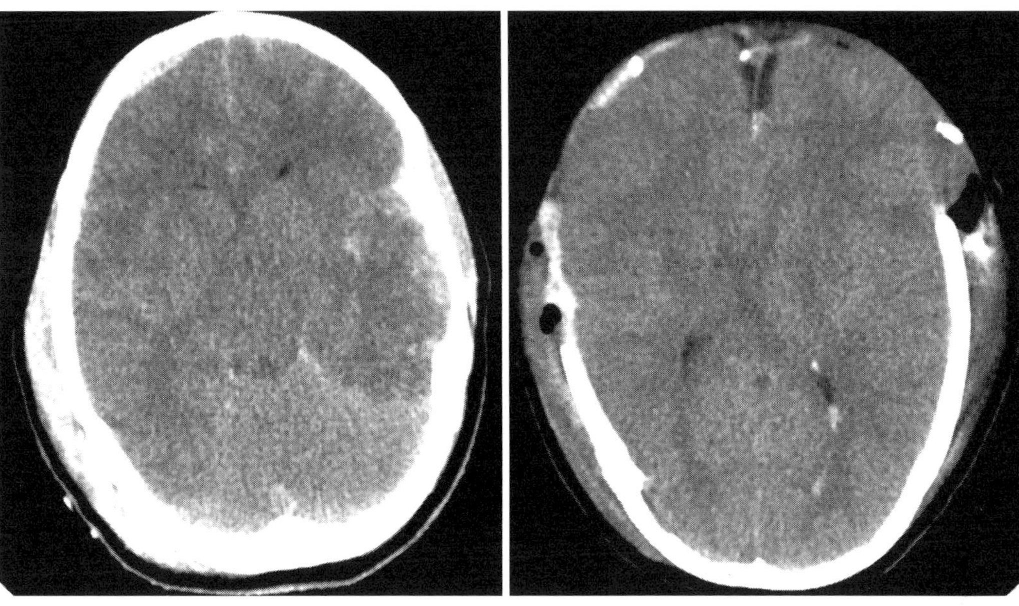

Fig. 12.6 Cerebral oedema. Day 1 and day 2 with bilateral craniectomy

decompression of epi- or subdural haematomas has been performed.

- A few days after the trauma, an oedema around the haematoma will occur.

Diffuse Axonal Injury (Fig. 12.5)

- Caused by shearing of the axons in rotational acceleration/deceleration closed head injuries.
- Most often not seen on the initial CT, or only as very small haemorrhages at the grey-white matter boundaries.
- Can appear during the next few days, but as over 50% are non-haemorrhagic, they will not appear on CT with certainty.

MRI is much more reliable for showing DAI. The patient's clinical condition will often be worse than expected from the first CT.

Cerebral Oedema (Fig. 12.6)

- Can be diffuse.
- Associated with DAI or hypoxia but can also develop without concomitant traumatic lesions.
- Develops during the first 24–48 h.
- Focal oedema can be associated with intra- or extra-axial haemorrhage.
- Can cause compression of blood vessels and eventually evolve into ischaemic areas of the brain.

Cerebral Herniations

- Occur secondary to intra- or extra-axial expansive lesions and/or oedema.
- Subfalcine herniation is radiologically the most common type. It involves displacement of the cingulated gyrus under the inferior margin of the falx, compression of the ipsilateral lateral ventricle, blocking of the foramen of Monro and dilatation of the opposite lateral ventricle and midline shift.
- The anterior cerebral artery can be compressed until occlusion with infarction following.
- Transtentorial herniation is most often descending, where the medial part of the temporal lobe is pressed downwards, narrowing the ipsilateral basal cisterns and compressing the oculomotor nerve and eventually posterior cerebral artery with infarction following.
- Can also be ascending with the vermis dislocated upwards, obliteration of the fourth ventricle and subsequent hydrocephalus.
- If the intracranial pressure increases, eventually herniation and incarceration at the foramen magnum will occur (Parizel et al. 2005).

12.2.3 Vascular Injuries

- Compression of vessels due to raised ICP can cause hypoperfusion and eventually infarction.
- Trauma can cause dissection or laceration of vessels either intra- or extra-cranially and hypoperfusion or thrombus (Fig. 12.7).

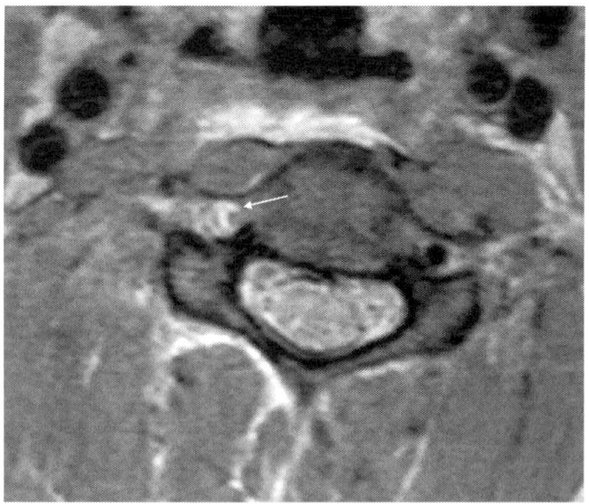

Fig. 12.7 Dissection of the right vertebral artery

- Subarachnoid haemorrhage can cause severe vasospasm and subsequent infarction.

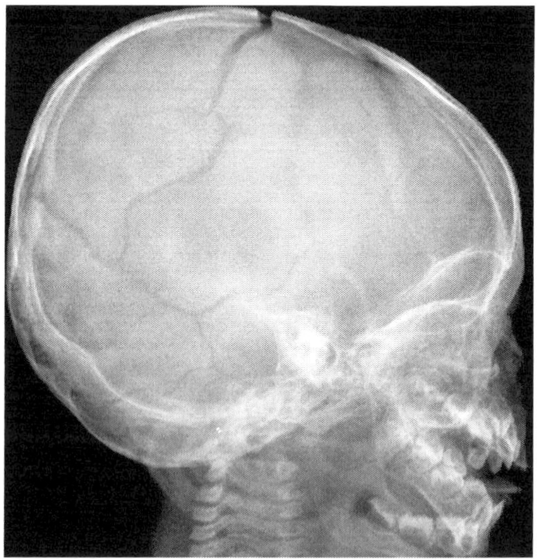

Fig. 12.8 Complex skull fracture in a child

12.2.4 Skull Fractures

Skull fractures will not be presented in detail. Facial fractures, however, represent the risk of respiratory problems and should be assessed on the first CT scan. One should pay particular attention to the orbits, especially the optic canal; the central skull base, especially the carotid canal and the temporal bone as fractures here may require immediate surgical intervention. Intracranial air bubbles imply fractures involving the nasal sinuses or temporal bone.

12.2.5 Specific Intracranial and Cervical Vascular Concerns

Suspected vascular injury and in particular vascular dissection requires MRI or CT angiography. A conventional angiography may be necessary.

Lack of cerebral circulation confirms brain death. In these cases, filling of the intracerebral vessels during conventional angiography is absent due to extremely increased intracranial pressure. Angiography is considered to be a confirmatory test in doubtful situations, where brain death has to be stated before possible organ donation (Yousem et al. 2010).

12.3 Specific Paediatric Concerns

In children with trauma, unilateral infarction is seen in association with acute subdural haematoma. Also, cerebral oedema is more common in children than in adults.

12.3.1 Non-accidental Injury (NAI) or 'Battered Child Syndrome'

Always consider NAI in young children with head trauma, particularly in those without appropriate trauma history. Most NAI head injuries occur under the age of 2 years. The neurological presentation is often non-specific. CT is the most appropriate acute imaging procedure (Lonergan et al. 2003).

Typical imaging findings in NAI are:

- Skull fractures (Fig. 12.8)
- Subdural haematomas, often of different age (Fig. 12.9)
- Cerebral oedema
- Hypoxic ischaemic encephalopathy (Figs. 12.9 and 12.10)
- Rarely intraventricular, intracerebral or epidural haematomas

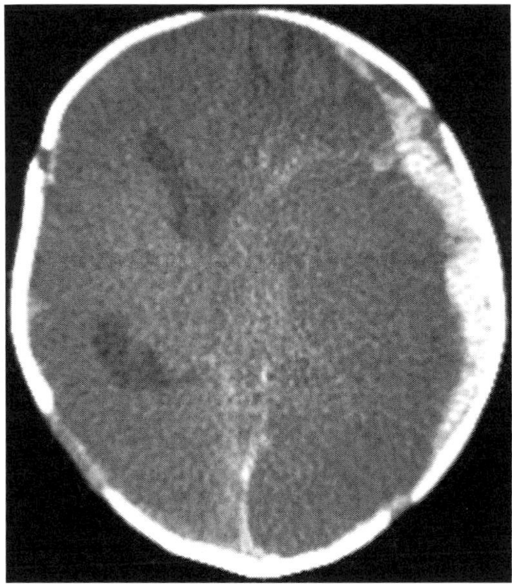

Fig. 12.9 Subdural haematoma, hypoxic ischaemic encephalopathy and subfalcine herniation

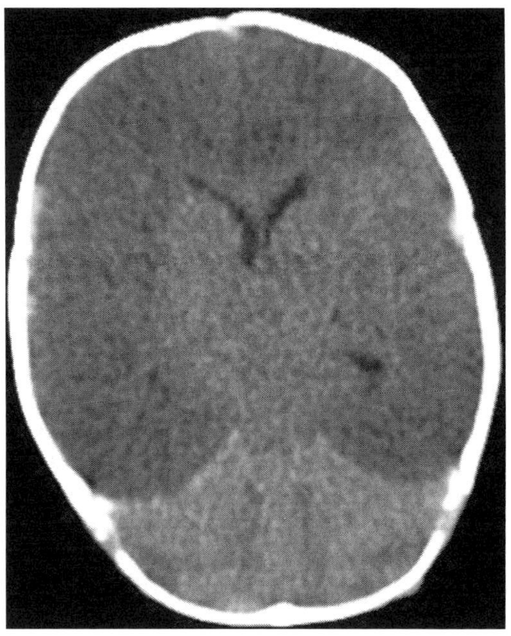

Fig. 12.10 Acute reversal sign ('white cerebellum') due to diffuse hypoxic brain injury

Tips, Tricks, and Pitfalls: Paediatric Head Traumas

- Accidental skull fractures are usually linear, unilateral, affect the parietal bones and do not cross sutures.
- Non-accidental fractures are often more complex.
- Linear skull fractures can be missed on axial CT scans!
- Accidental subdural haematomas are more often unilateral, non-accidental more often bilateral.
- Non-accidental subdural haematomas extend more often into the interhemispheric fissure.
- Acute reversal sign ('white cerebellum') + loss of white/grey matter differentiation + interhemispheric subdural haematoma are suggestive of NAI.
- Subdural haematomas become isodense after about a week (depends on size), but dating of subdural collections is very imprecise.
- MRI gives greater detail of subdural haematomas, may help to date the injury and is helpful to assess the extent of the parenchymal injury.
- Remember: None of the aforementioned features are pathognomonic!
- Remember also that children with temporal arachnoid cysts may get subdural and/or intra-cystic haematomas even after mild head traumas!

A child suspected for NAI should not be sent home! Contact the paediatrician on call! Refer to a complete skeletal survey if NAI is suspected in infants and young children. Occult injury is rare in children over 3 years of age.

References

Lonergan GJ et al (2003) From the archives of the AFIP. Child abuse: radiologic-pathologic correlation. Radiographics 23(4):811–845

Parizel PM et al (2005) New developments in the neuroradiological diagnosis of craniocerebral trauma. Eur Radiol 15:569–581

Yousem DM, Grossman RI (2010) Neuroradiology: the requisites. Mosby/Elsevier, Philadelphia, pp 576–584, Chapter 5 and 17

13 Radiological Evaluation of Cervical Spine Traumas

Helle Wulf Eskildsen, Anna Tietze, and Vibeke Fink-Jensen

Recommendations

Level I

Data are insufficient to support Level I recommendations for this subject.

Level II

A 3D CT of the cervical spine is superior to plain X-ray.

13.1 Overview

Radiographs (plain X-rays) can be the first step in evaluation of cervical spine injuries. However, C1, C2, C6 and C7 are often difficult to assess, frequently making supplementary CT necessary. CT therefore can be chosen as the examination of first choise, especially in adults.

H.W. Eskildsen (✉) • A. Tietze • V. Fink-Jensen
Department of Neuroradiology,
Aarhus University Hospital,
Noerrebrogade, 8000 Aarhus C, Denmark
e-mail: helleski@rm.dk; antz@cfin.dk; vibefink@rm.dk

Particularly, 3D reconstructions are valuable to visualize fractures and bone fragments.

Fractures of the cervical spine can be divided based on the mechanism of injury into *flexion*, *extension* or *compression* fractures, or according to stability into *stable* or *unstable* fractures, using the three-column model (Fig. 13.1).

Alternatively, as in this chapter, fractures can be classified according to their anatomical location.

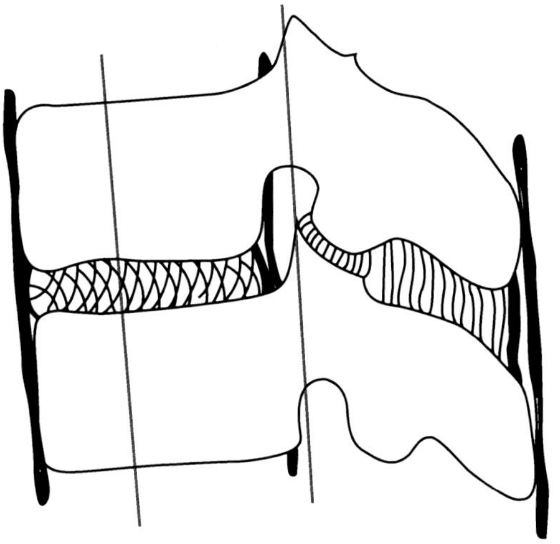

Fig. 13.1 The three-column model. Instability occurs when two of the three columns (anterior, middle or posterior) are injured

T. Sundstrøm et al. (eds.), *Management of Severe Traumatic Brain Injury*,
DOI 10.1007/978-3-642-28126-6_13, © Springer-Verlag Berlin Heidelberg 2012

Tips, Tricks, and Pitfalls: Cervical Spine Traumas

- Be systematic when evaluating cervical images; look for:
  - Maintained height of the vertebral bodies.
  - Alignment.
  - Normal distances and parallel surfaces between endplates in disc spaces, facet joints and spinous processes.
  - Continuous cortical margins.
  - Paraspinal haematomas.
- Alignment is evaluated along the lines of the anterior and posterior longitudinal ligament, the posterior margin of the spinal canal and along the posterior margin of the spinous processes.
- If performing CT, do always reconstruct and evaluate sagittal and coronal images!

13.2 Background

13.2.1 Atlanto-occipital Dislocation

Atlanto-occipital dislocation in anterior-posterior or longitudinal direction results in increased distance between the basion and the odontoid. This injury can be associated with odontoid or condylar fractures and results often in severe soft tissue damage and brain stem injury.

13.2.2 Atlanto-axial Distraction

Atlanto-axial distraction causes widening of the distance between C1 and C2 with concomitant prevertebral soft tissue swelling and ligamentous tears. Dislocation in the transverse plane with rupture of the transverse ligament and associated fractures results in increased distance between the anterior surface of the odontoid and the posterior surface of C1.

13.2.3 Jefferson's Fracture

Jefferson's fracture is a compression "burst" fracture of C1 and involves disruptions of the anterior and posterior arches of the atlas. Tears of the transverse ligament are associated. More often, a hyperextension injury is seen with compression of the posterior arch of C1, resulting in a stable posterior arch fracture (Fig. 13.2).

13.2.4 Hangman's Fractures

Hangman's fractures are fracture dislocations of C2 caused by hyperextension injuries. If there are bilateral neural arch fractures, anterior displacement of C2 on C3 occurs. The posterior ring is usually fixed by the inferior articular process, unless there is accompanying facet dislocation. However, most Hangman's fractures result only in minimal translation and angulation (Fig. 13.3).

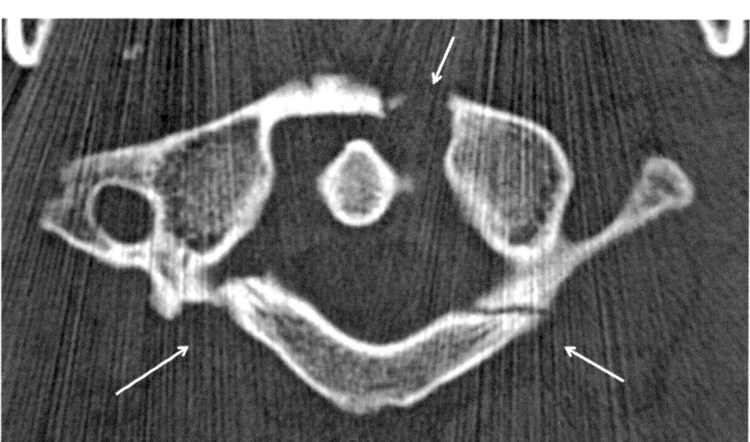

Fig. 13.2 Jefferson's fracture. *Arrows* indicate fractures disrupting anterior and posterior arches of C1

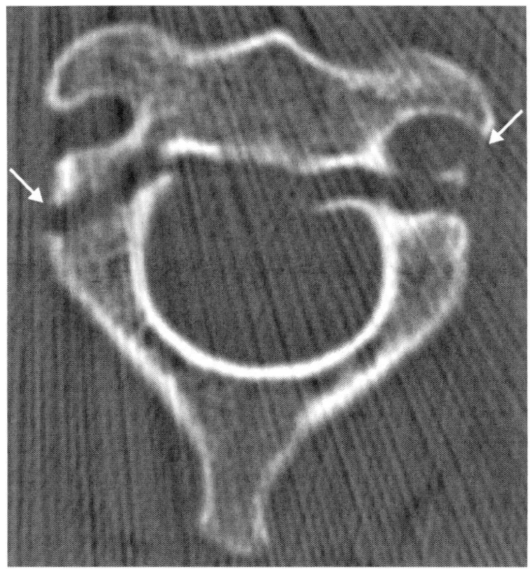

Fig. 13.3 Hangman's fracture: *Arrows* mark bilateral fracture through the posterior arch of C2.

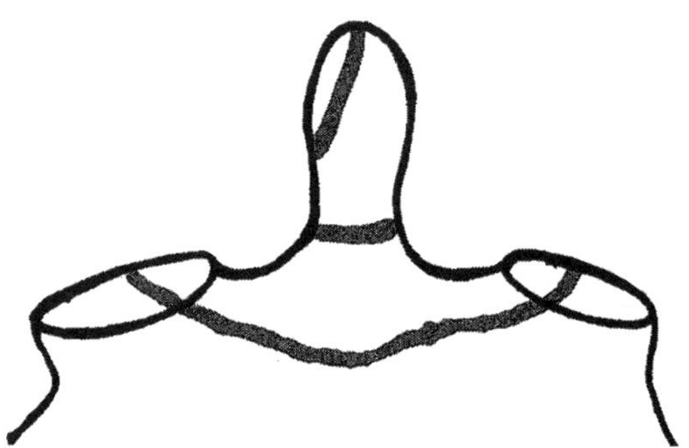

Fig. 13.4 Odontoid fractures. Type I: upper portion of the dens. Type II: junction of the dens with the body. Type III: through the body of the axis

13.2.5 Odontoid ('dens') Fractures

Odontoid ('*dens*') *fractures* are divided into three types with type II being unstable (Figs. 13.4 and 13.5).

13.2.6 Compression Fractures

Compression fractures of a vertebral body can involve one or both endplates. Most are wedge-shaped without involving the posterior cortex. Burst fractures also affect the posterior cortex of the vertebral body, and fragments can be displaced into the spinal canal.

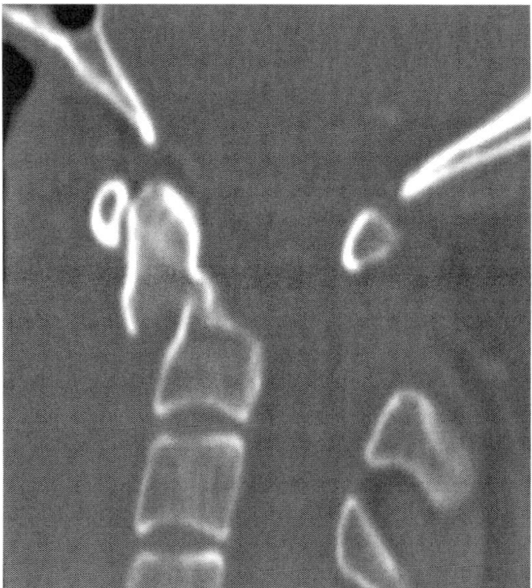

Fig. 13.5 Odontoid fracture, type II

13.2.7 Teardrop Fractures

Teardrop fractures can be caused by hyperflexion or hyperextension injuries (Fig. 13.6).

In hyperflexion injuries, a triangular fragment can be found at the anterior-inferior border of the vertebral body with reduction of the anterior body height and soft tissue swelling. Disruption of the anterior part of the disc and the posterior ligament complex results in posterior displacement of the fractured vertebra and diastasis of the interfacetal joints. These fractures are unstable.

Hyperextension injuries may also result in an avulsion of the anterior-inferior corner of the vertebral body but leaves the posterior columns intact and are stable.

13.2.8 Locked Facets

Locked facets are the result of anterior displacement with interfacetal dislocation and the articular mass of the vertebra above lying anterior to the articular mass of the vertebra below.

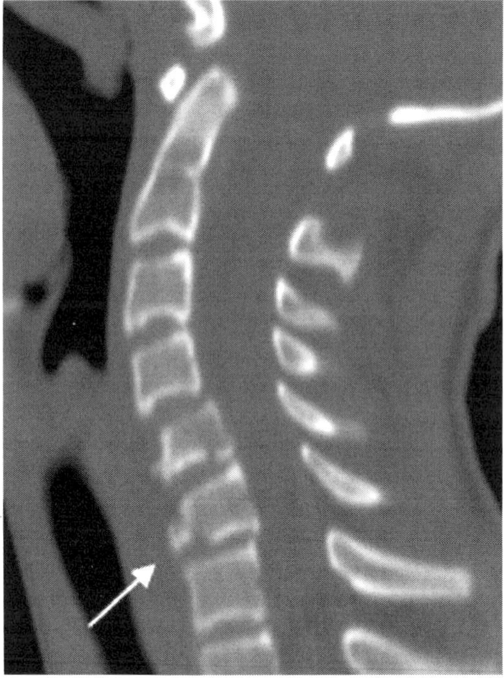

Fig. 13.6 Teardrop fracture C6 (*arrow*)

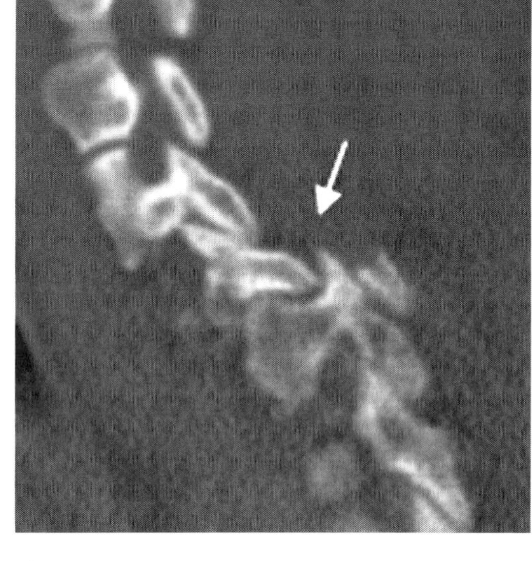

Fig. 13.7 Locked facets. Anterior displacement of inferior articular process is marked by the (*arrow*). Note the concomitant fracture of the articular process

This occurs uni- or bilaterally. The interosseous ligaments and discs are often disrupted (Fig. 13.7).

13.3 Imaging of Intraspinal Injuries

MRI is the modality of choice to visualize spinal soft tissue lesions such as spinal cord haemorrhage and oedema, transections, ligamentous tears, epidural haematomas, disc herniations and cord compression and also visualizes subluxations and fractures. Be aware that most of these lesions may occur without fractures or dislocations. Spinal cord oedema, ligamentous or disc lesions will appear bright on T2-weighted images (Fig. 13.8). Bright signal on T1-weighted images is related to acute haemorrhage.

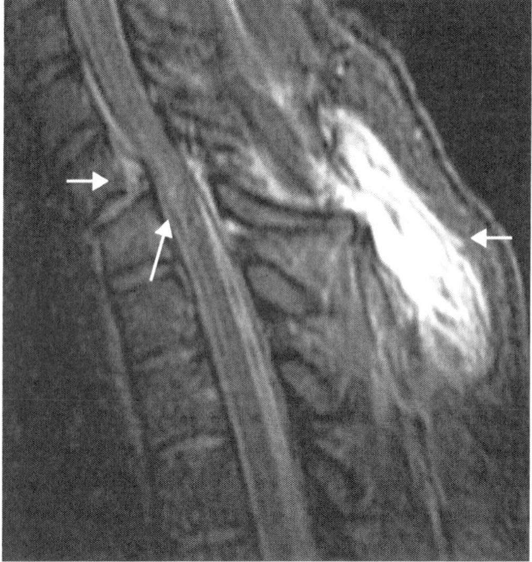

Fig. 13.8 T2-weighted STIR image. Cervical fracture (*short white arrow, anterior*) and dislocation with oedema of the spinal cord (*long white arrow*) and posterior soft tissue laceration (*bright areas, short white arrow, posterior*)

13.4 Specific Paediatric Concerns

In children under the age of 8 years, distraction and subluxation injuries (such as atlanto-occipital dislocation and rotatory subluxation of the atlas upon the axis) are more common than fractures and often involves the occipito-atlanto-axial segment. Keep the congenital variants in mind including absence of the posterior arch of C1 and the os odontoideum arising from the secondary ossification centre of the odontoid.

Suggested Reading

Grainger RD, Allison DJ et al (2001) Diagnostic radiology: a textbook of medical imaging. Churchill Livingstone, London, pp 1815–1833

Parizel PM et al (2005) New developments in the neuroradiological diagnosis of craniocerebral trauma. Eur Radiol 15:569–581

Yousem DM, Grossman RI (2010) Neuroradiology: the requisites. Mosby/Elsevier, Philadelphia, pp 576–584, Chapter 5 and 17

14 Blood Samples

Rasmus Philip Nielsen

Recommendations

Level I

Data are insufficient to support Level I recommendations for this subject.

Level II

Data are insufficient to support Level II recommendations for this subject.

Level III

Recommendations from other topics implicate the use of certain blood samples. There is level III evidence for avoiding hypoxia and hypo/hyperglycaemia. For this reason, measuring PaO_2 and blood glucose is evident.

14.1 Overview

Analysis of both venous and arterial blood is an important part of modern diagnostics. Basically, blood samples should only be performed if there is an adequate intervention to an abnormal laboratory value or if the parameter otherwise offers a help in diagnosis of the patient, in grading the severity of the disease, or in estimating the patient's prognosis.

Upon arrival of the patient with suspected severe traumatic brain injury, we suggest that the following blood samples should be taken:

- Arterial blood sample
  - Arterial pH, PaO_2, $PaCO_2$, base excess (BE) and/or bicarbonate
- Venous blood sample
  - Sodium, potassium, creatinine, haemoglobin, leucocytes, C-reactive protein (CRP), platelets, INR/PP, glucose, ethanol, ABO blood type, activated partial thromboplastin time (APTT), fibrinogen, myoglobin

If you already are monitoring the patient with arterial canula, all blood samples can be obtained from the artery.

Additional blood samples depend on the patient's premorbid condition and, on additional, extra-cranial injuries. Trauma against the abdomen suggests, for example, need for analysing liver enzymes and amylase. Haemorrhage indicates need for blood cross-matching in order to give blood transfusion. Suspected intake of alcohol or other toxic substances suggests additional samples for these toxic substances.

Normal values for adults (over 18 years) are seen in Table 14.1. There can be differences between laboratories and different equipment.

R.P. Nielsen
Anaestesi- Børne-og Kirurgicenter, Anaestesien 4. afd., Aalborg Hospital, Aarhus University Hospital, Hobrovej 18-22, Postboks 365, Aalborg 9100, Denmark
e-mail: rpn@dadlnet.dk

T. Sundstrøm et al. (eds.), *Management of Severe Traumatic Brain Injury*, DOI 10.1007/978-3-642-28126-6_14, © Springer-Verlag Berlin Heidelberg 2012

Table 14.1 Normal values for blood samples

pH	7.37–7.45	Haemoglobin	♂: 8.4–10.8 mmol/l ♀: 7.4–9.6 mmol/l
PaO_2	<40 years: 11.1–14.4 kPa >40 years: 9.6–13.7 kPa	Leucocytes	3.0–10.0 mia/l
$PaCO_2$	♂: 4.7–6.0 kPa ♀: 4.3–5.7 kPa	CRP	<8 mg/l
BE	−2.0 to +3.0 mmol/l	Platelets	150–450 mia/l
Bicarbonate	♂: 22.5–26.9 mmol/l ♀: 21.8–26.2 mmol/l	INR	0.9–1.1
Na+	137–145 mmol/l	PP	0.7–1.3
K+	3.5–4.6 mmol/l	Glucose	See Sect. 14.2
Creatinine	♂: 60–105 µmol/l ♀: 50–90 µmol/l	APTT	25–38 s
Fibrinogen	5.0–12.0 µmol/l		

Source: List of analysis, Clinical Biochemical Department, Aarhus University Hospital, Denmark, 2008.

Tips, Tricks, and Pitfalls

- In the acute setting, have a predefined list of routine blood samples to be taken.
- Take additional blood samples later, when the patient is stable and the patient's history is known.
- Evaluate the need for "routine" blood samples everyday.

14.2 Background

14.2.1 Arterial Blood Sample

The overall aim of the therapy of the patient with severe traumatic brain injury is to prevent secondary brain injury, which may be the consequence of hypotension and hypoxia (Cooke et al. 1995; Stocchetti et al. 1996). Hypoxaemia has been found to be significantly associated with increased morbidity and mortality (Chesnut et al. 1993; Marmarou et al. 1991). An arterial blood sample offers an easy and reliable picture of the arterial oxygenation, expressed by the PaO_2. At the same time, we get a picture of the acid–base balance in the arterial blood and of the ventilation, both of which are useful in the continued stabilization of the patient.

14.2.2 Haematology

Oxygenation is also dependent on the haemoglobin level, and therefore it is important to detect a possible anaemia. Nevertheless, blood transfusion is associated with significantly worse outcome in patients with TBI (Salim et al. 2008); therefore, a restrictive transfusion strategy is advisable. Infection parameters are important to detect complicating infectious disease.

14.2.3 Electrolytes

Hypertonic saline infusion bears the risk of inducing central pontine myelinolysis when given to a patient with chronic hypernatraemia (Kleinschmidt-DeMasters and Norenberg 1981). Giving mannitol in order to lower ICP will increase urinary output. Accurate balancing of fluid in- and output is essential and in that context also the serum concentrations of electrolytes. In addition, electrolytes is measured in order to correct possible acute abnormalities and to detect pre-existing deviations.

14.2.4 Coagulation

Abnormal coagulation can be due to pre-existing disease but is more often a consequence of tissue injury and hypoperfusion in the case of the trauma patient (Theusinger et al. 2009). To reveal these matters, basic coagulation parameters must be measured. A more useful description of the function of the coagulation system can be obtained by, for example, thrombelastography or rotation thrombelastometry, which describe the developing clot and can give advice of specific therapeutic interventions to correct possible abnormalities (Ganter and Hofer 2008; Kheirabadi et al. 2007).

14.2.5 Glucose

Data suggest that hyperglycaemia worsens ischemic brain injury and gives a poorer outcome (Cherian et al. 1997; Lam et al. 1991; Young et al. 1989). At the same time, hypoglycaemia is detrimental. Data from Jacka et al. (2009) suggest a non-significant increase in mortality and stay in intensive care unit for patients with brain injury. There is an on-going discussion between those who favour a tight blood glucose control (between 4.4 and 6.1 mmol/l) and those who suggests a more liberal approach to hyperglycaemia (Suarez 2009; Yoder 2009). We will leave this discussion to another chapter in this book and only state that blood glucose should never be less than 4 mmol/l and not over 12 mmol/l.

14.2.6 Myoglobin

In connection with trauma, there is often a release of myoglobin from injured tissue. Increased serum concentration of myoglobin leads to acute renal insufficiency and worsens the prognosis.

14.2.7 Pre-existing or Concomitant Disease and Differential Diagnosis

As mentioned above, additional blood samples may be necessary dependent on the patient's premorbid condition, additional injuries and suspicion of concomitant disease. This chapter does not leave space for further discussion on this matter.

14.3 Specific Paediatric Concerns

Blood samples should be obtained with microtechniques due to the reduced volume of circulating blood in children. Use of routine blood samples should be avoided due to risk of anaemia.

Some reference values will differ from the adult values.

References

Cherian L, Goodman JC, Robertson CS (1997) Hyperglycemia increases brain injury caused by secondary ischemia after cortical impact injury in rats. Crit Care Med 25:1378–1383

Chesnut RM, Marshall LF, Klauber MR, Blunt BA, Baldwin N, Eisenberg HM et al (1993) The role of secondary brain injury in determining outcome from severe head injury. J Trauma 34:216–222

Cooke RS, McNicholl BP, Byrnes DP (1995) Early management of severe head injury in Northern Ireland. Injury 26:395–397

Ganter MT, Hofer CK (2008) Coagulation monitoring: current techniques and clinical use of viscoelastic point-of-care coagulation devices. Anesth Analg 106:1366–1375

Jacka MJ, Torok-Both CJ, Bagshaw SM (2009) Blood glucose control among critically ill patients with brain injury. Can J Neurol Sci 36:436–442

Kheirabadi BS, Crissey JM, Deguzman R, Holcomb JB (2007) In vivo bleeding time and in vitro thrombelastography measurements are better indicators of dilutional hypothermic coagulopathy than prothrombin time. J Trauma 62:1352–1359; discussion 9–61

Kleinschmidt-DeMasters BK, Norenberg MD (1981) Rapid correction of hyponatremia causes demyelination: relation to central pontine myelinolysis. Science 211:1068–1070

Lam AM, Winn HR, Cullen BF, Sundling N (1991) Hyperglycemia and neurological outcome in patients with head injury. J Neurosurg 75:545–551

Marmarou A, Anderson RL, Ward JD, Choi SC, Young HF, Eisenberg HM et al (1991) Impact of ICP instability and hypotension on outcome in patients with severe head trauma. J Neurosurg 75:S59–S66

Salim A, Hadjizacharia P, DuBose J, Brown C, Inaba K, Chan L et al (2008) Role of anemia in traumatic brain injury. J Am Coll Surg 207:398–406

Stocchetti N, Furlan A, Volta F (1996) Hypoxemia and arterial hypotension at the accident scene in head injury. J Trauma 40:764–767

Suarez JIMD (2009) Tight control of blood glucose in the brain-injured patient is important and desirable. J Neurosurg Anesthesiol 21:52–54

Theusinger OM, Spahn DR, Ganter MT (2009) Transfusion in trauma: why and how should we change our current practice? Curr Opin Anaesthesiol 22:305–312

Yoder JMD (2009) Tight glucose control after brain injury is unproven and unsafe. J Neurosurg Anesthesiol 21:55–57

Young B, Ott L, Dempsey R, Haack D, Tibbs P (1989) Relationship between admission hyperglycemia and neurologic outcome of severely brain-injured patients. Ann Surg 210:466–473

15 Prognosis of Severe Traumatic Brain Injury: To Treat or Not to Treat, That Is the Question

Magnus Olivecrona

Recommendations

Level I

There are no data supporting an individual prognosis at this level.

Level II

There are no data supporting an individual prognosis at this level.

There is a prognostic value in age, GCS, GCS motor score, pupillary reactivity, hypotension, hypoxia, CT findings, blood glucose, serum sodium, and ethnic origin.

Level III

There are some data supporting an individual prognosis, prognosis calculators, at this level.

There seems to be a prognostic value in ICP and CPP.

There is insufficient evidence for the prognostic value of biomarkers and pressure reactivity.

M. Olivecrona
Department of Neurosurgery, University Hospital,
Umeå 901 85, Sweden
e-mail: magnus.olivecrona@neuro.umu.se

15.1 Overview

Prognosis, from Greek πρόγνωση – literally fore-knowing, foreseeing.

The prognosis of a disease can be used for discussing the seriousness or likely outcome of a disease. It can as such be used as an aid in the information process to the patient or her/his relatives. It also gives information to the treating physician about what she/he could expect.

The accuracy of prognosis on group or population level can be very precise but not at the level of the individual patient.

There are several factors that prognosticate for poor prognosis in severe traumatic brain injury, such as age, GCS, pupillary dilation with loss of light reflex, hypoxia, hypotension, mass lesions on CT, presence of subarachnoidal blood on CT, and others. These factors have been used in prognostic models of which two, IMPACT prognosis calculator and CRASH prognosis calculator, are available on the World Wide Web. They can be used for individual prognosis. None of these prognostic factors, alone, together, or as prognosis calculators, are strong enough to prognosticate outcome or even mortality at the individual level. They should therefore be used with caution. There is no prognostic factor or association of prognosis factors that with certainty can tell the treating physician not to initiate treatment. Development of such a criterion, as objective as possible, e.g. an initial CPP value, to make the decision to treat or not to treat possible, would be of great advantage.

T. Sundstrøm et al. (eds.), *Management of Severe Traumatic Brain Injury*,
DOI 10.1007/978-3-642-28126-6_15, © Springer-Verlag Berlin Heidelberg 2012

The ultimate way of using the prognosis would be to have the possibility to individualise the prognosis and so to use the prognosis for the prediction of the outcome in a specific individual and so to make treatment decision based on the prognosis possible.

The treating physician has to be aware of the limitations of the prognosis, and thus has to show great caution in using the estimated prognosis on an individual level, and/or to make treatment decisions based on this prognosis. There is a risk that prognostic factors, which are negative on the group level, will be used at the individual level and thus turn out to self-fulfilling, e.g. if the patient present with bilateral dilated and fixed pupils and the treating physician decides based on this prognostic factor not to treat.

Tips, Tricks, and Pitfalls

- There is no certain way of making a prognosis in an individual case.
- The presentation of poor prognostic factors such as bilateral dilated pupils does not necessarily mean that the patient will not survive or have a favourable outcome.
- In patients who initially are so bad that one suspect that they will not survive, the use of an objective measurement on which to base the initial treat or not-to-treat decision on, e.g. a first measured CPP of a certain level, could be very useful.

15.2 Background

Prognosis of outcome in head trauma has always interested man. In the ancient literature, references to the prognosis of head trauma are found, e.g. in the Edwin Smith Papyrus (Edwin 1600 B.C.) and in the writings of Hippocrates (1928).

Today, the prognosis of outcome of severe traumatic brain injury is mostly defined in relation to outcome measured as GOS (Jennett and Bond 1975). This can be in relation to every single level of GOS or to different dichotomisations, such as dead/alive and unfavourable/favourable. The influence of different prognostic factors on outcome can be analysed using statistical methods. The influence of a single factor on outcome can be analysed using univariate analysis. This result is of limited value. To adjust for confounders and/or the influence of other prognostic factors, more advanced statistical analysis such as logistic regression and multivariate analysis have to be used. Further statistical modelling can result in prognostic models, which even can try to make prognostication on the individual level.

Factors analysed for prognostic value can be of different kinds: patient characteristics (e.g. age, gender), admission data (e.g. GCS, type of injury, blood pressure), or data from the clinical course (e.g. episodes of high ICP, episodes of low CPP, seizures). These factors are then analysed against different kinds of outcome measures such as GOS, neuropsychological outcome, or functions of daily life. As stated above, GOS is the most commonly used outcome measure. The treatment protocol used has not been integrated in any prognosis analysis.

In modern times, the discussion about the prognosis in severe traumatic brain injury started with the introduction of the concept of secondary events by Miller in 1978 (Miller et al. 1978) and by the study of Chesnut and co-workers (Chesnut et al. 1993a).

During the last years, the 'International Mission for Prognosis and Clinical Trial design in TBI' study group (IMPACT) (Marmarou et al. 2007a) has published several papers on the prognosis in traumatic brain injury. They have pooled data from 11 international head injury studies and analysed data from 9,205 patients. Using these data, they have also designed a prognostic model, with a prognostic calculator (Steyerberg et al. 2008), which allows for estimation of the individual prognosis. The calculator, which is available on the IMPACT home page, gives the risk for mortality and unfavourable outcome (GOS 1–3) at 6 months (http://tbi-impact.org).

In 2008 the 'Medical Research Council Corticosteroid Randomisation After Significant Head Injury Study' (MRC CRASH) published a paper on the prognosis of head injury based on 10,008 patients enrolled in the study (Perel et al. 2008). They also constructed a prognosis calculator, which is available on their homepage (http://www.crash.lshtm.ac.uk), for the prognostication on the individual level. This calculator is based on the dichotomisation of the outcome in high-income countries (approximately one-fourth of the enrolled patients) and low-middle-income countries. The calculator gives the risk for mortality at 14 days and the risk for unfavourable outcome (GOS 1–3) at 6 months.

More than 15 other prognosis models have been published. The two prognosis models from IMPACT and CRASH have both been externally validated using large patient materials. Other models often lack such validation.

15.2.1 Prognostic Factors

15.2.1.1 Patient Characteristics

Sex: In severe traumatic brain injury, the majority of patients are men. There is no difference between the sexes in regard to prognosis (Ellenberg et al. 1996; Husson et al. 2010; Murray et al. 2007; Mushkudiani et al. 2007; Perel et al. 2008).

Age: Increasing age is a strong predictor of poorer outcome (Combes et al. 1996; Hukkelhoven et al. 2003; Mushkudiani et al. 2007; Perel et al. 2008). There seems in some studies to be a breaking point somewhere around 30–40 years of age (Hukkelhoven et al. 2003; Mushkudiani et al. 2007). The most head injury trials have an upper age limit, often 60–70 years of age. The relation between age and outcome in the paediatric and elderly populations are not very well studied.

Ethnic Origin: The IMPACT study group found poorer outcome in black patients compared with Caucasians (Mushkudiani et al. 2007).

15.2.1.2 Injury Severity, Clinical characteristics

Glasgow Coma Score, Glasgow Motor Score: GCS and GCS Motor Score are strong predictors for outcome (Husson et al. 2010; Marmarou et al. 2007b; Perel et al. 2008), irrespectively of time point for assessment. The assessment of GCS is time dependent in the course of severe traumatic brain injury (Arbabi et al. 2004; Stocchetti et al. 2004). The time point of assessment has to be taken into consideration if the assessment is done at the sight of the trauma, in the emergency room, after stabilisation, or even after intubation. In unconsciousness patients, the motor score has been claimed to be more reliable than the total GCS score (Healey et al. 2003). The modern care of severe traumatic brain injury includes early intubation and sedation, which has to be taken in consideration (Balestreri et al. 2004; Stocchetti et al. 2004). We have to bear in mind that a GCS score of 3 is an exclusion criterion in many studies, but papers reporting good outcome (GOS 4–5) in 8–33% of patients with an initial GCS of 3 have been published (Chamoun et al. 2009; Mauritz et al. 2009; Olivecrona et al. 2009b).

Pupillary Reaction: The absence of pupillary reactivity in one or both eyes is a strong prognostic factor (Marmarou et al. 2007b; Perel et al. 2008). This factor is claimed to be less sensitive for changes over time. In many studies of severe traumatic brain injury, dilated fixed pupil or pupils is an exclusion criterion. There are papers published with good outcome (GOS 4–5) in patients with unilateral or bilateral dilated fixed pupils (Clusmann et al. 2001; Mauritz et al. 2009; Olivecrona et al. 2009b). Also the loss of pupillary reactivity unilaterally is a poor prognostic sign, though not as bad a loss of bilateral reactivity. Marmarou et al. report an odds ratio for poorer outcome of around 7 for bilateral loss of pupil reactivity compared with an odds ratio of 3 for poorer prognosis by unilateral loss of pupil reactivity (Marmarou et al. 2007b).

Hypotension: Hypotension defined as systolic blood pressure <90 mmHg is a poor prognostic factor (Butcher et al. 2007; Chesnut et al. 1993b; Manley et al. 2001; McHugh et al. 2007; Miller et al. 1978; Murray et al. 2007; Walia and Sutcliffe 2002). The IMPACT study group found a bell-shaped curve for blood pressure, showing a better prognosis if the systolic blood pressure was between 120 and 150 mmHg, corresponding to mean arterial pressure of 85–110 mmHg (Butcher et al. 2007).

Hypoxia: Hypoxia is a factor for poor outcome (Chesnut et al. 1993b; Hukkelhoven et al. 2005; McHugh et al. 2007; Miller et al. 1978). The definition of hypoxia varies between studies (SaO_2 < 90/92% or PaO_2 < 60 mmHg).

15.2.1.3 Laboratory Parameters

Initial Blood Glucose: High blood glucose level correlates positively with poor outcome (Van Beek et al. 2007).

Initial Serum Sodium Levels: Low sodium levels are a poor prognostic factor, the same has been found for high sodium levels, but the findings are weaker (Van Beek et al. 2007). The use of hypertonic saline can be a confounding factor for the high sodium values.

Haemoglobin: Low haemoglobin is a factor for poor prognosis (Van Beek et al. 2007).

Biomarkers: Biomarkers such as S-100B, neuron specific enolase (NSE), and ApoE (ε) 4 have, during the last years, attracted much attention for their possible use in prognostication. The results are confounding. Some authors find prognostic value in the biomarkers (Nylen et al. 2008; Rainey et al. 2009; Rothoerl et al. 2000; Teasdale et al. 1997; Vos et al. 2004) and some authors do not (Alexander et al. 2007; Olivecrona et al. 2009a, 2010; Teasdale et al. 2005). No biomarker has been proven to have a strong predictive value. All series studying biomarkers are relatively small. Another issue of the use of biomarkers for prognostication is the question of which value should be used, the first measured, the highest measured value, or the sum of values over a certain time.

15.2.1.4 Structural Imaging

Computerised Tomography: In 1991, Marshall and collaborators introduced a system to classify CT scans; this system was initially designed as a descriptive method (Marshall et al. 1991). The Marshall classification, which focuses on the presence of mass lesions, has been correlated to the prognosis (Servadei et al. 2000). The importance of the CT scan features for prognosis was well established in the treatment guidelines published in 2000 (Chesnut et al. 2000). A combination of different CT features, such as midline shift, the presence of subarachnoid blood, epidural haematoma, or the compression of basal cisterns, increases the prognostic value (Maas et al. 2005, 2007). The presence of traumatic subarachnoid blood seems to one of the strongest predictors of poor outcome (Maas et al. 2005). The Rotterdam classification of the CT scan, introduced by Mass and collaborators in 2005, seems to have a stronger predictive value than the Marshall classification (Maas et al. 2005). There is another advantage of the Rotterdam classifications: it allows for the comparison of the CT scans over time.

15.2.1.5 Clinical Course

Intracranial Pressure: Intuitively, one would assume that ICP should be a prognostic factor. Some treatment concepts are focused on reducing the ICP (ICP-targeted therapy). Most authors report correlations between, e.g. the highest observed ICP and outcome, or the mean ICP over a certain time, often not very well defined, or the 'delivered' ICP over time (Farahvar et al. 2011; Vik et al. 2008). Most reported series are relatively small. The majority of authors do present a prognostic value of ICP (Balestreri et al. 2006; Farahvar et al. 2011; Marmarou et al. 1991; Vik et al. 2008). Strictly, the prognostic value of the ICP is difficult to interpret.

Cerebral Perfusion Pressure: Intuitively, the CPP should be a prognostic factor. CPP-targeted therapies have been one of the most used treatment concepts until the publication in 2007 of the third edition of the *American Guidelines* (Bratton et al. 2007). The same applies for CPP as for ICP: there have been many different ways trying to establish a prognostic correlation. Authors have reported of the prognostic value of CPP (Clifton et al. 2002; Juul et al. 2000; Kirkness et al. 2005), and others have reported of the non-prognostic value of CPP (Balestreri et al. 2006). Strictly, the prognostic value of the CPP is difficult to interpret.

Periods of Hypotension and Hypoxia: There are reports stating that the number and the duration of episodes of hypotension and/or hypoxia during the course of the treatment correlate negative to outcome (Sarrafzadeg 2001; Chesnut 1993a, b).

Pressure Reactivity, PR Index, and Intact Autoregulation: The PR, which is the regression coefficient of several MAP/ICP points, can be regarded as a surrogate measure for the auto-regulative state of the brain, with a negative to zero value of the PR regarded as an intact auto-regulation. There have been reports of poorer prognosis in patients with disturbed auto-regulation (Balestreri et al. 2005; Hiler et al. 2006; Howells et al. 2005; Zweifel et al. 2008).

15.3 Specific Paediatric Concerns

There are relatively few studies of severe traumatic brain injury in the paediatric population. Generally, one can assume that the severely injured child has a better prognosis than the adult with a corresponding trauma. This might be due to several factors such as a greater plasticity of the young brain, a general better healing capacity fewer concomitant diseases in the paediatric population. All major work on the prognosis of severe head injury has been done on adult populations. Generally, the recommendation must be to treat a child with severe traumatic brain injury aggressively.

References

Alexander S, Kerr ME, Kim Y et al (2007) Apolipoprotein E4 allele presence and functional outcome after severe traumatic brain injury. J Neurotrauma 24:790–797

Arbabi S, Jurkovich GJ, Wahl WL et al (2004) A comparison of prehospital and hospital data in trauma patients. J Trauma 56:1029–1032

Balestreri M, Czosnyka M, Chatfield DA et al (2004) Predictive value of Glasgow Coma Scale after brain trauma: change in trend over the past ten years. J Neurol Neurosurg Psychiatry 75:161–162

Balestreri M, Czosnyka M, Steiner LA et al (2005) Association between outcome, cerebral pressure reactivity and slow ICP waves following head injury. Acta Neurochir Suppl 95:25–28

Balestreri M, Czosnyka M, Hutchinson P et al (2006) Impact of intracranial pressure and cerebral perfusion pressure on severe disability and mortality after head injury. Neurocrit Care 4:8–13

Bratton SL, Chestnut RM, Ghajar J et al (2007) IX. Cerebral perusion thresholds. J Neurotrauma 24:S59–S64

Butcher I, Maas AI, Lu J et al (2007) Prognostic value of admission blood pressure in traumatic brain injury: results from the IMPACT study. J Neurotrauma 24: 294–302

Chamoun RB, Robertson CS, Gopinath SP (2009) Outcome in patients with blunt head trauma and a Glasgow Coma Scale score of 3 at presentation. J Neurosurg 111:683–687

Chesnut RM, Marshall SB, Piek J et al (1993a) Early and late systemic hypotension as a frequent and fundamental source of cerebral ischemia following severe brain injury in the Traumatic Coma Data Bank. Acta Neurochir Suppl (Wien) 59:121–125

Chesnut RM, Marshall LF, Klauber MR et al (1993b) The role of secondary brain injury in determining outcome from severe head injury. J Trauma 34:216–222

Chesnut RM, Ghajar J, Maas AI et al (2000) Computed tomography scan features. J Neurotrauma 17:597–628

Clifton GL, Miller ER, Choi SC et al (2002) Fluid thresholds and outcome from severe brain injury. Crit Care Med 30:739–745

Clusmann H, Schaller C, Schramm J (2001) Fixed and dilated pupils after trauma, stroke, and previous intracranial surgery: management and outcome. J Neurol Neurosurg Psychiatry 71:175–181

Combes P, Fauvage B, Colonna M et al (1996) Severe head injuries: an outcome prediction and survival analysis. Intensive Care Med 22:1391–1395

Edwin (1600 B.C.) Edwin Smith Surgical Papyrus. http://archive.nlm.nih.gov/proj/ttp/flash/smith/smith.html. Accessed 18 Apr 2011

Ellenberg JH, Levin HS, Saydjari C (1996) Posttraumatic amnesia as a predictor of outcome after severe closed head injury. Prospective assessment. Arch Neurol 53:782–791

Farahvar A, Gerber LM, Chiu YL et al (2011) Response to intracranial hypertension treatment as a predictor of death in patients with severe traumatic brain injury. J Neurosurg 114(5):1471–1478

Healey C, Osler TM, Rogers FB et al (2003) Improving the Glasgow Coma Scale score: motor score alone is a better predictor. J Trauma 54:671–678; discussion 678–680

Hiler M, Czosnyka M, Hutchinson P et al (2006) Predictive value of initial computerized tomography scan, intracranial pressure, and state of autoregulation in patients with traumatic brain injury. J Neurosurg 104:731–737

Hippocrates (1928) Hippocrates Volume III: on wounds in the head, in the surgery, fractures, joints, moclion translated by E.T. Withington Harvard University Press, Cambridge, MA, London England pp 7–51

Howells T, Elf K, Jones PA et al (2005) Pressure reactivity as a guide in the treatment of cerebral perfusion pressure in patients with brain trauma. J Neurosurg 102:311–317

Hukkelhoven CW, Steyerberg EW, Rampen AJ et al (2003) Patient age and outcome following severe traumatic brain injury: an analysis of 5600 patients. J Neurosurg 99:666–673

Hukkelhoven CW, Steyerberg EW, Habbema JD et al (2005) Predicting outcome after traumatic brain injury: development and validation of a prognostic score based on admission characteristics. J Neurotrauma 22:1025–1039

Husson EC, Ribbers GM, Willemse-van Son AH et al (2010) Prognosis of six-month functioning after moderate to severe traumatic brain injury: a systematic review of prospective cohort studies. J Rehabil Med 42:425–436

Jennett B, Bond M (1975) Assessment of outcome after severe brain damage. Lancet 1:480–484

Juul N, Morris GF, Marshall SB et al (2000) Intracranial hypertension and cerebral perfusion pressure: influence

on neurological deterioration and outcome in severe head injury. The Executive Committee of the International Selfotel Trial. J Neurosurg 92:1–6
Kirkness CJ, Burr RL, Cain KC et al (2005) Relationship of cerebral perfusion pressure levels to outcome in traumatic brain injury. Acta Neurochir Suppl 95:13–16
Maas AI, Hukkelhoven CW, Marshall LF et al (2005) Prediction of outcome in traumatic brain injury with computed tomographic characteristics: a comparison between the computed tomographic classification and combinations of computed tomographic predictors. Neurosurgery 57:1173–1182; discussion 1173–1182
Maas AI, Marmarou A, Murray GD et al (2007) Prognosis and clinical trial design in traumatic brain injury: the IMPACT study. J Neurotrauma 24:232–238
Manley G, Knudson MM, Morabito D et al (2001) Hypotension, hypoxia, and head injury: frequency, duration, and consequences. Arch Surg 136:1118–1123
Marmarou A, Anderson RL, Ward JD et al (1991) Impact of ICP instability and hypotension on outcome in patients with severe traumatic head trauma. J Neurosurg 75:S59–S66
Marmarou A, Lu J, Butcher I et al (2007a) IMPACT database of traumatic brain injury: design and description. J Neurotrauma 24:239–250
Marmarou A, Lu J, Butcher I et al (2007b) Prognostic value of the Glasgow Coma Scale and pupil reactivity in traumatic brain injury assessed pre-hospital and on enrollment: an IMPACT analysis. J Neurotrauma 24: 270–280
Marshall LF, Marshall SH, Klauber MR et al (1991) A new classification of head injury based on computerized tomography. J Neurosurg 75:s14–s20
Mauritz W, Leitgeb J, Wilbacher I et al (2009) Outcome of brain trauma patients who have a Glasgow Coma Scale score of 3 and bilateral fixed and dilated pupils in the field. Eur J Emerg Med 16:153–158
McHugh GS, Engel DC, Butcher I et al (2007) Prognostic value of secondary insults in traumatic brain injury: results from the IMPACT study. J Neurotrauma 24: 287–293
Miller JD, Sweet RC, Narayan R et al (1978) Early insults to the injured brain. JAMA 240:439–442
Murray GD, Butcher I, McHugh GS et al (2007) Multivariable prognostic analysis in traumatic brain injury: results from the IMPACT study. J Neurotrauma 24:329–337
Mushkudiani NA, Engel DC, Steyerberg EW et al (2007) Prognostic value of demographic characteristics in traumatic brain injury: results from the IMPACT study. J Neurotrauma 24:259–269
Nylen K, Ost M, Csajbok LZ et al (2008) Serum levels of S100B, S100A1B and S100BB are all related to outcome after severe traumatic brain injury. Acta Neurochir (Wien) 150:221–227; discussion 227
Olivecrona M, Rodling-Wahlstrom M, Naredi S et al (2009a) S-100B and neuron specific enolase are poor outcome predictors in severe traumatic brain injury treated by an intracranial pressure targeted therapy. J Neurol Neurosurg Psychiatry 80:1241–1247
Olivecrona M, Rodling-Wahlstrom M, Naredi S et al (2009b) Prostacyclin treatment in severe traumatic brain injury: a microdialysis and outcome study. J Neurotrauma 26:1251–1262
Olivecrona M, Wildemyr Z, Koskinen LO (2010) The apolipoprotein E epsilon4 allele and outcome in severe traumatic brain injury treated by an intracranial pressure-targeted therapy. J Neurosurg 112:1113–1119
Perel P, Arango M, Clayton T et al (2008) Predicting outcome after traumatic brain injury: practical prognostic models based on large cohort of international patients. BMJ 336:425–429
Rainey T, Lesko M, Sacho R et al (2009) Predicting outcome after severe traumatic brain injury using the serum S100B biomarker: results using a single (24 h) time-point. Resuscitation 80:341–345
Rothoerl RD, Woertgen C, Brawanski A (2000) S-100 serum levels and outcome after severe head injury. Acta Neurochir Suppl 76:97–100
Sarrafzadeh AS, Peltonen EE, Kaisers U et al (2001) Secondary insults in severe head injury–do multiply injured patients do worse? Crit Care Med 29(6): 1116–1123
Servadei F, Murray GD, Penny K et al (2000) The value of the "worst" computed tomographic scan in clinical studies of moderate and severe head injury. European Brain Injury Consortium. Neurosurgery 46:70–75; discussion 75–77
Steyerberg EW, Mushkudiani N, Perel P et al (2008) Predicting outcome after traumatic brain injury: development and international validation of prognostic scores based on admission characteristics. PLoS Med 5:e165; discussion e165
Stocchetti N, Pagan F, Calappi E et al (2004) Inaccurate early assessment of neurological severity in head injury. J Neurotrauma 21:1131–1140
Teasdale GM, Nicoll JA, Murray G et al (1997) Association of apolipoprotein E polymorphism with outcome after head injury. Lancet 350:1069–1071
Teasdale GM, Murray GD, Nicoll JA (2005) The association between APOE epsilon4, age and outcome after head injury: a prospective cohort study. Brain 128: 2556–2561
Walia S, Sutcliffe AJ (2002) The relationship between blood glucose, mean arterial pressure and outcome after severe head injury: an observational study. Injury 33:339–344
Van Beek JG, Mushkudiani NA, Steyerberg EW et al (2007) Prognostic value of admission laboratory parameters in traumatic brain injury: results from the IMPACT study. J Neurotrauma 24:315–328
Vik A, Nag T, Fredriksli OA et al (2008) Relationship of "dose" of intracranial hypertension to outcome in severe traumatic brain injury. J Neurosurg 109:678–684
Vos PE, Lamers KJ, Hendriks JC et al (2004) Glial and neuronal proteins in serum predict outcome after severe traumatic brain injury. Neurology 62:1303–1310
Zweifel C, Lavinio A, Steiner LA et al (2008) Continuous monitoring of cerebrovascular pressure reactivity in patients with head injury. Neurosurg Focus 25:E2

Potential Organ Donor: Organ Preservation

16

Silvana Naredi

Recommendations

Level I

Data are insufficient to support Level I recommendations for this subject.

Level II

Data are insufficient to support Level II recommendations for this subject.

Level III

Data are insufficient to support Level III recommendations for this subject.

Level of Evidence

There exists neither consensus nor scientific criteria for defining a potential organ donor.

Management strategies for the treatment of the organ donor and preservation of organ function are based on sparse scientific evidence.

S. Naredi
Department of Anesthesiology and Intensive Care, Umeå University Hospital, S90185 Umeå, Sweden
e-mail: silvana.naredi@anestesi.umu.se

16.1 Overview

Intensive care and organ donation have been related ever since the concept of brain death, i.e., death due to brain-related criteria was introduced. Even though the term potential organ donor is extensively used, there exists neither scientific evidence nor consensus criteria for defining a potential organ donor (Bell 2010).

The primary aim in a patient with a severe TBI is to give the patient full neurointensive care until treatment is regarded as futile. If all objective signs point towards that all functions of the brain are lost, procedures leading to the diagnosis of death is initiated. Organ donation and transplantation is based on the 'Dead Donor Rule'; death must be confirmed before organ donation is performed (Bernat 2005).

Diagnosis of death is regulated in national legal documents and is subject to modifications. The basis of diagnosis of dead is, in most western countries, the irreversible cessation of all functions of the entire brain, including the brainstem (Wijdicks et al. 2010).

When the diagnosis of death is completed, the critical care is changed towards maintenance of organ function. Death due to brain-related criteria leads to circulatory, pulmonary, hepatic and metabolic consequences that need attention in order to maintain sufficient organ function. The treatment strategies should aim at normalisation of organ physiology as far as possible (Shah 2008; Dictus et al. 2009). The use of an organ donor management protocol is recommended

T. Sundstrøm et al. (eds.), *Management of Severe Traumatic Brain Injury*,
DOI 10.1007/978-3-642-28126-6_16, © Springer-Verlag Berlin Heidelberg 2012

Table 16.1 Treatment of the organ donor

Parameter	Goal	Commentary
Systolic blood pressure	≥100 mmHg	Maintaining normovolemia with sufficient fluids, vasopressor support with dopamine and dobutamine (<10 μg/kg/min)
Urinary output	>1 mL/kg/h	Maintaining normovolemia with sufficient fluids, vasopressor support with dopamine and dobutamine (<10 μg/kg/min)
Haemoglobin	>100 g/L	Transfusion of red blood cells (RBC)
PaO_2	>12 kPa	Tidal volume (6–8 mL/kg), PEEP see below, recruitment manoeuvres
Fractional inspired oxygen (FiO_2)	<0.4	Tidal volume (6–8 mL/kg), PEEP see below, recruitment manoeuvres
Positive end expiratory pressure (PEEP)	<10 cmH_2O	High PEEP will impede venous return
$PaCO_2$	4.5–6.0 kPa	Normoventilation
Central venous pressure (CVP)	<10 mmHg	Maintain normovolemia
Body temperature	>35°C	Warming blankets, warm fluids
Blood glucose	<10 mmol/L	Short-acting insulin
Sodium	<155 mmol/L	Desmopressin, restricted use of sodium-containing fluids
pH	7.40–7.45	Maintaining normovolemia, sodium bicarbonate
Platelet count	$>50\times10^9$/L	Transfusion of platelets
PT/INR[a]	>1.5	Transfusion of fresh frozen plasma

[a]Prothrombin time/International Normalised Ratio

(DuBose and Salim 2008). For details regarding donor treatment, see Table 16.1.

We emphasise that organ donation from diseased persons is regulated by each country's legislation.

Tips, Tricks, and Pitfalls

- Maintain normovolemia.
- Use dopamine and dobutamine as first-line choices for vasopressor support.
- Use low tidal volume ventilation (6–8 mL/kg) and aim at normoventilation ($PaCO_2$, 4.5–6.0 kPa).
- Keep a neutral fluid balance and a urinary output >1 mL/kg/h.

16.2 Background

16.2.1 The Process of Herniation and Death

With a therapy resistant, increasing cerebral oedema, the ICP will continue to rise, until the CPP finally will become zero, resulting in cessation of perfusion of the brain and brainstem. Consequently, there will be a breakdown of the regulation of circulation; the blood pressure will fall to subnormal values due to the ultimate spinal cord sympathetic deactivation, which results in the loss of vasomotor tone followed by vasodilatation and hypotension (Dictus et al. 2009).

16.2.2 Circulatory Considerations

The hypotension, due to loss of vasomotor tone, aggravated by fluid loss due to diabetes insipidus, is the major problem in the care of an organ donator. Normovolemia and a systolic blood pressure ≥100 mmHg (MABP≥60 mmHg) and a CVP of 5–10 mmHg should be maintained in order to ensure an adequate organ perfusion. To keep the blood pressure at an acceptable level, sufficient fluids should be administered and, in addition, vasopressor support if necessary. There exists no scientific evidence regarding the preferable vasopressor to use. Dopamine (<10 μg/kg/min) and dobutamine (<10 μg/kg/min) are recommended, as first-line choices. Noradrenalin and adrenalin should be used with caution due to the risk of vasoconstriction and impaired organ function due to ischemia (Zaroff et al. 2002; Stoica et al. 2004; Brockmann et al. 2006; Shah 2008; Dictus et al. 2009; Schnuelle et al. 2009).

A shift from catecholamine use, towards taking advantage of the vasopressor properties of arginine vasopressin (antidiuretic hormone), has been proposed, especially in situations with an increasing demand for vasopressor support (Shah 2008; Dictus et al. 2009). For vasopressin analogues, a dose of >0.04 U/min should not be exceeded, in order to avoid coronary, renal and splanchnic vasoconstriction. The vasopressin analogue, 1-desamino-8-D-arginine vasopressin (desmopressin), traditionally utilised for the treatment of diabetes insipidus, has no significant vasopressor activity (Shah 2008; Dictus et al. 2009).

The secretion of antidiuretic hormone (ADH) is decreased after herniation and the urinary output increases. Left uncorrected, it will quickly lead to severe hypovolemia. Correction of hypovolemia can be made by crystalloids and colloids (albumin, RBC, fresh frozen plasma). Hydroxyethyl starch solutions should be used with caution, due to the possibility of negative effects on kidney function (Giral et al. 2007; Dictus et al. 2009). Normovolemia should always be maintained; both hypovolemia and hypervolemia have adverse effects concerning organ preservation.

16.2.3 Pulmonary Considerations

The organ with the highest probability to be unsuitable for transplantation is the lung; only 10–15% of multiorgan donors have lungs that can be used for transplantation (Pierre and Keshavjee 2005). The lungs can be subject to blunt trauma, and a systemic inflammatory response syndrome triggered by trauma can cause further damage. The fluid balance is especially important for lung preservation and should be kept neutral. The use of colloids has shown to be beneficial in minimising the development of pulmonary oedema (Dictus et al. 2009). Due to the risk of ventilator-associated pneumonia, antibiotics could be liberally administered; the contraindications to antibiotic therapy are limited, even though the benefits never have been evaluated in clinical studies. Performance of a bronchoscopy to obtain material for bacterial examination and culture could be considered. Ventilation strategies with low tidal volumes (6–8 mL/kg), normoventilation ($PaCO_2$ 4.5–6.0 kPa), peak inspiratory pressure <30 cmH_2O and PEEP of 5–10 cmH_2O, to reduce shear stress, should be employed. Recruitment manoeuvres and regular turning of the organ donor in order to avoid atelectasis are recommended. PaO_2 should be kept >12 kPa. FiO_2 should ideally be kept <0.4. It is preferable to increase FiO_2 before PEEP, since a high PEEP will impede venous return. If increased FiO_2 is required, the goal for PaO_2 could be decreased to >8–10 kPa (Brockmann et al. 2006; Shah 2008; Dictus et al. 2009). Administration of corticosteroids has become increasingly accepted in the management of lung donors and could be considered after contact with the transplantation centre (Kutsogiannis et al. 2006).

16.2.4 Renal Considerations

The urinary output should be kept >1 mL/kg/h. This is primarily achieved by adequate fluid administration and, if needed, vasopressor support. The systolic blood pressure should be ≥100 mmHg (MABP≥60 mmHg). Dopamine and/or dobutamine (<10 μg/kg/min) is primarily used to support a sufficient blood pressure level. Noradrenalin and/or adrenaline can be added in the lowest possible dose, and the use of vasopressin analogues can be considered (<0.04 U/min), if there is an increasing need for vasopressor support (Shah 2008).

Nephrotoxic drugs should be avoided. If the urinary output is <1 mL/kg/h, normovolemia and fluid balance should primarily be evaluated; secondarily, a small dose of diuretics can be used. Lack of ADH causes diabetes insipidus with increased urinary output leading to hypernatraemia; it is therefore important not to overuse sodium-containing crystalloids.

Clinically manifest diabetes insipidus (urinary output >300 mL/h, serum sodium >150 mmol/L, urinary sodium <20 mmol/L) is treated with volume replacement (glucose solutions 2.5–5%) and desmopressin in small repeated doses (0.4–1.0 μg intravenously). It is important to remember that the half-life of desmopressin is up to around 11 h.

16.2.5 Hepatic Consideration

Serum sodium should be kept <155 mmol/L, since high serum sodium concentration could cause impaired hepatic function (Shah 2008). CVP should be maintained between 5 and 10 mmHg, and PEEP should be kept as low as possible (<10 cmH_2O) to prevent hepatic congestion.

16.2.6 Metabolic Considerations

Dysfunction of the posterior pituitary is common, resulting in low levels of ADH, and administration of the vasopressin analogue desmopressin, in order to treat diabetes insipidus, is considered as standard procedure (Kutsogiannis et al. 2006; Shah 2008; Dictus et al. 2009). Hormonal replacement with thyroid hormones and corticosteroids remains controversial, due to sparse scientific evidence, but could be considered in specific cases (Zaroff et al. 2002; Brockmann et al. 2006; Kutsogiannis et al. 2006; Novitzky et al. 2006; Shah 2008; Dictus et al. 2009; Venkateswaran et al. 2009).

Hyperglycaemia is considered as a consequence of elevated levels of catecholamines, infusion of glucose and peripheral insulin resistance. Normoglycaemia should be maintained (Dictus et al. 2009).

In order to especially avoid cardiovascular complications, the body temperature should be kept >35°C, using warming devices and warm fluids (Dictus et al. 2009).

16.3 Specific Paediatric Concerns

Scientific data concerning donor management strategies are limited in adults and even more limited when it comes to children (Finfer et al. 1996; Mallory et al. 2009). Paediatric organ donors are rare in most hospitals. The diagnosis of death due to brain-related criteria is the same in paediatric patients as in adults, although the confirmation of death in infants may require specially trained staff. Consultation of specific expertise for advice and support should be liberally used, both for diagnosis of death and for management of the organ donor. The level of physiological and laboratory parameters must be adjusted for age, especially levels for blood pressure. A cuffed endotracheal tube is recommended even in small children due to the risk of aspiration (Mallory et al. 2009).

References

Bell MD (2010) Early identification of the potential organ donor: fundamental role of intensive care or conflict of interest? Intensive Care Med 36(9):1451–1453

Bernat JL (2005) The concept and practice of brain death. Prog Brain Res 150:369–379

Brockmann JG, Vaidya A et al (2006) Retrieval of abdominal organs for transplantation. Br J Surg 93(2): 133–146

Dictus C, Vienenkoetter B et al (2009) Critical care management of potential organ donors: our current standard. Clin Transplant 23(Suppl 21):2–9

DuBose J, Salim A (2008) Aggressive organ donor management protocol. J Intensive Care Med 23(6): 367–375

Finfer S, Bohn D et al (1996) Intensive care management of paediatric organ donors and its effect on post-transplant organ function. Intensive Care Med 22(12): 1424–1432

Giral M, Bertola JP et al (2007) Effect of brain-dead donor resuscitation on delayed graft function: results of a monocentric analysis. Transplantation 83(9): 1174–1181

Kutsogiannis DJ, Pagliarello G et al (2006) Medical management to optimize donor organ potential: review of the literature. Can J Anaesth 53(8):820–830

Mallory GB Jr, Schecter MG et al (2009) Management of the pediatric organ donor to optimize lung donation. Pediatr Pulmonol 44(6):536–546

Novitzky D, Cooper DK et al (2006) Hormonal therapy of the brain-dead organ donor: experimental and clinical studies. Transplantation 82(11):1396–1401

Pierre AF, Keshavjee S (2005) Lung transplantation: donor and recipient critical care aspects. Curr Opin Crit Care 11(4):339–344

Schnuelle P, Gottmann U et al (2009) Effects of donor pretreatment with dopamine on graft function after kidney transplantation: a randomized controlled trial. JAMA 302(10):1067–1075

Shah VR (2008) Aggressive management of multiorgan donor. Transplant Proc 40(4):1087–1090

Stoica SC, Satchithananda DK et al (2004) Noradrenaline use in the human donor and relationship with load-independent right ventricular contractility. Transplantation 78(8):1193–1197

Venkateswaran RV, Steeds RP et al (2009) The haemodynamic effects of adjunctive hormone therapy in potential heart donors: a prospective randomized double-blind factorially designed controlled trial. Eur Heart J 30(14):1771–1780

Wijdicks EF, Varelas PN et al (2010) Evidence-based guideline update: determining brain death in adults: report of the Quality Standards Subcommittee of the American Academy of Neurology. Neurology 74(23): 1911–1918

Zaroff JG, Rosengard BR et al (2002) Consensus conference report: maximizing use of organs recovered from the cadaver donor: cardiac recommendations, March 28–29, 2001, Crystal City, VA. Circulation 106(7):836–841

Part V

Acute Surgical Treatment

Basic Trauma Craniotomy

17

Terje Sundstrøm and Knut Wester

Recommendations

Level I

There are insufficient data to support a Level I recommendation for this topic.

Level II

There are insufficient data to support a Level II recommendation for this topic.

Level III

A basic trauma craniotomy is a large frontotemporoparietal craniotomy that provides access to the most common intracranial haematomas and bleeding sites.

As a rule, patients requiring surgery for brain trauma should be operated as soon as possible.

17.1 Overview

A basic trauma craniotomy is a large craniotomy (Bullock et al. 2006; Greenberg 2010; Narayan et al. 1995; Schmidek and Roberts 2006; Youmans and Winn 2011). This allows the surgeon to remove the most common types of acute intracranial haematomas, such as epidural, subdural and intracerebral haematomas and cerebral contusions. It also provides access to the most usual sources of bleeding. These include large draining veins near the superior sagittal sinus as well as contused tissue in the subtemporal and subfrontal areas and the temporal and frontal poles.

The fundamentals of surgical treatment have not changed much the last decades (Valadka and Robertson 2007). Basic trauma craniotomies should be large, and mass lesions should be evacuated without undue delay. Early surgical intervention is preferable to awaiting clinical deterioration, because ischemic brain damage is dependent on the duration of ischemia.

Tips, Tricks, and Pitfalls

- Always look at the patient.
- Do not hesitate if indication for surgery.

T. Sundstrøm (✉)
Department of Neurosurgery, Haukeland University Hospital, Jonas Lies Vei 65, 5021 Bergen, Norway

Department of Surgical Sciences and Department of Biomedicine, University of Bergen, Jonas Lies Vei 91, 5020 Bergen, Norway
e-mail: terje.sundstrom@gmail.com

K. Wester
Department of Surgical Sciences, University of Bergen, Jonas Lies Vei 65, 5021 Bergen, Norway

Department of Neurosurgery, Haukeland University Hospital, Jonas Lies Vei 65, 5021 Bergen, Norway
e-mail: knut.gustav.wester@helse-bergen.no

T. Sundstrøm et al. (eds.), *Management of Severe Traumatic Brain Injury*,
DOI 10.1007/978-3-642-28126-6_17, © Springer-Verlag Berlin Heidelberg 2012

- The best treatment for patients with very severe injuries can be to withhold surgery.
- Remember that cervical instability must be ruled out before positioning.
- Always remember: skin flap > bone flap.
- Make sure that scalp injuries do not interfere with the blood supply of your planned skin flap.
- If you believe that you have to remove the bone flap, make sure it is large enough to yield sufficient decompression.

17.2 How to Perform a Basic Trauma Craniotomy

Cervical instability must have been ruled out before positioning. The head of the patient is placed on a doughnut or similar headrest (Mayfield head holder can also be used, but be aware of cranial fractures), turned almost 90° to the opposite side and slightly elevated above the level of the heart. The craniotomy opening should be in the horizontal plane. A sandbag or pillow under the ipsilateral shoulder helps to prevent positional obstruction of cranial venous outflow. Such obstruction can be visualised by venous stasis on the neck. The patient should be placed in the lateral position if the cervical spine is not radiologically cleared. Unless deterioration is rapid, the scalp is shaved and prepared as for a standard operative procedure.

The skin incision is started 1 cm in front of the tragus at the zygomatic arch, then curved posteriorly and superiorly above the helix of the ear to the midline in the parietal region, further along the midline to the frontal region, and, if possible, ending at the hairline. Generally, the exposed cranial area must be sufficiently large to accommodate a craniotomy with 14–16 cm anteroposterior diameter (always remember: skin flap > bone flap).

Haemostasis of the skin margins is obtained with plastic clips or multiple curved forceps applied to the galeal layer. The superficial temporal fascia and the temporalis muscle are incised down to the bone, close to the margin of the skin opening. The myocutaneous flap is reflected and secured.

The following temporary measure should be reserved for epidural haematomas and only if it yields faster decompression than going straight for the craniotomy: in a patient who is rapidly deteriorating and has a known epidural haematoma in the temporal fossa, the temporal end of the incision is rapidly opened, and a burr hole is placed. A limited craniectomy is immediately performed using Leksell rongeurs with subsequent partial evacuation of the haematoma. This procedure will give a rapid reduction in ICP and decompression of the midbrain at the tentorial incisura, before continuing with the standard craniotomy.

Multiple burr holes (≥2; more holes in older patients) are placed in the parietal and frontal regions, preferably over suture lines. The burr holes are undermined, gently separating the dura and skull, and joined to form a large free bone flap. Special care is advised when operating near the superior sagittal sinus and in case of fractures crossing the sinus. The medial margin of the bone flap should be approximately 2 cm from the midline to avoid arachnoid granulations and large dural and cortical veins. The lateral sphenoid wing and temporal bone can be resected using Leksell rongeurs under direct visual control, thereby securing adequate exposure of the middle fossa. The temporal exposure should extend all the way to the skull base.

The dural opening is performed in a controlled manner to avoid massive external herniation, and care must be taken to avoid cortical lacerations. The opening begins over the area of maximal clot thickness or in the anterior temporal region, because relatively silent cortex will be affected here if the brain starts to herniate through the opening. The dura can be opened in a U-shaped manner going low over the frontal and temporal regions with the base towards the superior sagittal sinus, carefully avoiding damage to parasagittal bridging veins. This ensures safe access to the areas along the midline, as well as the middle and frontal fossa. There are also other ways to open the dura, for example, in a cruciate manner or by multiple individual slits. Intradural haematomas and cerebral contusions are evacuated, and the subdural space is explored, before careful haemostasis is obtained by bipolar electrocautery (caution is advised with respect to bridging veins) and haemostatic agents.

The dura is closed primarily when there is no present or anticipated significant brain swelling. The brain is otherwise simply covered with a dura substitute (artificial or periosteum) and sutureless adaptation of the dura. We do not recommend leaving the dura open with exposed brain if a craniectomy is indicated. Multiple dural tacking sutures are placed around the craniotomy margin, and one or two are placed centrally in the bone flap to prevent a postoperative epidural haematoma.

The bone flap is replaced and fixed, and the scalp is closed in two layers. Placement of a subgaleal drain can be considered. The wound is dressed, and a circular head bandage placed.

Considerations on primary and secondary decompressive craniectomy are described in another section.

17.3 Specific Paediatric Concerns

A craniotomy for the evacuation of an epidural or subdural haematoma in small children entails a risk of significant blood loss. A continuous and meticulous haemostasis therefore has to be exercised throughout the procedure. The anaesthesiologist in charge should keep the neurosurgeon continuously informed about the extent of blood loss. In infants, the bone flap may be removed, as it will be replaced spontaneously.

References

Bullock MR, Chesnut R, Ghajar J, Gordon D, Hartl R, Newell DW, Servadei F, Walters BC, Wilberger JE, Surgical Management of Traumatic Brain Injury Author Group (2006) Surgical management of traumatic brain injury. Neurosurgery 58:S2-1–S2-62

Greenberg MS (2010) Handbook of neurosurgery. Greenberg Graphics/Thieme Medical Publishers, Tampa/New York

Narayan RK, Wilberger JE, Povlishock JT (1995) Neurotrauma. McGraw Hill, New York

Schmidek HH, Roberts DW (2006) Schmidek & Sweet operative neurosurgical techniques: indications, methods, and results. Saunders/Elsevier, Philadelphia

Valadka AB, Robertson CS (2007) Surgery of cerebral trauma and associated critical care. Neurosurgery 61:203–220

Youmans JR, Winn HR (2011) Youmans neurological surgery. Saunders/Elsevier, Philadelphia

Surgical Management of Traumatic Intracranial Haematomas

18

Terje Sundstrøm and Knut Wester

Recommendations

Level I

There are insufficient data to support a Level I recommendation for this topic.

Level II

There are insufficient data to support a Level II recommendation for this topic.

Level III

In general, patients with intracranial haematomas and indications for surgery should be operated as soon as possible.

The reader must remember that the surgical recommendations are merely options when planning the treatment strategy for each individual patient. There is no defined threshold for whom surgery should be withheld, but the patient must have a possibility of a reasonable functional outcome. Patients with devastating brain injuries and/or high probability of a poor outcome should generally not be subjected to surgical treatment.

Indications and methods for surgery adapted from the Brain Trauma Foundation (Bullock et al. 2006)

- Epidural haematoma (EDH)
  - All EDHs > 30 cm^3
  - GCS < 9 and anisocoria
  - Observe if EDH < 30 cm^3, <15-mm thickness, <5-mm midline shift and GCS > 8 without neurological deficits
  - *Methods*: Craniotomy preferably providing complete exposure of the EDH and the bleeding source (consider initial small craniectomy with decompression if very rapid deterioration from a haematoma in the temporal fossa)
- Acute subdural haematoma (ASDH)
  - Thickness >10 mm or midline shift >5 mm, regardless of GCS score
  - Thickness <10 mm and midline shift <5 mm, if a GCS score <9 falls with ≥2 points, and/or asymmetric or fixed dilated pupils, and/or ICP > 20 mmHg
  - ICP monitoring if GCS < 9
  - *Methods*: Go straight for a large craniotomy with adequate exposure of the frontal and

T. Sundstrøm (✉)
Department of Neurosurgery, Haukeland University Hospital, Jonas Lies Vei 65, 5021 Bergen, Norway

Department of Surgical Sciences and Department of Biomedicine, University of Bergen, Jonas Lies Vei 91, 5020 Bergen, Norway
e-mail: terje.sundstrom@gmail.com

K. Wester
Department of Surgical Sciences, University of Bergen, Jonas Lies Vei 65, 5021 Bergen, Norway

Department of Neurosurgery, Haukeland University Hospital, Jonas Lies Vei 65, 5021 Bergen, Norway
e-mail: knut.gustav.wester@helse-bergen.no

T. Sundstrøm et al. (eds.), *Management of Severe Traumatic Brain Injury*, DOI 10.1007/978-3-642-28126-6_18, © Springer-Verlag Berlin Heidelberg 2012

temporal poles and the area along the superior sagittal sinus
- Intracerebral haematoma (ICH) and cerebral contusions
  - Any lesion >50 cm^3
  - GCS 6–8 with frontal or temporal contusions >20 cm^3, and midline shift ≥5 mm, and/or cisternal compression
  - Progressive neurological deterioration referable to the lesion, or refractory high ICP, or signs of mass effect on CT scan
  - *Methods*: Typically a standard trauma craniotomy because frequently associated with extracerebral haematomas
- Posterior fossa mass lesions
  - Mass effect on CT scan, neurological dysfunction or deterioration referable to the lesion (even a small volume can have profound effects!)
  - *Methods*: Midline suboccipital craniectomy or craniotomy with access to midline and both hemispheres (consider placing an EVD, either as an initial or closing manoeuvre)

18.1 Overview

The most important complication of a traumatic brain injury (TBI) is the development of an intracranial haematoma. Secondary brain injury can result and reduce the likelihood of a good outcome. In this context, an effective trauma care system with high-quality neurosurgery is essential, as intracranial haematomas occur in 25–45% of severe TBI patients, 3–12% of moderate TBI patients, and approximately 1/500 patients with mild TBI (Bullock et al. 2006).

Rates of mortality and morbidity after an acute subdural haematoma are the highest of all traumatic mass lesions, with an overall mortality rate of 40–60% (Bullock et al. 2006). This poor outcome results largely from associated parenchymal lesions and subsequent intracranial hypertension. About 50% of acute subdural haematomas have associated lesions (Bullock et al. 2006).

Patients with epidural haematomas have generally a favourable prognosis, and the overall mortality rate is about 10% (Bullock et al. 2006). It is not infrequent to observe excellent outcomes even in patients with ipsilateral mydriasis. However, less than one-third of patients with an epidural haematoma present with a GCS score below 9 and in the subgroup of patients with a GCS score of 3–5 mortality rates can approach 40% (Bullock et al. 2006).

The key factors in deciding whether to proceed with surgery of an intracranial haematoma are the overall clinical condition of the patient, the neurological status (including neurological deterioration), and the CT findings. Patients with a potential surgical lesion on the initial CT scan should, as a general rule, have a follow-up CT scan within 6–8 h or sooner if clinically indicated.

There are different attitudes towards indications for surgery of posttraumatic intracranial haematomas and decompressive craniectomy both in Europe (Compagnone et al. 2005) and in the USA (Bulger et al. 2002). Some of the most difficult questions are whether moderate-sized haematomas or contusions should be evacuated or simply observed (Valadka and Robertson 2007). Several courses of action are possible, and the decisions are often based on the judgement and experience of the responsible physicians.

Recently published evidence-based guidelines for the surgical management of brain injuries by the Brain Trauma Foundation (BTF) provide us with some directions (Bullock et al. 2006). All the recommendations are at the option level, supported only by Class III scientific evidence. The guidelines are, however, logical and clinically useful, and the recommendations on surgical indications, timing of operative treatment, and choice of operative methods are presented here.

The objective of the Scandinavian Neurotrauma Committee (SNC) with these guidelines is to give the young neurosurgeon a practical and basic manual of acute surgical management of brain injuries. Details on trauma surgery per se are not extensively covered in the otherwise comprehensive surgical guidelines from the BTF (Bullock et al. 2006). Our descriptions of relevant surgical techniques are therefore based on the expert opinion of the SNC and acknowledged textbooks in neurosurgery (Greenberg 2010; Narayan et al. 1995; Schmidek and Roberts 2006; Youmans and Winn 2011).

Rigorous surgical guidelines are difficult, perhaps impossible, to define due to the diversity of the intracranial lesions, the complexity of multi-traumatised patients, and a variety of individual patient characteristics. But, when doubt exists and consciousness is depressed, the neurosurgeon should always monitor intracranial pressure (ICP) and remove significant mass lesions without undue delay.

Tips, Tricks, and Pitfalls

- Always utilise all the information provided by the CT scan in the operative planning (e.g. scout view – see Fig. 18.2, fractures, reconstructions).
- When in doubt, operate! Surgery for epidural haematoma is a low risk procedure.
- Exploratory burr holes are not recommended.
- In general, place burr holes outside fracture lines.
- Be especially aggressive in the youngest children in order to prevent secondary brain injury.
- Intracranial haematomas in neonates and infants may present with symptoms of blood loss.
- Adults and children with temporal arachnoid cysts are prone to get subdural haematomas, even after minor head traumas.
- A craniotomy for the evacuation of an epidural or subdural haematoma in small children entails a risk of significant blood loss.
- In the absence of an adequate head trauma, always look for other injuries in infants with intracranial haematomas – child abuse?

18.2 Background

18.2.1 Epidural Haematoma

18.2.1.1 Pathogenesis

Epidural haematomas (EDHs) are primarily located in the temporal and temporoparietal regions (Fig. 18.1). The bleeding is often caused by a tear in an anterior or posterior branch of the middle meningeal artery and is frequently associated with a linear cranial fracture. The fracture is thought to initiate dural stripping, and as the EDH enlarges, the dura is progressively stripped from the inner table of the skull. EDHs have a peak incidence in the second decade of life. Due to the stronger dural adherence to the skull with increasing age, EDHs are a rare entity among older patients. Injuries to the middle meningeal veins, the diploic veins, or the venous sinuses are other possible sources of bleeding, and venous origin is not as infrequent as thought for many years. Venous bleeding is reported accountable for approximately one-third of EDHs in both adult and paediatric patients (Mohanty et al. 1995). An arterial focus is more often identified as a source of bleeding among adult than paediatric patients.

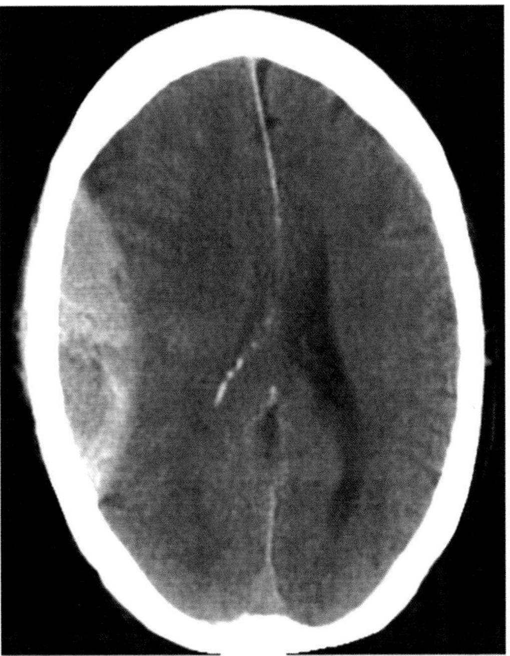

Fig. 18.1 Epidural haematoma with a typical biconvex appearance. This patient had a very rapid clinical deterioration. The *slightly darker area* in the posterior region of the haematoma is a sign of fresh bleeding

18.2.1.2 Treatment Options According to the Brain Trauma Foundation (Bullock et al. 2006)

An EDH greater than 30 cm^3 should be evacuated regardless of the Glasgow Coma Scale (GCS)

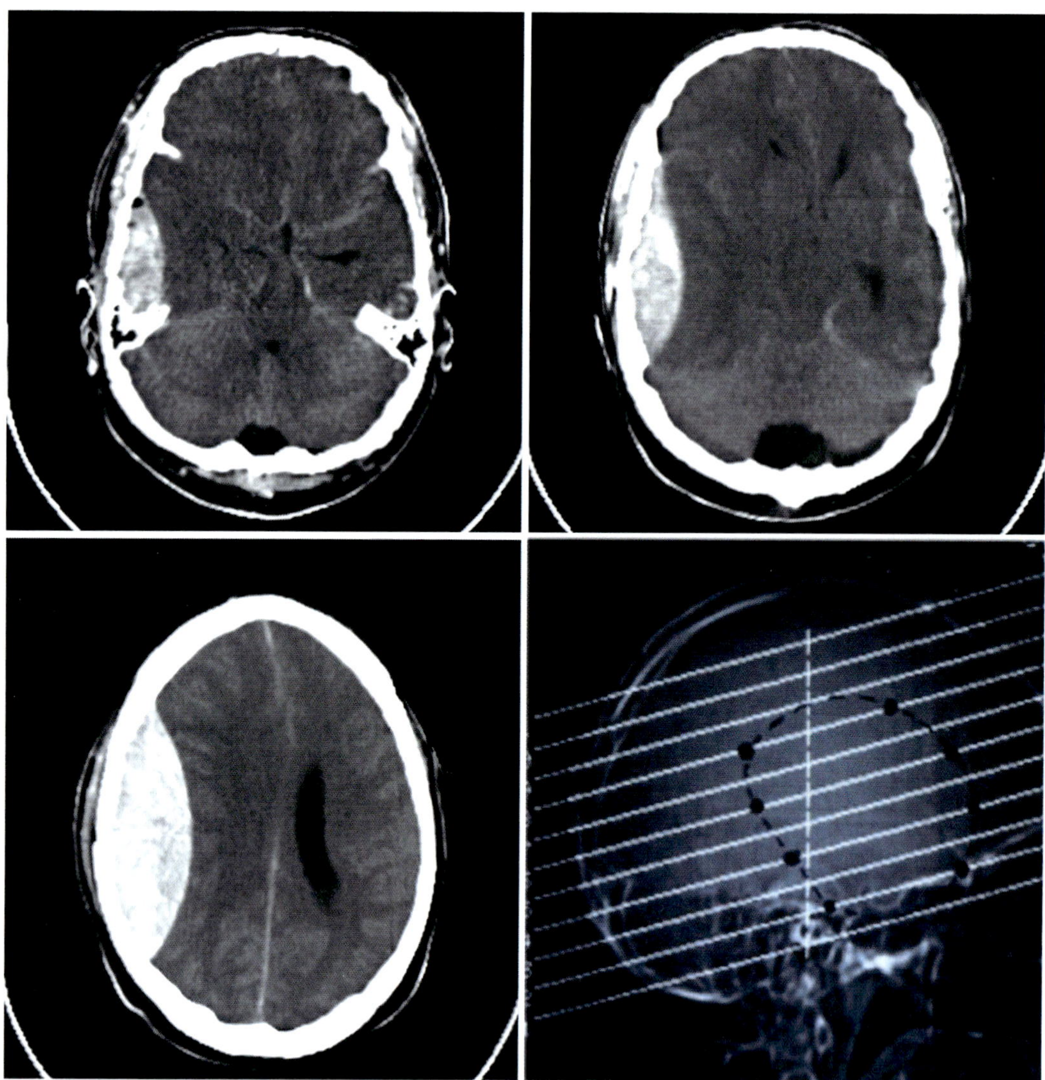

Fig. 18.2 Right-sided epidural haematoma with the equivalent extent delineated on a corresponding scout view. When planning the craniotomy, print the scout view and go through the series slice by slice, plotting the anterior and posterior margins of the haematoma

score. An EDH less than 30 cm^3, with less than 15-mm thickness, and with less than a 5-mm midline shift in patients with a GCS score greater than 8 without focal deficits can be managed conservatively with serial CT scans and close neurological observation in a neurosurgical centre.

It is strongly recommended that patients with an EDH, GCS of less than 9, and anisocoria undergo immediate surgical evacuation.

There are insufficient data to support one surgical treatment method. However, craniotomy provides a more complete evacuation of the haematoma.

18.2.1.3 Surgical Considerations

A craniotomy preferably providing complete exposure of the haematoma and the bleeding source is carried out using the preoperative CT scan as a guide (Fig. 18.2). After the information on the extent of the haematoma is visualised on the scout view, it can be readily transferred to the patient's head and the scalp incision, and craniotomy can be planned accordingly.

A standard frontotemporoparietal craniotomy as described earlier is typically appropriate. The EDH is usually clotted and removed with irrigation, suction, and cup forceps. If the neurological deterioration has been very rapid, an initial burr hole can be placed over or near the area of maximal clot thickness and consequently followed by a small craniectomy and evacuation of accessible haematoma before continuing with the standard craniotomy.

Thorough haemostasis is obtained by using bipolar electrocautery, haemostatic agents, bone wax, and tacking sutures. Bleeding from a branch of the middle meningeal artery can usually be controlled with bipolar electrocautery. EDHs arising from a tear in the main trunk of the middle meningeal artery in relation to a petrous bone fracture may necessitate packing of the foramen spinosum with haemostatic material (including bone wax). Bleeding from beyond the bony exposure may require additional bone removal but can often be controlled with dural tacking sutures. When haemostasis eventually is achieved in the epidural space, peripheral and bone flap tacking sutures are placed. An epicranial vacuum drain should be considered.

If the dura remains tense or has a bluish colour suggestive of intradural bleeding, and this was not expected from the preoperative CT scan, the subdural space should be inspected. A limited dural incision is initially made and expanded if necessary. Alternatively, intraoperative ultrasound can be used to look for underlying pathology.

18.2.2 Acute Subdural Haematoma

18.2.2.1 Pathogenesis

Acute subdural haematomas (ASDH) may arise from cortical contusions or lacerations or from torn surface or bridging veins (Fig. 18.3). With the latter, primary brain damage may be less severe. Approximately 50% of all patients have associated lesions, including contusions, haematomas, or cortical lacerations, with the majority occurring in the frontal and temporal lobes (Howard et al. 1989; Jamieson and Yelland 1972). ASDH are also frequently an important and potentially lethal complication of anticoagulant treatment (Mathiesen et al. 1995). If this is the case, there is usually a history of trauma, but the impact may have been minor. Lower mortality rates have been reported following warfarin-related intracranial haemorrhages (Mattle et al. 1989; Wintzen and Tijssen 1982). Be aware that individuals harbouring a temporal arachnoid cyst are especially prone to get a subdural haematoma, most often a chronic one, but also subacute ones after minor head traumas (Wester and Helland 2008).

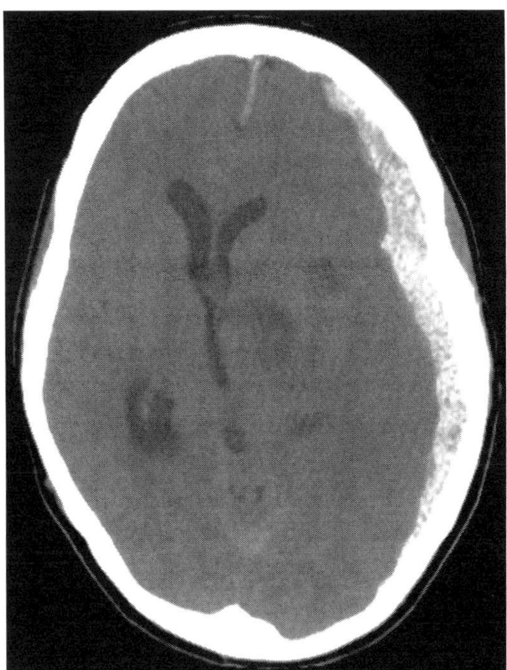

Fig. 18.3 Left-sided acute subdural haematoma with midline shift to the right. The patient herniated during transport to the hospital. Surgery required a large frontotemporoparietal craniotomy

18.2.2.2 Treatment Options According to the Brain Trauma Foundation (Bullock et al. 2006)

An ASDH with a thickness greater than 10 mm, or with a midline shift greater than 5 mm on a CT scan, should be evacuated, regardless of the GCS score. All patients with an ASDH, and a GCS score less than 9, should undergo intracranial pressure monitoring. A patient with a GCS score less than 9, with an ASDH less than 10 mm thick, and a midline shift less than 5 mm, should undergo evacuation of the lesion if the GCS score decreased between the time of injury and hospital admission by two or more points, and/or the patient presents with asymmetric or fixed dilated pupils, and/or the ICP exceeds 20 mmHg.

If surgical evacuation of an ASDH in a patient with a GCS score less than 9 is indicated, it should be performed using a craniotomy with or without bone flap removal and duraplasty.

18.2.2.3 Surgical Considerations

A large frontotemporoparietal craniotomy, as described earlier, is typically required to remove an ASDH and to address associated parenchymal lesions. Adequate exposure of the temporal and frontal poles and the area along the superior sagittal sinus is essential.

The blood clot is removed with irrigation, suction, and cup forceps. Care must be taken not to provoke any additional bleeding (especially towards the midline). The subdural space is widely inspected for additional haematoma, bleeding, and surface contusions. Expansion of the craniotomy margins is sometimes needed. Small amounts of clot that are not properly visualised and require undue brain retraction should be left undisturbed. Cortical bleeding points and avulsed bridging veins are coagulated with bipolar electrocautery, and haemostatic agents are used to control more diffuse cortical bleeding. Bleeding from the sinus wall should not be cauterised, as this only will enlarge the opening, and haemostatic agents combined with cottonoids should instead be used. A muscle patch may be needed if other measures prove inadequate.

Management of coexistent cortical contusions and intracerebral haematomas is described in Chap. 19.

Dural closure is considered when the haematoma is evacuated and haemostasis is obtained. If the dura can be closed easily and future brain swelling is deemed unlikely, the dura is sutured watertight following placement of multiple dural tacking sutures, and the bone flap is replaced. However, a duraplasty is often required, and replacement of the bone flap should then be avoided.

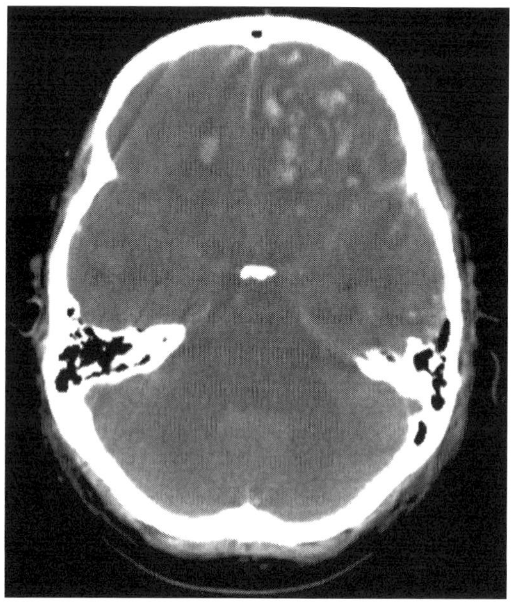

Fig. 18.4 Extensive cerebral contusions especially in the left frontal lobe. The patient also had a small acute subdural haematoma (not visualised on this image) and was operated with evacuation of the subdural haematoma followed by a duraplasty and craniectomy

18.2.3 Intracerebral Haematomas and Cerebral Contusions

18.2.3.1 Pathogenesis

Traumatic intracerebral haematomas (ICH) and cerebral contusions are often associated with epidural or subdural haematomas (Fig. 18.4). They occur most frequently in the frontal and temporal lobes, due to the brain impact against the skull. The areas most prone to haemorrhagic contusions are the inferior orbital aspects of the gyrus rectus and inferior frontal gyrus in the frontal lobes and the tips of the temporal lobes. Parietal and occipital lesions are less common and usually directly associated with the impact.

Subacute surgery may be required if ICH or contusions diagnosed by the initial CT scan evolve with perifocal oedema and/or enlargement of bleeding. The same applies for delayed traumatic intracerebral haematomas (DTICH). DTICH arise in areas of the brain that are described as normal in patients with otherwise abnormal initial CT scans (Gentleman et al. 1989). Please refer to the section on subacute surgery in Chap. 8.

Almost all patients with severe head injury and about 25% of those with moderate head injuries demonstrate surface contusions and small ICH on CT scans. However, only about 25% of trauma craniotomies are performed primarily for space-occupying contusions or ICH (Youmans and Winn 2011).

18.2.3.2 Treatment Options According to the Brain Trauma Foundation (Bullock et al. 2006)

Patients with parenchymal mass lesions and signs of progressive neurological deterioration referable to the lesion, medically refractory intracranial hypertension, or signs of mass effect on CT scan should be treated operatively. Patients with GCS scores of 6–8 with frontal or temporal contusions greater than 20 cm^3 in volume with a midline shift of at least 5 mm and/or cisternal compression on CT scan and patients with any lesion greater than 50 cm^3 in volume should be treated operatively. Patients with parenchymal mass lesions who do not show evidence of neurological compromise, who have controlled ICP and no significant signs of mass effect on CT scan, may be managed non-operatively with intensive monitoring and serial imaging.

Craniotomy with evacuation of mass lesions is recommended for those patients who have focal lesions and the surgical indications listed above.

18.2.3.3 Surgical Considerations

A standard trauma craniotomy is usually indicated because traumatic ICH and cerebral contusions are frequently associated with extra-axial haematomas. Special surgical considerations as specified for epidural or acute subdural haematomas should therefore be remembered.

Sizeable areas (>1–2 cm) of cerebral contusions with irreparably damaged brain, appearing purplish and mottled, can be removed. Ultrasound can be helpful in localising ICH at considerable depth from the cortex. The pia and bleeding superficial vessels are cauterized over the most traumatised area or in an otherwise non-eloquent area. A pial incision is made, and a subpial plane is established. Blood clots and adjacent contused brain are removed with gentle aspiration and bipolar electrocautery. A more limited resection of parenchymal lesions is prudent in eloquent areas, such as along the dominant superior temporal gyrus and the central sulcus. Avoid sacrifying non-bleeding arteries that traverse a traumatised area and that supplies healthy cortex.

Haemostasis after removal of ICH or cerebral contusions can be achieved with bipolar electrocautery, gentle tamponade with cottonoids soaked in saline, and lining the cavity with haemostatic agents. This is followed by routine closure.

A minimalistic approach through a small burr hole should only be considered in patients with an isolated traumatic ICH and no other associated lesions.

18.2.4 Posterior Fossa Mass Lesions

18.2.4.1 Pathogenesis

Traumatic lesions in the posterior fossa are rare and occur in less than 3% of all head injuries (Karasawa et al. 1997). The vast majority of published series deal with epidural haematomas. Subdural and intraparenchymal lesions are less frequent, but the more dangerous, as patients with mass lesions in the posterior fossa can undergo rapid clinical deterioration because of the limited space available and close relationship to vital centres in the brainstem. Timely recognition and surgical evacuation are therefore especially warranted. It is especially important to monitor the respiration if the patient is not already on a ventilator, as impaired lung ventilation will cause hypercapnia and vasodilatation and subsequently a rapidly developing vicious circle due to increased pressure on respiration regulating areas in the brainstem. The neurosurgeon must also be aware of any complicating hydrocephalus and be prepared to put in an external drainage.

18.2.4.2 Treatment Options According to the Brain Trauma Foundation (Bullock et al. 2006)

Patients with mass effect on the CT scan, or with neurological dysfunction, or deterioration referable to the lesion, should undergo operative intervention. Mass effect on the CT scan is defined as distortion, dislocation, or obliteration of the fourth ventricle; compression or loss of visualisation of the basal cisterns; or the presence of obstructive hydrocephalus. Close observation and serial imaging can be considered in patients with no significant mass effect on the CT scan and without signs of neurological dysfunction.

In patients with indications for surgical intervention, evacuation should be performed as soon as possible because patients can deteriorate rapidly, thus, worsening their prognosis.

Suboccipital craniectomy is the predominant method reported for evacuation of posterior fossa mass lesions and is therefore recommended.

18.2.4.3 Surgical Considerations

The patient is usually placed in the Concorde position, and a midline suboccipital craniectomy is performed. Access to the midline and both cerebellar hemispheres is ensured. The traumatic mass lesion is evacuated and haemostasis is obtained. Standard supratentorial ventricular drainage should be considered if there is a risk of the patient developing hydrocephalus, as an initial or closing manoeuvre.

Traumatic lesions in the posterior fossa are so infrequent that a detailed surgical description is not warranted in these basic guidelines on trauma surgery. The reader is referred to neurosurgical textbooks on operative procedures for further information.

18.3 Specific Paediatric Concerns

Most of the foundation for the medical and surgical treatment of children with severe head injuries is based on adult studies. This is a result of the lack of scientific data primarily dealing with children. Children involved in traffic accidents are just as likely to die from severe TBIs as adults (Johnson and Krishnamurthy 1998). Children do generally have a better overall outcome than adults, but younger children fare worse than older children, both with respect to mortality and long-term disability (Adelson 2000; Anderson et al. 2005). Moreover, the long-term deficits are often persistent and severe, even with aggressive management. It is therefore prudent to be very aggressive in preventing secondary brain injuries in children.

Young children have a more compressible brain and flexible skull than older children and adults. Because of this, there are fewer intracranial mass lesions and more white matter shear injuries in young children (Hahn et al. 1988; Zimmerman and Bilaniuk 1994). As the child gets older, the incidence of subdural and intracerebral haematomas becomes more similar to that of the adult (Luerssen et al. 1988; Zimmerman and Bilaniuk 1994). Epidural haematomas are more frequent among older children and adolescents than among neonates and infants. This is due to the relatively stronger attachment between the dura and the cranium but also because of a smaller risk of bony injury to the middle meningeal artery. A lower threshold for surgical treatment of epidural haematomas should be practised in children than in adults; only neurologically intact patients with a GCS score of 15 with or without headache should be considered candidates for observation.

In the absence of an adequate head trauma, always look for other injuries in infants with intracranial haematomas – "battered child syndrome"? Keep at the same time in mind that young children or even infants harbouring a temporal arachnoid cyst are especially prone to get subdural haematomas even after minor head traumas (Wester and Helland 2008). These haematomas may be of different ages and thus raise unjustified suspicion of child abuse.

References

Adelson PD (2000) Pediatric trauma made simple. Clin Neurosurg 47:319–335

Anderson V, Catroppa C, Morse S, Haritou F, Rosenfeld J (2005) Functional plasticity or vulnerability after early brain injury? Pediatrics 116:1374–1382

Bulger EM, Nathens AB, Rivara FP, Moore M, MacKenzie EJ, Jurkovich GJ, Foundation BT (2002) Management of severe head injury: institutional variations in care and effect on outcome. Crit Care Med 30:1870–1876

Bullock MR, Chesnut R, Ghajar J, Gordon D, Hartl R, Newell DW, Servadei F, Walters BC, Wilberger JE, Surgical Management of Traumatic Brain Injury Author Group (2006) Surgical management of traumatic brain injury. Neurosurgery 58:S2–1–S2–62

Compagnone C, Murray GD, Teasdale GM, Maas AI, Esposito D, Princi P, D'Avella D, Servadei F (2005) The management of patients with intradural post-traumatic mass lesions: a multicenter survey of current approaches to surgical management in 729 patients coordinated by the European Brain Injury Consortium. Neurosurgery 57:1183–1192

Gentleman D, Nath F, Macpherson P (1989) Diagnosis and management of delayed traumatic intracerebral haematomas. Br J Neurosurg 3:367–372

Greenberg MS (2010) Handbook of neurosurgery. Greenberg Graphics/Thieme Medical Publishers, Tampa/New York

Hahn YS, Chyung C, Barthel MJ, Bailes J, Flannery AM, McLone DG (1988) Head injuries in children under 36 months of age. Demography and outcome. Childs Nerv Syst 4:34–40

Howard MA, Gross AS, Dacey RG, Winn HR (1989) Acute subdural hematomas: an age-dependent clinical entity. J Neurosurg 71:858–863

Jamieson KG, Yelland JD (1972) Surgically treated traumatic subdural hematomas. J Neurosurg 37:137–149

Johnson DL, Krishnamurthy S (1998) Severe pediatric head injury: myth, magic, and actual fact. Pediatr Neurosurg 28:167–172

Karasawa H, Furuya H, Naito H, Sugiyama K, Ueno J, Kin H (1997) Acute hydrocephalus in posterior fossa injury. J Neurosurg 86:629–632

Luerssen TG, Klauber MR, Marshall LF (1988) Outcome from head injury related to patient's age. A longitudinal prospective study of adult and pediatric head injury. J Neurosurg 68:409–416

Mathiesen T, Benediktsdottir K, Johnsson H, Lindqvist M, von Holst H (1995) Intracranial traumatic and non-traumatic haemorrhagic complications of warfarin treatment. Acta Neurol Scand 91:208–214

Mattle H, Kohler S, Huber P, Rohner M, Steinsiepe KF (1989) Anticoagulation-related intracranial extracerebral haemorrhage. J Neurol Neurosurg Psychiatry 52:829–837

Mohanty A, Kolluri VR, Subbakrishna DK, Satish S, Mouli BA, Das BS (1995) Prognosis of extradural haematomas in children. Pediatr Neurosurg 23:57–63

Narayan RK, Wilberger JE, Povlishock JT (1995) Neurotrauma. McGraw Hill, New York

Schmidek HH, Roberts DW (2006) Schmidek & Sweet operative neurosurgical techniques: indications, methods, and results. Saunders/Elsevier, Philadelphia

Valadka AB, Robertson CS (2007) Surgery of cerebral trauma and associated critical care. Neurosurgery 61:203–220

Wester K, Helland CA (2008) How often do chronic extra-cerebral haematomas occur in patients with intracranial arachnoid cysts? J Neurol Neurosurg Psychiatry 79:72–75

Wintzen AR, Tijssen JG (1982) Subdural hematoma and oral anticoagulant therapy. Arch Neurol 39:69–72

Youmans JR, Winn HR (2011) Youmans neurological surgery. Saunders/Elsevier, Philadelphia

Zimmerman RA, Bilaniuk LT (1994) Pediatric head trauma. Neuroimaging Clin N Am 4:349–366

19 Surgical Management of Penetrating Brain Injuries

Terje Sundstrøm and Knut Wester

Recommendations

Level I

There are insufficient data to support a Level I recommendation for this topic.

Level II

There are insufficient data to support a Level II recommendation for this topic.

Level III

Patients with penetrating brain injuries that are otherwise stabilized and demonstrate neurological function or deterioration referable to a mass lesion should be considered for surgery.

19.1 Overview

Penetrating brain injuries (PBIs) have high fatality rates, but those who survive the initial phase can however demonstrate favourable outcomes. The primary injuries can entail a combination of scalp lesions, cranial fractures, intracranial haematomas, and cerebral lacerations. High energy PBIs frequently encompass distant lesions and are often followed by a detrimental increase in intracranial pressure (ICP).

There is no defined threshold for whom surgery should be withheld, but the patient must have a possibility of a reasonable functional outcome. Patients with devastating brain injuries and/or high probability of a poor outcome should generally not be subjected to surgical treatment.

Tips, Tricks, and Pitfalls

- Carefully consider ICP monitoring and/or EVD.
- Always carefully plan the way in and out (vascularity, exposure, wound closure).
- If you plan a skin flap, you have to take the wound into consideration: is it most suitable to incorporate the wound in the skin incision or is it better to place the incision around it, with a broad base to ensure a sufficient blood supply to the entire flap.

T. Sundstrøm (✉)
Department of Neurosurgery,
Haukeland University Hospital,
Jonas Lies Vei 65, 5021 Bergen, Norway

Department of Surgical Sciences and
Department of Biomedicine, University of Bergen,
Jonas Lies Vei 91, 5020 Bergen, Norway
e-mail: terje.sundstrom@gmail.com

K. Wester
Department of Surgical Sciences,
University of Bergen,
Jonas Lies Vei 65, 5021 Bergen, Norway

Department of Neurosurgery,
Haukeland University Hospital,
Jonas Lies Vei 65, 5021 Bergen, Norway
e-mail: knut.gustav.wester@helse-bergen.no

T. Sundstrøm et al. (eds.), *Management of Severe Traumatic Brain Injury*,
DOI 10.1007/978-3-642-28126-6_19, © Springer-Verlag Berlin Heidelberg 2012

- Perform a thorough debridement of all tissue layers.
- If possible, do not add foreign material.

19.2 Background

19.2.1 Pathogenesis

The majority of penetrating brain injuries in the civilian setting are caused by low-velocity gunshot wounds to the head (GSWH) (Potapov et al. 2001). These injuries have a high fatality rate, and mortality rates are often higher in self-inflicted injuries than in assaults. Siccardi and colleagues reported that 73% of patients with a GSWH died before reaching hospital and another 12% died within 3 h of injury (Siccardi et al. 1991). However, survivors do often experience a favourable outcome, with 74% having a good recovery or moderate disability (Levi et al. 1991).

Shrapnel, and not GSWH, is the major cause of PBIs in military conflicts. The prehospital management and modern resources in military hospitals are also very effective. The overall mortality rate is therefore lower; it is generally reported to be around 20% (Potapov et al. 2001).

A combination of soft tissue injuries, fractures, and parenchymal lesions may constitute the primary injuries from GSWH. The impact velocity of a projectile reflects the true wounding potential, and deformation and fragmentation of the missile enhance energy delivery to the tissue. Comminute fractures may injure the directly underlying structures, and bone fragments may be driven into the brain as secondary projectiles. Brain injuries can occur along the path of the projectile(s), as well as in more distant locations due to pressure waves and coup/contrecoup lesions. A rapid rise in ICP may follow a GSWH.

19.2.2 Treatment Options

No surgical intervention is generally warranted for patients with a post-resuscitation GCS score of 3, dilated and nonreactive pupils, and no significant mass lesion on the CT scan. Patients that are otherwise stabilized, and demonstrating some neurological function (motor or brain stem), or deterioration referable to a mass lesion, should be considered for urgent surgical treatment.

Small entrance bullet wounds to the head can be treated with local wound care and closure if the scalp is not devitalized and there are no surgical intracranial lesions. Treatment of more extensive wounds requires extensive debridement before primary closure to secure a watertight wound. In the presence of significant mass effect, debridement of necrotic brain tissue and safely accessible bone fragments, together with evacuation of intracranial hematomas with significant mass effect, is recommended. A minimal invasive approach is prudent in the absence of significant mass effect (Potapov et al. 2001).

If possible, any protruding part of a foreign body should not be removed before the patient is in the operating room.

Infection is an important secondary complication, and liberal use of antibiotics is recommended.

The neurosurgeon must carefully consider the need for intracranial pressure measurement and/or external ventricular drainage, in addition to the primary surgical treatment.

19.2.3 Surgical Considerations

The cranium is examined for external injuries. Thorough irrigation of the wound site(s) is performed. Consultation with a plastic surgeon may be warranted in selected cases. The skin incision must be carefully planned in order to, first, ensure vascularity and enable wound closure following excision of devitalized tissue and, second, to secure sufficient exposure of the bony defect and underlying haematomas. The cranial opening should extend well beyond the visible bone injury until intact dura is visualized.

Herniated brain tissue and the intracerebral penetration tract are flushed through the dural lesion, and accessible necrotic tissue, bone fragments, and foreign bodies are gently removed.

The dural opening may need to be enlarged to accommodate adequate debridement and haematoma evacuation. A thorough exploration must be performed, but preservation of viable brain tissue supersedes removal of deeply located fragments (Potapov et al. 2001). Haemostasis is preferably ensured by bipolar electrocautery and dural repair by autologous grafts (e.g. temporalis fascia or pericranium).

Bone replacement should be performed in case of no present or anticipated future significant brain swelling. High-velocity injuries are often associated with substantial oedema development, and it may be wise not to replace the bone in these cases. Before replacement of the bone flap or fragments, ample debridement and cleaning must be secured. Foreign materials must be utilized at a minimum, but miniplates, titanium wires, and craniofix devices are often needed to assemble multiple bony fragments. The importance of meticulous scalp closure is previously stated.

19.3 Specific Paediatric Concerns

There are no specific paediatric concerns. Please refer to Chaps. 17 and 18 for supplementary information.

References

Levi L, Linn S, Feinsod M (1991) Penetrating craniocerebral injuries in civilians. Br J Neurosurg 5:241–247

Potapov AA, Shahinian GG, Kravtchouk AD (2001) Surgical management of Penetrating brain injury. J Trauma 51:16–25

Siccardi D, Cavaliere R, Pau A, Lubinu F, Turtas S, Viale GL (1991) Penetrating craniocerebral missile injuries in civilians: a retrospective analysis of 314 cases. Surg Neurol 35:455–460

Decompressive Craniectomy

20

Pål André Rønning

Recommendations

Level I

There are insufficient data to support a Level I recommendation for this topic.

Level II

There are insufficient data to support a Level II recommendation for this topic.

Level III

Decompressive craniectomy is a surgical option in patients with refractory ICP not responding to first tier therapy.

20.1 Overview

According to the Monroe-Kelly doctrine the intracranial volume is constant and dictated by the confines of the scull. This volume contains under normal circumstances brain tissue, CSF and intracranial blood:

$$V_{IC} = V_{Br} + V_{Bl} + V_{CSF}$$

P.A. Rønning
Department of Neurosurgery, Oslo University Hospital, 4950 Nydalen, 0424 Oslo, Norway
e-mail: palronning@gmail.com

After a person sustains a head injury, this equation might be disturbed by increased volumes on the right-hand side of the equation due to oedema, hydrocephalus, mass lesions and/or hyperaemia. Due to the rigidness of the skull after closing of the sutures, this volume increase causes increased pressure after the compensatory mechanisms of reduced CSF and intracranial venous blood have been exhausted. When the standard measures for decreasing ICP have failed, an alternative is to increase the intracranial volume (V_{IC}) by removing a part of the scull (Hutchinson and Kirkpatrick 2004; Kakar et al. 2009).

Tips, Tricks, and Pitfalls

- There is conflicting scientific evidence as to when decompressive craniectomies might be helpful.
- The bone cuts are carried flush to the floor of the middle fossa.
- The dura should be opened.
- The bone must either be frozen or stored autologously.

20.2 Background

20.2.1 History

First advocated as a procedure to alleviate symptoms of increased ICP due to inoperable tumours in the beginning of the twentieth century by

T. Sundstrøm et al. (eds.), *Management of Severe Traumatic Brain Injury*,
DOI 10.1007/978-3-642-28126-6_20, © Springer-Verlag Berlin Heidelberg 2012

Kocher and Cushing, its use in head injuries was not documented until the 1960s. Its use in TBI has since been controversial but has seen a major revival in the last decade.

20.2.2 Indications

Results from the *DECRA* study were recently published, apparently demonstrating that patients with intractable intracranial hypertension and bi-frontotemporoparietal craniectomies have increased risk of poor outcome compared with patients who received conservative treatment (Cooper et al. 2011). However, the definition of intractable hypertension used in the study (>20 mmHg >15 min with first tier therapy), the number of crossovers from the conservative to the treatment arm (19/82 = 23%) and the fact that surgical lesions were excluded make us question the applicability of the conclusion in a normal clinical scenario. Thus, we still believe that decompressive craniectomy is a viable option in patients with intractable intracranial hypertension failing first tier therapy. In a recent Cochrane review, they find class I evidence to support the use of DC in children (Sahuquillo and Arikan 2006).

20.2.3 Operative Technique

The goal of surgery is to provide the brain with room for expansion; hence, a large craniectomy is preferred (Jiang et al. 2005). Usually, we divide the decompressive craniectomies into hemicraniectomies or bi-frontal craniectomies. The indications are unilateral or bi-frontal expansion, respectively.
Incision: A posterior bicoronal incision provides sufficient room for a bi-frontal craniectomy. A trauma flap can give decent exposure for a hemicraniectomy; however, the skin flap will depend on the frontal and parietal branches of the superficial temporal artery. By utilizing a T-incision, the skin flap might be better vascularised due to uninterrupted supply to the skin flap also from the occipital artery.
Craniectomy: It is imperative to decompress the middle fossa; hence, a hemicraniectomy should be flush with the floor of the middle fossa. In the bi-frontal craniectomy, there are two different methods: one leaving a small rim of bone above the superior sagittal sinus and the other removing this bone as well. In the latter approach, we advocate the use of two longitudinal burr holes across the sinus and thorough release of the sinus from the inside of the scull before turning the bone flap. Any bleeding from the sinus can usually be easily controlled by elevated head, pressure and haemostatic material. In case this is insufficient, rather large tears in the sinus can usually be controlled by the use of Tachoseal. There is a theoretical risk that the bi-frontal craniectomy (including the bone overlying sinus) might impede venous drainage secondary to the intracranial pressure pushing the sinus up against the posterior craniectomy edge. However, to our knowledge, there are no reports on this. On the contrary, we advocate that the medial border of the hemicraniectomies is placed 2 cm lateral to the sagittal suture since we have seen several patients with distended, raised bridging veins pressing against the lateral side of the remaining skull.
Duraplasty: The most important region to decompress is the temporal area. Theoretically, an inverse T-shaped incision centred on the temporal lobe is preferable to other incisions centred more superiorly due to the increased decompression of the temporal region. As to the duraplasty, some people leave the dura open, others use a synthetic suturable dura patch and others use a lay-on dura patch. It is claimed that the lay-on collagen dura substitutes produce less tissue reaction and easier dissection of the dura-galea interface when the time has come to reattach the bone flap (Horaczek et al. 2008; Biroli et al. 2008).
Closure: Due to the large surface area of the skin flap, an epidural drain is recommended. Suturing the temporal fascia should not be done due to the restrictive effect this can have on the brain expansion. Instead, the skin is closed by subcutaneous sutures and staples.
Complications: An early postoperative CT should be performed to assess blossoming of contusions and contralateral injuries that often increase postoperatively due to the tamponading coagulatory effect of preoperatively intracranial hypertension.

Furthermore, the CSF circulation is often influenced resulting in hygromas and ventriculomegaly. However, these abnormalities should be left untreated if at all possible since the reinsertion of the bone flap usually rectifies the problem (Stiver 2009).

Bone Storage: The bone flap can be frozen or it can be stored autologously. In the case of freezing, the bone flap is immediately dried off, marked and deep-frozen (at least −70°C). Otherwise, the bone can be implanted in the subcutaneous tissue of the abdomen. This has several advantages: reduced loss of osteoinductive proteins and logistical advantages (Kakar et al. 2009).

Reimplantation of the Bone Flap: There is a clear tendency for earlier reinsertion of the bone flap. As soon as the skin has healed and the brain is sufficiently slack to accommodate the bone flap, it should be reinserted (Kakar et al. 2009). This practice probably also reduces the incidence of motor-trephine syndrome and need for VP shunting (Stiver 2009).

20.3 Specific Paediatric Concerns

There are no specific paediatric concerns. However, meticulous perioperative haemostatis must be maintained due to the reduced blood volume in paediatric patients.

References

Biroli F, Fusco M, Bani GG, Signorelli A, Esposito F, de Divitiis O, Cappabianca P, Cavallo LM (2008) Novel equine collagen-only dural substitute. Neurosurgery 62:273–274

Cooper DJ, Rosenfeld JV, Murray L, Arabi YM, Davies AR, D'Urso P, Kossmann T, Ponsford J, Seppelt I, Reilly P, Wolfe R (2011) Decompressive craniectomy in diffuse traumatic brain injury. N Engl J Med. doi:10.1056/NEJMoa1102077

Horaczek JA, Zierski J, Graewe A (2008) Collagen matrix in decompressive hemicraniectomy. Neurosurgery 63:ONS176–ONS181

Hutchinson PJ, Kirkpatrick PJ (2004) Decompressive craniectomy in head injury. Curr Opin Crit Care 10: 101–104

Jiang JY, Xu W, Li WP, Xu WH, Zhang J, Bao YH, Ying YH, Luo QZ (2005) Efficacy of standard trauma craniectomy for refractory intracranial hypertension with severe traumatic brain injury: a multicenter, prospective, randomized controlled study. J Neurotrauma 22:623–628

Kakar V, Nagaria J, John KP (2009) The current status of decompressive craniectomy. Br J Neurosurg 23: 147–157

Sahuquillo J, Arikan F (2006) Decompressive craniectomy for the treatment of refractory high intracranial pressure in traumatic brain injury. Cochrane Database Syst Rev (1):CD003983

Stiver SI (2009) Complications of decompressive craniectomy for traumatic brain injury. Neurosurg Focus 26:E7. doi:10.3171/2009.4.FOCUS0965

Skull Fractures

21

Pål André Rønning

Recommendations

Level I

There are insufficient data to support a Level I recommendation for this topic.

Level II

There are insufficient data to support a Level II recommendation for this topic.

Level III

Open fractures, vault fractures depressed more than one bone width, and cosmetically disfiguring fractures should always be operated.

21.1 Overview

Fractures of the skull can be divided into fractures of the vault or the base of the skull. Such fractures are quite common and are important to acknowledge because in 70% they herald intracranial pathology; open fractures or fractures through the sinuses predispose to intracranial infections, and they can be cosmetically disfiguring.

P.A. Rønning
Department of Neurosurgery, Oslo University Hospital, 4950 Nydalen, 0424 Oslo, Norway
e-mail: palronning@gmail.com

Tips, Tricks, and Pitfalls

- Make a skin incision that offers good exposure of the fracture.
- The dura should be checked for lacerations, and a water tight dura seal should be accomplished in case of CSF leakage.
- Tack-up sutures should be placed surrounding the fracture site to prevent postoperative epidural haematomas.

21.2 Background

21.2.1 Vault Fractures

Vault fractures are common. They can be further divided into open or closed and depressed or non-depressed fractures. Fractures of the vault have a tendency to cause epidural haemorrhage. These epidural haematomas can be arterial or venous in nature. Usually, the arterial haematomas are caused by a bony spicula from the fracture tearing the middle meningeal artery. The venous haematomas are usually secondary to oozing from the fracture edges and have a tendency to expand slower than the arterial haematomas.

T. Sundstrøm et al. (eds.), *Management of Severe Traumatic Brain Injury*,
DOI 10.1007/978-3-642-28126-6_21, © Springer-Verlag Berlin Heidelberg 2012

The indications for surgery of vault fractures are based on the following (Bullock et al. 2006):

1. *Infection*: open fractures expose dura and/or the brain to microorganisms.
2. *Cosmetics*: fractures depressed more than one bone width have a tendency for disfiguration.
3. *Function*: depressed fractures (or haematomas secondary to the fracture) may cause neurological symptoms.

21.2.1.1 Operative Technique

Plan the incision to fully expose the fractured area. After exposure, access to the dura is essential; this can be obtained by lifting up a bone fragment with a periosteal elevator. If the fragments are wedged, a burr hole is placed clearly outside the fractured area and a craniotomy surrounding the fracture complex is performed. The fragments are carefully collected and saved. Any epidural haematoma is evacuated, and we also advise to create a small slit in the dura to check for any subdural haematoma that might have accumulated after the CT. Next, the dura is sewn watertight before tack-up sutures are placed between the dura and the bone edges. The fracture fragments are reassembled into a large bone flap by using plates and multiple microscrews or similar devices. The assembled bone flap is then reattached in a normal fashion.

In case of an open fracture, the skin edge needs thorough debridement before closure, and we advise for proper antibiotic prophylaxis.

In the case of comminute fractures where it is impossible to reassemble the bone, there are several options: make a split bone graft utilizing the contralateral skull with a similar curvature or use a material for bone replacement, e.g. hydroxyapatite, custom-made bone implants, etc. (Kakar et al. 2009).

21.2.2 Skull Base Fractures

Fractures through the base of the skull are divided into fractures through the anterior, middle, and posterior fossa. The latter entity will not be further discussed. The important factors to consider when dealing with skull base fractures are:

- *CSF leakage*: This can manifest as rhinorrhoea and/or otorrhoea. The fluid leak is a result of dural and arachnoid lacerations with fistula formation.
- *Infection*: CSF leaks represent a corridor for bacteria to gain access to the CSF space.
- *Vessel and nerve injury*: Vessels and nerves have an intimate relationship with the skull base; hence, fractures through the base of the skull can manifest with cranial nerve deficits (I, II, VI, VII, and VIII most often) and vessel injury.

The diagnosis of CSF leakage can be made by abundant clear discharge from the nose or ear in the presence of a known skull base fracture with pneumocephalus. When the leakage is less severe, the diagnosis can be much more difficult. CSF contains 60% of serum glucose; however, nasal discharge also has glucose present; hence, discharge with a positive glucose test has a high sensitivity but a low specificity for CSF leakage. Differentiating CSF from mucosal discharge can be made by the presence of beta-2-transferrin or beta-trace protein in the discharge, but the tests are not always readily available (Davies and Teo 1995). After having verified that the leaking fluid indeed is CSF, the site of leakage must be identified. If there is pneumocephalus and obvious fracture fragments tearing the dura, the leak site can usually be identified rather easily. It can, however, often be difficult to pinpoint the exact location of the CSF leakage. Usually, CT with thin cuts can provide a good idea about the site; further diagnosis requires either MR or CT cisternography.

In most cases of CSF leakage associated with skull base fractures, the leak spontaneously ceases within the first 10–12 days. Within this time frame, the risk of developing meningitis is rather low. A recently updated Cochrane review does not support the use of prophylactic antibiotics in patients with posttraumatic CSF leakage (Ratilal et al. 2011). At our institution , we routinely use lumbar drainage and bed rest in order to (hopefully) accelerate the resolution of leakage, but we pay close attention to CT scans and monitor for sufficient cisternal space around the brain stem.

Treatment of cranial nerve deficits secondary to skull base fractures and their management have a rather poor evidence base. Some advocate the use of steroids, whilst others advocate decompression of the affected nerve (Samii and Tatagiba 2002). The complexity of the anatomy also play an important role, and decompressive temporal bone facial nerve surgery is seldomly indicated, whilst decompression of the optic nerve has better documentation and is easier to perform.

In the acute setting, indications for surgery are:

1. CSF leaks and fractures where the prospect of resolution is deemed very unlikely.
2. CSF leaks that do not resolve within 10 days
3. Cranial nerve deficits in progression.

In the chronic setting, recurrent meningitis is also an indication for surgery.

21.2.2.1 Surgery

The basic goal is to achieve reasonable bony continuity, decompress neural structures, and patch the dura defect. In the case of a large comminute anterior skull base fracture with CSF leakage, a bi-coronal incision is planned. The periosteum is left intact with a vascularised pedicle so that it can be used later as a dura patch. Burr holes are placed over the superior sagittal sinus, and a large bi-frontal craniotomy is made, extending to the floor of the anterior fossa. The posterior wall of the frontal sinus is removed, and mucosa from the remaining sinus is removed. Instruments used for this purpose are contaminated by nasal pathogens and should be discarded. Next, the dura is dissected free from the anterior skull base (as far posterior as the planum sphenoidale), and the bony skull base is reconstructed if necessary. Most likely, this will entail tearing both olfactory nerves at the thin lamina cribrosa. Next, the dura is opened and the sagittal sinus and falx ligated and cut at the anteriormost end. Subfrontal dissection then allows basofrontal contusions to be removed, and the intradural floor can be carpeted using a dura substitute (artificial or fascia lata). Next, the dura is closed, and the epidural skull base can be glued with the pedicled periosteum flap or another dura substitute for a sandwich reconstruction of the basofrontal dura. Finally, the bone flap is reattached and the skin closed (Scholsem et al. 2008).

Postoperatively, the patient must not be ventilated using CPAP because of the risk of pneumocephalus. He/she should be covered prophylactically for upper respiratory tract microorganisms for the ensuing 5 days.

21.3 Specific Paediatric Concerns

Particular attention should be paid to children who sustain a diastatic fracture. Rarely, these fractures have a dura tear that subsequently can provide the nidus for a growing skull fracture whereby a leptomeningeal cyst with or without brain parenchyma protrudes through the bony opening. Symptoms and signs indicative of a growing fracture include a diastatic fracture that fails to fuse, progressive neurological symptoms, and/or seizures. Especially patients under the age of three with a cephalhematoma and a diastatic fracture should be followed up closely.

References

Bullock MR, Chesnut R, Ghajar J, Gordon D, Hartl R, Newell DW, Servadei F, Walters BC, Wilberger J (2006) Surgical management of depressed cranial fractures. Neurosurgery 58:S56–S60

Davies MA, Teo C (1995) Management of traumatic cerebrospinal fluid fistula. J Craniomaxillofac Trauma 1:9–17

Kakar V, Nagaria J, John KP (2009) The current status of decompressive craniectomy. Br J Neurosurg 23: 147–157

Ratilal BO, Costa J, Sampaio C, Pappamikail L (2011) Antibiotic prophylaxis for preventing meningitis in patients with basilar skull fractures. Cochrane Database Syst Rev CD004884. doi:10.1002/14651858.CD004884.pub3

Samii M, Tatagiba M (2002) Skull base trauma: diagnosis and management. Neurol Res 24:147–156

Scholsem M, Scholtes F, Collignon F, Robe P, Dubuisson A, Kaschten B, Lenelle J, Martin D (2008) Surgical management of anterior cranial base fractures with cerebrospinal fluid fistulae: a single-institution experience. Neurosurgery 62:463–469

22 Vessel Injuries

Pål André Rønning

Recommendations

Level I

There are insufficient data to support a level I recommendation for this topic.

Level II

There are insufficient data to support a level II recommendation for this topic.

Level III

The radiological investigation of choice is CT angiography. The goal of therapy is to prevent further neurological injury by sustaining sufficient cerebral blood flow and preventing embolic incidents.

22.1 Overview

Vessel injuries are uncommon but potentially devastating to the patient. Both blunt and penetrating trauma to the head can result in vessel injury. We will here divide vessel injuries into extracranial and intracranial vessel injuries. They are both difficult to diagnose without special contrast-enhanced radiological investigations, and a high index of suspicion must be entertained (Vertinsky et al. 2008). The vessel pathology itself can be divided into:

Dissection – a tear in the intima leaves a highly thrombogenic intima flap in the lumen of the vessel while at the same time a haematoma can develop in the vessel wall. Hence, the local blood flow can be impeded by both thrombosis and mural hematoma. Distal blood flow can be influenced due to embolic phenomena from the local thrombosis.

True aneurysms – focal outpouching from an injured vessel where at least one layer of the vessel wall is intact.

Pseudoaneurysms – focal outpouching from an injured vessel where all vessel wall layers are compromised, leaving just an organized haematoma as the barrier for further bleeding.

Both true and pseudoaneurysms have turbulent blood flow and can serve as a nidus for thrombosis and subsequent embolisation.

Tips, Tricks, and Pitfalls

- Maintain a high index of suspicion for vessel injury when there is:
  - Discrepancy between plain CT findings and the clinical state of the patient
  - Subarachnoid haemorrhage in the interhemispheric fissure
  - Fractures in close proximity to vessels

P.A. Rønning
Department of Neurosurgery, Oslo University Hospital, 4950 Nydalen, 0424 Oslo, Norway
e-mail: palronning@gmail.com

T. Sundstrøm et al. (eds.), *Management of Severe Traumatic Brain Injury*,
DOI 10.1007/978-3-642-28126-6_22, © Springer-Verlag Berlin Heidelberg 2012

22.2 Background

22.2.1 Extracranial Vessel Injury

The incidence of carotid or vertebral injury is 0.5–1% (Nedeltchev and Baumgartner 2005; Stein et al. 2009). These lesions carry high mortality rates (20–40%). In the face of blunt trauma, the usual mechanism is dissection. The interval from the injury itself to the formation of a thrombus of sufficient size to jeopardize flow is difficult to pinpoint but from 1 to 48 h has been documented. The dissection itself may also expand. In the meanwhile, the patient may be completely asymptomatic. Penetrating injuries more often transect the vessel or parts of the vessel and thereby expose the patient to compromised blood flow and significant blood loss. Explosions and ballistic injuries can cause dissections due to the shock wave resulting in an intima tear.

As already mentioned, these patients may be asymptomatic without any signs of overt trauma to the neck before they manifest with TIA, brain infarctions, or seizures. Physical findings that should entail further radiological investigations are Horner's syndrome, carotid bruits, or mandibular fractures. Also, comminute C1–C3 fractures, displacement, and affection of the intervertebral foramina are associated with vertebral injuries.

The radiological investigation of choice is CT angiography (Vertinsky et al. 2008). It is readily available, is fast, and easily performed in a trauma setting. Usually, this is sufficient to exclude extracranial vessel injury, but MRI can provide further confirmation and also information on possible infarction.

The goal of therapy is to prevent further neurological injury by sustaining sufficient cerebral blood flow and preventing embolic incidents. Therapeutic options are anticoagulation/platelet inhibition, surgical ligation, surgical resection and repair, bypass, and endovascular balloon occlusion or stent therapy. Both heparin/Low-molecular-weight heparin and/or platelet inhibitors are options for preventing further thrombosis and embolic events. There is insufficient documentation to recommend one over the other (Fusco and Harrigan 2011). A reasonable algorithm is to start with medical therapy in case of no contraindications and proceed with endovascular blood flow-sparing therapy in case of therapeutic failure on conservative treatment. In case of recurrent embolic episodes, vessel occlusion might be considered if the patient tolerate a balloon occlusion test. Treatment length for traumatic dissections has not been determined. We base this decision on ultrasound after 6 months and whether there are any rheological abnormalities in the offended vessel.

There are no randomised controlled trials on this subject. The natural history of these lesions shows a strong tendency towards spontaneous healing within the first couple of months. Intracranial haemorrhage constitutes a relative contraindication to anticoagulation, and other blood flow-sparing therapies should be considered, depending on the local expertise (endovascular or surgical).

Less often, patients present with an extracranial carotid or vertebral aneurysm. They can demonstrate symptoms secondary to embolisation, rupture, or local volume effect. These lesions are usually better visualized using MRI than CT. Therapy is controversial; their natural history shows a clear tendency towards regression. Hence, anticoagulation is often indicated to prevent embolisation in the meantime before spontaneous resolution. However, they should be subject to repeated radiological investigations. Enlargement, embolisation, and severe compressive symptoms should mandate consultation with expertise proficient in either flow-sparing therapy (suturing the aneurysm sac, resection and anastomosis, or endovascular stent therapy) or flow stopping-therapy (balloon occlusion test with subsequent ligation/coiling).

22.2.2 Intracranial Vessel Injury

These are divided into arteriovenous fistulas (AVF), traumatic aneurysms, thrombosis, and sinus injuries.

22.2.2.1 Arteriovenous Fistulas

The most common traumatic AVF is the carotid-cavernous fistula. Symptoms are related to arterialisation, volume, and increased venous pressure and include headache, chemosis, ptosis, ophthalmoplegia, and visual loss. CT angiography can give hints to the presence of an AVF, but DSA is mandatory to further elucidate the flow pattern. If it is a direct carotid-cavernous fistula (direct connection between ICA and the cavernous sinus), occlusion of the fistula is warranted to prevent neurological deterioration; however, if it is an indirect fistula (a fistula within the leaves of the cavernous sinus that are fed by intracavernous branches of the ICA), thrombosis of the fistula is common and conservative treatment is sufficient. Usually, endovascular embolisation of the fistula is the method of choice in treating the direct carotid cavernous fistulas.

22.2.2.2 Traumatic Aneurysms

These are rare, comprising less than 1% of all intracranial aneurysms (Semple 2004). Compared with 'spontaneous' aneurysms, they have a larger propensity for bleeding; 50% rupture within the first week. This can be explained by the fact that these aneurysms are pseudoaneurysms. They also have a clear predilection for more distal localisations than the spontaneous aneurysms, especially the A3+4 segments. They also show a clear tendency for rapid growth, and regular controls are warranted if indications for surgery have not already been made. A high index of suspicion must be maintained in patients admitted with penetrating injuries, where the offending object has been in close vicinity of the vessel, in patients with localized subarachnoid clots, in patients with large bleeds in the basal cisterns, in patients with fractures of the clivus, sphenoid sinus or medial temporal bone, and in patients exposed to shock waves. Data on the sensitivity of CT angiography compared with DSA is lacking. However, if there are any irregularities on the CTA, we recommend DSA, as it better reveals the hallmarks of traumatic aneurysms: delayed emptying and filling of the aneurysm, irregular contours, and absence of a neck. Obliteration of these aneurysms is usually recommended. The method of choice has traditionally been open surgery due to the lack of a neck and the poor strength of the aneurysm wall making traumatic aneurysms poor candidates for endovascular treatment. There are however now several reports claiming good results using combined endovascular stents and coils (Cohen et al. 2008). During surgery, these aneurysms have been notorious for their intraoperative tendency for rupture and difficult clip reconstruction, necessitating wrapping, ligation, or trapping with or without bypass (Semple 2004).

22.2.2.3 Traumatic Occlusion

The most common intracranial vessel to be occluded is the proximal intracranial ICA where the vessel is in intimate contact with bone. Fractures in the vicinity of the ICA should arouse concern and mandate an angiographic examination. Usually, CT angiography is reasonable, but if there are any irregularities, we advocate DSA. The occlusion is usually secondary to dissection with subsequent mural haematoma and thrombosis. The reported literature cite rates of 70–85% suffering from massive hemispheric infarction, but the patency of the circle of Willis clearly plays a role, and the selection bias in these reports has been clear. We advocate anticoagulation and perfusion studies to elucidate whether the cross-flow is adequate. In case of perfusion asymmetry, we increase the blood pressure and preferably utilise some form of metabolic surveillance in the affected hemisphere. There are also case reports on vascular augmentation procedures. In case of a patient already sustaining a massive infarction, we advocate hemicraniectomy if the clinical and radiological picture is concordant with a reasonable outcome.

22.2.2.4 Sinus Injury

Fractures extending across major dural sinuses can potentially tear the vessel wall and produce an extracerebral haemorrhage, usually an epidural. If an indication for evacuation is found, one should make arrangements for a potentially large haemorrhage when the bone flap is raised. Usually, the sinus tear is found and can be plugged with a finger while contemplating the next move. Depending on the size of the tear, a small piece of Tachosil® or similar material and slight pressure might be sufficient, but if large parts of the sinus are torn, reconstruction is recommended. Temporary occlusion using aneurysm clips to visualize the rent while reconstructing the vessel using sutures and an overlay of dura can be done, but depending on the sinus involved, occlusion can increase the pressure with subsequent herniation. A few case reports indicate that if the patient does not tolerate temporary sinus occlusion, a Fogarty® catheter can be inserted and used as a bypass vehicle while the sinus is reconstructed.

22.3 Specific Paediatric Concerns

There are no specific paediatric concerns for this subject.

References

Cohen JE, Gomori JM, Segal R, Spivak A, Margolin E, Sviri G, Rajz G, Fraifeld S, Spektor S (2008) Results of endovascular treatment of traumatic intracranial aneurysms. Neurosurgery 63:476–485; discussion 485–476. doi:10.1227/01.NEU.0000324995.57376.79

Fusco MR, Harrigan MR (2011) Cerebrovascular dissections: a review. Part II: blunt cerebrovascular injury. Neurosurgery 68:517–530. doi:510.1227/NEU.1220b1013e3181fe1222fda

Nedeltchev K, Baumgartner RW (2005) Traumatic cervical artery dissection. Front Neurol Neurosci 20:54–63

Semple P (2004) Traumatic aneurysms. In: LeRoux PD, Winn H, Newell DW (eds) Management of cerebral aneurysms. Saunders, Philadelphia, pp 397–408

Stein DM, Boswell S, Sliker CW, Lui FY, Scalea TM (2009) Blunt cerebrovascular injuries: does treatment always matter? J Trauma 66:132–143

Vertinsky AT, Schwartz NE, Fischbein NJ, Rosenberg J, Albers GW, Zaharchuk G (2008) Comparison of multidetector CT angiography and MR imaging of cervical artery dissection. AJNR Am J Neuroradiol 29:1753–1760

Insertion of Intracranial Monitoring Devices

23

Mikko Kauppinen

Recommendations

Level I

Data are insufficient to support a Level I recommendation for this topic.

Level II

A measuring device for intracranial pressure should be inserted in salvageable head injury patients with an abnormal computed tomography scan and a GCS score of 3–8.

Level III

Intracranial pressure should be monitored if two of the following features are noted at admission: age over 40 years, unilateral or bilateral motor posturing, and/or systolic blood pressure less than 90 mmHg.

Brain tissue oxygen monitoring can help to guide treatment towards improved brain oxygenation.

M. Kauppinen
Department of Neurosurgery,
Oulu University Hospital,
Kajaanintie 50, 90029 OYS, Finland
e-mail: mikko.kauppinen@ppshp.fi

23.1 Overview

The main objective of neurointensive monitoring is to maintain adequate cerebral perfusion and oxygenation, and to avoid secondary injury to the penumbra zone while the brain recovers. Cerebral perfusion is reduced, and poorer outcomes are associated with systemic hypotension and intracranial hypertension. Cerebral perfusion pressure (CPP), an indirect measure of cerebral perfusion, incorporates mean arterial blood pressure (MAP) and intracranial pressure (ICP): CPP=MAP−ICP The only way to reliably determine cerebral hypoperfusion is to continuously monitor ICP and blood pressure (Brain Trauma Foundation 2007).

The following two methods of measuring ICP are mostly used: parenchymal ICP probes or via an external ventricular drain (EVD).

Tips, Tricks, and Pitfalls

- When the map is different from the landscape, the landscape is right! Be aware of technical malfunction, and do not trust ICP values blindly.
- Always consider inserting an EVD in the early phase of treatment.

23.2 Background

ICP data can be used to predict the outcome and the worsening of intracranial pathology, to calculate and manage CPP, and restrict the potentially

T. Sundstrøm et al. (eds.), *Management of Severe Traumatic Brain Injury*,
DOI 10.1007/978-3-642-28126-6_23, © Springer-Verlag Berlin Heidelberg 2012

deleterious effects of ICP reduction therapies. ICP monitoring through an EVD also permits therapeutic drainage of CSF. Elevated ICP can be the first indicator of intracranial pathology. Intracranial hypertension is found in 40–60% of severely head-injured patients and is a major factor in 50% of all fatalities (Winn 2003). On the other hand, prophylactic treatment of ICP without ICP monitoring is not without risk (Brain Trauma Foundation 2007).

However, monitoring ICP gives only limited information regarding other factors known to be important to the pathophysiology of TBI, such as cerebral blood flow and metabolism.

Therapy following severe TBI is directed towards preventing secondary brain injury. Achieving this objective relies on assuring the delivery of an adequate supply of oxygen and metabolic substrates to the brain. Delivery of oxygen to the brain is a function of the oxygen content of the blood and the cerebral blood flow (CBF). Delivery of glucose and other metabolic substrates to the brain also depends on CBF (Brain Trauma Foundation 2007).

The development of additional monitoring systems to provide information regarding cerebral blood flow and metabolism has been a long-standing aim in neurocritical care. There are old techniques for measuring oxygen content in the cerebral venous outflow (jugular bulb catheter) and then indirectly calculate the oxygen saturation of the brain. In recent years, methods to continuously monitor cerebral perfusion have been developed. They can be divided into three subgroups: systems that measure CBF directly (thermal diffusion probes, transcranial Doppler), systems that measure delivery of oxygen (brain tissue oxygen monitors, near-infrared spectroscopy, jugular venous saturation monitors), and systems that assess the metabolic state of the brain (cerebral microdialysis) (Brain Trauma Foundation 2007). Of these subgroups, the brain oxygen delivery measuring devices are most widely used nowadays.

CBF probes, oxygen tension catheters, and microdialysis can be used to assess the events in a small region but possibly fail to detect harmful events in other parts of the brain. Conversely, more global approaches (venous oxygen saturation) fail to detect regional abnormalities (Maas et al. 2008).

Measuring different parameters is not without risk of complications. The obstruction (and therefore malfunction) risk of external ventricular drainage (EVD) is 6.3%. Malfunctions of parenchymal ICP catheters are reported as high as 16% (Brain Trauma Foundation 2007). The infection risk is substantially higher with EVD (about 10%) compared to plain ICP catheters (1%) (Winn 2003). The risk for hemorrhagic complications is about 1.1% with EVD but almost zero with parenchymal ICP catheter. However, clinically significant infections or haemorrhages associated with ICP devices causing patient morbidity are rare and should not deter the decision to monitor ICP (Brain Trauma Foundation 2007).

ICP measurement by parenchymal microstain gauge pressure transduction is similar to ventricular ICP. In contrast, fluid-coupled epidural devices or subarachnoid bolts and pneumatic epidural devices are less accurate than ventricular ICP monitors. Significant differences in readings have been demonstrated between ICP devices placed in the parenchyma versus the subdural space (Brain Trauma Foundation 2007).

23.2.1 Parenchymal ICP Catheter

An ICP catheter should be inserted in TBI patients with GCS of 3–8 and an abnormal CT finding (Winn 2003; Brain Trauma Foundation 2007). In addition, ICP monitoring is indicated in patients with severe TBI and normal CT findings when at least two of the following features are noted at admission: age over 40, unilateral or bilateral motor posturing, systolic blood pressure <90 mmHg because of elevated ICH risk. Their risk (53–63%) of ICH was similar to that of patients with an abnormal CT scan and severe TBI (Brain Trauma Foundation 2007). In contrast, a patient whose admission CT scan does not show a mass lesion, midline shift, or abnormal cisterns has a 10–15% chance of developing an ICH (Brain Trauma Foundation 2007).

Patients with GCS > 8 may benefit from ICP monitoring if CT demonstrates significant mass lesions or if treatment is required for associated injuries (Winn 2003). ICP monitoring should also be kept in mind during the evacuation of a hematoma when there is visible oedema at the end of the operation or when it is likely that intracranial hypertension is going to develop (practically always in cases when pre-op GCS is 3–8). Moreover, anesthetised TBI patients are ICP catheter candidates when it is not possible to follow neurological status reliably even if initial GCS would have been slightly over 8.

The operation can be done in ICU or in OR. It is possible to install an ICP catheter also without bolt after evacuation of a hematoma through a craniotomy opening (steps 10–11, 13–14). In that case, the catheter should be tunnelled under the skin and fixed with sutures.

Installation of a parenchymal ICP catheter with bolt:

1. Shave the hair.
2. Make a marking to the skin with a pen ca. 10–12 cm posterior from the nasion to mid-pupillary line (preferably right side, in some cases left side, for example, if haematoma is on left side).
3. Sterilise the operation area.
4. Cover the operation area.
5. Inject adrenalin-lidocaine mixture.
6. Make a little incision (4–6 mm) to the skin all the way to the skull.
7. Make a burr hole with a drill provided in the kit all the way through the skull.
8. Screw the ICP bolt to the burr hole.
9. Perforate the dura with a blunt instrument provided in the kit.
10. Calibrate the ICP catheter if the model requires it (there should be figure 0 mmHg in the screen after calibration) and save the reference number for later use.
11. Put the catheter into the brain parenchyma (2–3 cm deep).
12. Fix the catheter to the bolt by tightening the bolt's white screw and by using some adhesive tape.
13. Fix the catheter to the skin with tape/sutures or both.
14. Check the ICP reading on monitor.

23.2.2 Parenchymal PtO2 Catheter

There are studies (Stiefel et al. 2005; Brain Trauma Foundation 2007) which suggest that directing the treatment to improve brain oxygenation might benefit the patient more than plain traditional ICP-CPP treatment, which is still the golden standard in most centres. Most of these studies conclude that low (<10–15 mmHg over 30 min) PO_2 clearly increases both mortality and morbidity (Bardt et al. 1998; Valadka et al. 1998; Van den Brink et al. 2000). However, the present data is still only Level III evidence (Brain Trauma Foundation 2007).

Indications for installing PtO_2 catheters do not differ from regular ICP catheter installation indications. It should be considered in young patients when the probe is possible to install in a non-haemorrhagic area. The catheter costs more than a regular ICP catheter. Cost-effectiveness is still unknown. PtO_2 catheter is more prone to dysfunctions than regular ICP catheter. On the other hand, it gives valuable information of the actual O_2 situation in brain. Most catheters also produce information about the brain temperature. One must keep in mind, however, that the catheter should be placed into healthy, non-contused brain in order to gain reliable O_2 information.

The operation can be done in the ICU or in the OR. The catheter should be handled with care (do not bend the catheter to too tight curves) because of the fragile light cable inside it. It is possible to install a PtO_2 catheter also without bolt after evacuation of a hematoma through a craniotomy opening (steps 10–11, 13–15). In that case, the catheter should be tunnelled under the skin and fixed with sutures.

Installation of a parenchymal PtO_2 catheter with bolt:

1. Shave the hair.
2. Make a marking to the skin with a pen ca. 10–12 cm posterior from the nasion to midpupillary line (preferably right side; note that the PtO_2 probe should be always put to non-haemorrhagic area).
3. Sterilise the operation area.
4. Cover the operation area.
5. Inject adrenalin-lidocaine mixture.

6. Make a little incision (4–6 mm) to skin all the way to the skull.
7. Make a burr hole with a drill provided in the kit all the way through the skull.
8. Screw the ICP bolt to the burr hole.
9. Perforate the dura with a blunt instrument provided in the kit.
10. Connect the catheter to the monitor and check that the PtO_2 value (room air) is about 150–180.
11. Put the catheter into the brain parenchyma (2–3 cm deep) using white silicon tube around the catheter (a resistance should be felt when the silicon tube locks to ICP bolt).
12. Fix the catheter to the bolt by tightening gently bolt's screw (do not tighten the screw too tightly in order to prevent dysfunctions).
13. Put first a white butterfly around the catheter and lock it with a blue butterfly, then fix the butterflies to the skin with sutures (remember not to install the catheter too tightly curved).
14. Check the readings on monitor.
15. Note that it is possible that PtO_2 is not instantly correct (in case of blood around tip of the catheter). PtO_2 should be correct immediately after a possible blood clot has absorbed.

23.2.3 External Ventricular Drainage (EVD)

EVD is the most accurate, low-cost, and reliable method of monitoring ICP. It is also possible to recalibrate it in situ which is not always possible with the parenchymal catheters. It also allows therapeutic drainage of CSF. However, the external transducer must be constantly maintained at a fixed reference point relative to the patient's head to avoid measurement error (Brain Trauma Foundation 2007).

EVD should be considered in severe TBI patients when ICP is continuously over 20 mmHg (regardless of sedation and mannitol and hyperosmolar NaCl therapy), and there are not any other options for other surgical interventions. In some cases (young patients when it is likely that intracranial hypertension is going to develop later on), it is better to install an EVD instead of a parenchymal ICP catheter in the first place. However, it is often difficult to place the EVD in a TBI patient because of possibly shifted and/or small ventricles.

The operation can only be done in the OR. Be aware not to curve the catheter tightly and not to put sutures that obstruct the EVD when closing the incision. In order to prevent infections, it is recommended to tunnel the drain at least 5 cm under the skin.

Installation of an EVD:

1. Shave the hair.
2. Make a marking to the skin with a pen ca. 10–12 cm posterior from the nasion to mid-pupillary line (preferably right side, in some cases left side, for example, if hematoma is on left side).
3. Sterilise the operation area.
4. Cover the operation area.
5. Inject adrenalin-lidocaine mixture.
6. Make an incision (30–40 mm) to the skin all the way to the skull.
7. Haemostasis to skin arteries.
8. Remove the galea with a rasp.
9. Put a spreader to the incision.
10. Make a burr hole.
11. Use a hook and a Kerrison to clean the burr hole.
12. Use bone wax if needed.
13. Coagulate the dura and make an incision carefully through it.
14. Haemostasis.
15. Coagulate the arachnoidea and perforate it with a bipolar.
16. Install the EVD into the lateral ventricle (you should feel the resistance of the ependyma cells at the depth of 3–5 cm).
17. Immediately after you have punctured the ependyma cell layer and you have got some CSF, remove the mandrel and obstruct the flow of CSF.
18. Push the EVD without the mandrel a bit deeper (the optimum depth is 6–7 cm) and check that the EVD still works properly.
19. Tunnel the EVD under the skin and externalise it preferably >5 cm from the edge of the wound to prevent infections.

20. Close the wound preferably in two layers.
21. Cut the EVD a bit shorter if needed and install a luer tip provided in the kit (using also a back-up suture around the tip of the hose).
22. Fix the tip of EVD to skin with sutures.
23. Check that EVD is still working properly and connect it to the external hose system.

23.3 Specific Paediatric Concerns

Children have practically no extra intracranial space allowing room for haematomas or brain swelling after TBI. In paediatric cases, the ICP can rapidly reach dangerous levels with poor response to pressure-reducing medical therapy. Therefore, it is worth considering inserting an EVD instead of a regular ICP catheter before the ventricles are completely obliterated due to ensuing oedema. Implantation of a PtO_2 catheter is another good option for directing treatment. It is also possible to use dual probes (EVD and PtO_2) in some cases. In children, regular parenchymal ICP measuring devices are not the monitoring equipment of choice if other methods are available.

References

Bardt TF, Unterberg AW et al (1998) Monitoring of brain tissue PO2 in traumatic brain injury: effect of cerebral hypoxia on outcome. Acta Neurochir Suppl 71: 153–156

Brain Trauma Foundation (2007) Guidelines for the management of severe traumatic brain injury, vol 24 (Suppl 1), 3rd edn, Journal of neurotrauma. Mary Ann Liebert, Inc., New York

Maas A, Stocchetti N et al (2008) Moderate and severe traumatic brain injury in adults. Lancet Neurol 7:728–741

Stiefel MF, Spiotta A et al (2005) Reduced mortality rate in patients with severe traumatic brain injury treated with brain tissue oxygen monitoring. J Neurosurg 103:805–811

Valadka AB, Gopinath SP et al (1998) Relationship of brain tissue PO2 to outcome after severe head injury. Crit Care Med 26:1576–1581

Van den Brink WA, Van Santbrink H et al (2000) Brain oxygen tension in severe head injury. Neurosurgery 46:868–878

Winn RH (2003) Youmans neurological surgery, vol 1, 5th edn. Saunders (Elsevier), Philadelphia, pp 184–185

24 Maxillofacial Fractures

Ann Hermansson

Recommendations

Level I

There are insufficient data to support a level I recommendation for this topic.

Level II

There are insufficient data to support a level II recommendation for this topic.

Level III

The outcome of white blowout fractures is better if the entrapped soft tissue is freed within 48 h.

24.1 Overview

Many facial fractures do not need surgical reconstruction. If needed, it often should be performed after the acute phase. A thorough planning and investigation with imaging and control of the function and the mobility of the eyes, yaws and teeth should be undertaken. Some fractures lead to troublesome bleedings and/or airway problems and have to be addressed at once. Airway problems and surgical timing should be discussed at an early stage between neurosurgeon, anaesthesiologist and facial surgeon to decide the best approach.

A. Hermansson
ENT Department, University Hospital,
221 85 Lund, Sweden
e-mail: ann.hermansson@med.lu.se

Tips, Tricks, and Pitfalls

- Facial fractures might cause troublesome bleedings and airway obstruction.
- Skin lacerations in the face should be carefully stitched with consideration of structures under the skin that might be injured. Be aware of the facial nerve, the tear canals, the parotid glands and the structures in the eyelids and lips.
- Try to remove asphalt stains and dust from excoriations to avoid 'tattoos' after healing. A toothbrush might be helpful!
- Special considerations have to be made regarding timing of surgery and imaging in children.
- Early evaluation of eye movements and if possible function is important.
- Antibiotic treatment should be considered.
- Tetanus vaccination should be considered.
- Evaluation of sight and hearing is important and should be carried out as soon as possible.

T. Sundstrøm et al. (eds.), *Management of Severe Traumatic Brain Injury*,
DOI 10.1007/978-3-642-28126-6_24, © Springer-Verlag Berlin Heidelberg 2012

24.2 Background

Trauma to the skull often results in more or less obvious fractures extending into the facial bones. These will often result in disfiguration and, perhaps, disturbances in function in the orbit, mid-face and/or teeth and yaws and might be obvious already in the emergency room. However, some fractures are not that obvious and might be overlooked initially. It is therefore important to make an evaluation of both functional and aesthetic aspects of facial trauma. Below follows more detailed information on diagnosis, timing of surgery and follow-up. Especially interested readers are referred to textbooks (Zide 2006; Hammer 1995).

24.2.1 Diagnostics

CT scans of the facial bones (including the mandible) with or without 3D reconstructions can often be made from the initial trauma CT, but if not, it should be obtained. In some cases, mainly in children, an MRI might be helpful to map soft tissue in the orbit when white blowout fractures are suspected.

In some cases, one can see fractures in the mid-face but with very little dislocation. In most of these cases, no intervention is needed if there is no impaired function. Therefore, an early evaluation of eye movements and function will often be needed to decide whether to operate or not. Special considerations also have to be given to the function of the teeth and yaws.

24.2.2 Timing of Surgery

In most cases, facial fractures do not have to be addressed immediately, although this is often advantageous. If needed, they might be operated within 10–14 days or even later with good results. However, some fractures need to be addressed earlier. The naso-orbito-ethmoidal (NOE) fractures should be repositioned as soon as possible (Sargent and Rogers 1999). If a regular operation is not possible immediately, a closed reduction lifting the naso-orbito-ethmoidal complex in place should be considered as a first step to later reconstruction and is often effective.

If possible, white blowout fractures in children should be operated within 48 h, and thus should be recognised early. These orbital fractures are sometimes called trapdoor fractures; they are seen in children and young adults and are actually greenstick fractures of the orbit where the eye muscles get firmly entrapped and might be seriously damaged. It has been shown that the outcome of these fractures is better if the entrapped soft tissue is freed within 48 h (Grant et al. 2002).

The most obvious fractures needing immediate intervention are those causing airway obstruction and/or life-threatening bleedings. In some cases, endotracheal intubation is not possible and a coniotomy with a cannula placed through the cricothyroid membrane has to be performed early on, while in other cases, a regular tracheostomy should be considered both to facilitate the later reduction and osteosynthesis of facial fractures and the rehabilitation. If this is needed preoperatively, it is often wise to perform the tracheostomy as soon as possible to facilitate the patient care (Holmgren et al. 2007).

Skull base fractures can cause both bleeding and CSF leakage. While most leakages from the ear will cease spontaneously, liquorrhea from the nose must in many cases be patched operatively. This can be done either by open or endoscopic approach.

In most cases, it is thus wise to plan the surgery of maxillofacial trauma when appropriate evaluation has been made, often as a collaboration between ENT and/or plastic surgeons, maxillofacial surgeons and ophthalmologists. In some cases, the surgery has to be planned according to neurosurgical interventions, for instance, to address CSF leakages, which of course should be done *after* surgery including reposition of a NOE fracture! In most cases, surgery is best planned in one session.

24.2.3 Follow-Up

All cases of maxillofacial fractures have to be carefully followed. Not only must the aesthetic aspects be considered, but it is also important to make an evaluation of function. Both eyesight and hearing should be checked, and teeth and yaws should be evaluated by a dentist or a maxillofacial surgeon. It is often wise to inform the patient and his family that there often is need for additional operations or reconstructions during the years after a craniofacial trauma.

24.3 Specific Paediatric Concerns

Facial fractures are rare in children; when they do occur, special considerations have to be made. Fractures of the skull bones are much more common but might involve mid-face and yaws. However, most of these fractures will not show much dislocation and will heal without intervention. To keep radiation doses low, especially to the eyes, is even more important in children than in grown-ups. In some instances, MRI might be useful. Greenstick fractures in the orbit, so-called white blowout fractures, pose a special problem since they might cause entrapment of the periorbital structures and thereby severely restricted eye movements. These fractures are often hard to visualise both on CT scans and MRI. If there are clinical signs of entrapment, it is mandatory to explore the orbit even if imaging does not show a fracture. Thus, a forced duction test (testing the eye movements by trying to move the eye when gripping the muscles with a pair of forceps) might be needed to decide whether to operate or not. In most studies, intervention within 48 h is recommended to avoid permanent problems with double vision. Fractures of the maxilla and mandible in children should be given special consideration, keeping the possible damage to non-erupted teeth in mind.

References

Grant JH 3rd, Patrinely JR, Weiss AH, Kierney PC, Gruss JS (2002) Trapdoor fracture of the orbit in a pediatric population. Plast Reconstr Surg 109(2):482–489; discussion 490–495

Hammer B (1995) Orbital fractures: diagnosis, operative treatment, secondary corrections. Hogrefe & Huber Publishers, Seattle

Holmgren EP, Bagheri S, Bell RB, Bobek S, Dierks EJ (2007) Utilization of tracheostomy in craniomaxillofacial trauma at a level-1 trauma center. J Oral Maxillofac Surg 65(10):2005–2010

Sargent LA, Rogers GF (1999) Nasoethmoid orbital fractures: diagnosis and management. J Craniomaxillofac Trauma 5(1):19–27

Zide BM (2006) Surgical anatomy around the orbit: the system of zones. Lippincott Williams & Wilkins, Philadelphia

Part VI

Peroperative Anaesthesia

25 Choice of Anaesthesia Drugs and Medications

Bent Lob Dahl

Recommendations

Level I

There are insufficient data to support a Level 1 recommendation for this topic.

Level II

Prophylactic administration of barbiturates to induce burst suppression EEG is not recommended.

High-dose barbiturate administration is recommended to control elevated ICP refractory to maximum standard medical and surgical treatment. Hemodynamic stability is essential before and during barbiturate therapy.

Propofol is recommended for the control of ICP but not for improvement in mortality or 6-month outcome. High-dose propofol can produce significant morbidity.

Level III

All procedures should be aimed at preserving a normal ICP, cerebral circulation and oxygenation.

Use the drugs that you are most familiar with.

Titrate drugs carefully to avoid hypotension and changes in PaO_2 and $PaCO_2$.

Head should be in neutral position and elevated 10–15° to increase cerebral venous drainage without compromising CBF. It must be checked whether the venous drainage is compromised by a cervical collar.

B.L. Dahl
Department of Neuroanaesthesia and Neurocritical care, Aarhus University Hospital, Noerrebrogade 8000, Aarhus C, Denmark
e-mail: bentdahl@rm.dk

25.1 Overview

Most important in the treatment of patients with brain injury is to maintain oxygenation and blood pressure while securing airway and circulation in order to ensure the best outcome for the patients. Sedatives and analgesics are widely used to treat pain and agitation in prehospital setting as well as during operative procedures and intensive care.

The most widely used drugs are:

Sedatives	Thiopental, propofol, midazolam, dexmedetomidine, ketamine, clonidine
Analgesics	Morphine, fentanyl, remifentanil, sufentanil
Volatile anaesthetics	Sevoflurane, isoflurane, nitrous oxide
Muscle relaxants	Suxamethone, mivacurium, atracurium, cisatracurium, vecuronium, rocuronium
Inotropics	Dopamine, dopexamine, noradrenaline, phenylephrine, ephrine, adrenaline
NSAID	Ketorolac, paracetamol (acetaminophen)

T. Sundstrøm et al. (eds.), *Management of Severe Traumatic Brain Injury*,
DOI 10.1007/978-3-642-28126-6_25, © Springer-Verlag Berlin Heidelberg 2012

Tips, Tricks, and Pitfalls

- Use the drug you are most familiar with.
- A drop in blood pressure, or an unexpected high or low CO2, may create more havoc in the injured brain than use of a sub-optimal anaesthetic drug since the differences between the drugs detected in clinical trials are minor.
- Titrate your drugs. Remember many of the severely head-injured patients have additional injuries and are prone to be hypovolaemic and will require smaller doses of drugs.
- Muscle relaxants should be avoided.
- The acute patient has decreased intracranial compliance and hence decreased compensative ability for even minor changes in ICP. Anaesthesia and intubation should be performed according to this. All procedures should maintain normal ICP. Head should be in neutral position and elevated 10–15° to increase cerebral venous drainage without compromising CBF. It must be checked whether the venous drainage is compromised by a cervical collar.
- For acute intubation in a cardiorespiratory stable patient, propofol or thiopental can be used for sedation. Ketamine or dexmedetomidine can be used in cardiorespiratory unstable patients. All analgesics can be used. If relaxation is needed, suxamethone can be used for rapid induction intubation. Mivacurium, atracurium, cisatracurium and vecuronium eller rocuronium can also be used according to local instructions.
- 'Inotropics' such as norepinephrine, dopamine, dopexamine, phenylephrine and ephedrine can be used according to the clinical situation. Most TBI patients have a normal to increased cardiac output and vasodilatation and may benefit from norepinephrine infusion (2–20 µg/kg body weight/min).

25.2 Background

25.2.1 Propofol

Propofol has become widely used because of rapid onset and short duration, facilitating neurologic examination. Propofol has been shown to reduce cerebral metabolism and oxygen consumption, thereby providing a potential neuroprotective effect. One double-blind randomized controlled clinical trial (RCT) comparing morphine and propofol failed to show a significant difference in GOS or mortality. In a post hoc analysis, a significant increase in neurological outcome was observed in patients receiving high-dose propofol (Kelly et al. 1999).

Propofol infusion syndrome is a safety concern. The clinical features are hyperkalemia, hepatomegaly, lipemia, metabolic acidosis, myocardial failure, rhabdomyolysis and renal failure resulting in death. Doses exceeding 5 mg/kg/h, and any dose for more than 48 h, should be avoided.

25.2.2 Midazolam

Midazolam, a relatively short-acting benzodiazepine, is frequently used in neurointensive care units. Its use carries a significant risk of a decrease in MAP and a sustained increase in ICP resulting in a decrease in CPP. Midazolam can be reversed by flumazenil.

25.2.3 Barbiturates

Barbiturates have been used in two different situations: prophylactically and for treatment of refractory intracranial hypertension. Prophylactic use of barbiturates was investigated in two RCTs (Schwartz et al. 1984; Ward et al. 1985), which failed to demonstrate significant clinical benefit. In patients with diffuse injury, Swartz et al. observed a mortality of 77% compared with 43% in the mannitol control group. In both studies, an undesirable decrease in blood pressure was observed. Prophylactic use of barbiturates is not recommended.

The use of barbiturates for treatment of refractory intracranial hypertension was investigated by Eisenberg et al. (1988) in an RCT. The likelihood of survival for those patients whose ICP responded to barbiturates was 92% compared to 17% in non-responders. In patients with hypotension before randomization, barbiturates provided no benefit.

A Cochrane review (Roberts 2009) concluded: 'There is no evidence that barbiturate therapy in patients with acute severe head injury improves outcome. Barbiturate therapy results in a fall in blood pressure in one of four treated patients. The hypotensive effect will offset any ICP lowering effect on cerebral perfusion pressure'.

25.2.4 Ketamine

Ketamine has previously been contraindicated because of fear of increase in CBF and ICP. However, this effect is probably caused by an increase in $PaCO_2$. It is important to maintain blood pressure and oxygenation in these patients according to data from the Traumatic Coma Data Bank. The advantage of ketamine is that blood pressure and ventilation are better preserved. Ketamine can, for this reason, be used in patients with TBI.

25.2.5 Dexmedetomidine

Dexmedetomidine is an alpha-2 adrenergic receptor agonist with rapidly titratable sedative, sympatholytic and analgesic effects but almost without respiratory depression. Dexmedetomidine produces a decrease in CBF. The effect on cerebral metabolism in humans is unknown (Pasternak 2009). In a small series of healthy persons, an uncoupling of supply and demand in the brain was not found (Drummond et al. 2008). How it influences the injured brain is unknown. The possible benefit of attenuating the sympathetic response (decrease in heart rate and blood pressure to noxious stimuli and reduction in stress response and pulmonary vascular permeability) remains to be investigated.

25.2.6 Analgesics

25.2.6.1 Spontaneous Ventilation

Morphine and analogue drugs should be administered with extreme caution in the spontaneously breathing patient with exhausted intracranial compliance. Careful monitoring of conscious state, respiration, blood pressure and eventually gas analysis (PaO_2, $PaCO_2$), or capnometry/oximetry, is mandatory. Even a small dose of morphine (e.g. 3 mg IV) might provoke a decrease in $AVDO_2$, suggesting a state of hyperaemia.

25.2.6.2 Controlled Ventilation

Morphine, Fentanyl and Remifentanil

In the ventilator-treated patient, morphine and fentanyl do not increase CBF or ICP. On the contrary, a decrease in ICP is observed. This is caused by the sedative effect giving rise to a decrease in CO_2 production, and a decreased level of circulating catecholamines. An additive effect of hypnotics and analgesics on cerebral oxygen uptake may also play a role.

Sufentanil and Alfentanil

Sufentanil and alfentanil should be used with reservation because animal experiments indicate that sufentanil provokes a prolonged period of CBF and CBV increase (Milde et al. 1990). Comparative studies of fentanyl, alfentanil and sufentanil in patients subjected to craniotomy indicate that the use of the two latter drugs was accompanied by a decrease in CPP and an increase in CSF pressure. Cerebral autoregulation may play a role because correction of blood pressure normalized ICP. Both sufentanil and alfentanil elicit a decrease in blood pressure. As a consequence, a decrease in CVR and an increase in CBV may occur. Under these circumstances, an increase in ICP is observed.

Volatile Anaesthetics

There is an ongoing discussion of a neuroprotective effect of volatile anaesthetics and the clinical relevance of this effect. Isoflurane reduces neuron death in the early phase after head injury, but later on, this neuroprotective effect might increase apoptosis. Volatile anaesthetics can be used in patients with TBI.

Muscular Relaxation

Muscular relaxation can be necessary to facilitate ventilatory support but should be restricted because of a risk of hypoxemia in case of extubation, masking of seizures, association to myopathy and increased length of stay in ICU.

In experimental, as well as human studies, succinylcholine increases ICP. The rise in ICP is caused by activation from peripheral impulses from the muscles. Non-depolarising agents such as mivacurium, atracurium, cisatracurium, vecuronium and rocuronium do not increase ICP during controlled ventilation.

Inotropics

A sufficient blood pressure is important for outcome. If hypotension is observed and hypovolemia is excluded or treated, inotropics should be used. The effect of inotropics on CBF, $CMRO_2$ and ICP are not fully understood as there seems to be relatively few such receptors in cerebral vessels. The effect might depend on whether the BBB is broken or not. Inotropics must be used according to the clinical situation.

NSAID

Paracetamol (acetaminophen) might decrease the demand for morphine, and it lowers the body temperature. Ketorolac might also decrease the need for morphine. Often, it is not used because of adverse effects (bleeding and inhibition of bone healing). In a study by Casanelli et al. (2008) of 25 patients undergoing spine surgery, no bleeding was observed in the ketorolac group as compared to 3 patients in the placebo group.

25.3 Specific Paediatric Concerns

Sedatives, analgesics and neuromuscular blockers are widely used in children and infants with TBI. However, there are few studies on the paediatric consequences of these agents. For this reason, their use should be left to the treating doctor (Adelson 2003).

Adverse affects of propofol (increased mortality and the propofol infusion syndrome) have restricted the use of propofol for sedation and ICP control in paediatric patients with or without TBI. Other alternatives are available. Continuous infusion of propofol in intensive care is not recommended in paediatric patients as 'safety has not been established' (Center for Drug Evaluation and Research 2003).

References

Adelson PD, Bratton SL, Carney NA, et al (2003) Guidelines for the acute medical management of severe traumatic brain injury in infants, children and adolescents. Pediatric Crit Care Med 4(3 Suppl):S1–S491. http://tbiguidelines.org/glHome.aspx

Casanelli EH, Dean CL, Garcia RM et al (2008) Ketorolac use for postoperative pain management following lumbar decompression surgery: a prospective, randomized, double-blinded, placebo-controlled trial. Spine 33(12):1313–1317

Center for Drug Evaluation and Research. http://www.fda.gov/cder/pediatric/labelchange/htm. Accessed 5 May 2003

Drummond JC, Dao AV, Roth DM et al (2008) Effect of Dexmedetomidine on cerebral flow velocity, cerebral metabolic rate and carbon dioxide response in normal humans. Anesthesiology 108:225–232

Eisenberg HM, Frankowski RF, Contant CF et al (1988) High-dose barbiturate control of elevated intracranial pressure in patients with severe head injury. J Neurosurg 69:15–23

Kelly PF, Goodale LA, Williams J et al (1999) Propofol in the treatment of moderate and severe head injury: a randomized double-blinded pilot trial. J Neurosurg 90:1042–1057

Milde LN, Milde JH, Gallagher WJ (1990). Effects of sufentanil on cerebral circulation and metabolism in dogs. Anesth. Analog 70(2):138–146

Pasternak JJ, Lanier WL (2009) Neuroanesthesiology update. J Neurosurg Anesthesiol 21:73–97

Roberts I (2009) Barbiturates for acute traumatic brain injury (Review). Cochrane Libr (4):1–23

Schwartz M, Tator C, Towed D et al (1984) The University of Toronto head injury treatment study: a prospective randomized comparison of pentobarbital and mannitol. Can J Neurol Sci 11:434–440

Ward JD, Becker DP, Miller JD et al (1985) Failure of prophylactic barbiturate coma in the treatment of severe head injury. J Neurosurg 62:383–388

Blood Pressure, CO_2 and Oxygen Saturation

26

Bent Lob Dahl

Recommendations

Level I

There are insufficient data to support a level I recommendation for blood pressure, oxygenation and hyperventilation.

Level II

Blood pressure should be monitored and hypotension (systolic blood pressure <90 mmHg) avoided.

Level III

Normal oxygenation is recommended.

Oxygenation should be monitored and hypoxemia (PaO_2<60 mmHg (8 kPa) or O_2 saturation <90%) avoided.

26.1 Overview

Secondary insults after traumatic brain injury should be avoided. The injured brain is probably more prone to ischemia because of insufficient cellular oxygen delivery, when blood pressure and oxygen saturation is insufficient. Experimental studies indicate that cerebral hypoxia, apart from low arterial blood oxygen tension (PaO_2), is related to cerebral hypoperfusion.

Measurement of cerebral oxygenation has either temporal (MRI, Xe-CT) or spatial (jugular bulb oxygen saturation – $SjvO_2$, brain tissue partial pressure of oxygen – $PtiO_2$, microdialysis, near-infrared spectroscopy – NIRS and transcranial Doppler – TCD) limitations, especially in the initial acute treatment of TBI patients where such measurements have marginal value. The best possible way to ensure sufficient cerebral oxygenation in the acute setting is to control blood pressure, blood oxygen saturation and to maintain normocapnia.

Retrospective data of 717 patients with GCS<9 from the Traumatic Coma Data Bank showed that hypoxemia ($PaO_2 \leq 60$ mmHg) and hypotension (SBP≤90 mmHg) were independently associated with a significant increase in morbidity and mortality from severe head injury in the prehospital setting (Chesnut et al. 1993). Hypotension was associated with a doubling in mortality.

For ethical reasons, a prospective controlled study of the effect of hypoxemia and oxygenation has never been done and will probably never be done. However, clinical intuition and retrospective data indicate that correction of hypotension and hypoxia improves outcome.

B.L. Dahl
Department of Neuroanaesthesia and Neurocritical care, Aarhus University Hospital, Noerrebrogade 8000, Aarhus C, Denmark
e-mail: bentdahl@rm.dk

T. Sundstrøm et al. (eds.), *Management of Severe Traumatic Brain Injury*, DOI 10.1007/978-3-642-28126-6_26, © Springer-Verlag Berlin Heidelberg 2012

Tips, Tricks, and Pitfalls

- Vigorous evaluation and stabilisation of the patient according to ABC principles (American College of Surgeons 1997).
- Start with non-invasive monitoring of blood pressure, oxygen saturation and $ETCO_2$ and, when suitable, arterial blood gas and invasive measurement of blood pressure.
- Maintain SBP > 120 mmHg or MAP > 90 mmHg.
- Maintain oxygen saturation >95 or PaO_2 > 10 kPa.
- PEEP = 2–5 mmHg.
- Avoid hypotonic solutions (glucose).
- Hypertonic saline might correct hypotension (see individual chapter).
- Maintain normocapnia ($PaCO_2$ = 4.5–5.0 kPa).
- Maintain normothermia (36.5–38°C).
- In case of clinical signs of increased ICP (decrease in GCS ≥ 2, pupil abnormalities or paralysis of extremities), immediate hyperventilation ($PaCO_2$ 3.5–4.0 kPa), perhaps supplemented with mannitol (0.5–1 g/kg) or hypertonic saline (7.2%, 100–200 ml).
- In patients with possible hypovolaemia, hypertonic saline is preferable to mannitol to avoid osmotic diuresis and worsening of hypovolaemia.
- Reverse Trendelenburg position 0–15°.
- Head in neutral position.
- Indwelling catheter with the goal of a diuresis of 1 ml/kg/h.
- If volume treatment of the trauma patient only transiently or not at all stabilises vital parameters, ongoing bleeding must be suspected.
- Naso- or orogastric tube (nasogastric tube is contraindicated in suspicion of skull base fracture).

26.2 Background

TBI is divided in two separate events. The primary injury is the result of mechanical forces at the time of injury, resulting in damage to neurons, glia cells and vascular tissue. This leads to disruption of cell membranes and disturbance of ionic homeostasis (Stiefel et al. 2005) causing a neurotoxic cascade. Only preventive measures can avoid this. The secondary injury is the result of ischemia and possibly an acceleration of the initial events and calls for immediate and appropriate treatment. Hypotension and hypoxia might influence outcome in a negative direction. As it is unethical to perform randomised, prospective trials on the effect of hypotension and hypoxia, our recommendations are based on class II and III evidence.

26.2.1 Hypoxemia

The oxygen consumption of the brain ($CMRO_2$) is approximately 3–3.5 ml/100 g/min or 40–50 ml oxygen per minute. The oxygen reserve of the brain is very limited, and cessation of blood flow will lead to unconsciousness in 10–15 s.

In prospectively collected data from the Traumatic Coma Data Bank (TCDB), hypoxemia occurred in 22.4% of severe TBI patients and was significantly associated with increased morbidity and mortality (Chesnut et al. 1993). Duration of hypoxemia was studied in a subgroup of 71 in-hospital patients with TBI of varying degrees of severity. Duration of hypoxemia (defined as SaO_2 < 90%; median duration ranging from 11.5 to 20 min) was found to be an independent predictor of mortality, but not morbidity (Jones et al. 1994).

In patients with severe head injury (GCS 3–8), it is therefore important to administer high-flow oxygen, secure the airway under C-spine control and to ventilate the patient as soon as possible. Always consider the possibility of pneumo- or haemothorax in trauma patients. The effect of positive end-expiratory pressure (PEEP) has been controversial, as it might decrease MAP and increase ICP leading to a reduction in CPP. Mascia et al. (2005) found no increase in ICP during alveolar recruitment.

26.2.2 Hypotension

In patients with TBI, cerebral autoregulation, which normally secures CBF within a certain range of blood pressure, is compromised, leading to a linear correlation between blood pressure and CBF. Low blood pressure therefore might decrease CBF.

In the study from TCDB, a single observation of SBP<90 mmHg was an independent predictor of outcome and in fact was associated with increased morbidity and a doubling of mortality (Chesnut et al. 1993). Other studies show similar results (Gentleman 1992; Hill et al. 1993; Jeffreys and Jones 1981; Kohi et al. 1984; Miller and Becker 1982; Miller et al. 1978; Narayan et al. 1982; Pietropaoli et al. 1992; Rose et al. 1977; Seelig et al. 1986; Struchen et al. 2001).

Duration and number of hypotensive events might also influence outcome. Duration of episodes of hypotension was a significant, independent factor of mortality and morbidity (Jones et al. 1994).

In trauma patients, hypotension is caused by hypovolaemia until proven otherwise. However, one must always consider tension pneumothorax and cardiac tamponade. Other forms of shock in trauma patients are rare but might be the primary reason for the trauma (allergic, cardiogenic, neurogenic or septic shock).

Two i.v. lines must be inserted with rapid infusion of normotonic saline. Visible bleeding must be stopped immediately. Internal bleeding must be excluded or treated as soon as possible. According to ATLS, the response to volume treatment must be monitored continuously to guide volume therapy as well as the stability of the patient. If volume treatment only transiently or not at all stabilises vital parameters, ongoing bleeding must be suspected.

Until now, a positive effect of hypothermia as a neuroprotective measure in TBI patients has failed to be proven. In order to minimise haemorrhagic diathesis, it is important to avoid hypothermia.

26.2.3 CO_2

ET CO_2 should be monitored continuously, at least after intubation, and should be evaluated by serial arterial blood gas analyses. CO_2 reactivity averages a change in CBF of 2.5 ml/100 g/min/mmHg change in $PaCO_2$ (Cold 1990). The theoretical effects of hyperventilation are summarised in Fig. 26.1.

Hyperventilation is discussed in detail in Chap. 53. Prophylactic hyperventilation ($PaCO_2$ of 25 mmHg or less) is not recommended. Hyperventilation is recommended as a temporary measure for the reduction of elevated intracranial pressure (ICP). Hyperventilation should be avoided during the first 24 h after injury when cerebral blood flow (CBF) often is critically reduced. If hyperventilation is used, jugular venous oxygen saturation (SjO_2) or brain tissue oxygen tension ($PbrO_2$) measurements can be used to monitor oxygen delivery.

26.3 Specific Paediatric Concerns

Resuscitation and stabilisation of the cardiovascular and respiratory systems in the field, during transfer and in the hospital need to be emphasised in an effort to optimise outcome from severe paediatric brain injury (Adelson et al. 2003).

Children are more susceptible to trauma. They differ from adults in that they have shorter trachea, softer epiglottis, large occiput and a soft chest wall and abdomen. The spleen and liver are not protected by costae, and children have a large body surface area compared to body mass; this leads easily to hypothermia.

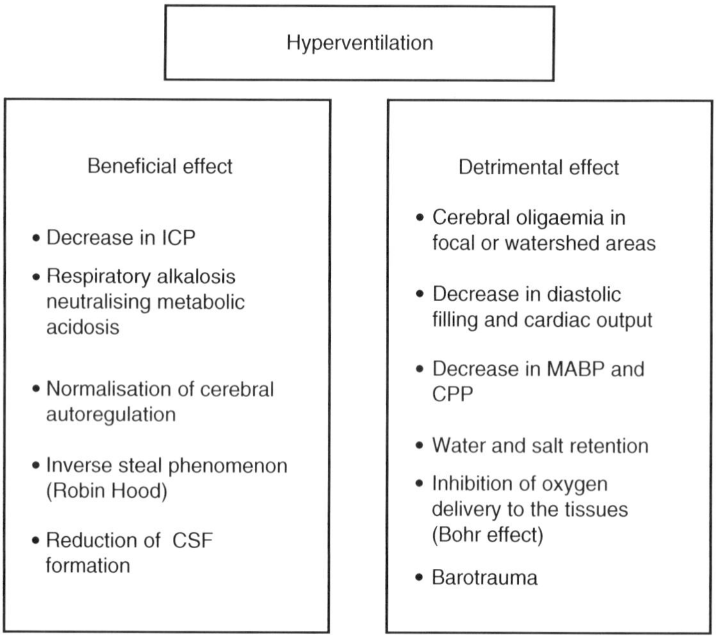

Fig. 26.1 Beneficial and detrimental effects of induced hyperventilation effects of hyperventilation (Cold 1990)

Table 26.1 Lower limits of normal systolic blood pressure at different ages

Age	Minimal systolic blood pressure
0–28 days	>60 mmHg
1–12 months	>70 mmHg
1–10 years	>70 + 2 × age in years mmHg
>10 years	>90 mmHg

Hypotension (Table 26.1) and hypoxemia should be avoided in children as well as in adults. Hypotension is a late sign of shock in children (>45% blood loss). Tachycardia, decreased urinary output and skin manifestations (cold, clammy, cyanotic, pale skin or increased capillary filling (>2 s)) are earlier signs of hypovolaemia (American College of Surgeons 1997).

Hypoxia in children is defined as $PaO_2 < 60–65$ mmHg (8–8.7 kPa) or O_2 saturation <90%. Desaturation occurs more rapidly in children than in adults, therefore oxygen saturation >95 or $PaO_2 > 10$ kPa is recommended.

Priorities in evaluation and treatment for traumatised patients (ABCDE) are the same for children and adults (American College of Surgeons 1997).

References

Adelson PD, Bratton SL, Carney NA et al (2003) Guidelines for the acute medical management of severe traumatic brain injury in infants, children and adolescents. Pediatric Crit Care Med 4(3 Suppl):S1–S491. http://tbiguidelines.org/glHome.aspx

Chesnut RM, Marshall LF, Klauber MR et al (1993) The role of secondary brain injury in determining outcome from severe head injury. J Trauma 34:216–222

Cold GE (1990) Cerebral blood flow in acute head injury. The regulation of cerebral blood flow and metabolism during the acute phase of head injury and its significance for therapy. Acta Neurochir Suppl 49:1–66

Gentleman D (1992) Causes and effects of systemic complications among severely head-injured patients transferred to a neurosurgical unit. Int Surg 77:297–302

Hill DA, Abraham KJ, West RH (1993) Factors affecting outcome in the resuscitation of severely injured patients. Aust N Z J Surg 63:604–609

Jeffreys RV, Jones JJ (1981) Avoidable factors contributing to the death of head injury patients in general hospitals in Mersey Region. Lancet 2:459–461

Jones PA, Andrews PJD, Midgely S et al (1994) Measuring the burden of secondary insults in head injured patients during intensive care. J Neurosurg Anesthesiol 6:4–14

Kohi YM, Mendelow AD, Teasdale GM et al (1984) Extracranial insults and outcome in patients with acute head injury – relationship to the Glasgow Coma Scale. Injury 16:25–29

Mascia L, Grasso S, Fiore T et al (2005) Cerebro-pulmonay interactions during the application of low levels of positive end-expiratory pressure. Intensive Care Med 31:373–379

Miller JD, Becker DP (1982) Secondary insults to the injured brain. J R Coll Surg Edinb 27:292–298

Miller JD, Sweet RC, Narayan R et al (1978) Early insults to the injured brain. JAMA 240:439–442

Narayan R, Kishore P, Becker D et al (1982) Intracranial pressure: to monitor or not to monitor? A review of our experience with head injury. J Neurosurg 56:650–659

Pietropaoli JA, Rogers FB, Shackford SR et al (1992) The deleterious effects of intraoperative hypotension on outcome in patients with severe head injuries. J Trauma 33:403–407

Rose J, Valtonen S, Jennett B (1977) Avoidable factors contributing to death after head injury. Br Med J 2:615–618

Seelig JM, Klauber MR, Toole BM et al (1986) Increased ICP and systemic hypotension during the first 72 hours following severe head injury. In: Miller JD, Teasdale GM, Rowan JO et al (eds) Intracranial pressure VI. Springer, Berlin, pp 675–679, 1996;40:764–767

Stiefel MF, Tomita Y, Marmarou A (2005) Secondary ischemia impairing the ion homeostasis following traumatic brain injury. J Neurosurg 103:707–714

Struchen MA, Hannay HJ, Contant CF et al (2001) The relation between acute physiological variables and outcome on the Glasgow Outcome Scale and Disability Rating Scale following severe traumatic brain injury. J Neurotrauma 18:115–125

Intracranial Pressure Reduction

27

Bent Lob Dahl

Recommendations

The Brain Trauma Foundation guidelines do not specifically deal with the peroperative period. In this chapter, however, the recommendations from the Brain Trauma Foundation concerning indications for intracranial pressure monitoring, intracranial pressure monitoring technology, and intracranial pressure thresholds are transferred to the peroperative setting. See Chap. 30 for details.

27.1 Overview

Elevated ICP should be anticipated in patients with traumatic brain injury. Peroperatively, ICP should be measured on wide indications and treatment should be instituted if ICP increases to more than 20 mmHg. The control of intracranial hypertension (ICP>20 mmHg) is based on the control of intracranial blood volume either via control of cerebral venous distension (central venous pressure, neck compression) or control by physiologic mechanisms including the chemical ($PaCO_2$, PaO_2, indomethacin, theophyllamine), neurogenic or hormonal (catecholamine), metabolic (hypnotics, analgesics, hypothermia), and autoregulatory control of cerebral circulation. Control of cerebral tissue water content is possible by osmotic-acting drugs like mannitol and hypertonic saline. During anaesthesia, it is important to have and apply a thorough understanding of the intracranial pathophysiology in order to avoid and treat intracranial hypertension in adults as well as in children.

B.L. Dahl
Department of Neuroanaesthesia and Neurocritical care, Aarhus University Hospital, Noerrebrogade 8000, Aarhus C, Denmark
e-mail: bentdahl@rm.dk

Tips, Tricks, and Pitfalls

- ICP control calls for preoperative planning, careful peroperative management in order to avoid ICP hypertension, and a treatment plan in case of ICP hypertension.

Anaesthesia planning:

- Planning of anaesthesia for patients with severe traumatic brain injury must always be in close collaboration with the neurosurgeon.
- Anticipate that increased ICP might occur during surgery.
- Measure ICP, if possible. Ask the neurosurgeon if the dura is tense before opening.
- Use trauma mechanism, clinical examination, age, GCS, motor posturing, and CT findings to evaluate the risk of increased intracranial pressure if actual measurement is not possible.
- Consider ICP measurement during anaesthesia for acute trauma surgery, even for patients with a normal cerebral CT scan.

T. Sundstrøm et al. (eds.), *Management of Severe Traumatic Brain Injury*,
DOI 10.1007/978-3-642-28126-6_27, © Springer-Verlag Berlin Heidelberg 2012

Anaesthesia basics:

- Normoventilation $PaCO_2$=4.5–5.5 kPa (35–40 mmHg).
- Always head in neutral position if possible.
- Always check cervical collar for neck pressure.
- Always reverse Trendelenburg position (rTP) 5–15° elevation of head.
- Keep ICP below 20 mmHg, CPP over 60 mmHg.
- Dura tension should be evaluated by the surgeon before opening of dura.
- Treat high dura tension or ICP immediately.

Anaesthesia ICP problems:

- Treat ICP above 20 mmHg:
  - Is anaesthesia deep enough?
  - Keep head in neutral position.
  - Increase rTP to 15°.
  - Increase ventilation to CO_2 approximately 4 kPa (30 mmHg) or 3.5 kPa (26 mmHg) very shortly.
  - Mannitol 0.25–1 g/kg (beware of osmotic diuresis especially in hypovolaemic patients).
  - Hypertonic saline 7.2%. Twenty millilitre to 100 ml in repeated doses (beware of existing hyponatremia). In the intensive care setting, small doses of 20–100 ml 7.2% NaCl usually control ICP.
  - Ask surgeon for surgical possibility to remove mass lesion.

27.2 Background

In the analysis of peroperative anaesthesia and ICP control, the guidelines from Brain Trauma Foundation are of much value, although these guidelines do not have anaesthesia as its primary aim. The basis of this chapter has to rely on scientific evidence, basic physiology, experience, and common sense in the absence of level I evidence. Therefore, it is imperative to understand the relationship between cerebral blood flow (CBF), mean arterial blood pressure (MABP), cerebral perfusion pressure (CPP), intracranial pressure (ICP), and the clinical examination.

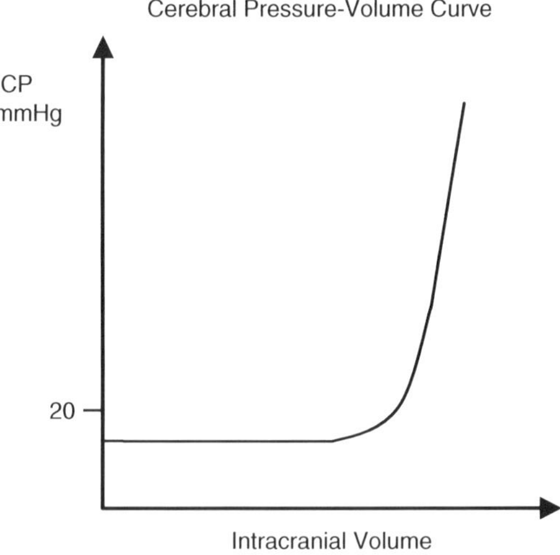

Fig. 27.1 Relationship between intracranial volume and intracranial pressure (*ICP*). During the initial intracranial volume increase, ICP is fairly constant because of compensatory mechanisms. When these mechanisms are exhausted, even small increases in volume lead to a marked increase in ICP

The Monro–Kellie doctrine, formulated in the 1820s, indicates that the cranium is a nonexpendable box containing the brain, cerebrospinal fluid (CSF), and arterial and venous blood volume. CSF is formed at a rate of 0.3 ml/min. The total amount of CSF is 140–200 ml, with 25–35 ml in the ventricular system and the rest in the cerebral and spinal subarachnoid spaces. ICP is fairly constant, as it is regulated by changes mainly in blood volume and CSF. In traumatic brain injury, an intracranial haemorrhage or oedema may develop. If the compensatory changes in blood volume and CSF are exhausted, ICP may increase rapidly even with minor changes in intracranial volume, as indicated in the pressure–volume curve (Fig. 27.1).

CPP is the difference between mean arterial blood pressure and ICP (CPP=MABP−ICP). Normally, cerebral autoregulation (Fig. 27.2) insures CBF of 50 ml/100 g brain/min (750 ml/min) within a range of MABP of approximately 50–160 mmHg. Below 50 mmHg CBF declines rapidly and EEG becomes iso-electric. At CBF

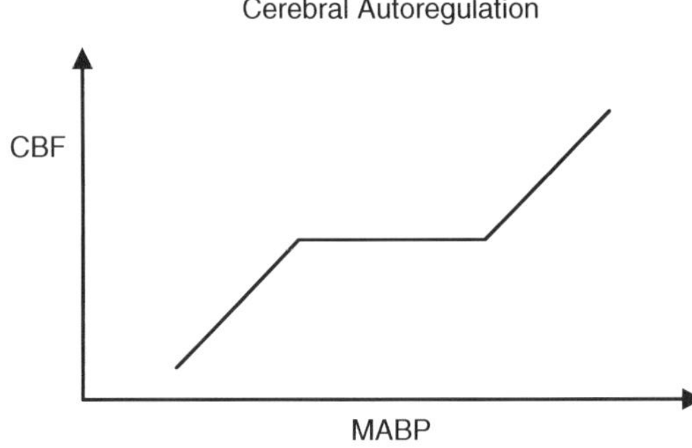

Fig. 27.2 Cerebral autoregulation. CBF of 50 ml/100 g/min are maintained in a range of MABP between 50 and 160 mmHg. Below 50 mmHg, CBF decreases, and above 160 mmHg, CBF increases

5 ml/100 g/min, irreversible cell death happens. MABP above 160 mmHg leads to an increase in CBF, which again increases cerebral blood volume and ICP and possibly adds to formation of cerebral oedema.

In the injured brain, cerebral autoregulation may be abolished, globally or locally. As a consequence, there will be a direct correlation between blood pressure and cerebral blood flow.

As a result of increased ICP, brain herniation might occur leading to further arterial compromise and pressure on brain tissue and nerves leading to a decline in GCS, pupillary abnormalities and/or paralysis. Cushing's response (increase in blood pressure and bradycardia in order to maintain CPP) is, compared to clinical changes, a late sign of high ICP.

Anaesthesiologists dealing with trauma patients must be aware that an increase in ICP might occur. In a prospective study of comatose patients with abnormal CT scans, the incidence of intracranial hypertension was 53–63%. If patients with normal CT scans demonstrated two or three adverse features (age >40 years, unilateral or bilateral posturing, or systolic blood pressure <90 mmHg), the risk of intracranial hypertension was similar to that of patients with abnormal CT scans. In patients with normal CT scans, intracranial hypertension was found in 13% of patients (Narayan et al. 1982). Before performing anaesthesia in a trauma patient, the demand for monitoring ICP must be evaluated. If there are signs of brain injury or intracranial hypertension, ICP must be monitored during surgery. In a retrospective study, Miller et al. (2004) found that even midline shift, basal cisterns, ventricular effacement, sulci compression, and grey/white matter contrast did not correlate with the initial ICP.

Intracranial hypertension is a leading cause of death in severe TBI. A randomized clinical trial of ICP monitoring with and without treatment will probably never be done; however, data suggest that normalisation of ICP improves outcome. It is generally accepted that intracranial hypertension must be treated regardless of whether it is actually monitored or diagnosed on clinical suspicion alone. Not monitoring ICP while treating for intracranial hypertension can be deleterious and result in poor outcome. How to measure ICP is described in Chaps. 23 and 30. A ventricular catheter connected to an external strain gauge transducer is the most accurate method of monitoring ICP. Parenchymal transducers are good alternatives, while subarachnoid or subdural fluid coupled devices and epidural devises are less accurate. The threshold for ICP is 20 mmHg, above which treatment to lower ICP generally is recommended.

27.2.1 Perioperative Management of ICP

Neuroanaesthesia is different from anaesthesia for other procedures in the way that both the surgeon and the anaesthesiologist work on the same organ – the brain. Removal of mass lesions might reduce the risk of intracranial hypertension but is not always possible if the main reason for intracranial hypertension is cerebral swelling due to oedema or increased cerebral blood volume. The control of intracranial hypertension under such circumstances is based on the control of intracranial blood volume; see Chap. 52 for details.

A large study on mainly tumour patients and subarachnoid haemorrhage patients gives a good picture of how intracranial hypertension is treated in clinical practice (Cold 2008). The ICP-reducing procedures most frequently used were (Table 27.1):

Table 27.1 In a study of 1,833 patients, the most frequently used measures to reduce ICP hypertension were reverse Trendelenburg position, hyperventilation, cyst puncture, and mannitol (Cold 2008)

Procedure	Number of patients	Percent of total
Reverse Trendelenburg position (rTP)	188	10.3
Hyperventilation	168	9.2
Decompression (drainage or cyst puncture)	74	4.0
Mannitol	56	3.1

Only 0.8% of the patients were treated for traumatic brain injury (TBI). However, there is no reason to believe that the treatment modalities are different in TBI. It is important to avoid hypotension, hypoxia, and ICP hypertension during the pre-, per-, and the postoperative period.

27.2.2 Pre- and Postoperative Period

In the pre- and postoperative period, it is important to anticipate ICP problems when planning premedication and pain management as sedation might induce hypoventilation leading to hypercapnia and increase in ICP. If ICP is not monitored, clinical symptoms and CT findings are used for evaluation of the risk of increased ICP.

27.2.3 Positive End-Expiratory Pressure (PEEP)

Adult respiratory distress syndrome develops in up to 20% of patients with severe head injury. Positive end-expiratory pressure (PEEP) is often required to maintain oxygenation; however, PEEP might influence ICP through decreased venous outflow as well as venous return and reduced arterial blood pressure. The effect of PEEP is mainly investigated in the ICU setting, and the results are conflicting. Coughing, Valsalva manoeuvre, application of PEEP and CPAP, and neck compression are supposed to increase ICP. Even application of a cervical collar for immobilization might increase ICP (Raphael and Chotai 1994).

Table 27.2 The effect of application of 5 and 10 cm H_2O PEEP on BP, ICP, and CPP (Duch and Cold 2008)

	5 cm H_2O		10 cm H_2O	
	Before	After	Before	After
BP	70.9	68.2	75.3	72.3
ICP	5.7	6.7	5.1	8.2
CPP	65.4	61.5	70.2	65.1

When patients are kept in the 30° head-up position (rTP), PEEP improves arterial oxygenation without increasing ICP (Frost 1977). In a study including patients with head injury, SAH, or hydrocephalus, PEEP at 5 cm H_2O did not alter ICP, and the clinical relevance of ICP increase at PEEP levels of 10 and 15 cm H_2O was questionable, as CPP did not change and remained greater than 60 mmHg. Application of PEEP at 10 and 15 cm H_2O has been shown to produce an increase in ICP without significant effect on CPP (Videtta et al. 2002). Generally, PEEP is considered as a valuable therapy for the comatose patient with pulmonary disorders such as pneumonia or pulmonary oedema (Frost 1977). Peroperatively, the effect of PEEP 5 and 10 cm H_2O on BP, ICP, and CPP has been investigated mainly in tumour patients ($N = 13$) (Table 27.2).

The application of PEEP had a minor negative effect on BP, ICP, and CPP (Duch and Cold 2008). However, the magnitude of these changes has to be weighed against the possibly positive effect of PEEP on atelectasis and oxygenation.

27.2.4 Patient Position

27.2.4.1 Head Elevation

In one study, the decrease in ICP during head elevation was smaller than the decline in blood pressure resulting in a decrease in CPP (Rosner and Coley 1986). In another study, head elevation was not accompanied by a change in CPP because the decrease in ICP corresponded to the decrease in BP (Feldman et al. 1992). In comatose patients, CBF decreases gradually, with head elevation from 0° to 45°, from 46 to 29 ml/min/100 g. During head elevation, the difference between arterial pressure and jugular pressure was the major determinant of CBF regardless of head Position (Moraine et al. 2000).

27.2.4.2 Head Flexion, Rotation, and Tilting

Changes in head position, including maximal flexion and lateral rotation, lead to an increase in ICP, and elevation of the head induces an ICP reduction. The most alarming increase in ICP is observed during head-down position (Schneider et al. 1993; Mavrocordatos et al. 2000). The mechanisms are intracranial venous distension and an increase in cerebral blood volume (Mchedlishvili 1988; Schreiber et al. 2002). Some studies indicate that moderate flexion of the head 15–30° is associated with a decrease in ICP due to the improved venous drainage.

27.2.4.3 Reverse Trendelenburg Position (rTP)

If ICP is not already monitored during craniotomy, subdural pressure can be measured after opening the cranium but before opening the dura (Cold et al 1996). An i.v. needle is introduced under the dura and connected to a pressure monitor. Repeated measurements of subdural pressure and CPP at neutral position and at varying degrees of rTP between 5° and 15° can thus be obtained within a few minutes and a decision concerning optimal positioning, as regards both the level of ICP and CPP, can be drawn. The optimal position is defined as the position in which subdural ICP was as low as possible, with CPP remaining greater than 60 mmHg or as high as possible. In patients operated for cerebral aneurysms, a considerable individual variation in the optimal position from zero to 15° rTP was found. The optimal position was 10–15° rTP (Juul and Cold 2008). It is recommended to optimise the position in trauma patients as well.

27.2.4.4 Hyperventilation

Hyperventilation lowers ICP significantly independent of anaesthetic method, but the effect differs. It is effective during propofol–fentanyl, propofol–remifentanil, isoflurane–fentanyl, and sevoflurane–fentanyl anaesthesia. The effect was most pronounced during isoflurane/sevoflurane–fentanyl anaesthesia and less effective during propofol–remifentanil/fentanyl anaesthesia. The reason for the low CO_2 reactivity during propofol anaesthesia might be that CPP in propofol anaesthesia is lower and close to the reflection point on the pressure–volume curve where compensatory mechanisms are exhausted (Juul and Cold 2008). However, even though jugular bulb oxygen tension ($SjvO_2$) was significantly lower during propofol anaesthesia, ischemia has never been described, probably because of the neuroprotective properties of propofol. For more detailed information on hyperventilation, see Chap. 53.

27.2.4.5 Mannitol or Hypertonic Saline (HS)

Mannitol is effective in reducing ICP in the management of traumatic intracranial hypertension in doses of 0.25–1.0 g/kg body weight. Current evidence is not strong enough to make recommendations on the use, concentration, and method of administration of hypertonic saline for the treatment of traumatic intracranial hypertension. Hyponatraemia should be excluded before administration of HS to avoid neurological symptoms such as central pontine myelinolysis. Osmotherapy is discussed in detail in Chap. 54.

27.3 Specific Paediatric Concerns

The general treatment threshold of ICP is 20 mmHg. However, the treatment approach should be individualised and modified by the response. The modalities are principally the same as in adults. The patients should be properly sedated and positioned with the head in neutral position, $PaCO_2$ in the lower end of eucapnia ($PaCO_2$ 4.5 kPa (35 mmHg)), and CPP should be maintained according to age. If increased ICP occurs in spite of this, apply rTP of up to 30° in normovolaemic patients under ICP and CPP control and consider neuromuscular blockade. Proceed to CSF drainage and hyperosmolar therapy with mannitol (<320 mOsm/l) or hypertonic saline (<360 mOsm/l). If surgery and ICP-reducing therapy is still ineffective, apply further hyperventilation ($PaCO_2$=4–4.5 kPa (30–35 mmHg)). Treatment should now be guided by the CBF, $SjvO_2$, or $PtiO_2$ in the brain. If ICP is not normalised, you must proceed to second-tier therapy at the discretion of the treating doctors (hyperventilation to CO_2 = 30 mmHg, barbiturate coma, decompressive craniectomy) (Adelson et al. 2003).

References

Adelson PD, Bratton SL, Carney NA, et al (2003) Guidelines for the acute medical management of severe traumatic brain injury in infants, children and adolescents. Pediatric Crit Care Med 4(3 Suppl):S1–S491. http://tbiguidelines.org/glHome.aspx

Cold GE, Tange M, Jensen TM, Ottesen S (1996) Subdural pressure measurement during craniotomy. Correlation with tactile estimation of dural tension and brain herniation after opening of dura. Br J Neurosurg 1:69–75

Cold GE (2008) Material included in the database. In: Gold GE, Juul N (eds) Monitoring of cerebral and spinal haemodynamics during neurosurgery. Springer, Berlin/Heidelberg, pp 59–66

Duch B, Cold GE (2008) Effect of positive end-expiratory pressure on subdural intracranial pressure in patients undergoing supratentorial craniotomy. In: Cold GE, Juul N (eds) Monitoring of cerebral and spinal haemodynamics during neurosurgery. Springer, Berlin/Heidelberg, pp 255–272

Feldman Z, Kanter MJ, Robertson CS et al (1992) Effect of head elevation on intracranial pressure, cerebral perfusion pressure, and cerebral blood flow in head-injured patients. J Neurosurg 76:207–211

Frost EA (1977) Effects of positive end-expiratory pressure on intracranial pressure and compliance in brain-injured patients. J Neurosurg 47:195–200

Juul N, Cold GE (2008) Method. In: Cold GE, Juul N (eds) Monitoring of cerebral and spinal haemodynamics during neurosurgery. Springer, Berlin/Heidelberg, p 70

Miller MT, Pasquale M, Kurek S et al (2004) Initial head computerized tomographic scan characteristics have a linear relationship with intracranial pressure after trauma. J Trauma 56:967–972

Moraine J-J, Berré J, Mélot C (2000) Is cerebral perfusion pressure a major determinant of cerebral blood flow during head elevation in comatose patients with severe intracranial lesions? J Neurosurg 92:606–614

Narayan RK, Kishore PR, Becker DP et al (1982) Intracranial pressure: to monitor or not to monitor? A review of our experience with severe head injury. J Neurosurg 56:650–659

Raphael JH, Chotai R (1994) Effects of cervical collar on cerebrospinal fluid pressure. Anaesthesia 49:437–439

Mavrocordatos P, Bissonnette P, Ravussion P (2000) Effects of neck position and head elevation on intracranial pressure in anaesthetized neurosurgical patients: preliminary results. J Neurosurg Anesthesiol 12: 10–14

Mchedlishvili G (1988) Pathogenetic role of circulatory factors in brain oedema development. Neursurg Rev 11:7–13

Schneider GH, von Helden GH, Franke R, Lanksch WR, Unterberg A (1993) Influence of body position and cerebral perfusion pressure. Acta Neurochir 59:107–112

Schreiber SJ, Lambert UKW, Doepp F, Valdueza JM (2002) Effects of prolonged head-down tilt on internal jugular vein cross-sectional area. Br J Anaesth 89:769–771

Rosner MJ, Coley IB (1986) Cerebral perfusion pressure, intracranial pressure, and head elevation. J Neurosurg 65:636–641

Videtta W, Villarejo F, Cohen M et al (2002) Effects of positive end-expiratory pressure on intracranial pressure and cerebral perfusion pressure. Acta Neurochir Suppl 81:93–97

Part VII

Monitoring in Neurointensive Care

28 Secondary Clinical Assessment

Jacob Bertram Springborg and Vagn Eskesen

Recommendations

Level I

Data are insufficient to support Level I recommendations for this subject.

Level II

Data are insufficient to support Level II recommendations for this subject.

Level III

Repeated evaluation of consciousness and neurological status should be conducted. Clinical changes in neurointensive care patients should be correlated with the more advanced monitoring systems.

28.1 Overview

Repeated neurological examinations should be performed as part of the monitoring of the neurological dysfunction in the neurointensive care unit, taking into consideration the pharmacological treatment of the patient. Deteriorations should be correlated to changes in the supplementary physiological monitoring, and together these observations should guide clinical decisions.

J.B. Springborg (✉) • V. Eskesen
University Clinic of Neurosurgery,
Copenhagen University Hospital, Blegdamsvej 9,
2100 Copenhagen, Denmark
e-mail: jacob.springborg@rh.regionh.dk;
vagn.eskesen@rh.regionh.dk

Tips, Tricks, and Pitfalls

- Always take into consideration the current medication of the patient when evaluating the neurological state of the patient.
- The brainstem can anatomically be considered as a three-floor system.
- Detailed motor and sensory examinations are most often not possible or necessary in the neurointensive care unit.
- Correlate the objective findings to information from the more technical, physiological monitoring.

28.2 Background

Patients with severe TBI are as part of their treatment in the neurointensive care unit frequently under the influence of various analgesics, sedatives or muscle relaxants. Moreover, many of these patients are intubated and mechanically ventilated. Together, these conditions limit the clinical examination normally used to evaluate neurological function. Nevertheless, some form of basic clinical monitoring should, together with the more technical, physiological monitoring described in the next chapters, be initiated in the neurointensive care unit, and these repeated observations should guide clinical decisions.

T. Sundstrøm et al. (eds.), *Management of Severe Traumatic Brain Injury*,
DOI 10.1007/978-3-642-28126-6_28, © Springer-Verlag Berlin Heidelberg 2012

28.2.1 Measures of Consciousness

The level of consciousness must repeatedly be evaluated to appreciate clinical improvement or deterioration, of course taking into consideration the level of analgesia and sedation. The Glasgow Coma Scale (GCS) was originally designed to evaluate the severity of brain dysfunction in the early posttraumatic period in patients with TBI and not as a monitoring tool (Teasdale and Jennett 1974). Nevertheless, the three modalities tested are useful to monitor the depth and duration of impaired consciousness but should however always be reported with the three separate scores to appreciate in which modalities the patient has deficits (King et al. 2000). In intubated patients, the verbal score is untestable and the added GCS score is not applicable. Models have been designed to estimate the verbal score from the eye opening score and the motor score (Rutledge et al. 1996; Meredith et al. 1998), but the use of such models have been questioned (Chesnut 1997).

28.2.2 Symptoms and Signs Involving the Eyes and the Brain Stem

More comprehensive evaluations of the brainstem function should also be conducted, and for didactic reasons, the brainstem can be considered a three-floor system consisting of the midbrain (mesencephalon), pons and medulla oblongata.

Detailed examinations of the pupils and eyes should be repeated, and changes in pupil light reaction or diameter should be considered a warning sign of pathology close to or in the upper or middle brainstem or oculomotor nerve. The distinct pupillary abnormalities seen in lesions in or near the mesencephalon (dilated fixed pupils) and pons (pinpoint pupils) should be recognisable, as should the different horizontal eye deviation patterns seen in lesions in the frontal cortical (deviation towards lesion), midbrain (deviation towards lesion) and pontine (deviation away from lesion) gaze centres. Lesions in the medial longitudinal fasciculus cause internuclear ophthalmoplegia, which in the comatose patient is only assessable by testing the oculocephalic reflexes. Vertical eye deviation (downwards) can be seen with lesions in the mesencephalon and in more pronounced brainstem lesions, which may also cause skew deviation. In the unconscious patient, spontaneous roving eye movements may be present if the upper and middle brainstem is intact, as they depend on normal function of the oculomotor nuclei and connections from these. Different forms of nystagmus can be seen with lesions in the cerebellum and brainstem.

The oculocephalic and oculovestibular reflexes are anatomically complex but are mainly driven by signals from the semicircular canals via the vestibular nuclei located between the pons and medulla oblongata. From here they extend to the abducens and oculomotor nuclei in the pons and mesencephalon, and from these to the lateral and medial rectus muscles of the eyes. Preserved oculocephalic reflexes (‘doll's eyes') are normally present in the unconscious patient, whereas absent reflexes (‘fixed eyes') are seen in upper and middle brainstem lesions. In the conscious patient, the oculocephalic reflex is repressed and the eyes appear ‘fixed'. Caloric testing of the oculovestibular reflex with cold water is a strong stimulus, which in the unconscious patient results in conjugated eye movements towards the ear that is rinsed. Ice water is normally only used as part of the examination of brain death.

Middle brainstem (pontine) impairment can be further tested by the examination of the ciliary and cornea reflexes, which have an afferent limb in the trigeminal nerve and an efferent limb in the facial nerve with a relay in the middle brainstem. The reflexes disappear in deep coma and with lesions in the pons.

Lower brainstem dysfunction can be tested by an examination of the gag reflexes with an afferent limb in the glossopharyngeal nerve and an efferent limb in the vagus nerve, and the cough reflex with both an afferent and efferent limb in the vagus nerve. A formal assessment of lower brainstem dysfunction in the unconscious patient is often reserved for patients where brain death is suspected.

Finally, evaluation of respiratory function is also a test of brainstem function as the respiratory regulatory centre is anatomically located in this area (reticular formation). However, with controlled mechanical ventilation, the spontaneous respiratory pattern is not recognisable.

As part of the evaluation of the best motor response, a brief evaluation of the motor function of all four extremities should be performed and recorded. Abnormal flexion implies that the lesion is located in the cerebral hemispheres or internal capsule with disinhibition above the midbrain, and abnormal extension implies midbrain to upper pontine dysfunction (Matis and Birbilis 2008). The muscle tone, deep tendon reflexes and plantar reflexes are of less importance in the unconscious patient, but assessment can serve as baseline for later comparison. Especially side differences are important to recognise, as they are indicative of focal pathology. Moreover, repetitive testing of these modalities may reveal spinal cord or peripheral nerve lesions not appreciated in the initial evaluation of the patient or disclose improvements or deteriorations in such lesions.

A comprehensive examination of sensory modalities is most often not possible or necessary in the neurointensive management of patients with severe traumatic brain injury but should of course be performed in patients with coexistent spinal cord or peripheral nerve lesions as soon as the patient is able to cooperate.

The neurointensive care unit nurses should be trained in GCS scoring, and evaluation of the pupils and motor response, and instructions for the actions that should be taken when deterioration is observed, should be available. How often the different examinations should be performed depends on the clinical condition of the patient, the time from injury and the current treatment of the patient, e.g. extensive stimulation is not meaningful in a patient deeply sedated as part of intracranial pressure management.

28.3 Specific Paediatric Concerns

Standard GCS scoring of non-verbal children is inapplicable. Take into consideration the normal development of the central nervous system in children when evaluation the current neurological state.

References

Chesnut RM (1997) Appropriate use of the Glasgow Coma Scale in intubated patients: a linear regression prediction of the Glasgow verbal score from the Glasgow eye and motor scores. J Trauma 42:345

King BS, Gupta R, Narayan RK (2000) The early assessment and intensive care unit management of patients with severe traumatic brain and spinal cord injuries. Surg Clin North Am 80:855–870

Matis G, Birbilis T (2008) The Glasgow Coma Scale – a brief review. Past, present, future. Acta Neurol Belg 108:75–89

Meredith W, Rutledge R, Fakhry SM, Emery S, Kromhout-Schiro S (1998) The conundrum of the Glasgow Coma Scale in intubated patients: a linear regression prediction of the Glasgow verbal score from the Glasgow eye and motor scores. J Trauma 44:839–844

Rutledge R, Lentz CW, Fakhry S, Hunt J (1996) Appropriate use of the Glasgow Coma Scale in intubated patients: a linear regression prediction of the Glasgow verbal score from the Glasgow eye and motor scores. J Trauma 41:514–522

Teasdale G, Jennett B (1974) Assessment of coma and impaired consciousness. A practical scale. Lancet 2:81–84

A Neurological Wake-Up Test in the Neurointensive Care Unit: Pros and Cons

29

Niklas Marklund

Recommendations

Level I

There is no evidence to support a Level I recommendation for the use or avoidance of the neurological wake-up test in neurointensive care.

In general intensive care, there is Level I evidence that daily interruption of continuous i.v. sedation reduces intensive care unit stay and improves the outcome of mechanically ventilated patients.

Level II

There are insufficient data to support a Level II recommendation for the use of the wake-up test in neurointensive care.

Level III

The neurological wake-up test may provide important clinical information not obtained with other neurointensive care monitoring tools.

The neurological wake-up test leads to a modest increase in ICP and CPP in sedated, mechanically ventilated patients with TBI.

The neurological wake-up test leads to a mild biochemical stress response in TBI patients.

In a small subset of patients, the neurological wake-up test leads to marked increases in ICP and/or decreases in CPP.

A subgroup analysis of a small number of patients with severe TBI implies that the benefits of daily interruption of sedation observed in general intensive care may not be observed in patients with severe TBI.

29.1 Overview

Traumatic brain injury (TBI) induces a marked systemic biochemical stress response with the release of several stress-related hormones including cortisol and the catecholamines. A major aim of using continuous sedation in the neurointensive care unit (NIC) unit is to attenuate the TBI-induced stress response via reduction of the cerebral energy metabolic demands. In the era of modern multimodality monitoring and neuroimaging for patients with severe TBI, what is the role for repeated neurological evaluation, using a neurological wake-up test (NWT), of patients on continuous sedation and mechanical ventilation? In particular, does the information obtained by the NWT outweigh the risk of inducing a substantial stress response? The use of NWTs in NIC is controversial and is not mentioned in any recent TBI guidelines. Although daily interruption of continuous sedation is suggested for patients in general intensive care, reasons for not using the NWT in NIC may be a fear of an NWT-induced stress response and uncertainty to the additional value of NWTs in patients

N. Marklund
Department of Neurosurgery, Uppsala University Hospital, Uppsala 751 85, Sweden
e-mail: niklas.marklund@neuro.uu.se

T. Sundstrøm et al. (eds.), *Management of Severe Traumatic Brain Injury*,
DOI 10.1007/978-3-642-28126-6_29,

monitored with multimodality monitoring and frequent neuroradiological examinations. A recent survey showed that the use of NWT varies markedly in Scandinavian NIC units where half of the evaluated centres never use the NWT, whereas others use the NWT up to six times daily. In a series of studies characterising the NWT-induced stress response, the NWT was found to induce a significant increase in ICP and CPP in severe TBI patients on controlled ventilation. Additionally, the NWT caused an increase in adrenocorticotrophic (ACTH) hormone, catecholamine and cortisol levels. In the absolute majority of patients, the ICP and CPP changes were modest and transient and the absolute increases in stress hormone levels were small. However, the stress response was marked in a small subset of patients. These studies suggest that the NWT is safe in the majority of patients but that the test should be individualised and avoided in patients reacting with markedly increased ICP and/or decreased CPP. Although important clinical information may be obtained from the NWT, future studies need to evaluate the risk-benefit ratio of the NWT in TBI management.

Tips, Tricks, and Pitfalls

- Propofol sedation is ideal when the neurological wake-up test is used for repeated neurological evaluation of TBI patients.
- The neurological wake-up test provides useful information on the neurological status on each patient not readily obtained by other methods.
- In a subset of patients, the wake-up test may lead to increased ICP and/or reduced CPP.
- When performing the test, stop the continuous intravenous sedation and evaluate if the patient obeys commands (squeeze a hand, move a foot, raise arms etc.) according to the RLS-85 and/or the motor component of the GCS. If the patient does not obey commands, a painful stimulus at the angle of the jaw is delivered and the best motor response is noted.

29.2 Background

The description of the Glasgow Coma Scale in 1974 (Teasdale and Jennett 1974) provided clinicians with a tool for the evaluation of the level of consciousness in patients with severe TBI. Since that time, the increasing use of prehospital sedation, paralysis and intubation has resulted in difficulties in appropriately evaluating the level of consciousness in TBI patients. Unconscious TBI patients are frequently managed in the neurointensive care (NIC) setting using endotracheal intubation and controlled ventilation, and the majority of these patients will require continuous sedation, mechanical ventilation and monitoring of ICP and CPP. The use of modern multimodality monitoring and neuroimaging provides much information useful for the management of the TBI patient, and rapid technical developments in NIC during recent decades has extended the possibility of neuromonitoring from basic ICP and CPP measurement to brain neurochemistry (intracerebral microdialysis), brain tissue oxygen monitoring ($PbtiO_2$) and jugular venous oxygen saturation ($SjvO_2$). These monitoring tools help to control and maintain intracranial dynamics with the aim to prevent, detect and treat secondary insults known to exacerbate the primary injury (Tisdall and Smith 2007). Evaluation of the level of consciousness using the 'neurological wake-up test' (NWT; Skoglund et al. 2009) may be used as an additional monitoring tool during NIC of TBI patients to reveal important changes in the neurological condition of the patients, changes that can only be detected by a neurological examination (Helbok and Badjatia 2009). The reason to use NWT is thus to detect neuroworsening and delayed neurological deficits, well-known clinical problems in the care of TBI (Maas et al. 2008). In awake TBI patients, such as those with mild and moderate injuries at risk for neurological deterioration, frequent neurological evaluations are routine standard of care. During NIC of severely brain-injured patients, continuous sedation helps achieving ICP and CPP control and reduces the cerebral energy metabolic demands (Rhoney and Parker 2001). Since the NWT requires interruption of continuous sedation with an associated risk for a stress response, its use is controversial.

It has been stated that a third of intensive care unit (ICU) patients worldwide are mechanically ventilated accompanied by large doses of sedatives associated with significant morbidity. Since it was repeatedly shown that continuous IV sedation in general intensive care may increase the risk of ventilator-associated pneumonias, prolong mechanical ventilation and cause a higher mortality, daily interruption of continuous sedation was evaluated in several reports (Kollef et al. 1998; Girard et al. 2008; Ostermann et al. 2000; Wittbrodt 2005). A protocol of daily interruption of sedation and spontaneous breathing trials reduced duration of mechanical ventilation and length of stay in intensive care without increasing complication frequency (Kress et al. 2000). Additionally, incorporation of a daily sedation interruption policy significantly reduced ICU stay and days of mechanical ventilation, opioid administration and ICU complications without inducing long-term cognitive, psychological and adverse functional outcomes (Schweickert et al. 2004; Wittbrodt 2005; Girard et al. 2008; Jackson et al. 2010). Thus, these data strongly indicate that daily interruption of sedation decreases the duration of mechanical ventilation and improves outcome in medical intensive care patients (Kress et al. 2000; Girard et al. 2008). Still, some uncertainty of patient safety and risk for agitation has led to limited use of this sedation strategy, estimated to be used only in 30–40% of intensive care units (see Girard et al. 2008).

So, since interruption of continuous sedation in general ICU likely positively influences outcome, what about NIC? Currently, there is no strong evidence guiding NIC clinicians. To date, the only study addressing this sedation strategy is a recent randomised control trial where a small subgroup of 21 TBI patients did not show decreased ventilation or ICU days following daily interruption of continuous sedation (Anifantaki et al. 2009). In a recent survey of NIC units in Scandinavia, the use of the NWT differed markedly among centres from up to six times daily, whereas about 50% never used the NWT (Skoglund et al. 2011; Strömgren and Marklund 2003). One reason may be that midazolam, used in many of the evaluated Scandinavian centres, makes repeated NWTs more difficult than when continuous propofol sedation is used. Likely, more important reasons include a fear of inducing a NWT-induced stress response carrying a risk of inducing an additional stress to the vulnerable brain and the questioned additional value of NWTs in modern multimodality NIC.

In a series of recent studies, an evaluation of the NWT with the aim of characterising a possible NWT-induced stress response has been performed. Initially, changes in ICP and CPP in patients with severe TBI on controlled ventilation were evaluated. The ongoing propofol sedation was interrupted and a total of 127 NWTs were evaluated and the main findings were that the NWT induced a significant yet modest and transient increase in mean arterial blood pressure, heart rate, ICP and CPP (Skoglund et al. 2009; see Fig. 29.1). However, in a small subset of patients, the changes in CPP and ICP were marked and may have resulted in a secondary insult to the injured brain (Fig. 29.2). It was concluded that the NWT was safe in the majority of patients but that the test should be individualised and avoided in patients reacting with markedly increased ICP and/or decreased CPP (Skoglund et al. 2009).

TBI induces a marked systemic biochemical stress response with the release of several stress-related hormones including cortisol and the catecholamines (Clifton et al. 1981; Mautes et al. 2001; Bondanelli et al. 2005; Dimopoulou and Tsagarakis 2005). In a subsequent study, NWT-induced changes in adrenocorticotrophic hormone, cortisol, norepinephrine and epinephrine were studied (Skoglund et al. 2012). The NWT significantly increased all evaluated hormone levels when compared to those obtained during ongoing (baseline) propofol sedation, although the absolute increases were small. These studies support the notion that the NWT causes a biochemical stress response, the consequences of which remain undetermined, that is mild in the majority of patients.

In NIC, we must be cautious of the cerebral energy metabolic consequences of the TBI-induced stress response that may likely be increased by the NWT. In our NIC unit, we have much experience in using the NWT, performed

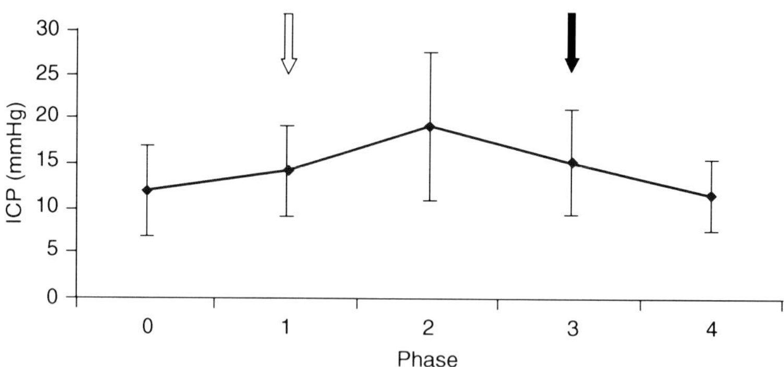

Fig. 29.1 Changes in ICP values during interruption of continuous propofol sedation and when performing the NWT. NWT-induced ICP changes in TBI patients (means ± SD). Compared to baseline values, the NWT procedure significantly increased ICP when propofol sedation was interrupted. *Phase 0*: baseline values; *phase 1*: continuous propofol sedation was interrupted (*white arrow*); *phase 2*: evaluation of the level of consciousness was performed; *phase 3*: propofol infusion was restarted (*black arrow*); *phase 4*: stable baseline levels were reached. A statistically significant difference, compared to phase 0 baseline values, is indicated with *asterisk* (Modified from Skoglund et al. (2009) and used with permission from the publisher)

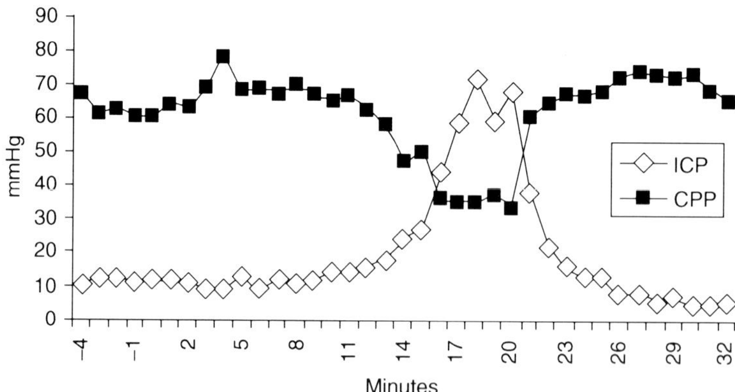

Fig. 29.2 An example with a marked ICP increase combined with a CPP decrease during the NWT is shown. This 19-year-old male sustained a severe TBI and presented in the emergency room with a Glasgow Motor Scale score of 2 and a dilated left pupil. Repeated CT scans showed minor contusion, a skull base fracture and diffuse brain swelling. The patient was treated in our NIC unit for 7 days using sedation, mechanical ventilation and ICP/CPP management. At long-term follow-up, the patient has made an excellent recovery (extended Glasgow outcome scale score of 8) (Used with permission from Skoglund et al. (2009))

by trained nurses and physicians on a regular basis, and the obtained information are key components of our clinical decision making. The central question is whether the (likely) minor risk of a detrimental stress response or metabolic distress in patients with severe TBI is counterbalanced by useful information gained by the NWT. Needless to say, medically unstable TBI patients with marked increases in ICP or decreases in ICP should not be evaluated using the NWT due to the risk of imposing a secondary insult. Although important information of the clinical condition of the patient can be obtained using the NWT, the benefits or risks associated with this test are yet unclear. Future studies may clarify the effects of the NWT on aspects of brain neurochemistry, blood flow and brain tissue oxygenation in addition to establishing the use of NWT in daily clinical decision making. To date, detailed evaluation of the stress response may help individualising the use and frequency of NWT and determine its role in the management of severe TBI.

29.3 Specific Paediatric Concerns

To date, there are no published data on the use of the NWT in paediatric TBI patients. Due to safety concerns, propofol is not approved for long-term continuous sedation in paediatric intensive care. Other sedative compounds frequently used for severe paediatric TBI (e.g. benzodiazepines, barbiturates) makes the NWT difficult or even impossible to perform. Although the NWT is not contraindicated in paediatric TBI, children may be more prone to react with marked ICP and/or CPP changes than adults. Thus, the NWT may be more difficult to implement as a monitoring tool in the routine management of severely injured paediatric TBI patients when compared to the adult setting.

References

Anifantaki S, Prinianakis G, Vitsaksaki E et al (2009) Daily interruption of sedative infusions in an adult medical-surgical intensive care unit: randomized controlled trial. J Adv Nurs 65:1054–1060

Bondanelli M, Ambrosio MR, Zatelli MC et al (2005) Hypopituitarism after traumatic brain injury. Eur J Endocrinol 152:679–691

Clifton GL, Ziegler MG, Grossman RG (1981) Circulating catecholamines and sympathetic activity after head injury. Neurosurgery 8:10–14

Dimopoulou I, Tsagarakis S (2005) Hypothalamic-pituitary dysfunction in critically ill patients with traumatic and nontraumatic brain injury. Intensive Care Med 31:1020–1028

Girard TD, Kress JP, Fuchs BD et al (2008) Efficacy and safety of a paired sedation and ventilator weaning protocol for mechanically ventilated patients in intensive care (Awakening and Breathing Controlled trial): a randomised controlled trial. Lancet 371:126–134

Helbok R, Badjatia N (2009) Is daily awakening always safe in severely brain injured patients? Neurocrit Care 11:133–134

Jackson DL, Proudfoot CW, Cann KF, Walsh T (2010) A systematic review of the impact of sedation practice in the ICU on resource use, costs and patient safety. Crit Care 14:R59

Kollef MH, Levy NT, Ahrens TS et al (1998) The use of continuous i.v. sedation is associated with prolongation of mechanical ventilation. Chest 114:541–548

Kress JP, Pohlman AS, O'Connor MF, Hall JB (2000) Daily interruption of sedative infusions in critically ill patients undergoing mechanical ventilation. N Engl J Med 342:1471–1477

Maas AI, Stocchetti N, Bullock R (2008) Moderate and severe traumatic brain injury in adults. Lancet Neurol 7:728–741

Mautes AE, Muller M, Cortbus F et al (2001) Alterations of norepinephrine levels in plasma and CSF of patients after traumatic brain injury in relation to disruption of the blood–brain barrier. Acta Neurochir (Wien) 143:51–57; discussion 57–58

Ostermann ME, Keenan SP, Seiferling RA, Sibbald WJ (2000) Sedation in the intensive care unit: a systematic review. JAMA 283:1451–1459

Rhoney DH, Parker D Jr (2001) Use of sedative and analgesic agents in neurotrauma patients: effects on cerebral physiology. Neurol Res 23:237–259

Schweickert WD, Gehlbach BK, Pohlman AS et al (2004) Daily interruption of sedative infusions and complications of critical illness in mechanically ventilated patients. Crit Care Med 32:1272–1276

Skoglund K, Enblad P, Marklund N (2009) Effects of the neurological wake-up test on intracranial pressure and cerebral perfusion pressure in brain-injured patients. Neurocrit Care 11:135–142

Skoglund K, Enblad P, Marklund N (2011) Monitoring and sedation differences in the management of severe head injury and subarachnoid hemorrhage in Scandinavian neurocritical care centers 1999–2009. EANN meeting, Blankenberge, 4–7 May 2011

Skoglund K, Enblad P, Marklund N (2012) Interruption of continuous sedation increases cortisol and ACTH levels in patients with severe TBI. Crit Care Med 40(1):216–222

Strömgren K, Marklund N (2003) The use of neurological examination in severely brain-injured patients – its use in Scandinavian Neurointensive Care Units and the influence on ICP and CPP. European Association of Neuroscience Nursing Congress (EANN), Copenhagen, 19–21 May 2003

Teasdale G, Jennett B (1974) Assessment of coma and impaired consciousness. A practical scale. Lancet 2:81–84

Tisdall MM, Smith M (2007) Multimodal monitoring in traumatic brain injury: current status and future directions. Br J Anaesth 99:61–67

Wittbrodt ET (2005) Daily interruption of continuous sedation. Pharmacotherapy 25:3S–7S

Intracranial Pressure (ICP) 30

Peter Reinstrup

Recommendations

Level I

There are insufficient data to support a Level I recommendation for this topic.

Level II

There are insufficient data to support a Level II recommendation for this topic.

Level III

ICP monitoring is recommended and even mandatory when manipulating the cerebral perfusion pressure (CPP) following traumatic brain injury (TBI) as well as in patients with subarachnoidal haemorrhage (SAH) and suspected hydrocephalus. On the other hand, there is a report claiming that the use of an ICP device by itself reduces outcome; this finding can however be due to the treatment in the ICP group.

P. Reinstrup
Department of Intensive and Perioperative Care, Skanes University Hospital, S221 85 Lund, Sweden
e-mail: peter.reinstrup@med.lu.se

30.1 Overview

Monitoring brain functions is difficult in comatose patients. Continuous ICP recording is of value in cases of severe head trauma since the therapy of head-injured patients aims at preventing secondary injuries due to an elevated ICP and/or a low cerebral perfusion pressure. Insertion of an ICP device should be considered following intracranial surgery if complications are estimated as probable and, in a limited number of cases, also for evacuation of CSF, as well as for the differentiation between normal and low-pressure states. In cases of a subarachnoidal bleeding, it is recommended to insert a ventricular catheter not only as a means for ICP measurements, but also since the possibility to drain ventricular fluid might be compulsory.

Under normal circumstances, the pressure is isobaric throughout the intrathecal fluid system when measured at a similar level, i.e. with the patient in a supine position. Pathological conditions like foramina Monroi cysts or limited flow in the aqueduct may lead to differences between ventricular and spinal pressures. Local changes may exist between the supratentorial and infratentorial parenchyma and even between different sites in the same compartment.

Gold standard for continuous ICP measurement is a ventricular catheter connected to an external pressure transducer, the alternative being a parenchymatous pressure device. Readings from the latter might however deviate from the true ICP values; knowing that even small changes in ICP can have a dramatic impact on the patient, these deviations may have clear consequences on outcome.

T. Sundstrøm et al. (eds.), *Management of Severe Traumatic Brain Injury*,
DOI 10.1007/978-3-642-28126-6_30, © Springer-Verlag Berlin Heidelberg 2012

Tips, Tricks, and Pitfalls

- If the ventricles are visible on the CT scan, insertion of a ventricular ICP device should always be considered.
- If a parenchymatous device is to be used, always assess the credibility of the reading by comparing with a recent CT scan.
- While most departments agree on an upper limit for a normal ICP of 20 mmHg, inter-centre differences in ICP zero point choices will influence this limit and hence the estimated CPP.
- Ventricular ICP recording curves should always oscillate. Should the amplitude diminish, the following causes have to be excluded: misplacement of the catheter tip, air in the tubings, clotting of the catheter, or a collapse of the entire ventricular system (Fig. 30.1).
- Is an elevated ICP as such deleterious for the brain? An upper limit for damages, solely related to an elevated ICP, has not been possible to establish, but it is generally accepted that an ICP higher than 20 mmHg is abnormal. An ICP above 40 mmHg is always associated with neurological symptoms such as impaired consciousness accompanied by abnormal electrical activity (EEG) as well as dilatation of the pupil. A persisting pressure above 60 mmHg is fatal.
- ICP and brain death? Supratentorial blood flow comes to an arrest when mean ICP approaches the systolic arterial blood pressure. Since clinical brain death criteria are based on the loss of function of the cranial nerves emanating from the infratentorial space, it is possible to have a supratentorial ICP indicating abolished circulation with preserved functions in these nerves.
- Transcranial Doppler (TCD) can be an aid in the decision whether an ICP device is necessary or not. Pulsatility index (PI) of the flow velocity correlates to some extent with the ICP.
- It is generally recommended to place the ICP device in the non-dominant hemisphere, but in cases of acute subdural hematomas, the highest, and therefore most relevant, pressure is found in the affected hemisphere (Chambers et al. 1998).

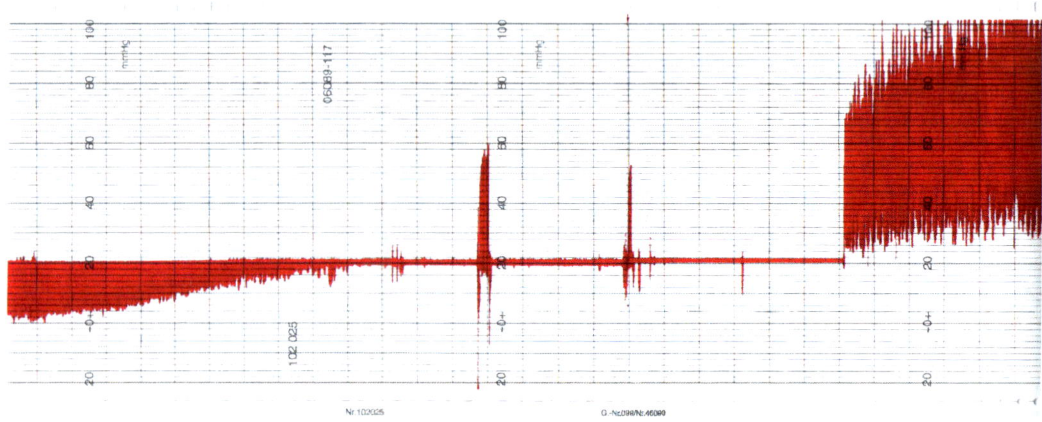

Fig. 30.1 ICP registration from a patient with an open ventricular pressure device shown in mmHg and with 5 min between *vertical lines*, events going from *left to right*. The amplitude of the ICP diminishes to zero around the drainage level of 20 mmHg. The drainage is closed at three occasions. During closure the correct ICP is registered. Following the two first closures, the drainage is again opened and the ICP curve follows the drainage level of 20 mmHg, whereas at the third closure on the *right side* of the registration, the line is kept closed and mean ICP approaches 60 mmHg

30.2 Background

Magendie observed already in 1,842 that the pressure in a meningocele sac in infants with spina bifida was transmitted to the fontanel and that a high pressure in this system caused loss of consciousness. Key and Retziug (1875) were the first to measure, and Knoll (1886) to record, ICP in animals. Quincke (1891) introduced lumbar puncture to the clinic, opening up for studies of ICP using this route. Our present knowledge of brain physiology and pathophysiology is, to a large extent, based on continuous measurements of ICP. Under normal circumstances, there is a uniform pressure in the intrathecal fluid (Koskinen) if measured at similar levels. However, local changes can exist in the parenchyma and differences in ICP exist between the infratentorial and supratentorial compartments, and this divergence is changing over time (Slavin and Misra 2003). ICP correlates to changes in tissue oedema (intracellular and/or interstitial), changes in the amount of liquor, and/or cerebral blood volume (CBV) (including bleeding) of a certain dignity.

30.2.1 Ventricular ICP Monitoring

The ventricular pressure was first measured in humans by Hodgson in 1928. Lundberg (1960) developed the equipment for continuous measurement of ventricular ICP in the late 1950s, and this is the technique still utilized for ventricular pressure measurements and drainage. This is considered the gold standard for measuring ICP, using tubing from the ventricular system to an extracranial pressure transducer which must be positioned at a fixed reference point on the head. The chosen reference point for the zero level of this pressure device differs between centres. The technique originally described by Lundberg builds on a reference zero point at the highest point of the head out of practical reasons. With such a set-up, the true ICP value is underestimated with approximately 5 mmHg as compared to when the zero reference point is positioned at the midhead or when compared to the various parenchymatous devices, which all have the zero point at the tip of the catheter. The parenchymatous ICP readings may therefore vary within small limits (0–10 mmHg), depending of the placement of the catheter tip and position of the head.

30.2.2 Complications with Non-parenchymatous Devices

The risk of infection is approximately 1% per day with an intraventricular ICP catheter. In the clinic, you get a feeling that it is the drainage of liquor per se that causes the ventriculitis (Rossi et al. 1998). Since drainage is most common in patients with blood in the ventricular system, the blood itself could act as a growth medium. Though rare, the insertion procedure of these catheters might also give rise to complications, such as intraparenchymatous bleedings and cerebrospinal fluid leakage (Guyott et al. 1998; Rossi et al. 1998); if possible, a normal coagulation screening test should be obtained before inserting a catheter.

In an attempt to overcome the drawbacks associated with ventricular ICP measurements, a variety of extraventricular devices has been developed, including subdural devices based on saline-filled transducers, e.g. Richmond screw or Leeds bolt, as well as extradural devices based on electrical impedance, e.g. Gaeltec and Ladd. Each of these devices suffers from problems associated with blockage of the lumen if the brain swells as well as baseline measurement drift over time.

30.2.3 Parenchymatous ICP Monitoring

In the early 1990s, microsensors opened up for catheters placed within the brain parenchyma for measurement of ICP. They were based on either fibre optics (Camino) or electrical impedance (Codman 'Microsensor', Spiegelberg). The readings are comparable with those of the intraventricular catheters; they are minimally invasive and have minimal baseline drift, but this drift unfortunately increases with time and can, in rare cases, reach 10 mmHg (Al-Tamimi et al. 2009). Hence, circumventing this drawback, Raumedic made a catheter with an air duct to the tip, but even these catheters have, so far, a drift over time (Citerio et al. 2008). Despite these shortcomings, microcatheters have become the standard method of measuring ICP in many neurosurgical centres worldwide. It is vital, though, to mention that a number of neurosurgical centres have reported on cases where these devices have given false values (Fernandes et al. 1998) and that they have no advantages concerning complications (Khan et al. 1998).

30.2.4 Lumbar Versus Supratentorial ICP Monitoring

There is a good correlation between mean lumbar and ventricular pressures in the supine patient, with a mean difference of 10 mm H_2O (0.75 mmHg) (Lenfeldt et al. 2007). However, wave amplitudes have been found to be 2 mmHg smaller in lumbar recordings (Eide and Brean 2006).

30.2.5 Infratentorial Versus Supratentorial Intracranial Pressure

Hitherto, the infratentorial volume down to the foramen magnum has not been thoroughly investigated. Slavin and Misra (2003) used external ventricular drainage placed in a lateral ventricle together with infratentorial ICP measurement using an intraparenchymal sensor inserted into the cerebellum. In patients with various infratentorial pathologies, a difference in ICP was found between the infratentorial and supratentorial compartments, a difference which in addition changed over time.

Following posterior fossa surgery, a parenchymatous pressure transducer was placed in the cerebellum and a Richmond bolt in the frontal area. During the first 12 h, the posterior fossa pressure was 50% higher than that in the supratentorial compartment in all patients. Over the next 12 h, the supratentorial pressures were 10–15% higher than those measured in the posterior fossa, but following 48 h of monitoring, the pressures had equilibrated (Rosenwasser et al. 1989).

30.2.6 Non-invasive Methods for Assessing ICP

ICP cannot be measured exactly by non-invasive means, but crude estimations can be made to give the clinician a clue as to what the ICP is likely to be. Such assessments are based on case history, clinical symptoms (headache, vomiting, nausea), and radiological investigations. It must be emphasized that a normal morphology of the brain as visualized by a CT or MR scan never exclude an elevated ICP, and a treating physician cannot rely solely on radiological features to interpret ICP. MR imaging–derived elastance index, on the other hand, correlates with ICP over a wide range of ICP values (Alperin et al. 2000). This method as such is unfortunately hampered with such a low sensitivity that it allows for differentiation only between normal and elevated ICP; in addition, it is quite complicated to perform. Last, but not least, transcranial Doppler (TCD) has been used to estimate ICP. The calculations in a mathematical model using arterial blood pressure and cerebral flow velocity predict ICP with good accuracy (Schmidt et al. 2002). A more straightforward method utilizes the correlation between pulsative index (PI) and ICP where $ICP = 10.9 \times PI - 1.3$ or $ICP \approx 10 \times PI$ (Bellner et al. 2004).

30.2.7 When to Monitor ICP

Monitoring brain functions is difficult in comatose patients. Since one aim of the therapy of head-injured patients is to prevent secondary injuries to the brain due to high ICP and/or low cerebral perfusion pressure, continuous recording of ICP has been found to be of value in cases of severe head trauma. Hence, in head-injured patients with intracranial mass lesions on the admission CT, a persistent high ICP was observed in 60% as compared to 13% in those with a normal CT, while the presence of at least two or more of the following factors increased the incidence of high ICP up to 60% in the group with normal CT: age above 40, systolic blood pressure below 90 mmHg, and motor posturing (Narayan et al. 1982).

Insertion of an ICP device should be considered following intracranial surgery if complications are estimated as probable, in the presence of establish elevated intracranial pressure, in a limited number of cases for the evaluation of CSF shunts, and for the purpose of differentiating between normal and low pressure states. Treatment of intracranial hypertension is also best guided by continuous intracranial pressure monitoring (Johnsson and Jennet 2005). In cases of a subarachnoidal bleeding, it is recommended to insert a ventricular catheter not only as a means for ICP measurements but also because drainage of ventricular fluid might be compulsory (Sakowitz et al. 2006).

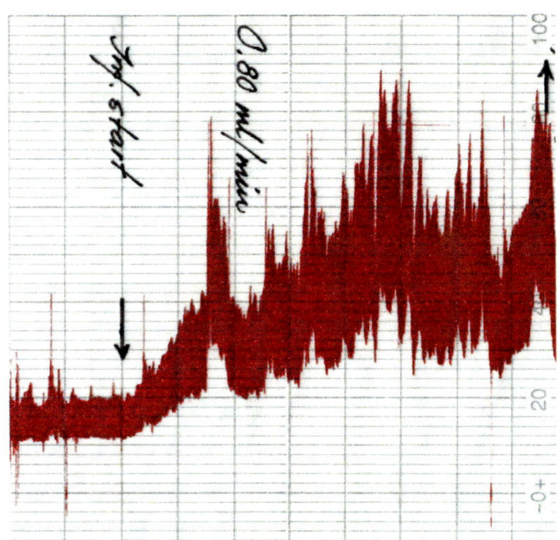

Fig. 30.2 ICP recording from a patient during a lumbar infusion of fluid (0.8 ml/min) showing a concomitant rise both in ICP and amplitude. The pressure is shown in mmHg, and there is 5 min between *vertical lines*, events going from *left to right*

30.2.8 ICP Waveform Analysis

Mean ICP has until recently been the sole information of interest obtained from the ICP devices, but the ICP recording can provide additional information. During rising ICP, the arterial pulse pressure wave of the ICP curve increases in amplitude as a sign of the decreased compliance in the CNS (Fig. 30.2), while conversely the ICP curve oscillations become minute after a craniectomy.

The ICP curve has variations superimposed on the arterial pulse pressure curve, one with a respiratory synchronicity and another with a slower frequency of 0.5–2/min seen during sedation or sleep, but of unknown origin (Fig. 30.3). On top of this, some TBI patients develop plateau waves as described already by Lundberg (1960) but still of unidentified origin even though one might suspect rapid changes in CBV (Fig. 30.4). Plateau waves have been considered a malignant sign but have recently been shown not to be associated with a worse outcome (Castellani et al. 2009).

The introduction of digital registration has facilitated analysis of the curve itself, but so far, it is mainly the amplitude which is used to interpret

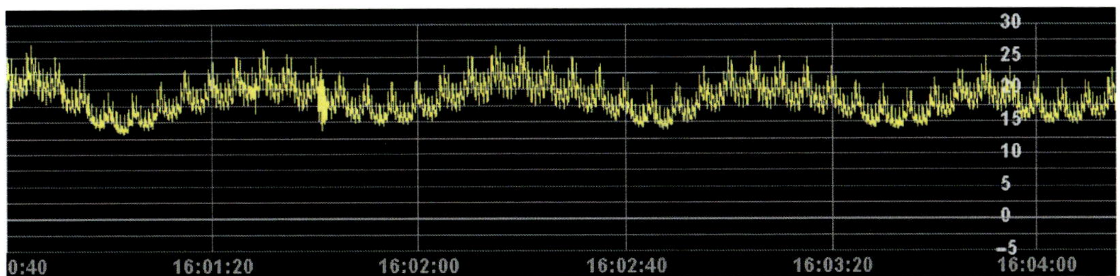

Fig. 30.3 An ICP tracing in a TBI patient during sedation and artificial ventilation. The pressure is shown in mmHg and between *vertical lines* passes 40 s. The fast undulation is due to the pulse pressure, and the slow part (12/min) is due to the ventilation. A slower wave of approx. 1/min, the so-called B wave, is seen in sedated or sleeping patients

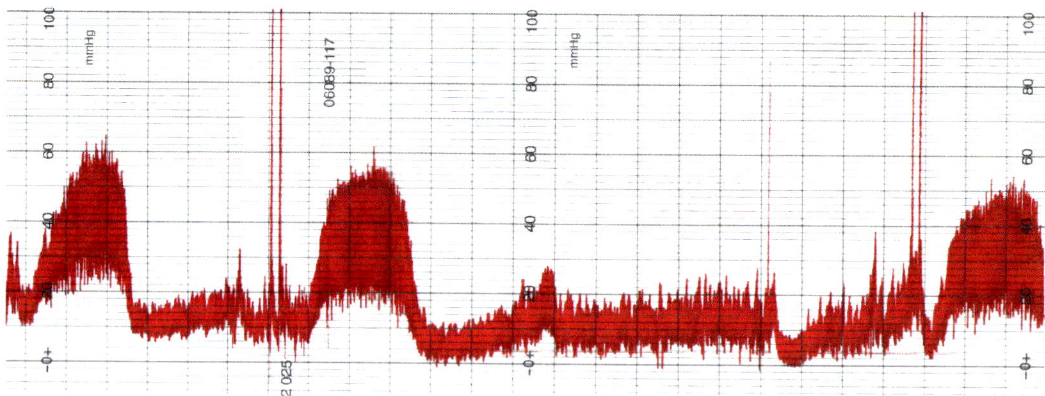

Fig. 30.4 ICP recording in a TBI patient showing plateau waves. The pressure is shown in mmHg, and there is 5 min between *vertical lines*, events going from *left to right*

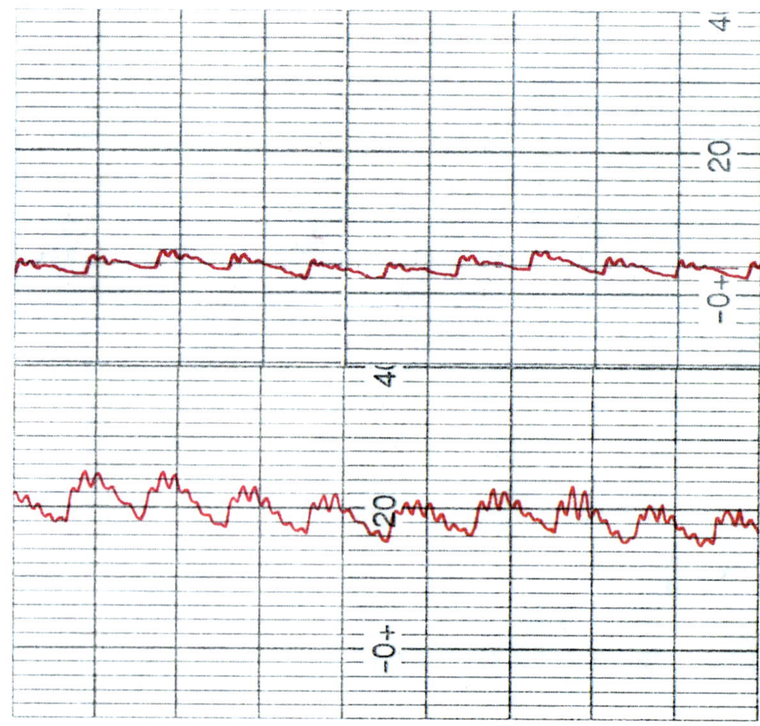

Fig. 30.5 Typical curve forms at normal (*left panel*) and slightly elevated (*right panel*) ICP from the same patient. The pressure is shown in mmHg, and the paper speed gives 1 s per *vertical line*, events going from *left to right*. The ICP curve created by the systolic pulse is usually tetrahumped, and the individual waves are called p_1–p_4. This can be seen very vaguely on the *left panel*, whereas in the *right panel* up to six humps can be located. The *curve* during low ICP has a prominent p_1 (*left panel*), but a prominent p_2 is seen in the *right panel* where the ICP is higher

the status of the brain (Eide and Kerty 2011); as of today, the appearance of the pressure curve in itself has not been thoroughly investigated.

The ICP curve is usually tetrahumped, and the individual waves are called p_1–p_4 respectively. The appearance of the curve differs; under conditions of normal ICP the p_1 has the greatest amplitude, whereas during states of elevated ICP the p_2 waves often becomes the highest (Fig. 30.5).

30.2.9 MR Compatibility

Provided no metal is used in connection with the ventricular ICP device, an MR scan can be performed without risks. Many centres have dedicated equipment for ABP monitoring in the scanning room, and these systems can be used also for ICP monitoring provided the pressure transducer is situated well away from the scanning site.

Generally, all parenchymatous ICP devices should be disconnected, and if placed via a bolt, this must be non-magnetic. The Raumedic catheter is said to be approved for use in the MR environment, although no legal obligations of such a statement has been presented. The Codman sensor is so far the only device approved for MR scanners of up to 1.5 T and with a radiofrequency below one SAR, provided the catheter is coiled and taped to the head in a special way to minimize thermogenesis (Newcombe et al. 2008).

30.3 Specific Paediatric Concerns

In infants, ICP can be assessed by measuring head circumference and palpating the fontanel, a method that is no longer available after closure of the cranial sutures, leaving fundoscopy as the remaining bedside non-invasive method. It is important to bear in mind that the lack of papilloedema does not exclude elevated ICP.

Neonates have slightly lower ICP, i.e. between 0 and 10 mmHg, as compared to 0 and 15 mmHg in grown-ups. On the other hand, the pressure-volume curve of a normal infant shows less ability to buffer increments of volume, resulting in a steeper volume-ICP slope as a sign of lower total compliance (Shapiro et al. 1994). Very high intracranial pressures are usually fatal if prolonged, but children can tolerate higher pressures for longer periods.

References

Alperin NJ, Lee SH, Loth F, Raksin PB, Lichtor T (2000) MR–Intracranial pressure (ICP): a method to measure intracranial elastance and pressure noninvasively by means of MR imaging: baboon and human study volume. Radiology 217(3):877–885

Al-Tamimi YZ, Helmy A, Bavetta S, Price SJ (2009) Assessment of zero drift in the Codman intracranial pressure monitor: a study from 2 neurointensive care units. Neurosurgery 64(1):94–98

Bellner J, Romner B, Reinstrup P, Kristiansson KA, Ryding E, Brandt L (2004) Transcranial Doppler sonography pulsatility index (PI) reflects intracranial pressure (ICP). Surg Neurol 62(1):45–51

Castellani G, Zweifel C, Kim DJ, Carrera E, Radolovich DK, Smielewski P, Hutchinson PJ, Pickard JD, Czosnyka M (2009) Plateau waves in head injured patients requiring neurocritical care. Neurocrit Care 11:143–150

Chambers IR, Kane PJ, Signorini DF, Jenkins A, Mendelow AD (1998) Bilateral ICP monitoring: its importance in detecting the severity of secondary insults. Acta Neurochir Suppl 71:42–43

Citerio G, Piper I, Chambers IR, Galli D, Enblad P, Kiening K, Ragauskas A, Sahuquillo J, Gregson B, BrainIT Group (2008) Multicenter clinical assessment of the Raumedic Neurovent-P intracranial pressure sensor: a report by the BrainIT group. Neurosurgery 63(6):1152–1158

Eide PK, Brean A (2006) Lumbar cerebrospinal fluid pressure waves versus intracranial pressure waves in idiopathic normal pressure hydrocephalus. Br J Neurosurg 20(6):407–414

Eide PK, Kerty E (2011) Static and pulsatile intracranial pressure in idiopathic intracranial hypertension. Clin Neurol Neurosurg 113:123–128

Fernandes HM, Bingham K, Chambers IR, Mendelow AD (1998) Clinical evaluation of the Codman microsensor intracranial pressure monitoring system. Acta Neurochir Suppl 71:44–46

Guyott LL, Dowling C, Diaz FG, Michael DB (1998) Cerebral monitoring devices: analysis of complications. Acta Neurochir Suppl 71:47–49

Johnston IH, Jennet B (1973) The place of continous intracranial pressure monitoring in neurosurgical practice. Acta Neurochir 29:53–63

Key A, Retzius G (1875) Studies in der Anatomie des Nerven system und der Bindesgewebes. Bd. I. Samson & Wallin. Stockholm

Khan SH, Kureshi IU, Mulgrew T, Ho SY, Onyiuke HC (1998) Comparison of percutaneous ventriculostomies and intraparenchymal monitor: a retrospective evaluation of 156 patients. Acta Neurochir Suppl 71:50–52

Knoll PH (1886) Uber die Druckschwankungen in der Cerebrospinalflussigkeit und den Wechsel in der Blutfulle des centralen Nervensystems. Sitzungsberichte der Kaiserlichen Akademie der Wissenschaften 217–246

Lenfeldt N, Koskinen LO, Bergenheim AT, Malm J, Eklund A (2007) CSF pressure assessed by lumbar puncture agrees with intracranial pressure. Neurology 68(2):155–158

Lundberg N (1960) Continuous recording and control of ventricular fluid pressure in neurosurgical practice. Acta Psychiatr Neurol Scand 1(Supplement 149):193

Narayan RK, Kishore PR, Becker DP, Ward JD, Enas GG, Greenberg RP, Domingues Da Silva A, Lipper MH, Choi SC, Mayhall CG, Lutz HA 3rd, Young HF (1982) Intracranial pressure: to monitor or not to monitor? A review of our experience with severe head injury. J Neurosurg 56(5):650–659

Newcombe VFJ, Hawkes RC, Harding SG, Willcox R, Brock S, Hutchinson PJ, Menon DK, Carpenter TA, Coles JP (2008) Potential heating caused by intracranial pressure transducers in a 3-tesla magnetic resonance imaging system using a body radiofrequency resonator: assessment of the Codman MicroSensor Transducer. J Neurosurg 109:159–164

Rosenwasser RH, Kleiner LI, Krzeminski JP, Buchheit WA (1989) Intracranial pressure monitoring in the posterior fossa: a preliminary report. J Neurosurg 71(4):503–505

Rossi S, Buzzi F, Paparella A, Mainini P, Stocchetti N (1998) Complications and safety associated with ICP monitoring: a study of 542 patients. Acta Neurochir Suppl 71:91–93

Sakowitz OW, Raabe A, Vucak D, Kiening KL, Unterberg AW (2006) Contemporary management of aneurysmal subarachnoid hemorrhage in Germany: results of a survey among 100 neurosurgical departments. Neurosurgery 58(1):137–145

Schmidt B, Czosnyka M, Klingelhöfer J (2002) Clinical applications of a non-invasive ICP monitoring method. Eur J Ultrasound 16(1–2):37–45

Shapiro K, Morris WJ, Teo C (1994) Intracranial hypertension: mechanisms and management. In: Cheek WR, Marlin AE, McLone DG et al (eds) Pediatric neurosurgery: surgery of the developing nervous system, 3rd edn. Saunders, Philadelphia, pp 307–319

Slavin KV, Misra M (2003) Infratentorial intracranial pressure monitoring in neurosurgical intensive care unit. Neurol Res 25(8):880–884

Quincke HI (1891) Verhandlungen des Congresses für Innere Medizin, Zehnter Congress, Wiesbaden. 10. pp. 321–331

Brain Tissue Oxygen Monitoring 31

Troels Halfeld Nielsen

Recommendations

Level I

There are insufficient data to support a Level I recommendation for this topic.

Level II

There are insufficient data to support a Level II recommendation for this topic.

Level III

Brain tissue oxygen below 5–15 mmHg is associated with higher mortality after severe TBI. There is insufficient data to support a Level III recommendation for brain tissue oxygen-guided therapy after severe TBI.

31.1 Overview

Monitoring of brain tissue oxygenation represents one of an array of regional cerebral monitors including microdialysis for measurement of regional metabolism, thermal diffusion probes for measurements of CBF and near-infrared spectroscopy that also measures brain tissue oxygenation. Common for all modalities is that they comprise a supplement to the routinely used ICP monitoring. These regional monitors have gained increasing interest over the last two decades because they open up possibilities to develop treatment strategies aiming at optimizing not only ICP but also cerebral blood flow, oxygenation and metabolism.

In the last decade, direct measurement of brain tissue oxygen tension ($PtiO_2$) has become the most frequently used technique for monitoring brain oxygenation because of its ease of use and continuous measurement. The technique provides online bedside information about the oxygen tension in a few mm^3 of brain tissue.

In spite of the wide distribution of the technique, it is not yet completely understood exactly what brain oxygen monitors measure. $PtiO_2$ is influenced by changes in FiO_2, PaO_2, $PaCO_2$ and MAP among others (Maloney-Wilensky and Le Roux 2010). Rosenthal et al. demonstrated that $PtiO_2$ primarily represent the product of CBF and the arteriovenous oxygen tension difference (Rosenthal et al. 2009), suggesting that $PtiO_2$ reflects the diffusion of oxygen across the blood-brain barrier and delivery more than cerebral oxygen metabolism.

Quite a few studies have tried to determine the normal values and the ischemic values of $PtiO_2$. Normal values range between 23 and 48 mmHg, but values as low as 9 mmHg have been observed in uninjured human brain (Meixensberger et al. 1993; Pennings et al. 2008). Ischemic values

T.H. Nielsen
Department of Neurosurgery,
Odense University Hospital,
Sdr. Boulevard 29, 5000 Odense, Denmark
e-mail: troels.nielsen@ouh.regionsyddanmark.dk

T. Sundstrøm et al. (eds.), *Management of Severe Traumatic Brain Injury*,
DOI 10.1007/978-3-642-28126-6_31, © Springer-Verlag Berlin Heidelberg 2012

range from 10 to 25 mmHg in different studies (Chang et al. 2009; Doppenberg et al. 1998; Kiening et al. 1996; Valadka et al. 1998; van den Brink et al. 2000; van Santbrink et al. 1996; Zauner et al. 1997). The wide range of both normal and ischemic values makes it difficult to establish an ischemic threshold. Further, the relationship to cerebral oxidative energy metabolism is not established. These factors should be kept in mind when interpreting $PtiO_2$ measurements.

Studies has been conducted to assess both the relationship between $PtiO_2$ levels and mortality after severe TBI (Bardt et al. 1998; Chang et al. 2009; Doppenberg et al. 1998; Kiening et al. 1996; Valadka et al. 1998; van den Brink et al. 2000; van Santbrink et al. 1996; Zauner et al. 1997) and the effect of a $PtiO_2$-guided therapy on outcome (Chang et al. 2009; Fletcher et al. 2010; Martini et al. 2009; Meixensberger et al. 2003, 2004; Tolias et al. 2004; van den Brink et al. 2000). Although there seems to be Level III evidence to support that episodes with hypoxia is associated with increased mortality, data does not support evidence of an effect of $PtiO_2$-guided therapy on outcome after severe TBI.

Tips, Tricks, and Pitfalls

- A low or decreasing $PtiO_2$ can reflect low or decreasing CBF as a result of high ICP/low CPP, hyperventilation or low PaO_2. Also, a low or decreasing $PtiO_2$ can reflect cerebral oedema and therefore diffusion-limited delivery of oxygen (diffusion limited hypoxia).
- Always allow at least one hour after implantation of the $PtiO_2$ catheter for stabilization. To ensure that the $PtiO_2$ probe is functioning correctly, always do an 'oxygen challenge test'. That is, $PtiO_2$ should increase >20 mmHg when increasing FiO_2 to 1.0 for 2–5 min.
- Bear in mind that $PtiO_2$ is a regional measurement, and the interpretation of the values should always be based on the location of the probe. The probe could be placed in a traumatic contusion, infarcted tissue, etc.

31.2 Background

A relatively large number of clinical studies have suggested a relation between measured $PtiO_2$ levels and mortality following TBI (Bardt et al. 1998; Chang et al. 2009; Doppenberg et al. 1998; Kiening et al. 1996; Valadka et al. 1998; van den Brink et al. 2000; van Santbrink et al. 1996; Zauner et al. 1997). In a prospective study of 22 patients with severe TBI, van Santbrink et al. demonstrated that episodes with $PtiO_2$<5 mmHg for at least 0.5 h were correlated to significant increased mortality (van Santbrink et al. 1996). In a prospective study including 34 patients, Bardt et al. reported a higher mortality rate after TBI in patients with $PtiO_2$ < 10 mmHg for more than 30 min (56% vs. 9%) (Bardt et al. 1998). In 1998, Valadka et al. reported in a prospective observational study an increased mortality after TBI with $PtiO_2$ values less than 15 mmHg (Valadka et al. 1998). Similarly, van den Brink et al. found, in 2000 in a prospective observational study of 101 patients with TBI an increasing mortality after TBI with $PtiO_2$ values less that 15 mmHg, the likelihood of death increasing with increasing duration of time below 15 mmHg (van den Brink et al. 2000). Accordingly, there is Level III evidence that brain tissue oxygen below 5–15 mmHg is associated with increased mortality.

The association between $PtiO_2$ levels after severe TBI and outcome raises the question whether a therapy focused on optimizing $PtiO_2$ ($PtiO_2$-guided therapy) can improve outcome. In 2004, Tolias et al. reported the effect of treatment of 52 patients with severe TBI with a FiO_2 of 1.0 and compared the results with a cohort of 112 matched historical controls (Tolias et al. 2004). All patients were monitored with $PtiO_2$ probes along with microdialysis to study cerebral metabolism. Although they found a decreased brain lactate and lactate/pyruvate ratio in the treatment group, no improvement in outcome in this group could be demonstrated. In total, Stiefel et al., Narotam et al. and Spiotta et al. have studied 234 patients with severe TBI managed according to a $PtiO_2$-optimizing protocol and compared them to a control group managed with ICP-/CPP-guided therapy only (Narotam et al. 2009; Spiotta et al. 2010; Stiefel et al. 2004). All three studies reported quite similar results decreasing the mortality from around 44% in the control group to around 25% in the treatment group. Furthermore, Narotam et al. found a significant higher GOS in the treatment group compared to the control group (3.55 vs. 2.71). However, all three studies relied on historical controls with a significant mortality compared to today's standard. Furthermore, Fletcher el al. found in a retrospective study of 41 patients that $PtiO_2$-guided therapy was associated with increased cumulative fluid balance, use of vasopressors and increased rate of refractory intracranial hypertension and pulmonary oedema (Fletcher et al. 2010). Also, Martini et al. found in a retrospective study comparing 506 patients managed by ICP-/CPP-guided therapy with 123 patients managed with $PtiO_2$-guided therapy a higher mortality rate in the $PtiO_2$ group, correcting for baseline differences in severity of brain injury (Martini et al. 2009). No RCT has been conducted addressing this topic. Accordingly, the diverging conclusions from different studies and the obvious limitations of these along with the lack of a RCT makes it impossible to give evidence-based recommendations regarding $PtiO_2$-guided therapy in patients with severe TBI.

31.3 Specific Paediatric Concerns

Studies of brain oxygen tension in paediatric TBI have shown that low $PtiO_2$ and the amount of time with reduced $PtiO_2$ are associated with poor outcome in children with severe TBI. The thresholds seem to be identical to those in the adult population. Further, episodes with reduced $PtiO_2$ might be seen without significant changes in normal physiological values (i.e. ICP, CPP, SaO_2, PaO_2, etc.) (Figaji et al. 2008; Figaji and Adelson 2009; Figaji et al. 2009a, b). However, the number of paediatric patients studied is small.

References

Bardt TF, Unterberg AW, Hartl R, Kiening KL, Schneider GH, Lanksch WR (1998) Monitoring of brain tissue PO2 in traumatic brain injury: effect of cerebral hypoxia on outcome. Acta Neurochir Suppl 71:153–156

Chang JJ, Youn TS, Benson D, Mattick H, Andrade N, Harper CR, Moore CB, Madden CJ, Diaz-Arrastia RR (2009) Physiologic and functional outcome correlates of brain tissue hypoxia in traumatic brain injury. Crit Care Med 37:283–290

Doppenberg EM, Zauner A, Watson JC, Bullock R (1998) Determination of the ischemic threshold for brain oxygen tension. Acta Neurochir Suppl 71:166–169

Figaji AA, Adelson PD (2009) Does ICP monitoring in children with severe head injuries make a difference? Am Surg 75:441–442

Figaji AA, Fieggen AG, Argent AC, Leroux PD, Peter JC (2008) Does adherence to treatment targets in children with severe traumatic brain injury avoid brain hypoxia? A brain tissue oxygenation study. Neurosurgery 63:83–91; discussion 91–92

Figaji AA, Zwane E, Thompson C, Fieggen AG, Argent AC, Le Roux PD, Peter JC (2009a) Brain tissue oxygen tension monitoring in pediatric severe traumatic brain injury. Part 1: relationship with outcome. Childs Nerv Syst 25:1325–1333

Figaji AA, Zwane E, Thompson C, Fieggen AG, Argent AC, Le Roux PD, Peter JC (2009b) Brain tissue oxygen tension monitoring in pediatric severe traumatic brain injury. Part 2: relationship with clinical, physiological, and treatment factors. Childs Nerv Syst 25:1335–1343

Fletcher JJ, Bergman K, Blostein PA, Kramer AH (2010) Fluid balance, complications, and brain tissue oxygen tension monitoring following severe traumatic brain injury. Neurocrit Care 13:47–56

Kiening KL, Unterberg AW, Bardt TF, Schneider GH, Lanksch WR (1996) Monitoring of cerebral oxygenation in patients with severe head injuries: brain tissue PO2 versus jugular vein oxygen saturation. J Neurosurg 85:751–757

Maloney-Wilensky E, Le Roux P (2010) The physiology behind direct brain oxygen monitors and practical aspects of their use. Childs Nerv Syst 26:419–430

Martini RP, Deem S, Yanez ND, Chesnut RM, Weiss NS, Daniel S, Souter M, Treggiari MM (2009) Management guided by brain tissue oxygen monitoring and outcome following severe traumatic brain injury. J Neurosurg 111:644–649

Meixensberger J, Dings J, Kuhnigk H, Roosen K (1993) Studies of tissue PO2 in normal and pathological human brain cortex. Acta Neurochir Suppl (Wien) 59:58–63

Meixensberger J, Jaeger M, Vath A, Dings J, Kunze E, Roosen K (2003) Brain tissue oxygen guided treatment supplementing ICP/CPP therapy after traumatic brain injury. J Neurol Neurosurg Psychiatry 74:760–764

Meixensberger J, Renner C, Simanowski R, Schmidtke A, Dings J, Roosen K (2004) Influence of cerebral oxygenation following severe head injury on neuropsychological testing. Neurol Res 26:414–417

Narotam PK, Morrison JF, Nathoo N (2009) Brain tissue oxygen monitoring in traumatic brain injury and major trauma: outcome analysis of a brain tissue oxygen-directed therapy. J Neurosurg 111:672–682

Pennings FA, Schuurman PR, van den Munckhof P, Bouma GJ (2008) Brain tissue oxygen pressure monitoring in awake patients during functional neurosurgery: the assessment of normal values. J Neurotrauma 25:1173–1177

Rosenthal G, Hemphill JC 3rd, Manley G (2009) Brain tissue oxygen tension is more indicative of oxygen diffusion than oxygen delivery and metabolism in patients with traumatic brain injury. Crit Care Med 37:379–380

Spiotta AM, Stiefel MF, Gracias VH, Garuffe AM, Kofke WA, Maloney-Wilensky E, Troxel AB, Levine JM, Le Roux PD (2010) Brain tissue oxygen-directed management and outcome in patients with severe traumatic brain injury. J Neurosurg 113(3):571–580

Stiefel MF, Heuer GG, Smith MJ, Bloom S, Maloney-Wilensky E, Gracias VH, Grady MS, LeRoux PD (2004) Cerebral oxygenation following decompressive hemicraniectomy for the treatment of refractory intracranial hypertension. J Neurosurg 101:241–247

Tolias CM, Reinert M, Seiler R, Gilman C, Scharf A, Bullock MR (2004) Normobaric hyperoxia–induced improvement in cerebral metabolism and reduction in intracranial pressure in patients with severe head injury: a prospective historical cohort-matched study. J Neurosurg 101:435–444

Valadka AB, Gopinath SP, Contant CF, Uzura M, Robertson CS (1998) Relationship of brain tissue PO2 to outcome after severe head injury. Crit Care Med 26:1576–1581

van den Brink WA, van Santbrink H, Steyerberg EW, Avezaat CJ, Suazo JA, Hogesteeger C, Jansen WJ, Kloos LM, Vermeulen J, Maas AI (2000) Brain oxygen tension in severe head injury. Neurosurgery 46:868–876; discussion 76–78

van Santbrink H, Maas AI, Avezaat CJ (1996) Continuous monitoring of partial pressure of brain tissue oxygen in patients with severe head injury. Neurosurgery 38:21–31

Zauner A, Doppenberg EM, Woodward JJ, Choi SC, Young HF, Bullock R (1997) Continuous monitoring of cerebral substrate delivery and clearance: initial experience in 24 patients with severe acute brain injuries. Neurosurgery 41:1082–1091; discussion 91–93

Measurement of Brain Temperature 32

Peter Reinstrup and Carl-Henrik Nordström

Recommendations

Level I

There are insufficient data to support a Level I recommendation for this topic.

Level II

There are insufficient data to support a Level II recommendation for this topic.

Level III

The brain temperature does not differ from core temperature.

32.1 Overview

The brain metabolism results in a vast heat production. In addition to the deliverance of nutrients and oxygen and the drainage of waste products such as CO_2, the very high cerebral blood flow (CBF) also acts as a heat sink, resulting in an equalisation of the temperature between brain and body.

P. Reinstrup (✉)
Department of Intensive and Perioperative Care,
Skanes University Hospital, S221 85 Lund, Sweden
e-mail: peter.reinstrup@med.lu.se

C.-H. Nordström
Department of Neurosurgery,
Odense University Hospital
Sdr. Boulevard 29, 5000 Odense Denmark
e-mail: carl-henrik.nordstrom@med.lu.se

Tips, Tricks, and Pitfalls

- Body temperature can be substituted for brain temperature.
- If the brain temperature is of specific interest, it can be obtained by placing a temperature probe through a ventricular catheter.
- A temperature probe placed in the jugular bulb can be utilised to indirectly measure brain temperature.

32.2 Background

Instruments designed for measuring temperature were manufactured in Italy already in beginning of the seventeenth century. Daniel Gabriel Fahrenheit probably performed the first measurement of human body temperature. Since then, body temperature has been measured at different sites, where rectal and vaginal temperatures (37.0°C) are regarded as the classic substitutes for the core temperature. In intensive care situations, these classic measuring points are often substituted by measurements from bladder, oesophagus, and central circulation, whereas obtaining armpit, ear, or oral temperature seems to be less encroaching means in the awake patient.

T. Sundstrøm et al. (eds.), *Management of Severe Traumatic Brain Injury*,
DOI 10.1007/978-3-642-28126-6_32,

For direct measurement of brain temperature, the skull needs to be opened and a temperature probe inserted. Temperature probes are commercially available for placement in the parenchyma as well as in the ventricles. Mellergård and Nordström (1990) presented the first direct measurement of human brain temperature in 1990. They inserted a temperature probe through a ventricular catheter utilised for routine intracranial pressure monitoring. This approach permitted recording of the temperature along the route of the ventricular catheter, giving information about temperature variations at various depths from the cortical surface.

Brain temperature can be recorded indirectly by measuring temperature in the blood leaving the brain, e.g. by placing a temperature probe in the jugular bulb. The ear (tympanic) temperature has been claimed to reflect the epidural temperature – a statement without solid scientific support. Ear temperature correlates – at least in the younger population – to orally measured temperature.

Brain temperature is generally slightly higher than the body core temperature: 0.3±0.3°C (range −0.7 to 2.3) (Mellergård and Nordström 1991; Rossi et al. 2001). The observation is probably explained by the exceptionally high-energy metabolism of the brain (Sakurai et al. 2006). The difference between cerebral and body core temperature has been reported to increase during fever and to decrease during induced hypothermia (Rossi et al. 2001). The temperature difference also decreases in patients treated with barbiturate coma and increases in situations with reduced cerebral blood flow (Rumana et al. 1998).

The adult human brain – weighing from 1 to 1.5 kg – has a global blood flow of nearly 750 ml/min, and the total cerebral blood volume is approximately 60–70 ml. Accordingly, cerebral blood volume is exchanged about ten times every minute. This high blood flow will counteract any major discrepancy between brain and body core temperature.

The rectal temperature is, hence, regarded to be sufficiently close to brain temperature for routine purpose during neurocritical care (Mellergård and Nordström 1991). For specific scientific purposes, total information of brain, jugular, and body core temperature might give additional information. There is a temperature gradient within the brain with the central parts being warmer than the surface. The temperature gradient between the lateral ventricle and the epidural space has been reported to be 0.4–1.0°C (Mellergård 1994). This gradient was studied thoroughly in euthermic patients by Fountas et al. (2004). In their study, the mean rectal temperature was 37.65±0.68°C, and the intraventricular temperature was 37.84±1.03°C. At 1 cm outward from the lateral ventricle, the mean intraparenchymal temperature was 38.21±0.32°C, 38.39±0.33°C at 2 cm, 38.27±0.31°C at 3 cm, 38.26±0.29°C at 4 cm, and finally, 37.9±0.50°C at 5 cm (close to the epidural space). The gradient with a lower temperature at the surface is probably due to heat radiation and convection through the calvarium. When opening the skull during neurosurgery, the most superficial layer down to 1 cm below the brain surface has a 1.4°C lower temperature as compared to the central parts (Stone et al. 1997).

32.2.1 Normal Temperatures

The most common factors influencing the body temperature are age and gender. Elderly persons' temperature will tend to be in the lower range, children's temperature at the high end. The temperature differs during the day with lowest temperature in the morning and highest in the evening. Women's temperature will rise during ovulation.

Brain: central 36.8±1.0°C, parenchyma 37.3±0.3°C, epidural 36.9±0.5°C
Rectal: 36.7±0.7°C
Axillary: 35.5–37.0°C
Oral: 33.2–38.2°C
Ear: 35.4–37.8°C

32.3 Specific Paediatric Concerns

See above.

References

Fountas KN, Kapsalaki EZ, Feltes CH, Smisson HF 3rd, Johnston KW, Robinson JS Jr (2004) Intracranial temperature: is it different throughout the brain? Neurocrit Care 1(2):195–199

Mellergård P (1994) Monitoring of rectal, epidural, and intraventricular temperature in neurosurgical patients. Acta Neurochir Suppl (Wien) 60:485–487

Mellergård P, Nordström CH (1990) Epidural temperature and possible intracerebral temperature gradients in man. Br J Neurosurg 4(1):31–38

Mellergård P, Nordström CH (1991) Intracerebral temperature in neurosurgical patients. Neurosurgery 28(5):709–713

Rossi S, Zanier ER, Mauri I, Columbo A, Stocchetti N (2001) Brain temperature, body core temperature, and intracranial pressure in acute cerebral damage. J Neurol Neurosurg Psychiatry 71(4):448–454

Rumana CS, Gopinath SP, Uzura M, Valadka AB, Robertson CS (1998) Brain temperature exceeds systemic temperature in head-injured patients. Crit Care Med 26(3):562–567

Sakurai A, Kinoshita K, Inada K, Furukawa M, Ebihara T, Moriya T, Utagawa A, Kitahata Y, Okuno K, Tanjoh K (2006) Brain oxygen metabolism may relate to the temperature gradient between the jugular vein and pulmonary artery after cardiopulmonary resuscitation. Acta Neurochir Suppl (Wien) 96:97–99

Stone JG, Goodman RR, Baker KZ, Baker CJ, Solomon RA (1997) Direct intraoperative measurement of human brain temperature. Neurosurgery 41(1):20–24

Monitoring Microdialysis

33

Peter Reinstrup and Carl-Henrik Nordström

Recommendations

Level I

There are insufficient data to support a Level I recommendation for this topic.

Level II

There are insufficient data to support a Level II recommendation for this topic.

Level III

With intracerebral microdialysis, it is possible to detect upcoming ischemia and cell death.

33.1 Overview

Microdialysis is an invasive technique based on placement of a small catheter into the brain parenchyma. The distal end of the catheter is a dialysis membrane. The lumen is perfused with Ringer acetate into which molecules are taken up by osmosis from the surrounding tissue. The irrigation fluid can be analysed online bedside (most commonly) or later at some convenient time. With the current technique, approximately 70% of the original parenchymal concentrations of the most commonly analysed substrates can be recovered in this fluid. By positioning the catheter in an area of interest, e.g. a contused area, the method can give consecutive samples of the extracellular fluid, thereby monitoring the ongoing metabolism of this tissue. The normally analysed substrates bedside is glucose, lactate, pyruvate, glycerol, and glutamate. It is recommended to use intracerebral microdialysis as a complement to intracranial pressure (ICP) and cerebral perfusion pressure (CPP) monitoring in severe cases of TBI subarachnoid haemorrhage and TBI. The lactate/pyruvate ratio is considered to be a sensitive marker for the development of ischemia, whereas glycerol is considered to reflect cell death (Fig. 33.1).

Tips, Tricks, and Pitfalls

- The microdialysis catheter can be placed either during a craniectomy in the OR or at the Neurointensive Care Unit using local anaesthetics. With an available CT or MR scan, a percutaneous implantation using a small twist-drill craniostomy makes for a precise placement of the microdialysis catheters.

P. Reinstrup (✉)
Department of Intensive and Perioperative Care,
Skanes University Hospital, S221 85 Lund, Sweden
e-mail: peter.reinstrup@med.lu.se

C.-H. Nordströ
Department of Neurosurgery,
Odense University Hospital,
Sdr. Boulevard 29, 5000
Odense, Denmark
e-mail: carl-henrik.nordstrom@med.lu.se

T. Sundstrøm et al. (eds.), *Management of Severe Traumatic Brain Injury*,
DOI 10.1007/978-3-642-28126-6_33, © Springer-Verlag Berlin Heidelberg 2012

Interpretation of bedside results

- *Ischemia* starts with decreasing concentrations of glucose and with a concomitant increase in the increase in lactate/pyruvate ratio followed by an increase in glycerol indicating cell membrane disintegration. If the lactate/pyruvate value is high, try to improve the circulation and/or the oxygenation of the area.
- *Infection* starts with an increase in glycerol.
- *Epilepsy* often starts with an increase in glutamate and a simultaneous decrease in glucose.

33.2 Background

Microdialysis (Gr. *mikros* small+*dia* through+*lysis* dissolution) is primarily a technique for extracting substances from a tissue in order to analyse the chemical composition of extracellular fluids, but the technique may be used also to deliver chemical substances to the tissue (e.g. drugs). The microdialysis method was developed almost 40 years ago for monitoring chemical events in the animal brain and is since long a regarded scientific technique. In the late 1980s, the possibilities for using microdialysis for the monitoring of the human brain were explored. In 1995, CMA Microdialysis (Stockholm, Sweden) introduced a sterile microdialysis catheter, a robust microdialysis pump, and a bedside

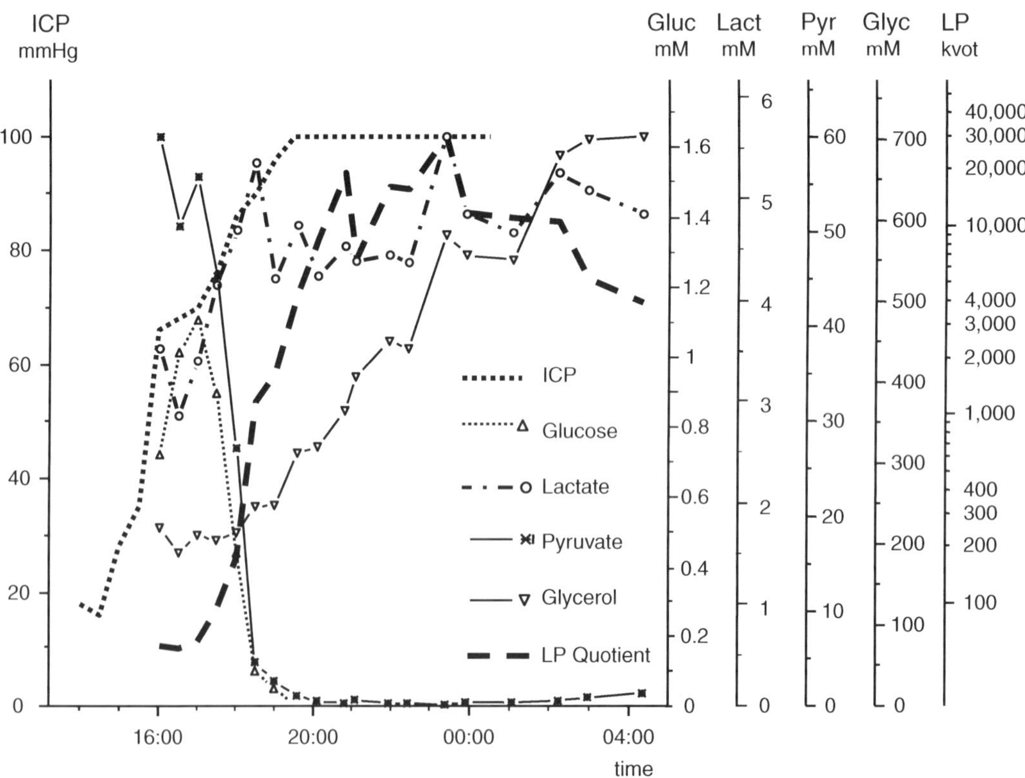

Fig. 33.1 The above microdialysis registration is from the 'better' hemisphere in a patient with increasing ICP due to an expanding epidural haematoma. The increased ICP attenuates the CBF, resulting in ischemia. The reduced delivery of substrates due to the decreased blood flow results in a reduction of glucose and pyruvate. The anaerobic metabolism with increased lactate production and a concomitant decrease in pyruvate is seen as an increase in the lactate/pyruvate quota (L/P Quotient). The escalating ischemia leads to a breakdown of cell membranes as seen as a rise in glycerol concentration emanating from the disintegration of the cell membranes liberating glycerol-phosphate

biochemical analyser. The instrumentation was originally intended for subcutaneous and intramuscular use, but with a slight modification of the microdialysis catheter, it has mainly been used intracerebrally as an integrated part of routine multimodality brain monitoring (Nordström 2010). Since microdialysis is a technique permitting sampling of stable biochemical compounds that traverse the dialysis membrane, it has rapidly been accepted for research purposes. The possibilities for scientific studies during intensive care are virtually unlimited.

Microdialysis presents an opportunity for continuous monitoring of metabolic changes in the tissue even before, if ever they are reflected in peripheral blood chemistry or in systemic physiological parameters. The currently used equipment is manufactured by CMA Microdialysis (Stockholm, Sweden) and consists of a small pump delivering a continuous flow of 0.3 μl/min as standard. The perfusion fluid is a Ringer solution adjusted to be iso-osmolar to the composition of cerebral interstitial fluid. From the pump, the fluid is lead through thin tubings to the 1-cm long microdialysis membrane at the end of the catheter. The diameter of the microdialysis probe is approximately 0.6 mm. At the tip of the probe, a small gold thread is implanted in order to be identifiable on CT- or MR-scanning, but small enough not to obscure the images. After having passed through the microdialysis membrane, the perfusion fluid passes into a thin inner tube positioned within the tip of the microdialysis catheter. The microdialysis perfusate is finally collected into microvials, which are routinely exchanged every 30 or 60 min after which the perfusate is analysed at once bedside, utilising enzymatic techniques. The chemicals usually monitored during routine neurocritical care are: glucose, pyruvate, lactate, glutamate, and glycerol. The biochemical analysis usually takes 6–10 min. With the microdialysis technique used as described perfusion rate 0.3 μl/min, membrane length 10 mm, and membrane permeability cut-off at 20 kDa, a recovery of approximately 70% of the true interstitial concentrations is obtained. When microdialysis is performed as a clinical routine technique, this difference is without significance whereas, on the other hand, for the interpretation of results, a stable extraction rate is mandatory. For scientific purposes, it is possible to obtain true interstitial concentration levels.

Substances usually analysed bedside (normal value in brackets)

- Glucose (1.7–0.9 mmol/l) reflects CBF, brain consumption and systemic plasma glucose concentration. Low values can be due to hypoperfusion or low-plasma glucose.
- Lactate (2.9–0.9 mmol/l) and pyruvate (160–50 mol/l) are markers for ischemia and hypoxia. In practice, it is only the lactate/pyruvate ratio (23–0.4) that is used. Glycerol (80–40 mol/l) is a marker for lipolysis and high values can be due to breakdown of cell membranes. Glutamate (16–16 mol/l) is a marker of cytotoxicity in brain tissue.

33.3 Specific Paediatric Concerns

CPP appears to be lower in children than in adults, although the actual lowest threshold for normal brain function has not been determined accurately and may also vary with age. Hence, in anti-oedema therapy using the route of lowering the CPP, it is mandatory to be guided by intracerebral microdialysis. However, there are no studies so far that define the normal values during different ages and even less during TBI.

References

Hillered L, Persson L, Nilsson P, Ronne-Engstrom E, Enblad P (2006) Continuous monitoring of cerebral metabolism in traumatic brain injury: a focus on cerebral microdialysis. Curr Opin Crit Care 12(2):112–118

Nordström CH (2010) Cerebral energy metabolism and microdialysis in neurocritical care. Childs Nerv Syst 26(4):465–472

Jugular Bulb Measurements ($SJVO_2$) 34

Bo-Michael Bellander and Peter Reinstrup

Recommendations

Level I

There are insufficient data to support a Level I recommendation for this topic.

Level II

There are insufficient data to support a Level II recommendation for this topic.

Level III

Jugular venous saturation measurements can be used to monitor cerebral oxygenation where a jugular venous saturation ($SjvO_2$) below 50% should be considered as a treatment threshold (Bratton et al. 2007).

34.1 Overview

Jugular bulb venous oxygen saturation ($SjvO_2$) is the percentage of oxygen bound to haemoglobin in the blood returning from the brain. This reflects the residue of oxygen in blood having passed the brain tissue. $SjvO_2$ can give information about global hypoperfusion or hypoxemia, but there are many concerns when looking at focal brain pathologies.

Tips, Tricks, and Pitfalls

- $SjvO_2$ is a global monitor that not necessarily unmasks focal or even regional ischemia.
- The jugular venous blood is not truly mixed; an ischemic area might be drained by the opposite jugular vein.
- Tissue with limited capacity for oxygen extraction, e.g. re-perfused infarcted tissue or tissue with mitochondrial dysfunction, will give false normal or even high $SjvO_2$.
- The tip of the catheter has to be situated in the jugular bulb in order to avoid contamination from extracerebral blood (Fig. 34.2).
- A radiographic check, lateral skull X-ray or CT, is necessary before jugular venous samples are used. The tip of the catheter should be located slightly medial to the mastoid bone at the level of the mastoid base.
- Fast evacuation (≥10 mL/min) from a jugular bulb catheter increases the risk for contamination of extracerebral blood in the sample.

B.-M. Bellander, (✉)
Department of Clinical Neuroscience, Section for Neurosurgery, Karolinska University Hospital, Building R3:02, 171 76 Solna, Stockholm, Sweden
e-mail: bo-michael.bellander@karolinska.se

P. Reinstrup
Department of Intensive and Perioperative Care, Skanes University Hospital, Lund, S221 85 Lund
e-mail: peter.reinstrup@med.lu.se

T. Sundstrøm et al. (eds.), *Management of Severe Traumatic Brain Injury*,
DOI 10.1007/978-3-642-28126-6_34, © Springer-Verlag Berlin Heidelberg 2012

- A rapid injection of fluid in the retrograde catheter does not affect the brain. Even in situations of low CBF, a rapid injection of contrast only reach up to the sinus confluens and drains again through the contralateral sinus transversus (Fig. 34.2).

34.2 Background

The main part of the cerebral blood flow (CBF) leaves through the internal jugular vein. The blood from the left and right sinus transversus flowing into the two internal jugular veins is not evenly distributed (Fig. 34.1). It is important to emphasise that the blood leaving through one internal jugular vein can, but does not necessarily emanate from the ipsilateral hemisphere; it may be more or less polluted from the contralateral side (Fig. 34.1). An ischemic area might therefore, to varying degrees, be drained by the opposite jugular vein.

Access to the jugular bulb, the conjunction between the transverse sinus and the intern jugular vein, offers an opportunity to analyse blood leaving the brain. Blood chemistry from this site provides an insight into the correlation between the global cerebral blood flow (CBF_{global}) and the cerebral metabolic rate of O_2 ($CMRO_2$). The measuring is based on the insertion of a catheter in retrograde direction in the internal jugular vein to the jugular bulb (Fig. 34.2), the ideal set up being a catheter which can provide continuous measurements in real time.

The method was introduced in the mid-1980s (Garlick and Bihari 1987) and is today regarded as an important part of modern multimodal monitoring in the NICU (Gopinath et al. 1994) even though contradictory opinions have been presented (Latronico et al. 2000).

34.2.1 Adequate Catheter Positioning

A radiographic check, skull X-ray (Fig. 34.2) or CT, is necessary before jugular venous samples are used. The tip of the catheter should be located slightly medial to the mastoid bone at the level of the mastoid base (Jakobsen and Enevoldsen 1989).

34.2.2 Contamination with Extracerebral Blood

Approximately 2.7% (0–6.6%) of the blood in the internal jugular vein is of extracerebral ori-

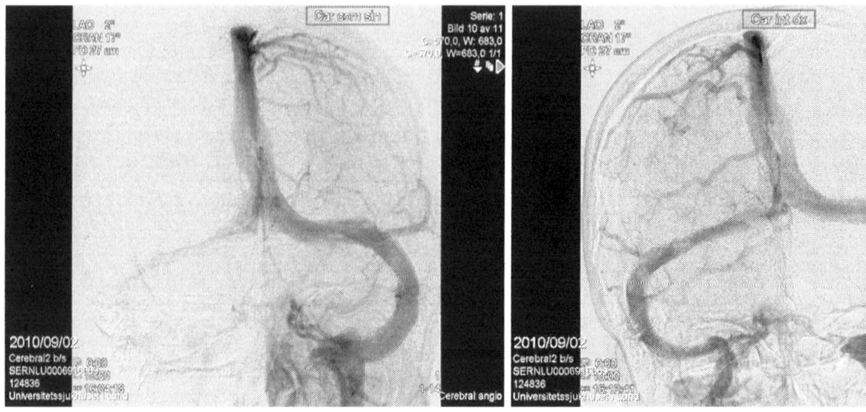

Fig. 34.1 Cerebral angiograms showing the sinuses and the internal jugular veins. The *left picture* is taken after injection in the left internal carotid artery (ICA), and in this patient the blood from the left hemisphere leaves mainly through the left internal jugular vein. The *right picture*, from the same patient, is taken after injection of contrast in the right ICA. The blood from this hemisphere leaves through both internal jugular veins

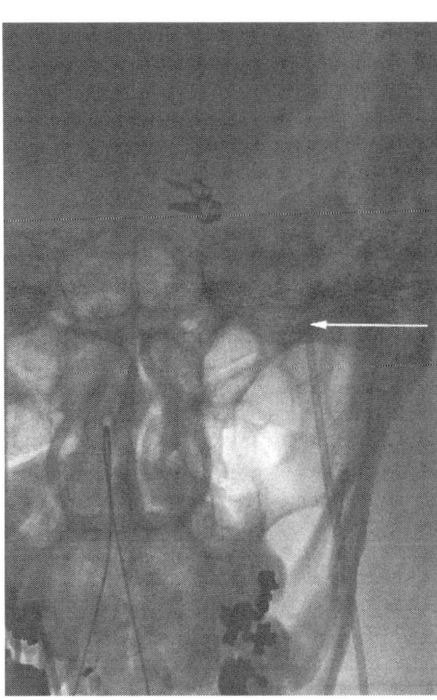

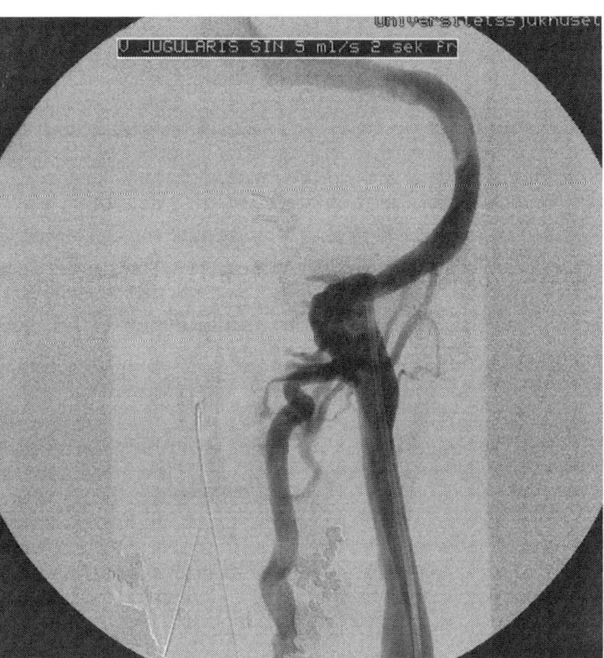

Fig. 34.2 Both pictures are from the same patient. On the *left side*, a plain X-ray of the skull where the *arrow* is pointing at the tip of the catheter. On the *right side*: a plain X-ray during a 5-mL/s contrast injection, thereby visualising the sinus transversus up to sinus confluens, the bulb in the middle of the picture, and the internal jugular vein going down out of the picture. A catheter is seen in the internal jugular vein and just below the jugular bulb: the extracerebral veins

gin (Shenkin et al. 1948). A jugular bulb catheter retracted more than 2 cm below the skull base shows an increase in $SjvO_2$ of more than 10% in 33% of the patients (Jakobsen and Enevoldsen 1989) indicating increased contamination. Rapid evacuation (10 mL/min) of jugular venous blood tends to present with higher $SjvO_2$ values than slow evacuation (2 mL/min), again indicating contamination with extracerebral blood (Matta and Lam 1997). Furthermore, a decrease in CBF and thereby reduced flow out through the internal jugular vein may lead to an increased proportion of extra cerebral blood and, thus, a false high $SjvO_2$.

34.2.3 Normal Values of $SjvO_2$

Normal values for $SjvO_2$ were established by Gibbs and co-workers as early as in 1942 (Gibbs et al. 1942), reporting on average values of 62% (range between 55% and 71%) (Woodman and Robertson 1995). In a recent report, the average $SjvO_2$ was 61% with the upper limit at 71% (Henson et al. 1998) even though others have used 75% as an upper limit (Cormio et al. 1999). A lower limit for $SjvO_2$ has been suggested to 55% (Cormio et al. 1997; Cruz 1993), but lower limits, down to 45%, has also been suggested (Chan et al. 2005).

34.2.4 Factors Lowering $SjvO_2$

Decreased Oxygen Delivery: One reason for a decreased oxygen delivery is a reduced CBF. There are several factors attenuating CBF, one being increased cerebral vascular resistance (CVR) as during increased ICP, hyperventilation, vasospasm (Schneider et al. 1995), or by endogenous or exogenous cerebral vasoconstrictors. A decrease in oxygen delivery can also be of extracerebral origin as in hypotension, hypoxia, or anaemia (Robertson et al. 1995).

Increased Cerebral Metabolism: Fever and seizures increase oxygen consumption. Fever increases the body's metabolic rate by 10–13% per centigrade. In piglets, a rise in temperature from 38°C to 42°C increases CBF by 97% and $CMRO_2$ by 65% (Busija et al. 1988). The uncoupling between CMR and CBF with an increased CBF will in this situation counteract a lowering of the $SjvO_2$. Seizures in rats increase $CMRO_2$ by 150–250% (Meldrum and Nilsson 1976), and it is often difficult for the circulation to cope with such an increase, resulting in a lowering of $SjvO_2$.

34.2.5 Factors Increasing $SjvO_2$

Decreased Cerebral Metabolism: Hypothermia decreases $CMRO_2$ approximately 5% per centigrade (Woodman and Robertson 1995). Barbiturate coma treatment may reduce cerebral oxygen consumption with up to 50% (Pierce et al. 1962). With the CBF-CMR coupling, $SjvO_2$ might not be changed, but since barbiturates have a vasoconstrictive effect in low concentrations and in high act as vasodilatators, the $SjvO_2$ can change in any direction. Anaemia has been shown to result in low $SjvO_2$ values underestimating the reduction in CBF (Cruz et al. 1993).

34.2.6 $SjvO_2$ Versus CBF

If CMR as well as arterial blood pressure, arterial oxygen saturation, and haemoglobin content is stable, changes in $SjvO_2$ corresponds to changes in CBF (Robertson et al. 1989). However, alkalosis, e.g. induced by hyperventilation, makes the tissue less able to extract oxygen such that a normal $SjvO_2$ might occur despite a low tissue pO_2 and an ischemic cerebral metabolism. However, provided pH < 7.6, the tissue extraction of O_2 is not impaired resulting in a $SjvO_2$ adequately reflects a tissue pO_2 (Cruz et al. 1992). This multitude of factors involved makes it an unreliable method to estimate CBF with other than in special cases.

34.2.7 TBI Patients

In head trauma, patients' $SjvO_2$ has been reported to average 68% (range: 32–96%) (Woodman and Robertson 1995).

34.2.8 Jugular Venous Desaturation ($SjvO_2 \leq 50\%$)

Jugular venous desaturation has been shown to occur on at least one occasion during the observation time in 39% (Robertson et al. 1995) of severely brain injured patients. Approximately half of the episodes are due to cerebral causes (intracranial hypertension, or vascular spasm), and the rest had systemic causes (hypotension, hypoxia, hypocarbia, or anaemia) (Robertson et al. 1995). Microdialysis used in concert with jugular bulb measurements have shown increased concentrations of lactate and glutamate to occur in conjunction with $SjvO_2$ < 50% in 7 out of 22 patients (Robertson et al. 1995).

34.2.9 Early Episodes of Desaturation

Jugular venous desaturation was identified in 6 out of 8 patients during evacuation of a traumatic intracranial hematoma in the emergency operating room. In all 6 cases, $SjvO_2$ increased from 47 ± 10% to 63 ± 5% after the evacuation of the hematoma (Robertson et al. 1995). Spontaneous episodes of desaturation have been shown to occur frequently during the acute phase (<48 h) of TBI, SAH, and ICH (Schneider et al. 1995). Approximately one third of severe TBI patients presents with cerebral desaturation immediately after admission (Vigue et al. 1999). Many episodes of desaturation are attributed to hyperventilation, insufficient cerebral perfusion pressure (CPP), and severe, therapy-resistant vasospasm (Schneider et al. 1995). In a study including 25 severe TBI patients, a total of 42 episodes of jugular bulb oxygen desaturation (<50% > 10 min) were observed. The majority of incidences, 83%, occurred within 48 h following injury. Of the major associated secondary insults, hypocapnia was involved in 45% of the episodes, hypoperfusion in 22%, raised ICP in 9%, and a combination of the above in 24% (Lewis et al. 1995).

34.2.10 $SjvO_2 \leq 50\%$ and Outcome

Episodes of desaturation among patients suffering from severe TBI (GCS ≤ 8) have a strong association to poor outcome (Robertson et al. 1995). Mortality 3 months post-trauma increased from 21% in the group of no incidence of desaturation to 37% if one episode of desaturation occurred and 69% if multiple episodes of desaturation occurred during the NICU stay (Robertson et al. 1995). In accordance concerning good recovery or moderate disability (GOS 4–5), the opposite was found, with incidences at 44%, 30%, and 15% respectively.

34.2.11 $SjvO_2 \geq 75\%$ and Outcome

In a study including 450 severely head injured patients, an increased mortality 6 months post trauma was found among patients presenting with high $SjvO_2 > 75\%$ (Cormio et al. 1999). Patients with high $SjvO_2$ due to O_2 extraction problems or regional ischemia was found to present with unfavourable outcome, while patients with high $SjvO_2$ due to excessive cerebral blood flow in relation to the metabolic demands, hyperaemia, had a decent outcome (Cormio et al. 1999).

34.2.12 $AVD_{lactate}$

An arteriovenous difference in lactate exceeding 0.3 mmol/L with the higher lactate in the jugular bulb indicates ischemia as long as the peripheral serum level of lactate is <2.1 mmol/L (Artru et al. 2004).

34.3 Specific Paediatric Concerns

There are no specific paediatric concerns due to the lack of specific paediatric data.

References

Artru F, Dailler F, Burel E, Bodonian C, Grousson S, Convert J et al (2004) Assessment of jugular blood oxygen and lactate indices for detection of cerebral ischemia and prognosis. J Neurosurg Anesthesiol 16:226–231

Bratton SL, Chestnut RM, Ghajar J, McConnell Hammond FF, Harris OA, Hartl R, Manley GT, Nemecek A, Newell DW, Rosenthal G, Schouten J, Shutter L, Timmons SD, Ullman JS, Videtta W, Wilberger JE, Wright DW (2007) Guidelines for the management of severe traumatic brain injury. J Neurotrauma 24:S65–S70

Busija DW, Leffler CW, Pourcyrous M (1988) Hyperthermia increases cerebral metabolic rate and blood flow in neonatal pigs. Am J Physiol 255:H343–H346

Chan MT, Ng SC, Lam JM, Poon WS, Gin T (2005) Re-defining the ischemic threshold for jugular venous oxygen saturation – a microdialysis study in patients with severe head injury. Acta Neurochir Suppl 95:63–66

Cormio M, Robertson CS, Narayan RK (1997) Secondary insults to the injured brain. J Clin Neurosci 4:132–148

Cormio M, Valadka AB, Robertson CS (1999) Elevated jugular venous oxygen saturation after severe head injury. J Neurosurg 90:9–15

Cruz J (1993) On-line monitoring of global cerebral hypoxia in acute brain injury. J Neurosurg 79:228–233

Cruz J, Gennarelli TA, Hoffstad OJ (1992) Lack of relevance of the Bohr effect in optimally ventilated patients with acute brain trauma. J Trauma 33:304–310

Cruz J, Jaggi JL, Hoffstad OJ (1993) Cerebral blood flow and oxygen consumption in acute brain injury with acute anemia: an alternative for the cerebral metabolic rate of oxygen consumption? Crit Care Med 21:1218–1224

Garlick R, Bihari D (1987) The use of intermittent and continuous recordings of jugular venous bulb oxygen saturation in the unconscious patient. Scand J Clin Lab Invest Suppl 188:47–52

Gibbs EL, Lennox WG, Nims LF, Gibbs FA (1942) Arterial and cerebral venous blood: arterial-venous differences in man. J Biol Chem 144:325–332

Gopinath SP, Robertson CS, Contant CF, Hayes C, Feldman Z, Narayan RK et al (1994) Jugular venous desaturation and outcome after head injury. J Neurol Neurosurg Psychiatry 57:717–723

Henson LC, Calalang C, Temp JA, Ward DS (1998) Accuracy of a cerebral oximeter in healthy volunteers under conditions of isocapnic hypoxia. Anesthesiology 88:58–65

Jakobsen M, Enevoldsen E (1989) Retrograde catheterization of the right internal jugular vein for serial measurements of cerebral venous oxygen content. J Cereb Blood Flow Metab 9:717–720

Latronico NMD, Beindorf AEMD, Rasulo FAMD, Febbrari PMD, Stefini RMD, Cornali CMD et al

(2000) Limits of intermittent jugular bulb oxygen saturation monitoring in the management of severe head trauma patients. Neurosurgery 46:1131–1139

Lewis SB, Myburgh JA, Reilly PL (1995) Detection of cerebral venous desaturation by continuous jugular bulb oximetry following acute neurotrauma. Anaesth Intensive Care 23:307–314

Matta BF, Lam AM (1997) The rate of blood withdrawal affects the accuracy of jugular venous bulb. Oxygen saturation measurements. Anesthesiology 86:806–808

Meldrum BS, Nilsson B (1976) Cerebral blood flow and metabolic rate early and late in prolonged epileptic seizures induced in rats by bicuculline. Brain 99:523–542

Pierce EC Jr, Lambertsen CJ, Deutsch S, Chase PE, Linde HW, Dripps RD et al (1962) Cerebral circulation and metabolism during thiopental anesthesia and hyperventilation in man. J Clin Invest 41:1664–1671

Robertson CS, Narayan RK, Gokaslan ZL, Pahwa R, Grossman RG, Caram P Jr et al (1989) Cerebral arteriovenous oxygen difference as an estimate of cerebral blood flow in comatose patients. J Neurosurg 70:222–230

Robertson CS, Gopinath SP, Goodman JC, Contant CF, Valadka AB, Narayan RK (1995) SjvO2 monitoring in head-injured patients. J Neurotrauma 12:891–896

Schneider GH, von Helden A, Lanksch WR, Unterberg A (1995) Continuous monitoring of jugular bulb oxygen saturation in comatose patients–therapeutic implications. Acta Neurochir (Wien) 134:71–75

Shenkin HA, Harmel MH, Kety SS (1948) Dynamic anatomy of the cerebral circulation. Arch Neurol Psychiatry 60:240–252

Vigue B, Ract C, Benayed M, Zlotine N, Leblanc PE, Samii K et al (1999) Early SjvO2 monitoring in patients with severe brain trauma. Intensive Care Med 25:445–451

Woodman T, Robertson SC (1995) Jugular venous oxygen saturation monitoring. In: Narayan RK, Wilberger JE Jr, Povlishock JT (eds) Neurotrauma. McGraw-Hill, New York, pp 519–553

Cerebral Blood Flow (CBF) and Cerebral Metabolic Rate (CMR)

35

Peter Reinstrup and Eric L. Bloomfield

Recommendations

Level I

There are insufficient data to support a Level I recommendation for this topic.

Level II

There are insufficient data to support a Level II recommendation for this topic.

Level III

Individualized treatment of traumatic brain injury (TBI) can be guided by cerebral blood flow (CBF) measurements.

35.1 Overview

Over time, we have come to understand the concepts of cerebral blood flow and its relationship to pH changes and metabolism of the brain. Current evidence tells us that insufficient flow can lead to ischemic regions of the brain with poor clinical outcome. The challenge today is to find an economical hands-on method to measure CBF bedside. With such techniques, one could hope to foster better outcome for patients with TBI. Present methods still remain in the research realm; hopefully, future will see new avenues for CBF measurements that are specific, economical and easy to utilize at the bedside.

Tips, Tricks, and Pitfalls

- Measurement of CBF and CMR in TBI patients can give information about how to optimize the cerebral circulation.
- MR, CT and some of the SPECT techniques are not accurate in absolute blood flow values, but gives excellent information about the relative distribution.
- A crude estimation of the absolute blood flow can be obtained by comparing the relative CBF picture with the blood flow through cerebellum. Cerebellum does under normal circumstances have a constant high flow.
- Appropriate safety measures must be taken to minimize radiation exposure to medical staff and patients. In handling 133Xe, care should be taken to avoid

P. Reinstrup (✉)
Department of Intensive and Perioperative Care, Skanes University Hospital, S221 85 Lund, Sweden
e-mail: peter.reinstrup@med.lu.se

E.L. Bloomfield
Department of Anesthesiology, Mayo Clinic, 200 First Street SW, Rochester Mn. 55905 USA
e-mail: bloomfield.eric@mayo.edu

T. Sundstrøm et al. (eds.), *Management of Severe Traumatic Brain Injury*, DOI 10.1007/978-3-642-28126-6_35, © Springer-Verlag Berlin Heidelberg 2012

direct contact with any part of the body. Our safety rules involve 0.6 rad/min of exposure time for the surgeon and less than 5 μrad/min exposure to surrounding personnel.

- Concerning information about 133Xenon, the emitted photons from 133Xenon are of low energy and, as such, can be absorbed by 0.1 mm of lead to reduce exposure by 90%. The physical half-life of 133Xe is 5.27 days.

35.2 Background

35.2.1 Normal Brain

The brain weight is only 2% of body mass, but it receives 20% of the cardiac output. The reason for this is the high cerebral metabolic rate (CMR) demanding a constant delivery of oxygen and nutrients and the removal of waste products such as CO_2. CMR changes with activity and during deep sleep and sedation; anaesthesia can reduce O_2 consumption down to 50% from the normal (3.3 ml O_2/100-g brain/min or 29-mmol glucose/100-g brain/min) (Reinstrup et al. 2008; Alkire et al. 1995, 1997; Madsen et al. 1991; Kaisti et al. 2002). Metabolism increases in areas with increased neuronal activity as in normal movement-thinking (Ingvar and Philipson 1977; Paradiso et al. 1999; Buxton 2002; Qiu et al. 2008). During pathological circumstances, as in epilepsy, O_2 metabolism can increase up to 200%. In these local areas with elevated metabolism, there will be a concomitant increase in the local CBF. Under normal circumstances, this coupling keeps a constant relationship between the CMR and CBF (Qiu et al. 2008; Buxton 2002). The CBF_{global} through the brain is determined by the CPP and the cerebrovascular resistance (CVR) with CBF=CPP/CVR. Within normal limits of mean arterial blood pressure (MAP) (60–150 mmHg), the CPP does not affect the CBF due to the cerebral auto-regulation (Paulson et al. 1990).

CVR is under neuronal and chemical control. The reason for the increase in CBF during increased metabolism is mainly due to the increased CO_2 production lowering the perivascular pH (Kontos et al. 1977; Reinstrup et al. 1992). A relaxation of the cerebral arteries can also be attained due to the small extracellular potassium increase as a result of the neuronal membrane depolarization. The cerebral arteries also react to global changes in CO_2, which creates uniform changes in CBF as during hyperventilation (Reinstrup et al. 1994), the normal response being 1–2 ml/100-g brain/mmHg change in $pACO_2$ or 7–10 ml/100-g brain/kPa change in $pACO_2$, depending on the measurement technique. The Kety and Schmidt (1948) technique, which investigates global CBF, describes a CO_2 response of 1 ml/100-g brain/min. Another investigation, looking at the response in the cortical grey substance, reports on a CO_2 response of 1.8 ml/100-g brain/min (Messeter et al. 1986). Lowering the CO_2 as in hypocapnic hyperventilation therefore results in a vasoconstriction with a lowering of the CBF. If the CMR and hence the CO_2 production is constant, such a lowering of the blood flow results in a gradual increase in the perivascular CO_2. The concomitant lowering of the perivascular pH may thus counteract the effect of the arterial hypocapnia, resulting in a reduced vasoconstrictive effect over time.

The neuronal tropic centres for metabolism are in the cell bodies situated in the grey substance of the brain. With the strict coupling between CMR and CBF (Buxton 2002; Qiu et al. 2008), local differences in CMR creates a similar uneven but geographically correlated distribution of the CBF (see Fig. 35.1).

35.2.2 CMR and CBF

35.2.3 Traumatic Brain Injury

Traumatic brain injury (TBI) affects the cerebral circulation. The metabolic reactions to brain trauma fuel the production and liberation of a variety of biochemical substances including

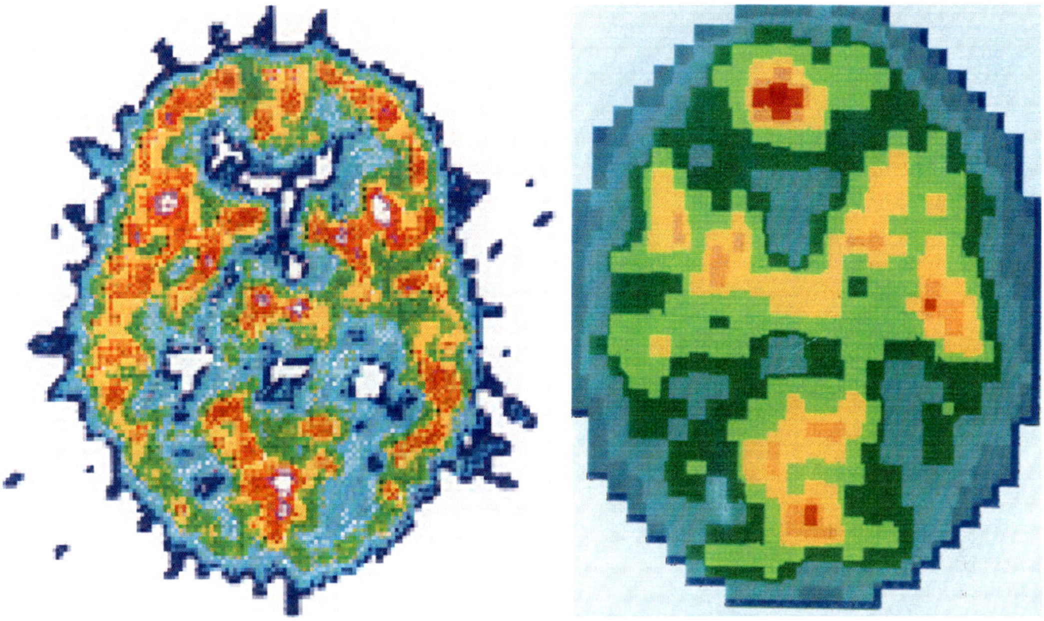

Fig. 35.1 A slice 2 cm above the orbitomeatal line representing the brain metabolism on the left and the corresponding CBF (right ^{133}XenonSPECT). The $CMR_{glu\text{-}Global}$ was 27 mmol/100-g brain/min, and the CBF_{global} was 55 ml/100-g brain/min (The *left picture* has been published in *Br J Anaesthesiol*. The *right* has been published in *Anesthesiology*)

vasoactive ones (Golding et al. 1999). This might be the reason for the change in CBF_{global} over time. Generally after a brain trauma, CMR_{global} is reduced to 50%; the reduction on CMR seems to correlate to the severity of the brain trauma (Obrist et al. 1984). Not all but many patients follow a specific pattern (Obrist et al. 1984). In the hyperacute phase after the injury, CMR_{global} is low with a similar reduction as the CBF_{global}. After approximately 12 h, the hyperaemic phase starts and CBF_{global} increases to normal awake values. If there is a low CMR, one could invoke relative hyperaemia. Three days after the trauma, the CBF_{global} is back to the same low level as in the immediate phase after the trauma, but now there may be signs of vasospasm in many patients (Martin et al. 1997). Beside this, auto-regulation (Enevoldsen and Jensen 1978; Jünger et al. 1997) and the CO_2 response (Obrist et al. 1984; Enevoldsen and Jensen 1978; Schalén et al. 1991) has been impaired which had lead to hyperaemia. The 3D picture of CMR and even more the 3D CBF picture do often show a patchy picture due to local changes in metabolism and local changes in vasoactive substances (Fig. 35.2). In TBI patients, 3D investigations have indeed revealed that ischaemia occurs on a local level (Abate et al. 2008; Werner and Engelhard 2007; Bouma et al. 1992; Coles et al. 2004; Inoue et al. 2005) and that the presence of such ischaemia is associated with poor neurological outcome (Werner and Engelhard 2007; Bouma et al. 1992).

35.2.4 Measuring CBF

For many neurologic or neurosurgical patients, an ideal brain monitoring would be a non-invasive, continuous 3D measurement of cerebral blood flow and metabolism in real time. Our present monitoring capacity is far from this situation. CBF measurements are still cumbersome and involve remedies limiting such investigations in daily usage. Prior to the Kety–Schmidt method, attempts to get information of the CBF were based on probes placed into the jugular vein to

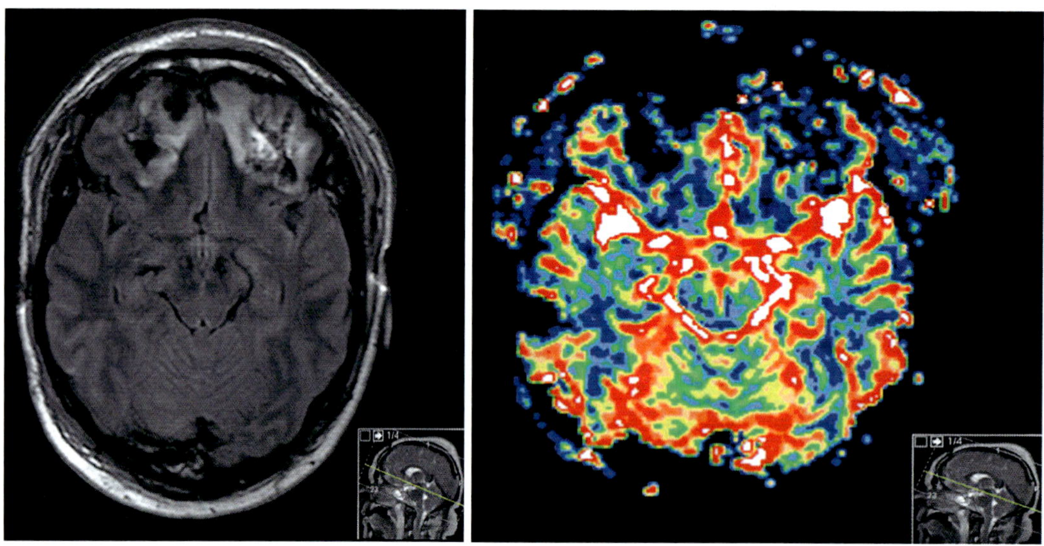

Fig. 35.2 A traumatic brain injury with frontal contusions seen on the MR Flair on the *left picture*. On the *right hand* is the corresponding CBF showing low perfusion in and adjacent to the contusions

detect physiologic changes in cerebral blood flow. Over the years, a number of techniques have been utilized to measure blood flow in the arteries of the neck. The measurement of cerebral venous outflow can include heat clearance techniques in blood vessels and in brain tissue, hydrogen clearance, angiography, ultrasonography, diffusible and non-diffusible tracer-based measurements of cerebral flow, laser Doppler, positron emission tomography (PET), magnetic resonance imaging (MRI) and computerized tomography (CT). Some of the important methods are briefly described below.

35.2.5 Measuring the Global CBF (CBF_{global}) (Kety–Schmidt)

The Fick principle is used to calculate blood flow through different organs where blood flow is equal to the quantity of a substance removed or added in time, divided by the difference between arterial and venous concentrations of the substance. This method for measuring organ blood flow was first applied to the brain in 1944 by C. F. Schmidt and S. S. Kety.

They used inhalation of a highly diffusible, inert gas (nitrous oxide (N_2O)) and frequent measurements of the arterial N_2O. To represent output of blood leaving the brain, N_2O concentration is measured in the jugular bulb. N_2O uptake in the brain per unit time is equal to the amount of N_2O brought to the brain by the arterial blood minus the amount carried away in the cerebral venous blood. Thus, at a time when the N_2O content of the brain and its cerebral venous blood reached equilibrium in approximately 10–15 min, the brain content of nitrous oxide and CBF could be estimated. Kety and Schmidt (1946) found that the CBF_{global} was 54 ml/100-g brain/min in young healthy males.

35.2.6 Measuring Global CMR (CMR_{global})

By combining the CBF measurements with arterial and jugular venous oxygen measurements, it was possible to calculate the $CMRO_2$ by the following equation:

$$CMRO_2 = CBF \times (CaO_2 - CjvO_2)$$

CaO_2 is the arterial content of O_2, and $CjvO_2$ is the O_2 content from the blood leaving the brain at the jugular bulb.

The arterial or venous content of O_2 (C_xO_2) is dependent on the O_2 amount dissolved in plasma and the O_2 bound to haemoglobin. Since PaO_2 reflects only free oxygen molecules dissolved in plasma and not those bound to haemoglobin, PaO_2 alone does not give the C_xO_2 in the blood; for that, you need also to know how much oxygen is bound to haemoglobin. The SaO_2 and haemoglobin give this. Many factors influence on these amounts, but in general:

$$C_xO_2 / 100 \text{ ml} = O_{2\text{-plasma}} + O_{2\text{-haemoglobin}}$$
$$= (K_{\text{plasma}} \times pO_2) + (\text{Hb} \times K_{\text{haemoglobin}} \times SO_2)$$
$$\text{If } pO_2 \text{is in mmHg}, K_{\text{plasma}} = 0.003$$
$$\text{If } pO_2 \text{is in kPa}, K_{\text{plasma}} = 0.023$$
$$\text{If Hb is in g} / 100 \text{ ml}, K_{\text{haemoglobin}} = 1.36$$
$$\text{If Hb is in mmol} / \text{l}, K_{\text{haemoglobin}} = 2.18$$

35.2.7 Alternative Methods to Measure CBF_{global}

35.2.7.1 Double-Indicator Dilution Technique

The transcerebral double-indicator dilution technique is a rather new method to measure CBF_{global}. It is based on bolus injection of ice-cold indocyanine-green dye with a simultaneous recording of thermo- and dye-dilution curves in the aorta and the jugular bulb using combined fibre-optic thermistor catheters. CBF was calculated from the mean transit times of the dye and thermal indicator through the brain. However, the authors conclude that, at present time, the accuracy and resolution of this technique is not high enough to detect the effect of minor changes of physiological variables (Mielck et al. 2004).

35.2.8 Ultrasound

This method is a simple technique performing Doppler ultrasound examination of the extracranial arteries in the neck. Several articles describe flow and flow volume measurements in the internal carotid artery and vertebral artery (Scheel et al. 2000; Albayrak et al. 2007; Yazici et al. 2005). The examination is performed in supine position with the head slightly to the opposite side. The vessel lumen diameter is measured at systole, and the cross-sectional area of each vessel is calculated. Angle-corrected blood flow velocity is measured with the pulsed Doppler and sample volume expanded to encompass the entire vessel diameter (Fig. 35.3). The volume blood flow of each artery is calculated as time-averaged maximum flow velocity and multiplied with the area. In theory, it is a simple technique, which is not the case in practice; it has never been evaluated against the classic standard techniques as previously described.

35.2.9 Local–Regional CBF

Kety proceeded in his laboratory and developed techniques to present local CBF in animals by inhalation of a diffusible radioactive gas (trifluoroiodomethane). Kety could obtain post-mortem slices of the brain showing relative CBF in different brain regions, and this is in fact the beginning of the later 3D CMR–CBF visualizations.

In 1961, Lassen and Ingvar (1961) introduced the intra-carotid ^{85}krypton method introducing radioisotopes into CBF measurements in vivo. By rapid injection of this radioactive ß-emitter and multiple (Geiger–Müller) ionization detectors placed directly on the brain surface, they were able to look at regional CBF in animals. The washout curves of ^{85}Krypton recorded on the different detectors was predominantly influenced by the CBF in the tissue closest to the detectors. In order to penetrate the skull bone, Harper et al. (1963) substituted ^{85}Krypton for ^{133}Xenon and started to use collimators for a higher resolution. Mallet and Veall (1963) started with the inhalation of ^{133}Xenon, thereby making the method less invasive. Obrist (Obrist et al. 1975) applied the Kety–Schmidt equations so that intravenously injected ^{133}Xenon became a clinical method for investigating CBF and CMR. These methods gave excellent information of the cortical structures, but no information of deeper structures warranting 3D systems.

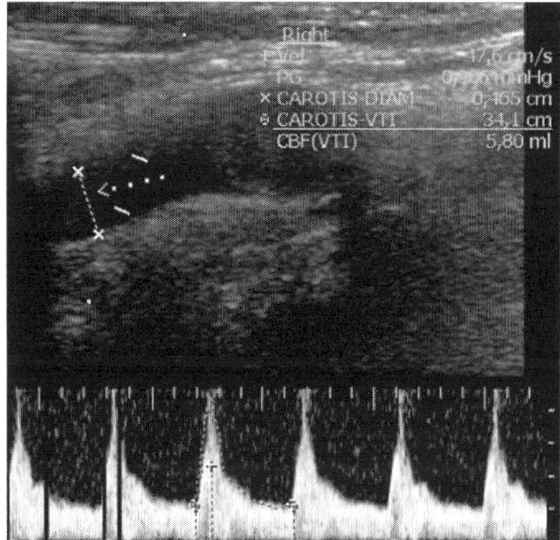

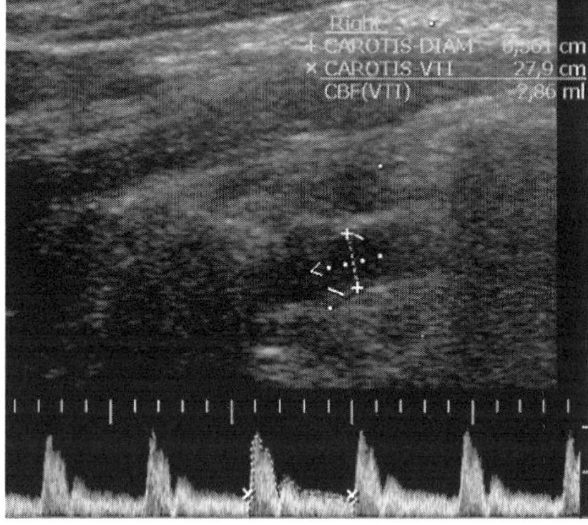

Fig. 35.3 Measurement of CBF with ultrasound at the neck. *Left picture* is measurement in the internal carotid artery, and *right* is the vertebral artery (even though the text in the picture states it should be carotid artery). The vertebral artery is found in between two vertebras that can be seen as *dark shadows* on each side

35.2.10 Thermal Diffusion Flow Probes

This is an invasive procedure that measures flow by estimating the temperature gradient between two plates on the surface of the brain. It measures the blood flow only in the one area of cortex underlying it. The technique yields continuous values and has been used intraoperatively. The microprobe provides a sensitive, continuous and real-time assessment of intraparenchymal regional cerebral blood flow (rCBF) in absolute flow values that is in good agreement with sXe–rCBF measurements (Vajkoczy et al. 2000). However, it can yield false estimations if it is even slightly displaced.

35.2.10.1 3D Brain Investigations

Positron emission tomography (PET) and single-photon emission computed tomography (SPECT).

In PET, the radioisotope decay creates emission of positrons resulting in production of gamma photons moving in opposite directions. This fact makes it possible to pinpoint the exact location of the decay of the radioisotope. In SPECT, the tracer emits gamma rays making it more difficult to determine its exact origin, and the spatial resolution is therefore much better with PET. This can be seen in the figure above (see Fig. 35.1). The left picture being a CMR-PET study and the right a CBF-SPECT study presenting slices through the same brain areas. The basic technique requires injection of a radioisotope (radionuclide) where individual differences in binding sites and attachments allows for investigations of different brain structures and brain functions. The foundation of these techniques is based on the detection of radioisotopes emitted by an emission-computed tomography. A computer calculates the three dimensions of the isotope distribution, which allows for imaging of the investigated volume into thin slices. In modern scanners, the correlation to brain structures is often accomplished with the aid of a CT X-ray scan performed on the patient during the same session.

The concept of emission tomography was started in the late 1950s, and clinical useful apparatus came in the 1970s and 1980s. The scanners are based on the placement of multiple scintillation detectors in a ring around the head.

35.2.11 Stable Xenon CT

Development of the stable Xenon CT method came shortly after the introduction of the CT in the mid 1970s. Xenon, with its high atomic number, attenuates X-rays, and thus in the CT scan, one can directly measure its concentration in the brain. Determination of the outflow or venous concentration is therefore not required when utilizing the Fick principle. The input or arterial concentration was established by Kelcz et al. (1978), determining the solubility of xenon in tissue and blood; this was the basis for converting end-tidal xenon values to arterial concentrations. The concentration of xenon in arterial blood could therefore be determined from end-tidal xenon measured by a thermo-conductivity analyzer. Now, by measuring the concentration of xenon in the blood and brain, the time for which xenon has been administered and knowing the blood–brain partition coefficient for xenon, the CBF can be calculated, using a modified Kety–Schmidt formula for xenon.

Xenon in high concentrations is an anaesthetic, and in the beginning, it was necessary to inhale it in such concentrations, but the improvements in CT scan technology in combination with the modern computer capabilities have made the process of Xe/CBF more user-friendly. The Xe/CBF measurement can be repeated after an interval of 20 min, making it useful for investigating also auto-regulation and CO_2 response. Another advantage is that the Xe/CT CBF is directly coupled to a CT scan thereby showing the anatomy.

35.2.12 CT Perfusion

Perfusion CT was first described by Axel (1980, 1983), but it has taken many years to develop the technique to be used in clinical practice. To obtain information about cerebral blood flow with the CT, an amount of intravenous contrast medium is injected. The CT scanning and contrast injection is started simultaneously. The CT scanner runs the same slices over and over again while the contrast medium passes the brain. The examination is based on the indicator dilution theory. Following administration of the intravenous bolus of contrast medium, the X-ray density of the vessels and brain temporarily increases. In basic terms, the method is based on the determination of the speed by which the blood is traversing the brain or in other words the mean transit time (MTT) as well as the cerebral blood volume (CBV). Conclusions about these parameters are drawn from the extent and course over time of the increase in density due to the contrast medium over time. These estimations requires the use of software-employing complex deconvolution algorithms, but when the MTT and CBF is found, the CBF=CBV/MTT (Hoeffner et al. 2004). Some controversies exist concerning the accuracy of the quantitative results and their reproducibility. Despite this, many clinics use CT perfusion in evaluating their neurological patients as it is the most convenient method, and some correlation to the PET methodology has been found (Shinohara et al. 2010).

35.2.13 MR Perfusion

The way of measuring CBF with MR is essentially the same as the CT perfusion method. The use of dynamic susceptibility contrast magnetic resonance imaging (DSC-MRI) for assessment of perfusion-related parameters is promising (Wirestam et al. 2009), but the concept is hampered by a number of methodological complications. For example, an accurate registration of the arterial input function, i.e. the concentration-versus-time curve in an appropriate tissue-feeding artery is interfered by different factors (Østergaard et al. 1996; Wirestam et al. 2009). Attempts to achieve absolute quantification of perfusion parameters by standard DSC-MRI have typically been characterized by overestimated values of CBV and CBF (Knutsson et al. 2007; Wirestam et al. 2009), which is due to a correspondingly underestimated arterial concentration time integral. Hence, the majority of existing implementations of DSC-MRI provide only relative perfusion parameters (Kaneko et al. 2004) even though it clearly reflects absolute changes due to CO_2 variations (Wirestam et al. 2009).

In 1992, Williams et al. (1992) found an alternative to the above method using contrast injection called arterial spin labelling. Arterial spin labelling uses magnetically labelled water protons as an endogenous tracer. The overall goal of all-existing arterial spin labelling is to produce a flow-sensitized image or 'labelled' image and a 'control' image in which the static tissue signals are identical. At the same time, one has to see that the magnetization of the inflowing blood differs. Despite the remarkable progress in this technique, arterial spin labelling has still not overtaken traditional invasive methods (Petersen et al. 2006).

35.3 Specific Paediatric Concerns

At birth, cortical rCBFs are lower than in adults. CBF increases and reaches a maximum at the fifth year of 50–85% higher than those for adults and thereafter decreased reaching adult levels after the 15 year. The time needed to reach normal adult values differed for each cortical region. The shortest time was found on the primary cortex, and the longest, on the associative cortex. Cognitive development of the child seems to be related to changes in blood flow of the corresponding brain regions (Chiron et al. 1992).

References

Abate MG, Trivedi M, Fryer TD, Smielewski P, Chatfield DA, Williams GB, Aigbirhio F, Carpenter TA, Pickard JD, Menon DK, Coles JP (2008) Early derangements in oxygen and glucose metabolism following head injury: the ischemic penumbra and pathophysiological heterogeneity. Neurocrit Care 9:319–325

Albayrak R, Degirmenci B, Acar M, Haktanır A, Colbay M, Yaman M (2007) Doppler sonography evaluation of flow velocity and volume of the extracranial internal carotid and vertebral arteries in healthy adults. J Clin Ultrasound 35:27–33

Alkire MT, Haier RJ, Barker SJ, Shah NK, Wu JC, Kao YJ (1995) Cerebral metabolism during propofol anesthesia in humans studied with positron emission tomography. Anesthesiology 82:393–403

Alkire MT, Haier RJ, Shah NK, Anderson CT (1997) Positron emission tomography study of regional cerebral metabolism in humans during isoflurane anesthesia. Anesthesiology 86:549–557

Axel L (1980) Cerebral blood flow determination by rapid-sequence computed tomography. Radiology 137:679–686

Axel L (1983) Tissue mean transit time from dynamic computed tomography by a simple deconvolution technique. Invest Radiol 18:94–99

Bouma GJ, Muizelaar JP, Stringer WA, Choi C, Fatouros P, Young HF (1992) Ultra-early evaluation of regional cerebral blood flow in severely head-injured patients using xenon-enhanced computerized tomography. J Neurosurg 77:360–368

Buxton RB (2002) Coupling between CBF and CMRO2 during neuronal activity. Int Congr Ser 1235:23–32

Chiron C, Raynaud C, Maziere B, Zilbovicius M, Laflamme L, Masure MC, Dulac O, Bourguignon M, Syrota A (1992) Changes in regional cerebral blood flow during brain maturation in children and adolescents. J Nucl Med 33:696–703

Coles JP, Fryer TD, Smielewski P et al (2004) Defining ischemic burden after traumatic brain injury using 15O PET imaging of cerebral physiology. J Cereb Blood Flow Metab 24:191–201

Enevoldsen EM, Jensen FT (1978) Autoregulation and CO2 responses of cerebral blood flow in patients with acute severe head injury. J Neurosurg 48(5):689–703

Golding EM, Robertson CS, Bryan RM Jr (1999) The consequences of traumatic brain injury on cerebral blood flow and autoregulation: a review. Clin Exp Hypertens 21(4):299–332

Harper AM, Glass HI, Steven JL, Granat AH (1964) The measurement of local blood flow in the cerebral cortex from the clearance of xenon. J Neurol Neurosurg Psychiatry 27:255

Hoeffner EG, Case I, Jain R, Gujar SK, Shah GV, Deveikis JP, Carlos RC, Thompson BG, Harrigan MR, Mukherji SK (2004) Cerebral perfusion CT: technique and clinical applications. Radiology 231(3):632–644, Epub 2004 Apr 29

Ingvar DH, Philipson L (1977) Distribution of cerebral blood flow in the dominant hemisphere during motor ideation and motor performance. Ann Neurol 2:230–237

Inoue Y, Shiozaki T, Tasaki O et al (2005) Changes in cerebral blood flow from the acute to the chronic phase of severe head injury. J Neurotrauma 22:1411–1418

Jünger EC, Newell DW, Grant GA, Avellino AM, Ghatan S, Douville CM, Lam AM, Aaslid R, Winn HR (1997) Cerebral autoregulation following minor head injury. J Neurosurg 86:425–432

Kaisti KK, Metsähonkala L, Teräs M, Oikonen V, Aalto S, Jääskeläinen S, Hinkka S, Scheinin H (2002) Effects of surgical levels of propofol and sevoflurane anesthesia on cerebral blood flow in healthy subjects studied with positron emission tomography. Anesthesiology 96(6):1358–1370

Kaneko K, Kuwabara Y, Mihara F, Yoshiura T, Nakagawa M, Tanaka A, Sasaki M, Koga H, Hayashi K, Honda H (2004) Validation of the CBF, CBV, and MTT values by perfusion MRI in chronic occlusive cerebrovascular disease: a comparison with 15O-PET. Acad Radiol 11(5):489–497

Kelcz F, Hilal SK, Hartwell P, Joseph PM (1978) Computed tomography measurement of the xenon brain–blood partition coefficient and implications for the regional cerebral blood flow: a preliminary report. Radiology 127:358–392

Kety SS, Schmidt CF (1946) Measurement of cerebral blood flow and cerebral oxygen consumption in man. Fed Proc. Jun;5:264

Kety SS, Schmidt CF (1948) The effect of altered arterial tension of carbon dioxide and oxygen on cerebral oxygen consumption of normal young men. J Clin Invest 27:484–492

Knutsson L, Börjesson S, Larsson EM, Risberg J, Gustafson L, Passant U, Ståhlberg F, Wirestam R (2007) Absolute quantification of cerebral blood flow in normal volunteers: correlation between Xe-133 SPECT and dynamic susceptibility contrast MRI. J Magn Reson Imaging 26:913–920

Kontos HA, Wei EP, Jarrel Raper A, Patterson JL (1977) Local mechanism of CO2 action on cat pial arterioles. Stroke 8:226–229

Lassen NA, Ingvar DH (1961) The blood flow of the cerebral cortex determined by radioactive krypton. Experientia. Jan 15;17:42–3

Madsen PL, Schmidt JF, Wildschiødtz G, Friberg L, Holm S, Vorstrup S, Lassen NA (1991) Cerebral O2 metabolism and cerebral blood flow in humans during deep and rapid-eye-movement sleep. J Appl Physiol 70(6): 2597–2601

Mallett BL, Veall N (1963) Investigation of cerebral blood-flow in hypertension, using radioactive-xenon inhalation and extracranial recording. Lancet. May 18;1(7290):1081–2

Martin NA, Patwardhan RV, Alexander MJ, Africk CZ, Lee JH, Shalmon E, Hovda DA, Becker DP (1997) Characterization of cerebral hemodynamic phases following severe head trauma: hypoperfusion, hyperemia, and vasospasm. J Neurosurg 87(1):9–19

Messeter K, Nordström CH, Sundbärg G, Algotsson L, Ryding E (1986) Cerebral hemodynamics in patients with acute severe head trauma. J Neurosurg 64(2): 231–237

Mielck F, Bräuer A, Radke O, Hanekop G, Loesch S, Friedrich M, Hilgers R, Sonntag H (2004) Changes of jugular venous blood temperature associated with measurements of cerebral blood flow using the transcerebral double-indicator dilution technique. Eur J Anaesthesiol 21(4):289–295

Obrist WD, Thompson HK, Wang HS, Wilkinson WE (1975) Regional cerebral blood flow estimated by 133Xenon inhalation. Stroke 6:245–256

Obrist WD, Langfitt TW, Jaggi JL, Cruz J, Gennarelli TA (1984) Cerebral blood flow and metabolism in comatose patients with acute head injury. J Neurosurg 61: 241–253

Østergaard L, Weisskoff RM, Chesler DA, Gyldensted C, Rosen BR (1996) High resolution measurement of cerebral blood flow using intravascular tracer bolus passages. Part I: mathematical approach and statistical analysis. Magn Reson Med 36:715–725

Paradiso S, Johnson DL, Andreasen NC, O'Leary DS, Watkins GL, Boles Ponto LL, Hichwa RD (1999) Cerebral blood flow changes associated with attribution of emotional valence to pleasant, unpleasant, and neutral visual stimuli in a PET study of normal subjects. Am J Psychiatry 156:1618–1629

Paulson OB, Strandgaard S, Edvinsson L (1990) Cerebral autoregulation. Cerebrovasc Brain Metab Rev 2(2): 161–192

Petersen ET, Zimine I, Ho Y-CL, Golay X (2006) Non-invasive measurement of perfusion: a critical review of arterial spin labelling techniques. Br J Radiol 79: 688–701

Qiu M, Ramani R, Swetye M, Rajeevan N, Constable RT (2008) Anesthetic effects on regional CBF, BOLD, and the coupling between task-induced changes in CBF and BOLD: an fMRI study in normal human subjects. Magn Reson Med 60(4):987–996

Reinstrup P, Uski T, Messeter K (1992) Modulation by carbon dioxide and pH of the contractile response to potassium and prostaglandin F2α in isolated pial arteries. Br J Anaesth 69:615–620

Reinstrup P, Ryding E, Algotsson L, Berntman L, Uski T (1994) Effects of nitrous oxide on human regional cerebral blood flow and isolated pial arteries. Anesthesiology 81(2):396–402

Reinstrup P, Ryding E, Ohlsson T, Sandell A, Erlandsson K, Ljunggren K, Salford LG, Strand S, Uski T (2008) Regional cerebral metabolic rate (positron emission tomography) during inhalation of nitrous oxide 50% in humans. Br J Anaesth 100(1):66–71, Epub 2007 Nov 23

Schalén W, Messeter K, Nordström CH (1991) Cerebral vasoreactivity and the prediction of outcome in severe traumatic brain lesions. Acta Anaesthesiol Scand 35(2):113–122

Scheel P, Ruge C, Schoning M (2000) Flow velocity and flow volume measurements in the extracranial carotid and vertebral arteries in healthy adults: reference data and the effects of age. Ultrasound Med Biol 26:1261–1266

Shinohara Y, Ibaraki M, Ohmura T, Sugawara S, Toyoshima H, Nakamura K, Kinoshita F, Kinoshita T (2010) Whole-brain perfusion measurement using 320-detector row computed tomography in patients with cerebrovascular steno-occlusive disease: comparison with 15O-positron emission tomography. J Comput Assist Tomogr 34(6):830–835

Vajkoczy P, Roth H, Horn P, Lucke T, Thomé C, Hubner U, Martin GT, Zappletal C, Klar E, Schilling L, Schmiedek P (2000) Continuous monitoring of regional cerebral blood flow: experimental and clinical validation of a novel thermal diffusion microprobe. J Neurosurg 93:265–274

Werner C, Engelhard K (2007) Pathophysiology of traumatic brain injury. Br J Anaesth 99:4–9

Williams DS, Detre JA, Leigh JS, Koretsky AP (1992) Magnetic resonance imaging of perfusion using spin inversion of arterial water. Proc Natl Acad Sci U S A 89:212–216

Wirestam R, Engvall C, Ryding E, Holtås S, Ståhlberg F, Reinstrup P (2009) Change in cerebral perfusion detected by dynamic susceptibility contrast magnetic resonance imaging: normal volunteers examined during normal breathing and hyperventilation. J Biomed Sci Eng 2:210–215

Yazici B, Erdoğmuş B, Tugay A (2005) Cerebral blood flow measurements of the extracranial carotid and vertebral arteries with Doppler ultrasonography in healthy adults. Diagn Interv Radiol 11:195–198

Transcranial Doppler (TCD) 36

Peter Reinstrup, Jan Frennström, and Bertil Romner

Recommendations

Level I

There are insufficient data to support a Level I recommendation for this topic.

Level II

There are insufficient data to support a Level II recommendation for this topic.

Level III

TCD is useful for the detection of vasospasm and cerebral haemodynamic impairment following spontaneous and traumatic subarachnoid haemorrhage. TCD gives an indication as to whether the ICP is normal or high.

P. Reinstrup
Department of Intensive and Perioperative Care, Skanes University Hospital, S221 85 Lund, Sweden
e-mail: peter.reinstrup@med.lu.se

J. Frennström
Department of Neurosurgery, Skanes University Hospital, S221 85 Lund, Sweden
e-mail: jan.frennstrom@gmail.com

B. Romner (✉)
Department of Neurosurgery 2092, Rigshospitalet, 2100 Copenhagen, Denmark
e-mail: bertil.romner@rh.regionh.dk

36.1 Overview

By using a 1–2-MHz pulsed Transcranial Doppler (TCD), it is possible to penetrate the skull bone at special sites (windows) and register the flow velocity (FV) in the insonated artery at well-defined depts. In this way, the FV can be registered in the central arteries as well as in some of the veins. A normal FV in an artery normally indicates an adequate circulation to the territory it supplies. High and low FV does not necessarily have correlations to the CBF since the diameter of the measured vessel is unknown. If the FV is high, a differentiation between hyperaemia and vasospasm can be obtained by performing a Lindegaard Index (LI) which is the correlation between the FV in the middle cerebral artery and the internal carotid artery.

The shape of the FV curve can in addition give an indication of increased intracranial pressure.

Tips, Tricks, and Pitfalls

- For a TCD investigation, it is best to stand on the patient's right side. Let the left wrist rest on the patient's forehead and insonate the MCA through the posterior temporal window. By this approach, you will have your right hand free to adjust the equipment.
- The normally high CBF is to a great extent due to a low mean resistance in the cerebral circulation. This is seen in

T. Sundstrøm et al. (eds.), *Management of Severe Traumatic Brain Injury*,
DOI 10.1007/978-3-642-28126-6_36, © Springer-Verlag Berlin Heidelberg 2012

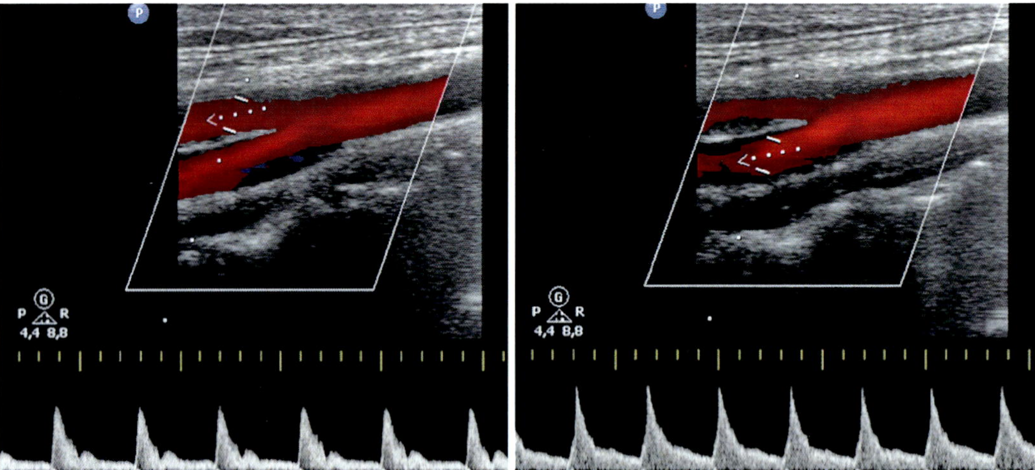

Fig. 36.1 Shows the carotid arteries in the neck. The common carotid artery is seen to the *right* in both pictures and the FV curves at the *bottom*. The *left curve* shows the FV in the external carotid artery (ECA), whereas the internal carotid artery (ICA) is on the *right*

the high FV during diastole as compared to non-cerebral arteries of similar size (Fig. 36.1).

- Start insonating the middle cerebral artery at a depth of 50 mm and proceed inwards until you find a flow which moves away from the probe, at which point you have reached the anterior communicating artery (ACA). This finding strengthens that it is the MCA. Then, follow the vessel out again and register the highest FV value.

36.2 Background

Ultrasound is sound with frequencies greater than the upper limit of the human hearing, i.e. above 20 kHz. Within medicine, ultrasound has been used during the last 50 years to penetrate into the human body measuring the reflections, reflections that can be used for the imaging of soft tissues in the body. Superficial structures are visualized at frequencies ranging from 7 to 18 MHz, but in order to penetrate into deeper structures such as the liver or the kidneys, the frequency has to be lowered down to between 1 and 6 MHz. Unfortunately, the lower the frequency you use, the lower resolution of the picture you get. Also, the higher the density of a tissue, the less penetration of the sound wave and, hence, the mature skull bone is blocking for ultrasound penetration into the brain. After the age of 1 year, it is already impossible to identify individual structures within the brain. However, in a brain-traumatized patient upon whom a craniectomy has been performed, there is an artificial window through which it is possible to investigate the brain rather than using a CT scan. On youngsters, the fontanel can be utilized in a similar manner for improved resolution (Fig. 36.2).

There are many advantages of utilizing TCD. It is non-invasive, inexpensive, can be performed bedside, is easily repeated and can be used for continuous monitoring. TCD ultrasound was introduced in 1982 by Aaslid et al. (1982). A Doppler ultrasound beam of 2 MHz produced from a piezoelectric crystal is bounced back from the erythrocytes in an individual artery. The ultrasound examination of a blood vessel by these means is referred as to insonate the vessel. The TCD probe is placed over different 'acoustic windows', i.e. specific areas of the skull where the bone layer is thin or through the foramen magnum. In order to help the investigator to insonate the artery, the signal is presented as a

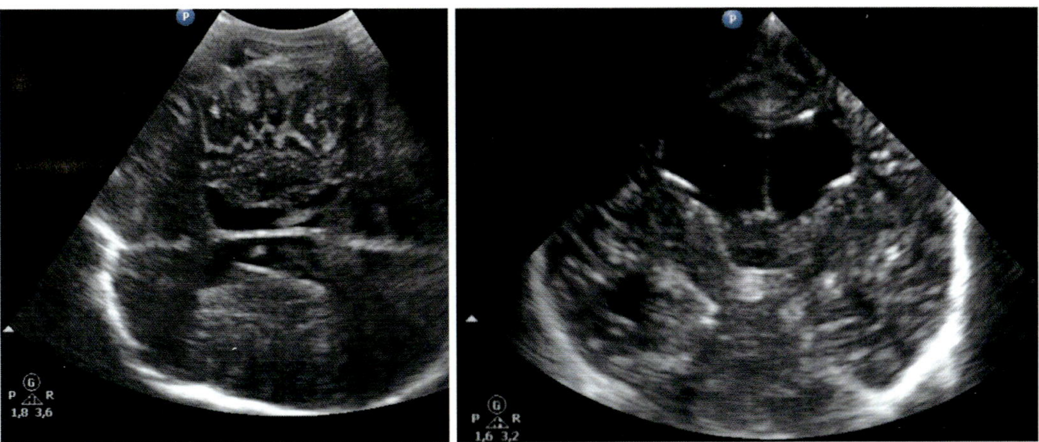

Fig. 36.2 Ultrasound pictures of the brain. On the *left hand* is an axial slice showing highly detailed brain anatomy in a craniotomized patient. On the *right hand* is a similar detailed coronary view through the fontanel in a 6 months old child with hydrocephalus

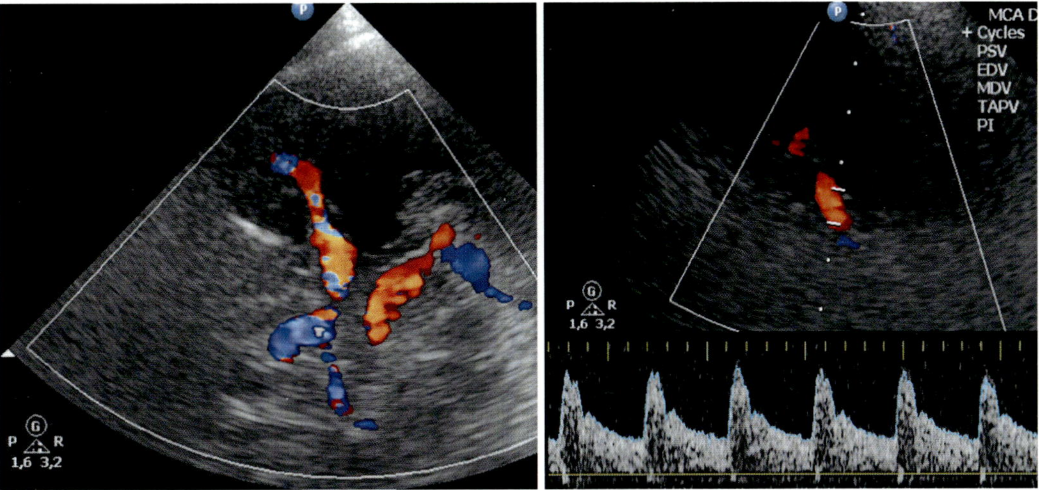

Fig. 36.3 *Left picture* is a Colour Doppler visualization of the cerebral arteries showing the middle cerebral artery (MCA) pointing upward toward the Doppler probe, the anterior cerebral artery (ACA) in the *left side* of the picture and the posterior cerebral artery (PCA) in the *right side*. The *right picture* shows a TCD recording in the MCA

sound through a loudspeaker as well. The reflected signal is received by the transducer and converted to an electric signal after the subtraction of the original emission. The signal is pulsed, making it possible to register from different distances or depths from the probe. A computer converts the resulting signal into a graph that provides information about the speed and direction of blood flow through the blood vessel being examined (Fig. 36.3).

36.2.1 Temporal Window

Finding the thin bony layer of the temporal bone, 'the temporal window', can be difficult; it varies in size and location with each patient and may also differ individually from the one side to the other. Furthermore, such a transtemporal window is absent in up to 10% of the adult population, and it is most difficult to find in older individuals, females and Africans. There are usually two possible sites

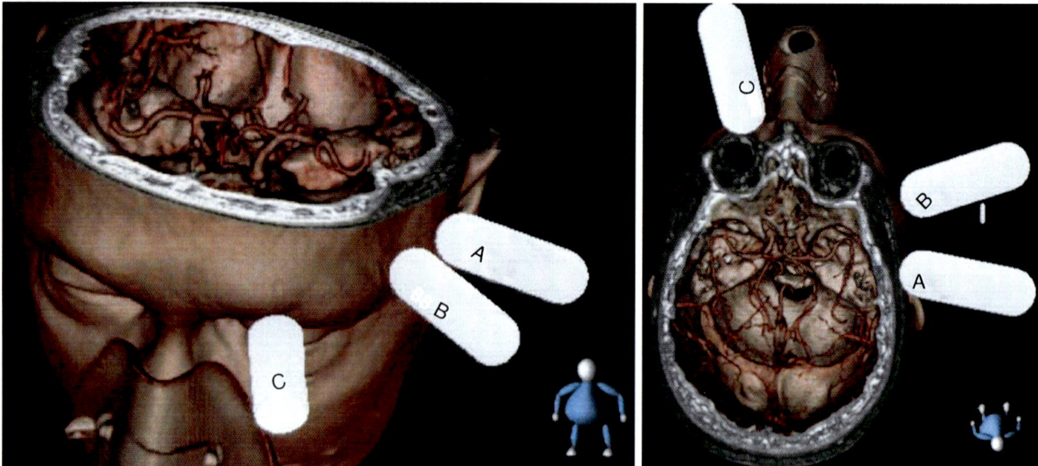

Fig. 36.4 The figures indicate the position and angle to insonate the MCA and ACA. *A* is the posterior temporal window and *B* is the anterior. MCA signal is found 3–6 cm below the skin. Following the MCA inward, the bifurcation with the anterior and posterior artery is eventually found as an additional flow directed away from the probe, i.e. a negative curve component. *C* anterior cerebral artery is found at a depth of 6–8 cm

to penetrate with the ultrasound wave in the temporal window; one situated approximately 1 cm behind the corner of the eye, the other one a cm up and in front of the ear meatus (Fig. 36.4). The transducer's orientation should be pointed in a slightly upward direction pointing in between these two centres. The transducer should be tilted and moved slowly over the skin to pinpoint the best signal and highest flow velocity. The temporal window can be used to insonate the middle cerebral artery (MCA), the anterior cerebral artery (ACA), the posterior cerebral artery (PCA) and the terminal portion of the internal carotid artery (ICA), just prior to its bifurcation.

36.2.2 Transorbital Window

The transorbital window gives access to the ophthalmic artery (OA) as well as the internal carotid artery at the siphon level. The transducer is gently placed on the closed eyelid. The transducer should be pointed slightly medial (Figs. 36.4 and 36.5). Damage to the eye has never been reported, but not every equipment is approved for the use of this approach, and it is important to start the investigation at a low power setting.

36.2.3 Suboccipital Window

The occipital or foraminal window allows for insonating the distal vertebral arteries (VA) and the basilar artery (BA). When evaluating the vertebrobasilar system, the best results are obtained with the patient lying on the side with the head forward extended to open up the gap between the atlas and the cranium. The transducer is placed in the nuchal crest (Fig. 36.5). The orientation should be towards the bridge of the patient's nose. The BA is found in the midline and the VA slightly at each side. The depth of the anatomic structures will vary with each patient depending upon the thickness of the sub occipital soft tissue.

Depths to investigate and the cerebral arteries together with their respective typical flow velocities (FV (cm/s))

3–6 cm	Middle cerebral artery	*MCA*	55 ± 12
6–8 cm	Anterior cerebral artery	*ACA*	50 ± 11
6–7 cm	Posterior cerebral artery	*PCA*	40 ± 10
3.5–7 cm	Vertebral artery	*VA*	40 ± 10
7.5–12 cm	Basilar artery	*BA*	40 ± 10

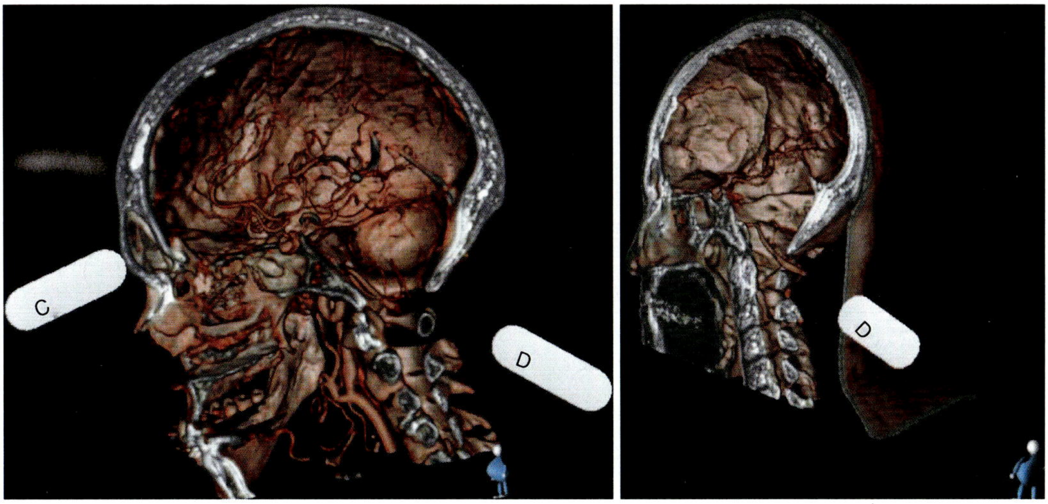

Fig. 36.5 In the *left* picture, *C* shows the horizontal angle to insonate the ofthalmic artery (OA), the anterior cerebral artery (ACA) and the internal carotid artery (ICA) whereas *D* indicates the angle by which to investigate the vertebral artery (VA) and basilar artery (BA). *Right* picture shows the placement of the probe on the skin in the nuchal crest

36.2.4 TCD Flow Velocity (FV) Correlation to Cerebral Blood Flow (CBF)

TCD FV is measured in the basal arteries of the brain. If CBF is altered, with an unchanged tone in these large arteries i.e. by changing the tone only in the peripheral pial resistance arteries, there should be a direct positive correlation between the FV in the basal arteries and the CBF. However, this direct correlation will be altered if similar changes are taking place simultaneously in basal arteries and peripheral resistance arteries. If the CBF regulating change in arterial tone only occurs in the basal arteries, there is a direct negative correlation between CBF and TCD FV readings, as described by Giller et al. (1998) in the formula FV = cerebral blood flow/vessel diameter in the insonated artery. Unfortunately, no general correlation has been found between absolute CBF and FV (Bishop et al. 1986; Clark et al. 1996). However, despite the limitation of the above-mentioned assumption, the simplicity of the TCD technique and its lack of invasiveness warrants for further evaluations to determine whether it can replace considerably more complicated CBF measurements for the evaluation of the cerebral circulation.

36.2.5 CO_2 Response

In healthy individuals, blood flow velocities in the large intracranial arteries are in direct relation to the arterial CO_2-concentrations ($pACO_2$), reflecting global cerebral vasoconstriction and relaxation due to changes in $pACO_2$ (Markwalder et al. 1984). Despite this, no correlation was found between the absolute values of CBF and FV during CO_2 provocation (Bishop et al. 1986; Clark et al. 1996). Furthermore, this TCD/CBF correlation is absent in patients with various brain pathologies, such as after subarachnoid haemorrhage (Romner et al. 1991) or following traumatic brain injury (Reinstrup et al. 2011).

36.2.6 Cerebrovascular Autoregulation

Cerebral autoregulation is the self-adjustments of the cerebrovascular tree in order to maintain a sufficient cerebral blood flow during alterations in mean arterial blood pressure (MAP). TCD is valid for determination of the lower limit of CBF autoregulation, and changes in CBF can be evaluated by TCD during changes in cerebral perfusion pressure in normal subjects (Larsen et al. 1994). TCD measurements of FV and pulsative index (PI)

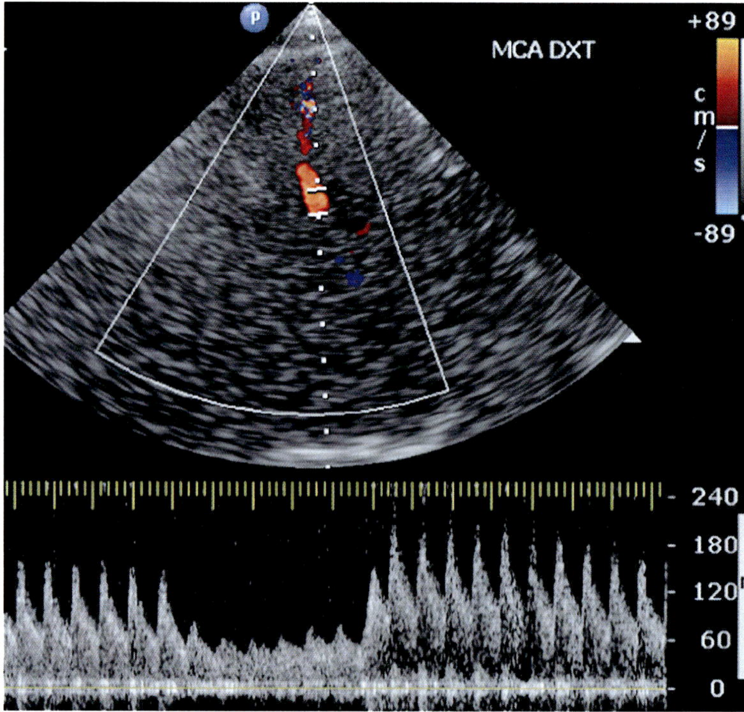

Fig. 36.6 Test of the cerebral vasoreactivity during TCD of the MCA. Following onset of the carotid artery compression, there is an immediate fall in ipsilateral MCA FV followed by a gradual rise due to autoregulation. On release, there is a brief overshoot due to the compensatory vasodilation

before and during pharmacological or mechanical manipulation of MAP, and hence autoregulation, can be used to monitor the reactivity of the intracranial vasculature tree (Aaslid et al. 1989; Mahony et al. 2000). The easiest and now widely used approach is the transient hyperaemic response test (THR) first described in 1991 by Giller (1991). It involves a continuous recording of the MCA FV during which a 3- to 10-s compression of the ipsilateral common carotid artery is performed. This results in a sudden reduction in the MCA FV, which in turn provokes a vasodilatation in the vascular bed distal to the MCA if the autoregulation is intact (Fig. 36.6). Thus, following the release of the compression a transient increase, well above the previous base level, is seen in MCA FV due to the autoregulatory compensatory dilatation and later this reply will return to normal.

36.2.7 High Flow Velocity (FV) and the Lindegaard Index (LI)

Increased FV is found in vasospastic parts of an artery. The vasospasm can be very local, affecting only millimetre long segments of the artery; hence, it is important to investigate as much of the artery as possible. High FV can also be caused by hyperaemia, and there is nothing in the curveform that can be used to differentiate between these two sources for a high FV. The ICA feeds the MCA, ACA and PCA. In case of vasospasm in MCA, ACA and PCA, resulting in a reduced flow through some or all of them, the effect in the feeding artery is a reduced flow as measured on the neck in the ICA. Contrary to this, the flow through the ICA increases during hyperaemia. The ICA lumen is usually unchanged during different intracranial pathologies, resulting in a direct relationship between FV and flow. Lindegaard et al. (1988) used the MCA/ICA FV relationship to discriminate between hyperaemia and vasospasm and to assess the severity of vasospasm. The MCA/ICA ratio is normally around two with some age and sex variations (Krejza et al. 2005).

Generally, a flow velocity above 120 cm/s is indicative of a vasospasm. However, if the FV increases slowly over days to this level, it seldom gives rise to clinical symptoms.

If MCA FV rises to between 120 and 150 cm/s with a LI at 3–5, the vasospasm is considered moderate.

If MCA FV is 150–220 cm/s and LI is >6, the vasospasm is generally severe and if MCA increases above 200 cm/s with LI > 6, the vasospasm is usually critical.

Hyperaemia increases flow velocities in both MCA and ICA keeping LI unchanged <3, whereas in cases of escalating vasospasm FV is increased in the intracranial arteries with an attenuated FV in the ICA, showing up as an elevated LI.

In order to evaluate the flow in the BA, one has to look at the intracranial/extracranial FV ratio in the posterior circulation, i.e. the ratio between BA and one of the vertebral arteries measured extracranially on the neck in analogy with the MCA/ICA ratio. An FV threshold of 80 cm/s is indicative of BA vasospasm. A normative value of a BA/extracranial VA FV ratio (BA/EVA) is 1.7. The BA/EVA is >2 in all patients with BA vasospasm and generally <2 in patients without. Furthermore, the BA/EVA ratio shows a close correlation with BA diameter and is >3 in all patients with severe vasospasm (Soustiel et al. 2002). EVA should be insonated at a depths ranging from 45 to 55 mm.

36.2.8 TCD, ICP and Pulsative Index (PI)

Pulsative index PI = systFV – diastFV/meanFV was originally thought to describe the cerebrovascular resistance, but this is probably not the case since hyperventilation with vasoconstriction does not increase PI (Czosnyka et al. 1996). However, an artificially increased ICP, brought about by increasing the pressure in the epidural space, brings about a more pronounced reduction of flow velocities in the diastolic phase than in the systolic phase, i.e. increasing the pulse peak between systole and diastole. Furthermore, there is a lowering of the mean FV (Nagai et al. 1997). Looking at the PI equation, it should therefore be sensitive to increases in ICP, and such a correlation has indeed been found in children with hydrocephalus (Goh and Minns 1995; Govender et al. 1999; Nadvi et al. 1994) even though not all findings have been positive (Hanlo et al. 1995; Figaji et al. 2009). In adults, with various brain pathologies and equipped with ventricular ICP devices with a reference zero at the forehead level, a strong relationship was found between ICP and PI, with $ICP = 10.93 \times PI - 1.28$ or $ICP \approx 10 \times PI$ (Bellner et al. 2004). It must be emphasized, however, that PI cannot be used as a substitute for an ICP device but rather may be utilized as one additional tool in the evaluation of patients with suspected brain pathologies in the guidance whether the patient might gain from an ICP device.

36.3 Brain Trauma

36.3.1 Absolute FV

In comatose TBI patients, cerebral metabolic rate (CMR) is reduced with up to 50%, and compared to the normal coupling between CMR and CBF, these patients have normal to supranormal CBF values (Obrist et al. 1984). Most patients present with CBF changes over time, starting with low CBF values shortly after the trauma (Bouma and Muizelaar 1992), evolving to a hyperaemic phase, again substituted for a state of low CBF but now due to vasospasm. It takes around 3 weeks before the CBF returns to normal (Inoue et al. 2005). This development would be expected to show up as changes in the TCD FV, but the FV starts initially at normal values with a normal LI and hence do not reflect the low absolute CBF. The FV typically rises during the following 3 days up towards 100 cm/s and stay elevated for the next 14 days (Martin et al. 1997). LI remains low and thus the first increase in FV is due to hyperaemia. LI increases slowly over time indicating that the reason for the high FV goes from hyperaemia to vasospasm.

The infratentorial vascular territory is seldom investigated following TBI despite the fact that Soustiel and Shik found that one third of such patients presented with high FV in the BA as a sign of vasospasm (2004).

36.3.2 CO_2 Response

Arterial reactivity in brain-damaged areas is impaired so that a reduced CO_2 reactivity as measured with CBF correlates not only to the extent of damaged tissue and thereby to the severity of the brain injury but also to outcome (Cold et al. 1977; Schalén et al. 1991; Poon et al. 2005). In healthy subjects, blood flow velocities in the basal intracranial arteries are directly related to the $pACO_2$ (Markwalder et al. 1984). However, this correlation is absent in patients with subarachnoid haemorrhage (Romner et al. 1991). On the other hand, following TBI there is a more pronounced change in TCD FV than in CBF upon changes in $pACO_2$ (Reinstrup et al. 2011). A relationship of individual reactivity indices between the two parameters concerning CO_2 reactivity is therefore not established and CBF and mean FV are hence not exchangeable in patients with severe brain trauma.

36.3.3 Autoregulation

The correlation between CBF, as measured indirectly with changes in arteriovenous oxygen difference ($AVDO_2$), and TCD during autoregulation provocations has been established in healthy volunteers (Larsen et al. 1994). However, the classic correlation between CBF and TCD autoregulation has so far not been investigated for TBI patients. Autoregulatory capacity, as measured simultaneously in the basal arteries by TCD FV and in the pial arteries by laser Doppler flowmetry, was more severely impaired in the cortex than in the MCA during conditions of rising ICP and falling CPP. However, providing CPP was kept above 60 mmHg, cortical autoregulatory capacity was on level with that of the MCA (Zweifel et al. 2010). In an investigation of TCD-measured autoregulations in TBI patients, a correlation between impaired autoregulation and outcome was found (Sorrentino et al. 2011). In patients with minor head injuries, autoregulation is impaired in 28% (Jünger et al. 1997).

36.3.4 Brain Death (Cerebral Circulatory Arrest)

TCD FV measurement is not approved legally as a means to establish cerebral circulatory arrest, but it can give some useful information of the status of the circulation. In this context, it is mandatory to investigate both the supratentorial and the infratentorial spaces. As described above, an increasing ICP brings about a reduction in flow velocity mainly in the diastolic phase, finally leaving only the systolic peak in the basal arteries of the brain (Petty et al. 1990). Further elevation of the ICP leads to a FV reverberating or oscillating around zero, ending up with a brief peak in systole, called the 'systolic spike' and with a close to zero net flow through the brain (Langfitt et al. 1964). The final stage in intracranial hypertension results in a no-flow situation as well as no Doppler signal as investigated in animals (Nagai et al. 1997).

When using TCD to guide the appropriate time for performing a 4-vessel angiogram in cases where clinical diagnostics are inappropriate, we usually start the angiography procedure when the FV is reverberating or only showing a systolic spike both supra- and infratentorially, and so far all angiograms have shown cerebral circulatory arrest using such an approach. However, so far no investigation has been performed in order to correlate the TCD with angiography during upcoming circulatory arrest.

36.4 Specific Paediatric Concerns

Children between the age of 2 and 10 years have a mFV of 95 cm/s and a PI of 0.95. After the tenth year, the mFV are declining over the years to 85 cm/s and the PI to 0.80 at the age of 20. Girls do generally have a higher mFV than boys (Brouwers et al. 1990).

References

Aaslid R, Markwalder TM, Nornes H (1982) Noninvasive transcranial Doppler ultrasound recording of flow velocity in basal cerebral arteries. J Neurosurg 57: 769–774

Aaslid R, Lindegaard KF, Sorteberg W, Nornes H (1989) Cerebral autoregulation dynamics in humans. Stroke 20:45–52

Bellner J, Romner B, Reinstrup P, Kristiansson KA, Ryding E, Brandt L (2004) Transcranial Doppler sonography pulsatility index (PI) reflects intracranial pressure (ICP). Surg Neurol 62:45–51

Bishop CC, Powell S, Rutt D, Browse NL (1986) Transcranial Doppler measurement of middle cerebral artery blood flow velocity: a validation study. Stroke 17:913–915

Bouma GJ, Muizelaar JP (1992) Cerebral blood flow, cerebral blood volume, and cerebrovascular reactivity after severe head injury. J Neurotrauma 9(Suppl 1): S333–S348

Brouwers PJAM, Vries EM, Musbach M, Wieneke GH, Van Huffelen AC (1990) Transcranial pulsed doppler measurements of blood flow velocity in the middle cerebral artery: reference values at rest and during hyperventilation in healthy children and adolescents in relation to age and sex. Ultrasound Med Biol 16(1):1–8

Clark JM, Skolnick BE, Gelfand R, Farber RE, Stierheim M, Stevens WC, Beck G Jr, Lambertsen CJ (1996) Relationship of 133Xe cerebral blood flow to middle cerebral arterial flow velocity in men at rest. J Cereb Blood Flow Metab 16:1255–1262

Cold GE, Jensen FT, Malmros R (1977) The effects of pACO2 reduction on regional cerebral blood flow in the acute phase of brain injury. Acta Anaesthesiol Scand 21:359–367

Czosnyka M, Richards HK, Whitehouse HE, Pickard JD (1996) Relationship between transcranial Doppler-determined pulsatility index and cerebrovascular resistance: an experimental study. J Neurosurg 84:79–84

Figaji AA, Zwane E, Fieggen AG, Siesjo P, Peter JC (2009) Transcranial Doppler pulsatility index is not a reliable indicator of intracranial pressure in children with severe traumatic brain injury. Surg Neurol 72:389–394

Giller CA (1991) A bedside test for cerebral autoregulation using transcranial Doppler ultrasound. Acta Neurochir (Wien) 108:7–14

Giller CA, Hatab MR, Giller AM (1998) Estimation of vessel flow and diameter during cerebral vasospasm using transcranial Doppler indices. Neurosurgery 42: 1076–1081

Goh D, Minns RA (1995) Intracranial pressure and cerebral arterial flow velocity indices in childhood hydrocephalus: current review. Childs Nerv Syst 11: 392–396

Govender PV, Nadvi SS, Madaree A (1999) The value of transcranial Doppler ultrasonography in craniosynostosis. J Craniofac Surg 10:260–263

Hanlo PW, Gooskens RH, Nijhuis IJ, Faber JA, Peters RJ, van Huffelen AC, Tulleken CA, Willemse J (1995) Value of transcranial Doppler indices in predicting raised ICP in infantile hydrocephalus. A study with review of the literature. Childs Nerv Syst 11:595–603

Inoue Y, Shiozaki T, Tasaki O, Hayakata T, Ikegawa H, Yoshiya K, Fujinaka T, Tanaka H, Shimazu T, Sugimoto H (2005) Changes in cerebral blood flow from the acute to the chronic phase of severe head injury. J Neurotrauma 22:1411–1418

Jünger EC, Newell DW, Grant GA, Avellino AM, Ghatan S, Douville CM, Lam AM, Aaslid R, Winn HR (1997) Cerebral autoregulation following minor head injury. J Neurosurg 86:425–432

Krejza J, Szydlik P, Liebeskind DS, Kochanowicz J, Bronov O, Mariak Z, Melhem ER (2005) Age and sex variability and normal reference values for the V(MCA)/V(ICA) index. AJNR Am J Neuroradiol 26: 730–735

Langfitt TW, Weinstein JD, Kassell NF (1964) Cerebral vasomotor paralysis as a cause of brain swelling. Trans Am Neurol Assoc 89:214–215

Larsen FS, Olsen KS, Hansen BA, Paulson OB, Knudsen GM (1994) Transcranial Doppler is valid for determination of the lower limit of cerebral blood flow autoregulation. Stroke 25:1985–1988

Lindegaard KF, Nornes H, Bakke SJ, Sorteberg W, Nakstad P (1988) Cerebral vasospasm after subarachnoid haemorrhage investigated by means of transcranial Doppler ultrasound. Acta Neurochir Suppl (Wien) 42:81–84

Mahony PJ, Panerai RB, Deverson ST, Hayes PD, Evans DH (2000) Assessment of the thigh cuff technique for measurement of dynamic cerebral autoregulation. Stroke 31:476–480

Markwalder TM, Grolimund P, Seiler RW, Roth F, Aaslid R (1984) Dependency of blood flow velocity in the middle cerebral artery on end-tidal carbon dioxide partial pressure–a transcranial ultrasound Doppler study. J Cereb Blood Flow Metab 4:368–372

Martin NA, Patwardhan RV, Alexander MJ, Africk CZ, Lee JH, Shalmon E, Hovda DA, Becker DP (1997) Characterization of cerebral hemodynamic phases following severe head trauma: hypoperfusion, hyperemia, and vasospasm. J Neurosurg 87:9–19

Nadvi SS, Du Trevou MD, Van Dellen JR, Gouws E (1994) The use of transcranial Doppler ultrasonography as a method of assessing intracranial pressure in hydrocephalic children. Br J Neurosurg 8:573–577

Nagai H, Moritake K, Takaya M (1997) Correlation between transcranial Doppler ultrasonography and regional cerebral blood flow in experimental intracranial hypertension. Stroke 28:603–637

Obrist WD, Langfitt TW, Jaggi JL, Cruz J, Gennarelli TA (1984) Cerebral blood flow and metabolism in comatose patients with acute head injury. Relationship to intracranial hypertension. J Neurosurg 61:241–253

Petty GW, Mohr JP, Pedley TA, Tatemichi TK, Lennihan L, Duterte DI, Sacco RL (1990) The role of transcranial Doppler in confirming brain death: sensitivity, specificity, and suggestions for performance and interpretation. Neurology 40:300–303

Poon WS, Ng SC, Chan MT, Lam JM, Lam WW (2005) Cerebral blood flow (CBF)-directed management of ventilated head-injured patients. Acta Neurochir Suppl. 95:9–11

Reinstrup P, Ryding E, Asgeirsson B, Hesselgard K, Unden J, Romner B (2011) Cerebral blood flow (CBF) and transcranial doppler sonography (TCD) measurements of cerebraovascular CO2-reactivity in patients with acute severe head injury. J Cereb Blood Flow Metab

Romner B, Brandt L, Berntman L, Algotsson L, Ljunggren B, Messeter K (1991) Simultaneous transcranial Doppler sonography and cerebral blood flow measurements of cerebrovascular CO2-reactivity in patients with aneurysmal subarachnoid haemorrhage. Br J Neurosurg 5:31–37

Schalén W, Messeter K, Nordström CH (1991) Cerebral vasoreactivity and the prediction of outcome in severe traumatic brain lesions. Acta Anaesthesiol Scand 35:113–122

Sorrentino E, Budohoski KP, Kasprowicz M, Smielewski P, Matta B, Pickard JD, Czosnyka M (2011) Critical thresholds for transcranial Doppler indices of cerebral autoregulation in traumatic brain injury. Neurocrit Care 14:188–193

Soustiel JF, Shik V (2004) Posttraumatic basilar artery vasospasm. Surg Neurol 62:201–206

Soustiel JF, Shik V, Shreiber R, Tavor Y, Goldsher D (2002) Basilar vasospasm diagnosis: investigation of a modified "Lindegaard Index" based on imaging studies and blood velocity measurements of the basilar artery. Stroke 33:72–77

Zweifel C, Czosnyka M, Lavinio A, Castellani G, Kim DJ, Carrera E, Pickard JD, Kirkpatrick PJ, Smielewski P (2010) A comparison study of cerebral autoregulation assessed with transcranial Doppler and cortical laser Doppler flowmetry. Neurol Res 32:425–428

Near Infrared Spectroscopy (NIRS) or Cerebral Oximetry

37

Peter Reinstrup and Bertil Romner

Recommendations

Level I

There are insufficient data to support a Level I recommendation for this topic.

Level II

There are insufficient data to support a Level II recommendation for this topic.

Level III

NIRS can be used to detect upcoming intra- and extracerebral hematomas.

37.1 Overview

Near infrared spectroscopy (NIRS) measures the oxygenation of the haemoglobin in the cerebral tissue lying just underneath a probe. The probe is most often placed on the forehead since hair follicles affect the readings. Some doubts have been raised whether NIRS specifically measures the cerebral tissue or is contaminated by signals from extracerebral tissue it passes through. Furthermore, as haemoglobin absorbs infrared light, NIRS is affected by underlying blood of extravascular origin, such as in subdural haematomas, contusions, subarachnoid blood, as well as changes in cerebral blood volume (CBV). These factors are difficult to decipher, and at present the use of NIRS in TBI patients is controversial. However, by using more than one sensor and by focusing on trends, NIRS readings might be of value in this patient group.

Tips, Tricks, and Pitfalls

- NIRS probes can be placed over hair follicles but the melatonin in the hair affects the absorption of infrared light.
- NIRS from one single probe is too difficult to interpret.
- In patients with unilateral brain pathologies, a symmetrically placed contralateral probe should be placed and used as reference.

P. Reinstrup
Department of Intensive and Perioperative Care, Skanes University Hospital, S221 85 Lund, Sweden
e-mail: peter.reinstrup@med.lu.se

B. Romner (✉)
Department of Neurosurgery 2092, Rigshospitalet, 2100 Copenhagen, Denmark
e-mail: bertil.romner@rh.regionh.dk

T. Sundstrøm et al. (eds.), *Management of Severe Traumatic Brain Injury*,
DOI 10.1007/978-3-642-28126-6_37, © Springer-Verlag Berlin Heidelberg 2012

- Do never use the NIRS reading as the only monitoring device; changes in a NIRS reading should be controlled with other techniques.
- Remember that patients with total brain infarctions can still have a normal NIRS value.

37.2 Background

Oxymetry is a method for monitoring the oxygenation of haemoglobin. Near infrared spectroscopy (NIRS) is able to measure oxygen saturation (SO_2). Jobsis (1977) was the first to report on this and in 1985 came the first report on cerebral oxymetry in humans (Ferrari et al. 1985). The fact that when near infrared (NIR) light passes through a tissue, a proportion of this is absorbed, underlying the detection of changes in the concentration of oxy- and deoxyhaemoglobin. The absorption of light relates to the properties and amount of the material through which the light is travelling, based on the Beer–Lambert law. Tissues such as skin, bone, and brain are transparent to the NIR spectrum, whereas the two chromophores oxy- and deoxyhaemoglobin are not. Since the absorption characteristics of oxy- and deoxy-haemoglobin are different at different wavelengths, it is possible to quantify the cerebral oxygenation of the blood with its venous/arterial relationship of 70%/30% by choosing two or more wavelengths where the absorption of oxy- and deoxyhaemoglobin is maximally separated, i.e. between 700 and 850 nm.

At 810 nm, the absorption of NIR is equal for oxy- and deoxyhaemoglobin, and hence it is theoretically possible to measure the total amount of haemoglobin at this wavelength. With knowledge of the amount of haemoglobin, it is possible to calculate the CBV continuously at the bedside when knowing the haemoglobin concentration. However, so far, this technique is too unstable to be used in clinical practice (Canova et al. 2011).

An infrared beam penetrating into a tissue scatters in such a way that some of it is reflected back to the surface from where it is emitted. To this end, most apparatus use reflectance-mode NIRS in which the optical sensors are placed ipsilateral to the transmitter and exploit the fact that photons transmitted through a sphere will traverse an elliptical path in which the mean depth of penetration is proportional to the separation of the transmitter and the optical sensor.

Though small, some absorption does occur both in normal cerebral and extracerebral tissue. Since extracerebral tissue is not a homogenous layer, but a composite of all the layers of the scalp, bone, and dura, each of these layers with individual optical absorption characteristics may affect the results in a non-foreseeable manner. Especially, melatonin in hair and hair follicles absorbs NIR light to a high degree. The effect on the oximeter reading from these extracerebral layers is hence poorly understood (Young et al. 2000), and in adults the infrared beam has to pass a thick layer of extracranial tissue twice. In order to minimise the influence of the extracerebral tissue and extracerebral circulation, different algorithms has been applied and a number of techniques have been developed, but still without complete success (Al-Rawi and Kirkpatrick 2006).

37.2.1 Normal Values of NIRS

The normal value for cerebral oximetry is 58–82% (Kim et al. 2000). The wide normal range makes it more optimal to follow the trend in the particular patient and compare it with contralateral measurements.

37.2.2 Factors Affecting NIRS

An oximeter reading using NIRS is highly influenced by the venous blood giving an indication of the relationship between cerebral blood flow (CBF) and cerebral metabolism (CMR). The change in cerebral venous oxygenation is described in detail in Sects. 34.2.4 and 34.2.5.

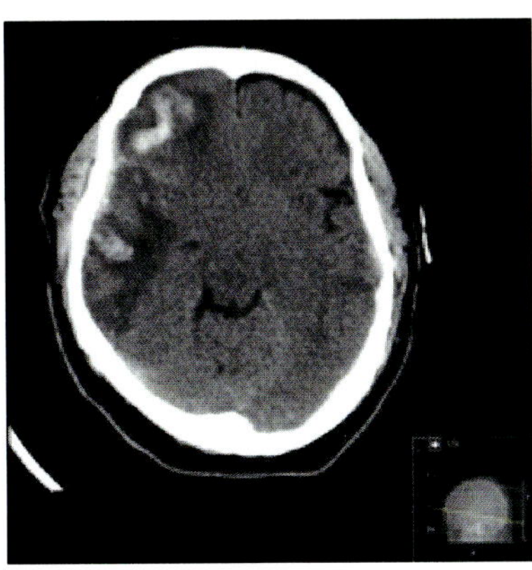
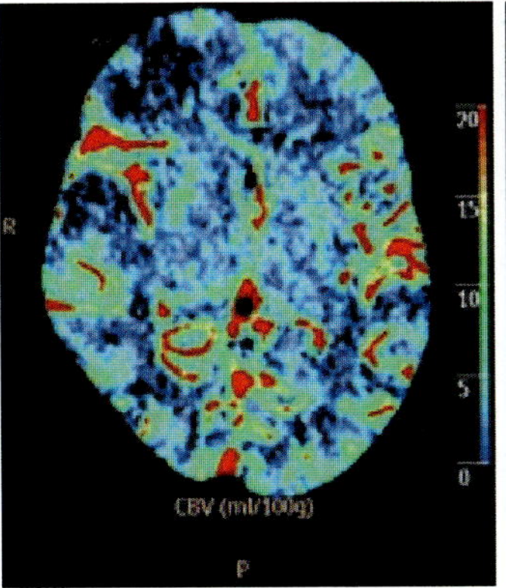

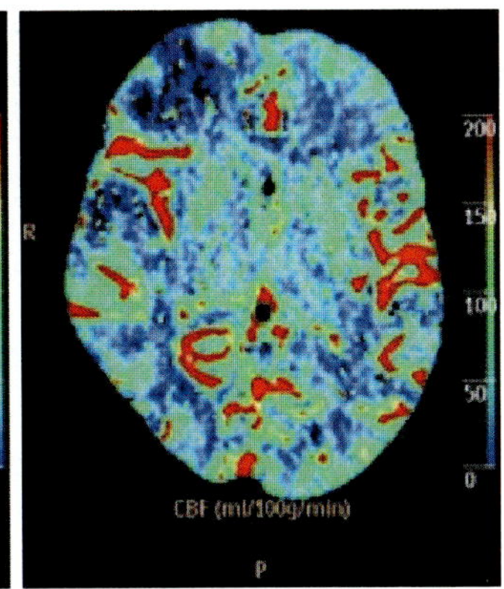

Fig. 37.1 A CT scan showing contusions in the right frontal and temporal regions (*left picture*). CBF (*middle picture*) and CBV (*left picture*) were measured simultaneously with CT perfusion. Cerebral oximetry probes were placed in a symmetrical manner bifrontally where the right sensor was placed over the frontal contusion (*left picture*). The reading was 94% over the contusion and 71% over the left side. The local CBF was low in the contused area (*middle picture*) as was the CBV (*left picture*). The reason for the high saturation in the contusion is most probably due to the extravasated blood, but can also be influenced by the non-metabolising tissue in the contusioned area, even though both CBF and CBV were low

37.2.3 TBI and Pathologic Brain

A major problem with NIRS is the influence of underlying brain pathologies. In dead or non-metabolising tissue, the NIRS can show either high or low values (Dunham et al. 2002), depending on the status of the sequestered blood. Extravasated blood can contain a varying degree of oxyhaemoglobin, whereas in cerebral contusions the non-metabolising tissue does not affect the oxyhaemoglobin content even though the flow through such a region is low (see Fig. 37.1). In fact, NIRS has been used to detect the development of intra- and extracerebral haematomas using a wavelength of 760 nm at which the absorption is increased at the haematoma side compared to the normal side (Gopinath et al. 1995), resulting in an increased NIRS reading at the haematoma side.

37.2.4 CBF Measurements with NIRS

By using a contrast medium and looking at its passage and amount, it is possible to calculate the Mean Transit Time (MTT) and CBV and thereby calculate the local CBF under the probe. Indocyanine green is an ideal contrast medium in conjunction with NIRS, as it has an absorption peak at 805 nm. However, a correlation to CBF has been found in some (Kuebler et al. 1998; Keller et al. 2003) but not all studies (Newton et al. 1997), and the method is not widely used.

37.3 Specific Paediatric Concerns

In healthy children, the normal range for cerebral oximetry is 60–80% (95% confidence interval, average is 68%). There are no studies investigating NIRS and TBI in children.

References

Al-Rawi PG, Kirkpatrick PJ (2006) Tissue oxygen index: thresholds for cerebral ischemia using near-infrared spectroscopy. Stroke 37:2720–2725

Canova D, Roatta S, Bosone D, Micieli G (2011) Inconsistent detection of changes in cerebral blood volume by near infrared spectroscopy in standard clinical tests. J Appl Physiol 110(6):1646–55, Epub 2011 Apr 7

Dunham CM, Sosnowski C, Porter JM, Siegal J, Kohli C (2002) Correlation of noninvasive cerebral oxymetry with cerebral perfusion in the severe head injured patient: a pilot study. J Trauma 52:40–46

Ferrari M, Giannini I, Sideri G, Zanette E (1985) Continous non invasive monitoring of human brain by near infrared spectoscopy. Adv Exp Med Biol 191: 873–882

Gopinath SP, Robertson CS, Contant CF, Narayan RK, Grossman RG, Chance B (1995) Early detection of delayed traumatic intracranial hematomas using near-infrared spectroscopy. J Neurosurg 83(3):438–444

Jobsis FF (1977) Noninvasive infrared monitoring of cerebral and myocardial oxygen sufficiency and circulatory parameters. Science 198:1264–1267

Keller E, Nadler A, Alkadhi H, Kollias SS, Yonekawa Y, Niederer P (2003) Noninvasive measurement of regional cerebral blood flow and regional cerebral blood volume by near-infrared spectroscopy and indocyanine green dye dilution. Neuroimage 20:828–839

Kim MB, Ward DS, Cartwright CR, Kolano J, Chlebowski S, Henson LC (2000) Estimation of jugular venous O2 saturation from cerebral oximetry or arterial O2 saturation during isocapnic hypoxia. J Clin Monit Comput 16(3):191–199

Kuebler WM, Sckell A, Habler O, Kleen M, Kuhnle GE, Welte M, Messmer K, Goetz AE (1998) Noninvasive measurement of regional cerebral blood flow by near-infrared spectroscopy and indocyanine green. J Cereb Blood Flow Metab 18:445–456

Newton CR, Wilson DA, Gunnoe E, Wagner B, Cope M, Traystman RJ (1997) Measurement of cerebral blood flow in dogs with near infrared spectroscopy in the reflectance mode is invalid. J Cereb Blood Flow Metab 17(6):695–703

Young AER, Germon TJ, Barnett NJ, Manara AR, Nelson RJ (2000) Behaviour of near-infrared light in the adult human head: implications for clinical near-infra red spectroscopy. Br J Anaesth 84:38–42

38 Clinical Neurophysiology: Evoked Potentials

Birger Johnsen

Recommendations

Level I

There are insufficient data to support a Level I recommendation for this topic.

Level II

The presence of ERPs (P300 or MMN) in comatose TBI patients predicts a favourable prognosis and justifies continuation of intensive therapy. Bilateral absent SEP indicate only 5% awakening, which may be considered in the decision on continuation of intensive therapy.

Level III

Results from EPs should always be interpreted in the actual clinical setting and combined with clinical findings.

38.1 Overview

Evoked potentials (EP) are objective non-invasive tests that may assess brain stem damage and detect cognitive functions in comatose patients; EPs are therefore of predictive value in TBI patients.

B. Johnsen
Neurofysiologisk Afdeling, Aarhus Universitetshospital, Nørrebrogade 44, 8000 Aarhus C, Denmark
e-mail: birgjohn@rm.dk

EPs are electrical signals recorded from the brain in response to different kind of sensory stimuli, for example, auditory or somatosensory stimuli. These responses directly track the afferent volleys and appear with latencies less than 25 ms and are therefore also named short-latency EPs. Event-related potentials (ERP) are EPs with longer latencies (up to 300 ms), and these EPs reflect higher cortical functions (Duncan et al. 2009).

EPs assess functional aspects of brain damage in addition to the clinical examination and in addition to the assessment of structural lesions by imaging techniques.

EPs of different modalities are of prognostic value in TBI patients, with some modalities predictive for a favourable prognosis and others predictive for an unfavourable prognosis. Absence of short latency EPs predicts an unfavourable outcome (Guérit et al. 2009), while the strongest predictor for a good prognosis is the presence of ERPs (Daltrozzo et al. 2007).

Tips, Tricks, and Pitfalls

- EPs performed too early may show over-optimistic results due to the risk of secondary damage in TBI patients (Guérit et al. 2009).
- Drugs may have a pronounced influence on ERPs (Duncan et al. 2009).
- EPs should be performed by experienced neurophysiology technicians and interpreted by clinical neurophysiologists.

T. Sundstrøm et al. (eds.), *Management of Severe Traumatic Brain Injury*,
DOI 10.1007/978-3-642-28126-6_38, © Springer-Verlag Berlin Heidelberg 2012

- The predictive power of EPs should, together with clinical findings and results of imagining techniques, be taken into consideration in the handling of TBI patients.

38.2 Background

The different EP modalities are easily performed, often in less than 15 min in comatose patients. Significant abnormalities of EPs include the absence of responses, increases in latencies, or increases in inter-peak latencies. The absence of responses or the presence of normal responses are the most reliable predictors, although an increase in latencies, an increase in inter-peak latencies, or amplitude changes may also be valuable.

38.2.1 BAEP

Brainstem auditory-evoked potentials (BAEP) are signals generated in the brainstem and recorded by scalp electrodes in response to click stimulation of the ears. Responses from the ear and the neural pathways in the pons are recorded with latencies less than 10 ms. BAEPs are present in about 50% of TBI patients (Guérit 2005). There are some controversies about the prognostic ability of BAEPs, and some of these controversies are probably caused by differences in timing of the examinations and differences in criteria for BAEP abnormalities. There is, however, rather good agreement on the fact that absence of BAEPs is a bad prognostic sign; for example, in a study of 64 TBI patients, Tsubokawa et al. (1980) found that all 23 cases with absence of the later BAEP waves died or went into a permanent vegetative state. On the other hand, the presence of BAEPs in TBI patients is not a useful predictor for a favourable outcome, as damage to brain regions outside the brainstem will not affect the BAEPs.

38.2.2 SEP

Somatosensory-evoked potentials (SEP) are recorded after electrical stimulation of the skin of the limbs. When used as a prognostic tool in comatose patients, the most used technique is to stimulate the median nerve at the wrist while recording responses from the peripheral nerve at the elbow or at Erb's point, over the spine at level C7 and over the primary sensory cortex. A systematic review of 41 articles on SEP as a prognostic marker for awakening from coma in TBI patients showed only 5% awakening in case of bilateral absent SEPs, 70% awakening in case of present but abnormal SEPs, and 89% awakening in case of normal SEPs (Robinson et al. 2003). Amantini et al. (2005) found that SEP showed a good predictive value both for good and bad prognosis.

38.2.3 VEP

Visual-evoked potentials (VEP) are recorded after visual light stimuli. VEPs are only rarely used as a prognostic tool in comatose patients (Guérit 2005).

38.2.4 ERP

Event-related potentials (ERP), also called cognitive-evoked potentials, reflect higher cortical functions. ERPs are elicited by occasional different stimuli within a repetitive standard stimulation, the so-called oddball paradigm. P300 is a positive response with a latency of about 300 ms that can be measured as a response to infrequent randomly presented stimuli, for example, a different tone in a sequence of frequently presented tones. Some attention or vigilance is required in order to obtain a P300 response, and it cannot be elicited in all normal subjects, which limits its sensitivity in predicting coma outcome. Another kind of ERP, the mismatch negativity (MMN) potential, is the brain's automatic response to change in auditory stimulation, and it has the great advantage of not being dependent on patient attention, as it can be recorded in comatose patients (Näätänen 2000). The MMN response occurs as a negative peak in the ERP 100–250 ms after stimulation change. Kane et al. (1996) reported that the presence of a MMN response in serial studies of TBI patients has specificity of 100% and a sensitivity of 89.7% for awakening.

In a meta-analysis very high positive predictive values for a favourable outcome were found for P300 (89%) and MMN (93%) when present. However, the sensitivity was not very high (76% for P300 and 34% for MMN) (Daltrozzo et al. 2007). This meta-analysis showed equal predictive power of P300 and MMN, and both techniques are recommended (Daltrozzo et al. 2007).

On the other hand, the absence of ERPs has no predictive value for a bad prognosis, as these components are not always present in normal subjects and they are sensitive to other factors, for example, sedatives.

38.2.5 Combinations of EP Modalities

Some authors combine findings from different EP modality studies in indices for global cortical function and for brainstem conduction, which is of prognostic value (Guérit 2005). Kane et al. (1996) suggest that when short-latency EPs are normal, ERPs may be performed in order to directly check brain function related to cognitive processes.

38.2.6 Influence of Drugs

Drugs interfering with EEG do also interfere with EPs, and drugs may have large influence on EPs, in particular ERPs. Halogenated gases, propofol, and thiopental (membrane interference) may cause latency increase due to interference with subcortical conduction. In contrast, short-latency EPs are very resistant.

38.2.7 Timing of Examinations

EPs performed too early after the trauma may give false optimistic results if secondary brain damage occurs and some authors suggest serial examinations. Facco et al. (1988) suggest that EPs have the best predictive value when performed 3–6 days post injury.

38.3 Specific Paediatric Concerns

There are only sparse results regarding the use of EPs in children. Robinson et al. (2003) found a higher chance for awakening and less disability in children with absent SEPs compared with adults. In general, there is insufficient evidence of an age limit above which the same interpretation criteria can be used as those used in adults (Guérit et al. 2009), and interpretations should therefore be made more cautiously in children.

References

Amantini A, Grippo A, Fossi S, Cesaretti C, Piccioli A, Peris A, Ragazzoni A, Pinto F (2005) Prediction of 'awakening' and outcome in prolonged acute coma from severe traumatic brain injury: evidence for validity of short latency SEPs. Clin Neurophysiol 116:229–235

Daltrozzo J, Wioland N, Mutschler V, Kotchoubey B (2007) Predicting coma and other low responsive patients outcome using event-related brain potentials: a meta-analysis. Clin Neurophysiol 118: 606–614

Duncan CC, Barry RJ, Connolly JF, Fischer C, Michie PT, Näätänen R, Polich J, Reinvang I, Van Petten C (2009) Event-related potentials in clinical research: guidelines for eliciting, recording, and quantifying mismatch negativity, P300, and N400. Clin Neurophysiol 120:1883–1908

Facco E, Munari M, Casartelli Liviero M, Caputo P, Martini A, Toffoletto F, Giron G (1988) Serial recordings of auditory brainstem responses in severe head injury: relationship between test timing and prognostic power. Intensive Care Med 14:422–428

Guérit JM (2005) Evoked potentials in severe brain injury. Prog Brain Res 150:415–426

Guérit JM, Amantini A, Amodio P, Andersen KV, Butler S, de Weerd A, Facco E, Fischer C, Hantson P, Jäntti V, Lamblin MD, Litscher G, Péréon Y (2009) Consensus on the use of neurophysiological tests in the intensive care unit (ICU): electroencephalogram (EEG), evoked potentials (EP), and electroneuromyography (ENMG). Neurophysiol Clin 39:71–83

Kane NM, Curry SH, Rowlands CA, Manara AR, Lewis T, Moss T, Cummins BH, Butler SR (1996) Event-related potentials – neurophysiological tools for predicting emergence and early outcome from traumatic coma. Intensive Care Med 22:39–46

Näätänen R (2000) Mismatch negativity (MMN): perspectives for application. Int J Psychophysiol 37:3–10

Robinson LR, Micklesen PJ, Tirschwell DL, Lew HL (2003) Predictive value of somatosensory evoked potentials for awakening from coma. Crit Care Med 31:960–967

Tsubokawa T, Nishimoto H, Yamamoto T, Kitamura M, Katayama Y, Moriyasu N (1980) Assessment of brainstem damage by the auditory brainstem response in acute severe head injury. J Neurol Neurosurg Psychiatry 43:1005–1011

39 Clinical Neurophysiology: Continous EEG Monitoring

Birger Johnsen

Recommendations

Level I

There are insufficient data to support a Level I recommendation for this topic.

Level II

There are insufficient data to support a Level II recommendation for this topic.

Level III

Continuous EEG monitoring can be used to detect epileptic seizures, in particular non-convulsive seizures in sedated TBI patients.

39.1 Overview

Electroencephalography (EEG) is the standard diagnostic tool when there is clinical suspicion of epileptic seizures, in particular non-convulsive seizures (NCS), which most often can only be diagnosed by EEG. By the use of continuous EEG monitoring (cEEG) performed over one to several days, it has been found that 11–18% of TBI patients had NCSs and 8% non-convulsive status epilepticus (NCSE) (Claassen et al. 2004; Vespa 2005). Prolonged seizure activity may be harmful by causing secondary brain damage. The aim of cEEG is to diagnose these subclinical seizures and to guide the clinician in the antiepileptic treatment.

Tips, Tricks, and Pitfalls

- Neurointensivists should be trained in detection of suspect EEG patterns and recognizing usual EEG artefacts. Clinical neurophysiologists should perform further analyses remotely by use of telemedicine.
- Without cEEG, the neurointensivists should be aware of subtle signs of NCSs: lowering of level of consciousness, myoclonia, nystagmus, eye deviation, pupil abnormalities, autonomic instability, or confusion (Friedman et al. 2009).
- Drugs, especially sedatives, may have profound effect on the EEG.

39.2 Background

39.2.1 EEG Diagnosis

EEG is used in TBI patients to diagnose NCS, to differentiate epileptic and non-epileptic movements, to identify other toxic or metabolic concurrent factors in coma, and to diagnose locked-in

B. Johnsen
Neurofysiologisk Afdeling, Aarhus Universitetshospital, Nørrebrogade 44, 8000 Aarhus C, Denmark
e-mail: birgjohn@rm.dk

T. Sundstrøm et al. (eds.), *Management of Severe Traumatic Brain Injury*,
DOI 10.1007/978-3-642-28126-6_39, © Springer-Verlag Berlin Heidelberg 2012

state. EEG is most often the only way to diagnose NCSs and NCSE (Friedman et al. 2009). cEEG monitoring in different groups of neurointensive patient has shown that a large fraction of patients have NCS or NCSE, which could only be diagnosed by EEG.

39.2.2 Incidence of Seizures

For TBI patients, a smaller material showed 5 of 13 TBI patients (38%) had NCE and 2 of those were in NCSE (Bergsneider et al. 1997). Convulsive seizures within the first week of TBI have been estimated to occur in 4–14% of untreated patients (Annegers et al. 1980; Temkin et al. 1990; Lee et al. 1995), and if NCSs are also taken into consideration, the incidence of seizures is higher (Friedman et al. 2009). Claassen et al. (2004) found NCSs in 18% of 51 TBI patients of which 8% were NCSE. Vespa (2005) found 22% of patients with seizures of which half were NCSs. These figures may have been affected by prophylactic anticonvulsant treatment. Sutter et al. (2011) showed that cEEG monitoring increases the frequency of NCSE diagnosis in ICU patients.

39.2.3 Are Non-convulsive Seizures Harmful?

Data from human (Lowenstein and Alldredge 1993; Towne et al. 1994; Young et al. 1996) and animal studies (Meldrum et al. 1973; Krsek et al. 2004; DeGiorgio et al. 1992, 1996) suggest that prolonged seizure activity may cause damage to the brain. An association between duration of status epilepticus and a bad prognosis has been found (Young et al. 1996), and the chance of successful treatment is higher, and mortality is lower if fast treatment is instituted (Lowenstein and Alldredge 1993; Towne et al. 1994). Wang et al. (2008) found that the presence of early seizures in TBI patients is an independent risk factor for poor outcome. Another study has shown that seizures in TBI patients result in increases in intracranial pressure and microdialysis lactate/pyruvate ratio (Vespa et al. 2007). On the other hand, aggressive antiepileptic treatment is not without risk as shown in a population of critically ill elderly patients (Litt et al. 1998), emphasizing that a correct diagnosis is important. Controlled outcome studies of effects of cEEG and subsequent antiepileptic treatment of NCSs and NCSE have, however, not been done.

39.2.4 Technical Aspects

Sedatives as propofol cause EEG changes such as progressive slowing, burst-suppression, and suppression. Neurophysiology technicians should be available for applying the electrodes and starting the monitoring. Bedside nurses and neurointensivists should be trained in detection of suspicious EEG patterns and recognition of usual artefacts and be able to prevent some of these, for example, by fixating an electrode. Clinical neurophysiologists can perform further analyses remotely by use of telemedicine at another department or at home. Analyses of the raw EEG from the huge amount of data generated by days of monitoring are not possible, and data analysing methods presenting compressed data in the time or frequency domain are necessary. These methods should allow the clinical neurophysiologist to detect suspicious areas and subsequently analyse the raw EEG of that area.

39.3 Specific Paediatric Concerns

NCSs and NCSE have also been described in children with TBI (Jette et al. 2006). The technique can be used in the paediatric population.

References

Annegers JF, Grabow JD, Groover RV, Laws ER Jr, Elveback LR, Kurland LT (1980) Seizures after head trauma: a population study. Neurology 30:683–689

Bergsneider M, Hovda DA, Shalmon E, Kelly DF, Vespa PM, Martin NA, Phelps ME, McArthur DL, Caron MJ, Kraus JF, Becker DP (1997) Cerebral hyperglycolysis following severe traumatic brain injury in humans: a positron emission tomography study. J Neurosurg 86:241–251

Claassen J, Mayer SA, Kowalski RG, Emerson RG, Hirsch LJ (2004) Detection of electrographic seizures with continuous EEG monitoring in critically ill patients. Neurology 62:1743–1748

DeGiorgio CM, Tomiyasu U, Gott PS, Treiman DM (1992) Hippocampal pyramidal cell loss in human status epilepticus. Epilepsia 33:23–27

DeGiorgio CM, Gott PS, Rabinowicz AL, Heck CN, Smith TD, Correale JD (1996) Neuron-specific enolase, a marker of acute neuronal injury, is increased in complex partial status epilepticus. Epilepsia 37:606–609

Friedman D, Claassen J, Hirsch LJ (2009) Continuous electroencephalogram monitoring in the intensive care unit. Anesth Analg 109:506–523

Jette N, Claassen J, Emerson RG, Hirsch LJ (2006) Frequency and predictors of nonconvulsive seizures during continuous electroencephalographic monitoring in critically ill children. Arch Neurol 63: 1750–1755

Krsek P, Mikulecká A, Druga R, Kubová H, Hlinák Z, Suchomelová L, Mares P (2004) Long-term behavioral and morphological consequences of nonconvulsive status epilepticus in rats. Epilepsy Behav 5:180–191

Lee ST, Lui TN, Wong CW, Yeh YS, Tzaan WC (1995) Early seizures after moderate closed head injury. Acta Neurochir (Wien) 137:151–154

Litt B, Wityk RJ, Hertz SH, Mullen PD, Weiss H, Ryan DD, Henry TR (1998) Nonconvulsive status epilepticus in the critically ill elderly. Epilepsia 39:1194–1202

Lowenstein DH, Alldredge BK (1993) Status epilepticus at an urban public hospital in the 1980s. Neurology 43:483–488

Meldrum BS, Vigouroux RA, Brierley JB (1973) Systemic factors and epileptic brain damage. Prolonged seizures in paralyzed, artificially ventilated baboons. Arch Neurol 29:82–87

Sutter R, Fuhr P, Grize L, Marsch S, Rüegg S (2011) Continuous video-EEG monitoring increases detection rate of nonconvulsive status epilepticus in the ICU. Epilepsia 52:453–457

Temkin NR, Dikmen SS, Wilensky AJ, Keihm J, Chabal S, Winn HR (1990) A randomized, double-blind study of phenytoin for the prevention of post-traumatic seizures. N Engl J Med 323:497–502

Towne AR, Pellock JM, Ko D, DeLorenzo RJ (1994) Determinants of mortality in status epilepticus. Epilepsia 35:27–34

Vespa P (2005) Continuous EEG monitoring for the detection of seizures in traumatic brain injury, infarction, and intracerebral hemorrhage: "to detect and protect". J Clin Neurophysiol 22:99–106

Vespa PM, Miller C, McArthur D, Eliseo M, Etchepare M, Hirt D, Glenn TC, Martin N, Hovda D (2007) Nonconvulsive electrographic seizures after traumatic brain injury result in a delayed, prolonged increase in intracranial pressure and metabolic crisis. Crit Care Med 35:2830–2836

Wang HC, Chang WN, Chang HW, Ho JT, Yang TM, Lin WC, Chuang YC, Lu CH (2008) Factors predictive of outcome in posttraumatic seizures. J Trauma 64: 883–888

Young GB, Jordan KG, Doig GS (1996) An assessment of nonconvulsive seizures in the intensive care unit using continuous EEG monitoring: an investigation of variables associated with mortality. Neurology 47:83–89

Radiological Follow-Up

40

Leif Hovgaard Sørensen

Recommendations

Level I

There is insufficient data to support a Level I recommendation for this topic.

Level II

There is insufficient data to support a Level II recommendation for this topic.

Level III

Plain CT is the most efficient imaging modality in acute neurotrauma and for follow-up examinations.

40.1 Overview

After a moderate to severe head trauma, neuroimaging is mandatory for visualising the degree of traumatic brain injury (TBI) as well as the nature and location of the lesions in the acute phase and in the follow-up period as well (Duhaime et al. 2010). Imaging is important in triaging patients for acute intervention, for follow-up, and for evaluation of the long-term outcome. In acute and subacute follow-up, imaging plain computed tomography (CT) is the most important modality. The need for MRI in the acute phase is generally of less importance, but MRI can be of value and should be utilised whenever a clinical situation remains unclear after CT. Also, digital subtraction angiography (DSA) should be utilised when-

Tips, Tricks, and Pitfalls

- Early follow-up imaging should be guided by the severity of the initial trauma and serial clinical examinations, primarily with CT.
- MRI should not be performed in the acute phase.
- Consider MRI whenever there is discrepancy between the clinical status and CT imaging.
  - SWI or T2* for DAI and other haemorrhagic lesions
  - Axial T1 or T2 weighted imaging for arterial dissection
  - T2* and T2 FLAIR for SAH
- DSA should be reserved for cases where endovascular therapy is indicated.
- Pitfalls.
  - Not all acute extracerebral haematomas are of high density on CT: in severely anaemic patients and patients with disseminated intravascular coagulation, subdural (SDH) and epidural (EDH) haematoma can be iso- or hypodense relative to the brain.

L.H. Sørensen
Department of Neuroradiology,
Aarhus University Hospital,
Nørrebrogade 44, DK-8000 Aarhus C, Denmark
e-mail: leisoere@rm.dk

T. Sundstrøm et al. (eds.), *Management of Severe Traumatic Brain Injury*,
DOI 10.1007/978-3-642-28126-6_40, © Springer-Verlag Berlin Heidelberg 2012

ever a vascular injury needs to be elucidated, especially if endovascular therapy is indicated.

40.2 Background

Traditionally, TBI has been classified into primary and secondary injuries, where primary injuries are defined as those occurring at the moment of impact like contusions and lacerations including deep lesions such as diffuse axonal injuries (DAI). The primary lesions are in general untreatable. Secondary injuries are those occurring after the primary injury, and if detected in due time, they are potentially preventable. Secondary lesions include local or generalised cerebral oedema, herniation syndromes, hydrocephalus, ischemic lesions secondary to venous compression and dissection of the internal carotid artery or vertebral artery, venous thrombosis, secondary haemorrhages, infections, and leakage of cerebrospinal fluid. As the secondary injuries are potentially reversible or even preventable if triage and proper treatment is initiated and maintained, all efforts should be aimed at stabilisation and thorough observation with brain imaging playing a pivotal role. Dividing injuries in primary and secondary lesions is in many ways arbitrary, as TBI rather should be seen as a dynamic situation in which the need for radiological follow-up is individual (Gean and Fischbein 2010). So far, there is lack of consensus in the literature regarding indications for follow-up imaging. Instead of routinely performing serial CT or MRI scanning, it is recommended that follow-up imaging should be based on the results of the initial scans and repeated clinical examinations (Smith et al. 2007). Routinely use of CT follow-up without a clear indication should be avoided, as transportation from the ICU will expose these often critically ill patients to a significant risk for complications like hemodynamic changes, desaturation, and increased intracranial pressure (Lee et al. 1997). Risk factors for progression of traumatic intracerebral haemorrhage on the initial CT scans are presence of subarachnoid haemorrhage (SAH), the size of the intracerebral haemorrhage, and the presence of a subdural haematoma. Patients with these pathologies and patients with mental deterioration should be rescanned early. Also, patients with basal SAH, midline shift of >5–10 mm, or with coagulation abnormalities should be observed closely, and follow-up imaging should be performed early. It has been shown that delayed injury developed in as many as 45% and that it was associated with a significantly higher mortality, slower recovery, and poorer outcome at 6 months follow-up (Smith et al. 2007; Chang et al. 2006; White et al. 2009; Stein et al. 1992, 1993).

A follow-up scanning is mandatory whenever the clinical status of a TBI patient is worsening, as this might be due to an expanding subdural (SDH) or epidural haematoma (EDH), which in combination with traumatic cerebral oedema might lead to increased intracranial pressure exceeding the limits for normal brain function or even risk of incarceration, thus indicating the need for intervention. Development of hydrocephalus is important to detect, as early shunting is important in order to avoid herniation. Delayed intracerebral haemorrhage is a frequent complication that might lead to clinical deterioration and thus indicating an acute CT.

Today, CT is regarded as the mainstay of imaging for TBI patients, as it has a high sensitivity and specificity regarding the detection of skull fractures and significant brain injuries. In the management of TBI patients, CT can precisely identify progression of an intracranial haemorrhage and early signs of secondary injury such as cerebral oedema, hydrocephalus, or herniation. Moreover, CT scanners are widely available; scan time is very short, and CT is compatible with all necessary equipment needed for life support and monitoring.

MRI has a higher sensitivity and specificity for detecting non-haemorrhagic lesions and shear-strain injuries, i.e. diffuse axonal injuries, especially when utilising special MRI sequences like susceptibility-weighted (SWI) imaging, which is important to be aware of, as up to 80% of DAI are non-haemorrhagic. The burden of DAI on SWI correlates with duration of coma and the long-term functional disability of TBI patients (Tong et al. 2004).

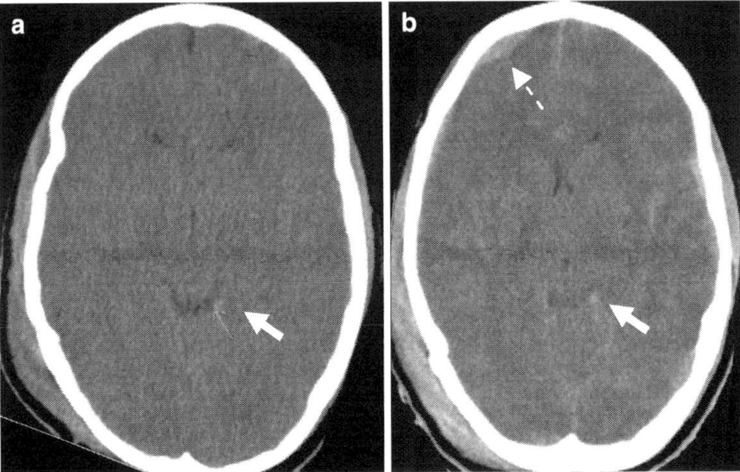

Fig. 40.1 (**a**) CT 1 h after a severe head injury. (**b**) 12 h later. The basal cistern is increasingly compressed (*fat arrows*). Note occurrence of a small EDH (*thin arrow*)

Although digital subtraction angiography (DSA) does not play a major role in the majority of TBI cases, it is of diagnostic value in cases with suspected vascular injury, but where CT or MRI fell short of visualising the lesion. DSA is of therapeutic importance when acute endovascular therapy is indicated.

40.2.1 CT (Including CT Angiography and CT Perfusion)

Plain CT is the primary imaging modality in TBI patients. It has a very high sensitivity and specificity for detection of significant cranial and intracranial injuries both in the acute and subacute phase. CT angiography (CTA) should be an option in all major trauma centres. With modern multidetector scanners, CTA is easy and fast to perform. Although clinically important vascular injuries are found in only 0.18–1.55% (Krings et al. 2008) of patients with head and neck injury, CTA should be performed in cases with increased risk of vascular lesions. Neurovascular lesions like dissection, pseudoaneurysm, arteriovenous fistula, and lacerations are strongly associated with fractures in the skull base, especially when clivus, the sphenoid sinus, and sella turcica are involved. In the neck, there is increased risk of artery lesions in situations with cervical fractures, fracture of a transverse foramen, and subluxations. Vascular lesions are also fairly common in penetrating traumas (Feiz-Erfan et al. 2007).

Traumatic subarachnoid haemorrhage (tSAH) is seen in as much as 60–80% after severe head trauma and is mainly located in sulci adjacent to contusions, but may also be found in the basal cisterns as in aneurysmal SAH. In these situations, it is important to find out whether a TBI with SAH is secondary to an aneurysm rupture or it is a true tSAH. This problem is easily solved with CTA, which should be used as a screening method reducing the need for catheter angiography. Head trauma is the most frequent reason for SAH. The panorama of complications after tSAH is the same as for SAH following aneurysm rupture, such as vascular spasms and obstruction of CSF by a blood clot or compromised resorption of CSF with subsequent development of hydrocephalus. Serial CT scans can show most pathologies that need neurosurgical intervention. Imaging signs of deterioration are progressing obliteration of the cortical sulci and the basal cisterns, which are early signs of incarceration (Fig. 40.1).

Subdural haematoma (SDH) is seen in 10–20% of severe TBI. It is a bleeding in the space between the dura and the arachnoid after rupture of bridging veins. SDH can cover a whole hemisphere and cross the cranial sutures, but not dural attachments and thus a SDH can never cross the midline. SDH is typically crescent shaped and hyperintense relative to the brain cortex in the acute phase. At follow-up CT after days to a few weeks, it becomes increasingly isodense with the cerebral cortex, and in weeks to months it becomes hypodense and will eventually reach attenuation values close to CSF, i.e. dark. Large SDHs with mass effect and midline shift are usually removed as soon as possible with a control CT the following day. Small SDH with limited mass effect will often be treated conservatively, where serial follow-up scans are indicated as the SDH will be surrounded by a thin capsule with small, fragile vessels with risk of rebleeding even after mild traumas. On CT, it is seen as more compartments with collections with different attenuation, Fig. 40.2.

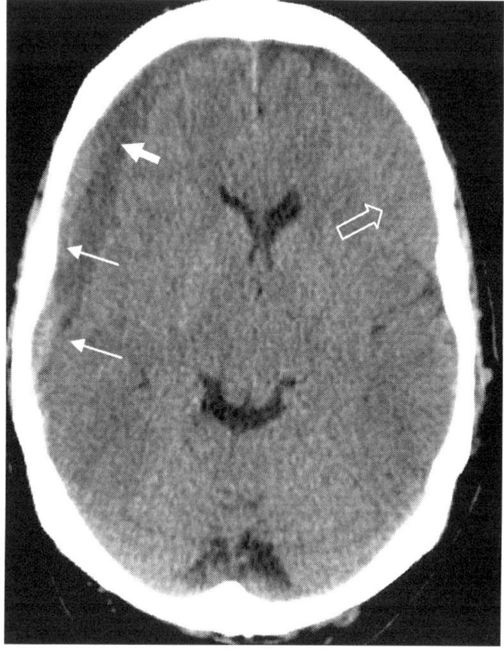

Fig. 40.2 Acute SDH (*thin arrows*), chronic SDH (*fat arrow*), and subacute SDH (*open arrow*)

EDHs are found in about 4% of TBI patients and are nearly always associated with a skull fracture. EDHs are most often seen in the temporal and frontal regions. It is a bleeding between the skull and dura, most often from a lacerated meningeal artery. They are typically biconcave and do not cross the cranial sutures, but can cross dural attachments and the midline. In the acute phase, EDHs are hyperintense, but if CT is performed in the hyperacute phase with an ongoing bleeding, the fresh blood will appear dark, giving the EDH a mixed density. This finding indicates a hyperacute situation, and if the haematoma is not removed, early and repeated CT follow-up is mandatory, as EDH can expand to a life-threatening size within a very short time, Fig. 40.3. Some guidelines (Marion 2006) recommend that EDH over 30 ml should be surgically removed regardless of the GCS, whereas EDH between 15 and 30 ml, GCS over 8 and a midline shift less than 5 mm can be treated non-surgically with repeated CT scanning and close clinical follow-up.

In the recent years, CT perfusion imaging (CTP), which is a bolus tracking technique, has developed into a useful and fairly user-friendly technology, which can provide valuable information in the evaluation of tissue viability as it can help to distinguish between patients with

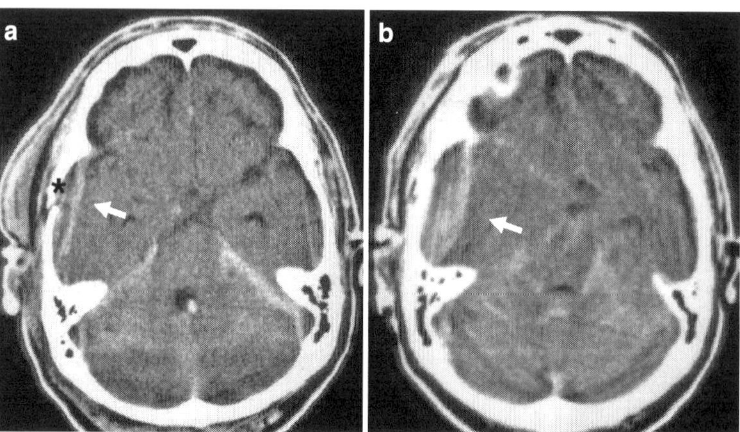

Fig. 40.3 Acute EDH, (**a**) CT 35 min after injury. (**b**) 10 min later. Note the skull fracture (*asterisk*)

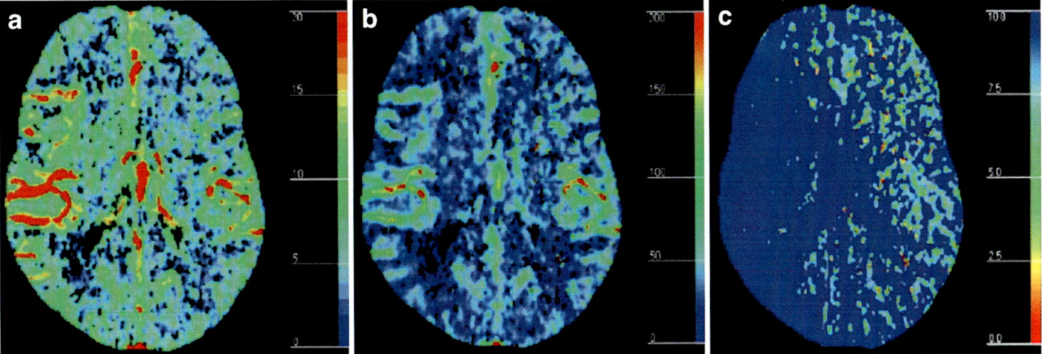

Fig. 40.4 CT perfusion after a moderate head trauma. (**a**) Cerebral blood flow (CBF). (**b**) Cerebral blood volume (CBV). (**c**) Mean transit time (MTT)

preserved and impaired autoregulation. It is possible to measure cerebral blood flow (CBF) and cerebral blood volume (CBV), and the mean transit time (MTT) can be calculated. Typically, CBV and CBF are low and MTT significantly prolonged in traumatic cerebral contusions (Soustiel et al. 2008), Fig. 40.4. CTP can visualise focal and diffuse brain injury and help in the prediction of progressing brain contusions and outline areas at risk of secondary injuries.

40.2.2 MRI

Already in 1986, Jenkins et al. proved that even low-field MRI can visualise nearly twice as many abnormalities as CT after TBI (Jenkins et al. 1986), e.g. diffuse axonal injuries (DAI) and small extra-axial collections. In spite of this, it has not been proven that early MRI will improve the long-time outcome after severe TBI (Manolakaki et al. 2009). On the other hand, MRI can in a later phase add important information regarding rehabilitation and the long-time outcome and disability (Lescot et al. 2009; Scheid et al. 2007; Solacroup and Tourrette 2003), especially with advanced MR technologies like MR spectroscopy (MRS), diffusion tensor imaging or tractography (DTI), and fMRI. There are some drawbacks regarding the use of MRI in TBI: it is difficult to observe and also to treat critically injured patients in the MR scanner. Even with modern equipment and the use of fast sequences, MR scanning is more time-consuming than CT. A complete whole body CT scan, which is routine in major traumas today, can be completed in less than a minute with a modern multidetector CT, while even an optimised MR scanning will take at least 10–15 min just covering the brain and upper neck. The longer imaging times can be a significant problem in uncooperative and claustrophobic patients. However, in the subacute and chronic setting, MRI has several advantages (Bigler et al. 1999; Hoelper et al. 2000; Hofman et al. 2001). Because of a better spatial and contrast resolution, MRI is far more sensitive than CT, especially in the detection of diffuse axonal injuries (DAI) and lesions in the brainstem, because these lesions are partly haemorrhagic and clearly visible on certain MRI sequences such as T2 FLAIR, DWI, and T2*. T2* and SWI are gradient echo sequences, both of which are highly sensitive for paramagnetic and diamagnetic substances, such as methaemoglobin, deoxyhaemoglobin, haemosiderin, and other blood products, Fig. 40.5.

SWI is a high-resolution, velocity-compensated, 3D gradient echo sequence based on both magnitude and phase data. SWI is highly sensitive and can reveal four to six times more microhaemorrhages than T2*, mainly because SWI include phase information (Gean and Fischbein 2010; Sehgal et al. 2005; Tong et al. 2003). Parenchymal lesions in the brainstem and small extra-axial haematomas in the posterior fossa and in regions adjacent to bone are easily visualised on MRI, but often obscured by bony artefacts on CT (Gentry 1994),

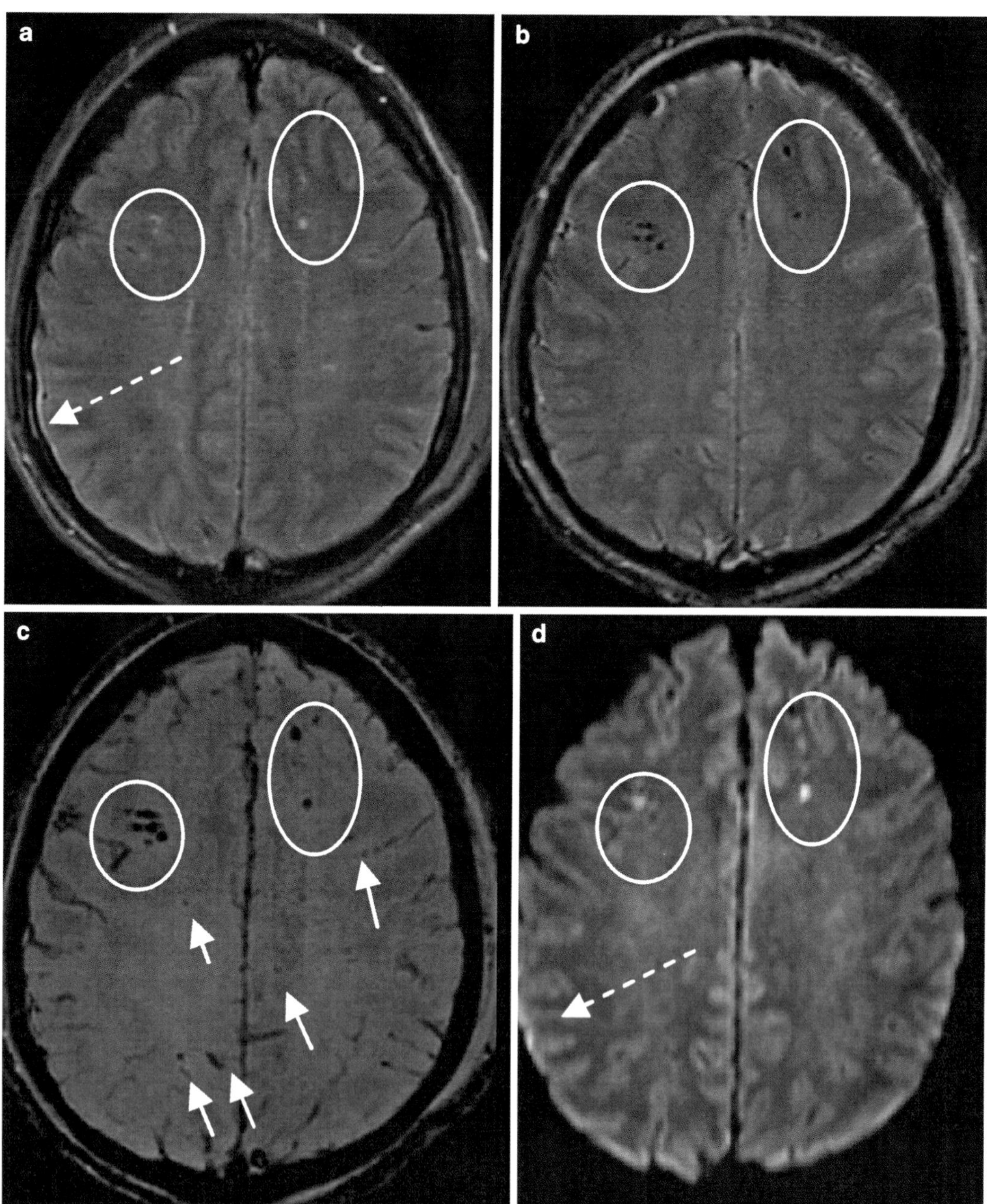

Fig. 40.5 MRI after a severe head trauma with Glasgow coma scale score of 4. (**a**) T2 FLAIR. (**b**) T2*. (**c**) SWI. (**d**) DWI. DAI, which are visible on all the shown MR sequences, are marked with rings. On the SWI image (**c**), additional DAI are marked with *small arrows*. Note the small SDH (*dashed arrows*) not visible on CT

Fig. 40.5. SAH can be seen on MRI weeks to months after the ictus, i.e. as long as there are blood products remaining in the subarachnoid space, where T2* and T2 FLAIR are the most usable sequences. MRI angiography is important in situations with suspected dissections in the carotid and vertebral arteries. The subintimal haematoma will organise to a clot, clearly visible on MRI as a crescent-shaped, bright structure, best seen on axial T1- or T2-weighted images, Fig. 40.6.

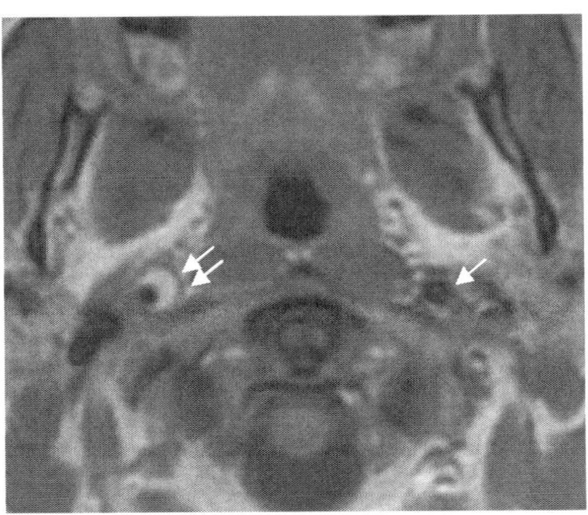

Fig. 40.6 ICA dissection. On this axial T1-weighted image, the false lumen is visible as a crescent-shaped, white structure (*double arrow*). The *left* ICA is normal (*single arrow*)

Traumatic venous complications like thrombosis can be seen in TBI following compression of a sinus or a laceration, where sinus thrombosis can give rise to intracranial hypertension and increased intracranial pressure with papillary oedema and sometimes intraparenchymal haemorrhage. Venous thrombosis can be visualised on MRI using phase-contrast angiography, where a normal, patent sinus can be seen with hyperintense (bright) signal, while a thrombus has low-signal intensity.

Generally, MRI should be performed whenever a clinical situation cannot be explained by CT (Cihangiroglu et al. 2002). It is also worth mentioning that CT, as opposed to MRI, is based on radiation and therefore associated with an increased risk of provoking cancer. It is especially problematic in this context with a majority of children and younger patients of whom many will be exposed to serial CT scans. No risks are associated with MRI provided all recommended safety measures be respected.

40.2.3 Digital Subtraction Angiography (e.g. Dissection)

Catheter angiography or digital subtraction angiography (DSA) plays a minor role in the routine diagnostic workup in the acute phase of head and neck trauma. The reported incidence of cerebral vascular trauma is up to 1.55% (Krings et al. 2008). Arterial dissection is the most frequent cerebrovascular sequelae after head and neck trauma followed by vascular transections, arteriovenous fistulas, formation of pseudoaneurysms, incarcerations with a vessel trapped between bony fragments, and thrombosis. Dissection is defined as an intramural haematoma mainly associated with an intimal tear allowing the arterial blood to pass under the intima and propagate distally resulting in stenosis, irregularity of the vessel lumen, and in some cases arterial dilatation (Zhao et al. 2007). On CTA and DSA, the typical dissection will present as a stenosis followed by a tapering of the vessel lumen. Sometimes, an intimal flap indicating a true and a false lumen is visible. Traumatic arterial dissection will improve or resolve spontaneously in only 55% compared to 85% in spontaneous dissections (Sturzenegger 1995). There is a risk of total occlusion in 20% (Rao et al. 2011). The primary treatment is anticoagulation therapy in order to avoid thromboembolic complications. It is also important to preserve the patency of the vessel. Endovascular therapy with stenting, vessel occlusion, or surgery is indicated in patients that remain symptomatic on medical therapy or where anticoagulation is contraindicated; the latter might be the case in trauma patients.

Traumatic aneurysms represent only 1% of all intracranial aneurysms (20% in paediatric cases), with ICA aneurysms in the cavernous segment as the most frequent type, representing nearly 50%; they are often associated with skull base fractures (Krings et al. 2008). An aneurysm can give rise to compression of the cranial nerves running in the cavernous sinus – most often the abducens nerve, as it is located in the same compartment as ICA, Fig. 40.7.

If the aneurysm ruptures, it can give rise to a carotid-cavernous fistula (CC-fistula), which is a direct communication between the intracavernous part of the ICA and the venous cavernous sinus. This can happen immediately or after a delay of days to weeks. The clinical findings are related to increased venous pressure with pulsating exophtalmos, vascular bruit, impaired motility of the eye, glaucoma, dilated veins,

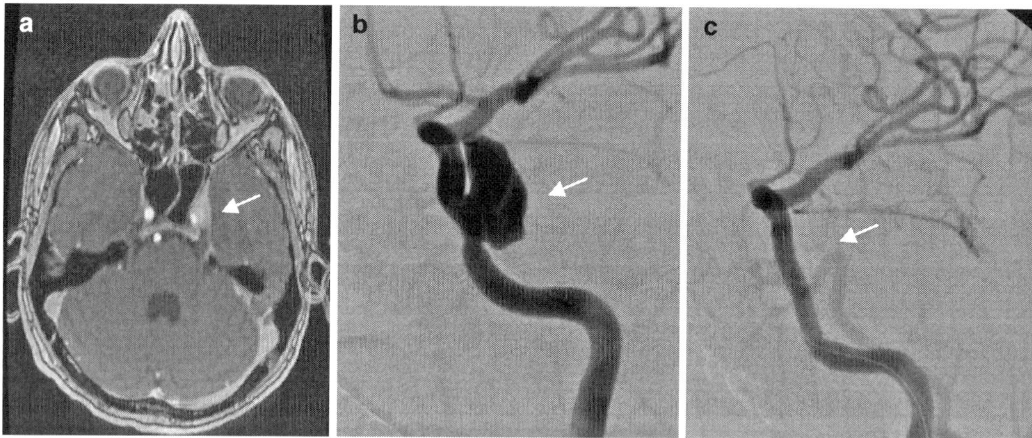

Fig. 40.7 Pseudoaneurysm following a severe head trauma. The patient presented with right sided abducens palsy. (**a**) MR angio showing a pseudoaneurysm (*arrow*). (**b**) DSA before endovascular treatment and (**c**) after treatment with a closed stent. The patient is without any symptoms post-stenting

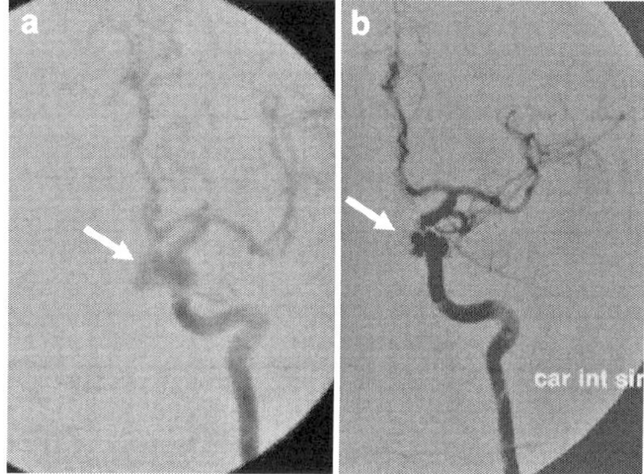

Fig. 40.8 A traumatic intracavernous aneurysm presenting with severe epistaxis 2 weeks after a traffic accident. (**a**) Before endovascular treatment with coils (*arrow*). (**b**) After coiling

and chemosis. DSA can provide the definitive diagnosis as it will show early opacification of the cavernous sinus and dilated veins draining like the superior ophthalmic vein and the superior and inferior sinus petrosus. If an aneurysm ruptures into the sphenoid sinus, it can result in a life-threatening epistaxis, Fig. 40.8.

Endovascular therapy is the preferred method in the treatment of traumatic aneurysms. One possibility is trapping of the aneurysm using coils or balloons, thereby sacrificing the parent artery. This is an effective and fairly safe procedure, provided that there are sufficient collaterals. ICA aneurysms in the cavernous sinus can also be treated using a closed stent, as that segment of ICA is without branches. A CC fistula can also be treated endovascularly by placing coils or balloons in the fistula. If the embolic material cannot be placed safely, trapping of the fistula can treat the lesion.

40.3 Specific Paediatric Concerns

During many years, there has been research on the indications and value of CT scanning after head-trauma in paediatric patients. Presently, recommendations for children older than 2 years for CT scanning include altered mental status, focal neurologic deficits, signs of skull base fracture, seizures, or injury patterns that are the result of major insults (Quayle et al. 1997; Schutzman et al. 2001). Children younger than 1 year need special attention, as their neurologic status is more difficult to assess. In this age group, the following symptoms indicate need of a CT scanning: any loss of consciousness, protracted vomiting, and irritability (Avarello and Cantor 2007). In other aspects, the general imaging recommendations are also valid for children. A drawback regarding CT is the radiation exposure, which is an important issue to be aware of, especially in young patients, as repeated CT scanning often are necessary. It is therefore recommended that MRI should be utilised more frequently in the monitoring of paediatric neurotrauma patients, although MRI is a more complicated procedure.

References

Avarello JT, Cantor RM (2007) Pediatric major trauma: an approach to evaluation and management. Emerg Med Clin North Am 25:803–836

Bigler ED, Johnson SC, Blatter DD (1999) Head trauma and intellectual status: relation to quantitative magnetic resonance imaging findings. Appl Neuropsychol 6:217–225

Chang EF, Meeker M, Holland MC (2006) Acute traumatic intraparenchymal hemorrhage: risk factors for progression in the early post-injury period. Neurosurgery 58:647–656

Cihangiroglu M, Ramsey RG, Dohrmann GJ (2002) Brain injury: analysis of imaging modalities. Neurol Res 24:7–18

Duhaime AC et al (2010) Common data elements in radiologic imaging of traumatic brain injury. Arch Phys Med Rehabil 91:1661–1666

Feiz-Erfan I, Horn EM, Theodore N et al (2007) Incidence and pattern of direct blunt neurovascular injury associated with trauma to the skull base. J Neurosurg 107:364–369

Gean AD, Fischbein NJ (2010) Head trauma. Neuroimaging Clin N Am 20:527–556

Gentry LR (1994) Imaging of closed head injury. Radiology 191:1–17

Hoelper BM et al (2000) Effect of intracerebral lesions detected in early MRI on outcome after acute brain injury. Acta Neurochir Suppl 76:265–267

Hofman PA et al (2001) MR imaging, single-photon emission CT, and neurocognitive performance after mild traumatic brain injury. Am J Neuroradiol 22:441–449

Jenkins A, Teasdale G, Hadley MD et al (1986) Brain lesions detected by magnetic resonance imaging in mild and severe head injuries. Lancet 2:445–446

Krings T, Geibprasert S, Lasjaunias PL (2008) Cerebrovascular trauma. Eur Radiol 18:1531–1545

Lee TT et al (1997) Follow-up computerized tomography (CT) scans in moderate and severe head injuries: correlation with Glasgow Coma Scores (GCS), and complication rate. Acta Neurochir (Wien) 139:1042–1047

Lescot T, Galanaud D, Puybasset L (2009) Exploring altered consciousness states by magnetic resonance imaging in brain injury. Ann N Y Acad Sci 1157:71–80

Manolakaki D et al (2009) Early magnetic resonance imaging is unnecessary in patients with traumatic brain injury. J Trauma 66:1008–1012

Marion DW (2006) Evidenced-based guidelines for traumatic brain injuries. Prog Neurol Surg 19:171–196

Quayle KS, Jaffe DM, Kuppermann N et al (1997) Diagnostic testing for acute head injury in children: when are head computed tomography and skull radiographs indicated? Pediatrics 99:E11

Rao AS, Makaroun MS, Marone LK et al (2011) Long-term outcomes of internal carotid artery dissection. J Vasc Surg 54(2):370–374, Epub ahead of print

Scheid R et al (2007) Comparative magnetic resonance imaging at 1.5 and 3 Tesla for the evaluation of traumatic microbleeds. J Neurotrauma 24:1811–1816

Schutzman SA, Barnes P, Duhaime AC et al (2001) Evaluation and management of children younger than two years old with apparently minor head trauma: proposed guidelines. Pediatrics 107:983–993

Sehgal V, Delproposto Z, Haacke EM et al (2005) Clinical applications of neuroimaging with susceptibility-weighted imaging. J Magn Reson Imaging 22:439–450

Smith JS et al (2007) The role of early follow-up computed tomography imaging in the management of traumatic brain injury patients with intracranial hemorrhage. J Trauma 63:75–82

Solacroup JC, Tourrette JH (2003) Assessing and predicting recovery from a coma following traumatic brain injury: contribution of neuroradiological data. Ann Readapt Med Phys 46:104–115

Soustiel JF et al (2008) Perfusion-CT for early assessment of traumatic cerebral contusions. Neuroradiology 50: 189–196

Stein SC et al (1992) Delayed brain injury after head trauma: significance of coagulopathy. Neurosurgery 30:160–165

Stein SC et al (1993) Delayed and progressive brain injury in closed-head trauma: radiological demonstration. Neurosurgery 32:25–30

Sturzenegger M (1995) Spontaneous internal carotid artery dissection: early diagnosis and management in 44 patients. J Neurol 242:231–238

Tong KA, Ashwal S, Holshouser BA et al (2003) Hemorrhagic shearing lesions in children and adolescents with posttraumatic diffuse axonal injury: improved detection and initial results. Radiology 227:332–339

Tong KA, Ashwal S, Holshouser BA et al (2004) Diffuse axonal injury in children: clinical correlation with hemorrhagic lesions. Ann Neurol 56:36–50

White CL, Griffith S, Caron JL (2009) Early progression of traumatic cerebral contusions: characterization and risk factors. J Trauma 67:508–514

Zhao WY, Krings T, Alvarez H et al (2007) Management of spontaneous haemorrhagic intracranial vertebrobasilar dissection: review of 21 consecutive cases. Acta Neurochir (Wien) 149:585–596

Neuromarkers

41

Ramona Åstrand, Johan Undén, Peter Reinstrup,
and Bertil Romner

Recommendations

Level I

There is insufficient data to support Level I recommendation for this topic.

Level II

There is insufficient data to support Level II recommendation for this topic.

Level III

Several biomarkers for brain injury are under active investigation and may have potential use in severity classification, prognostic evaluation and prediction of secondary brain injury.

R. Åstrand
Department of Neurosurgery,
2092, Rigshospitalet, 2100 Copenhagen,
Denmark
e-mail: raastrand@gmail.com

J. Undén (✉)
Department of Anesthesia and Intensive Care,
Skåne University Hospital Malmö,
205 02 Malmö, Sweden
e-mail: dr.johan.unden@gmail.com

P. Reinstrup
Department of Anesthesiology,
Skåne University Hospital Lund,
Lund 22185, Sweden
e-mail: peter.reinstrup@med.lu.se

B. Romner
Department of Neurosurgery, 2092, Rigshospitalet,
2100 Copenhagen, Denmark
e-mail: bertil.romner@rh.regionh.dk

41.1 Overview

Traumatic brain injury (TBI) is a significant cause of mortality and morbidity in adults and a leading cause of death in childhood. The diagnostic process includes clinical examination and in more severe cases neuroimaging, such as computed tomography of the head (CT) or magnetic resonance imaging (MRI). Biochemical markers are constantly being used as diagnostic tools for injuries in specific organs, such as troponin for myocardial infarction, creatinine for renal dysfunction and pancreas amylase and lipase for acute pancreatitis. A biomarker detectable in serum, and easily analysed, would be preferable as a complement to clinical assessment after TBI.

In 1983, Bakay and Ward suggested that an ideal serum marker should have high specificity for the brain, high sensitivity for brain injury, be released only after irreversible destruction of brain tissue, have rapid appearance in serum and be released in a time-locked sequence with the injury. They also stated that the marker should have a low variability regarding age and gender, that there should be reliable and accessible assays for analysis and that there should be a clinical relevance (Bakay and Ward 1983). None of the present biomarkers have so far been accepted as an ideal marker for brain injury.

During the last 15–20 years, research around brain biomarkers has accelerated. Most of the

T. Sundstrøm et al. (eds.), *Management of Severe Traumatic Brain Injury*,
DOI 10.1007/978-3-642-28126-6_41, © Springer-Verlag Berlin Heidelberg 2012

work has implicated the protein S100B as a promising surrogate marker for brain injury. Various biochemical markers in both cerebrospinal fluid (CSF) and serum have been investigated, and some are still under investigation.

Tips, Tricks, and Pitfalls

- Due to extracranial sources of S100B, multi-trauma patients with fresh long-bone fractures can also show highly elevated levels during the first 24 h, hence lowering the possibility of predicting patient outcome after severe TBI (STBI).
- Alcohol does NOT influence serum S100B levels.

41.2 Background

The potential use of neuromarkers in severe head injury has mainly been in regard of severity and outcome prediction. The clinical presentation of an unconscious patient, most often sedated and/or with external mechanical ventilation, makes traditional clinical evaluation difficult. Initial level of consciousness (GCS score), CT classifications (Marshall), pupil response and events of intracranial hypertension or hypoperfusion/hypoxia are some of the traditional clinical tools for estimating clinical progress and outcome. The prediction of secondary complications in a neurointensive care patient is also an interesting application of a potential brain biomarker.

41.2.1 Protein S100B

Protein S100B is the neuromarker that has been most extensively investigated and that has shown most promising results in head injury management. It is a small (21 kDa) calcium-binding protein expressed mainly in astroglial cells and Schwann cells in the central nervous system. It exerts both intracellular and extracellular effects, and depending on the concentration, it can be either neurotrophic or neurotoxic (Donato 2003). Protein S100B can be detected in both CSF and blood. The biomarker concentration has been shown to increase in CSF and/or serum after a vast number of cerebral diseases, e.g. traumatic brain injury (Ingebrigtsen et al. 1999), cerebral infarction (Herrmann et al. 2000) and subarachnoid haemorrhage (Moritz et al. 2010). Its median concentration in blood in healthy adults has been found to be 0.005 μg/L (Wiesmann et al. 1998). The half-life is estimated to be between 30 and 120 min, and it is excreted through the kidneys (Jonsson et al. 2000).

41.2.1.1 Outcome Measures

During the past decades, studies have found a correlation between serum S100B levels and clinical outcome according to Glasgow Outcome Scale (GOS) after severe head injury (Nylen et al. 2006; Raabe et al. 1999a). Patients with poor outcome (vegetative state or death) have significantly higher levels of S100B than those with favourable or severely disabled outcomes (da Rocha et al. 2006; Wiesmann et al. 2010). In a study on 79 severe TBI patients, a 2.1-fold increase of serum S100B was found in those with unfavourable compared to those with favourable outcome (Vos et al. 2010), and the authors suggested an admission S100B cut-off at 1.13 μg/L for prediction of unfavourable outcome at 6 months. The sensitivity for this was 0.88 and specificity 0.43.

In earlier studies, Raabe et al. found strong association between a cut-off level of 2.5 μg/L (any time) and unfavourable outcome (Raabe et al. 1999a, b), and Woertgen et al. found that serum levels above 2 μg/L (drawn within 6 h after trauma) predicted unfavourable outcome (positive predictive value 87%; negative predictive value 77%) (Woertgen et al. 1999). Somewhat differently, Mussack et al. found a lower cut-off level of 0.59 μg/L for 12-h post-injury samples, predicting unfavourable outcome at 1 year, to a specificity of 100% and Nylén et al. reported a cut-off of 0.55 μg/L (at admission) with a 100% specificity for predicting unfavourable outcome 1 year post-injury (Mussack et al. 2002; Nylen et al. 2008).

41.2.1.2 Repeated Measurements

Sampling is in most studies performed at admission and within 24 h post-injury. Some studies have made attempts of daily measurements for correlation to outcome. Nylén et al. correlated maximal serum S100B levels to outcome and found a significant difference in S100B concentrations between patients with favourable and unfavourable outcome (Nylen et al. 2008). Böhmer et al. collected daily CSF samples in 20 STBI patients and found that early elevations of S100B (up to 3 days) predicted deterioration to brain death (Bohmer et al. 2011). Dimopoulou et al. also reported elevated median serum S100B levels of 2.32 μg/L in those progressing to brain death, while survivors had significantly lower median values at 1.04 μg/L (Dimopoulou et al. 2003). A few studies have investigated the prediction of secondary insults after severe TBI and found a secondary S100B elevation over 24 h before clinical deterioration (Pelinka et al. 2003; Raabe et al. 1999).

Petzold et al. also reported that initial serum S100B was able to predict mortality 3–4 days before ICP readings did (Petzold et al. 2002). Olivecrona et al. investigated in a prospective, double-blind, randomized study the prognostic value of biomarkers and found that mean S100B values correlated with mean ICP during the first 12 h after trauma as well as when measured for 5 consecutive days (Olivecrona et al. 2009). They concluded that serum is a poor predictor of secondary insults.

Contrary to previous studies, some of the more recent studies have shown no significant correlation between early CSF-S100B or serum S100B and GOS or other outcome scales (Bellander et al. 2011), nor between dichotomized GOS (Olivecrona et al. 2009; Unden et al. 2007). They concluded that there is no clinical significant value of the marker as predictor of clinical outcome (Olivecrona et al. 2009).

41.2.1.3 Multi-trauma

One drawback of S100B is the presence of extracranial sources, especially bone marrow and adipose tissues (Unden et al. 2005). Pelinka et al. found that all patients studied with multiple organ trauma demonstrated raised S100B levels whether or not TBI was present, and they concluded that serum levels drawn during the first 24 h did not reliably predict clinical outcome in these patients. Daily measurements were advocated. However, another study by da Rocha did not find any correlation between higher S100B values and the presence of multi-trauma (da Rocha et al. 2006).

41.2.2 Glial Fibrillary Acidic Protein (GFAP)

This is one of the brick-stones in glial filaments, hence a cytoskeleton structure in astrocytes. It was first isolated in 1971 by Eng et al., and its molecular mass is between 40 and 53 kDa (Eng 1985; Eng et al. 2000). GFAP in CSF is increased in disorders causing astrogliosis and in e.g. stroke causing leakage from damaged cells to CSF. The CSF concentration correlates to the extent of damage and is seen to be extremely high in e.g. herpes encephalitis and large cerebral infarcts. Serum levels of GFAP have also shown to be highly elevated in severe TBI and are related to increased mortality and poor outcome. The major concern for this marker has, however, been the lack of reliable commercially available assays.

GFAP is the marker most specific for the brain, and it is only released in blood after cell death. Its characteristics suggest that GFAP may be a better biomarker for prediction of brain damage in TBI patients than S100B. Research was for quite long time limited to CSF measurements, but after the development of a relatively sensitive serum assay, research on GFAP has vastly increased (Missler et al. 1999; van Geel et al. 2002). It has been found that GFAP correlates with the severity of CT findings and clinical neurologic outcome (Lumpkins et al. 2008; Nylen et al. 2006; Pelinka et al. 2004). Lumpkins et al. found an excellent specificity for brain injury on CT when the cut-off level was set to 1.0 μg/L (Lumpkins et al. 2008). Nylén et al. found a 10- to 100-fold increase in serum GFAP after severe TBI and peak values above 6.98 μg/L (on day 1–4 after trauma) was not seen in any patients with favourable outcome. None of the survivors had serum GFAP above 15.04 μg/L (Nylen et al. 2006). Pelinka et al. found that GFAP (as well as S100B) levels were elevated for days in patients who did not survive. GFAP was a slightly better predictor of mortality after TBI when sampled <12 h after TBI (cut-off 1.5 μg/L; area under the curve, AUC 0.84, a measure of the accuracy of prediction with 0.5 being by chance and 1.0 being 100% sensitive/specific). S100B was, however, a more accurate predictor after 12 h (Pelinka et al. 2004). Wiesmann et al. also found a correlation between serum GFAP and neurological outcome (GOS) but only if GFAP was measured within 6 h after trauma, which is a notable difference from the previously mentioned studies (Wiesmann et al. 2010). Vos et al. also confirmed that elevated level of initial GFAP of 1.5 μg/L (sampled within 6 h) was a stronger predictor of death or unfavourable outcome than the traditional clinical signs (Vos et al. 2010).

Although GFAP has all the potential of being a better marker than S100B for TBI, especially due to its higher specificity, the large discrepancies of the present study results still call for further studies. The relatively new methods of analysing serum GFAP still have poor reproducibility and recovery.

41.2.3 Neuron Specific Enolase (NSE)

This is a cytoplasmic enzyme of glycolysis with a subunit consisting of $\gamma\gamma$-enolase or $\alpha\gamma$-enolase (Marangos and Schmechel 1987). It has a molecular mass of 78 kDa, and its biological half-life is over 20 h. It is normally found in neurons and neuroectodermal cells. NSE can be detected in both CSF and serum and has therefore been a potential biochemical marker under investigation. Serum concentration of NSE is known to increase in small-cell lung carcinoma and other neuroendocrine tumours (Gerbitz et al. 1986; Ishiguro et al. 1983; Velasco et al. 1985). The marker has also been investigated as a predictive marker of neurological outcome after cardiac arrest and cardiac surgery (Johnsson et al. 2000), as well as after TBI (Dauberschmidt et al. 1983).

Previous studies have shown promising results for CSF-NSE and serum NSE correlating to clinical outcome in severe head injury and to pathological findings on CT (Guzel et al. 2008; Meric et al. 2010; Ross et al. 1996; Vos et al. 2004). A recent study by Böhmer et al. on 20 severe TBI patients found that early elevations of CSF-NSE (within 1–3 days) predicted deterioration to brain death, even better than CSF-S100B (Bohmer et al. 2011).

There are however conflicting results from other studies, finding no correlation to outcome or other parameters such as CT results or GCS score (Bellander et al. 2011; Naeimi et al. 2006). There is also a disagreement around NSE's temporal course (Olivecrona et al. 2009; Raabe et al. 1999). Another major drawback of NSE is its prevalence in erythrocytes and its release in the blood by haemolysis (Johnsson et al. 1995).

41.2.4 Other Biomarkers

Several other biomarkers, such as neurofilament protein (NF), myelin basic protein (MBP), interleukin-1, interleukin-6 and tau, have been and some are still under investigation, but none have yet had any breakthrough as a diagnostic or prognostic marker in TBI. Currently, the methods of proteomics are constantly being refined for finding novel putative biomarkers diagnostic of brain injury.

41.3 Specific Paediatric Concerns

Data on biomarkers in the paediatric population are scarce and difficult to interpret due to the vulnerability of patient age blood sampling time and extracranial release.

References

Bakay RA, Ward AA Jr (1983) Enzymatic changes in serum and cerebrospinal fluid in neurological injury. J Neurosurg 58:27–37

Bellander BM, Olafsson IH, Ghatan PH, Bro Skejo HP, Hansson LO, Wanecek M, Svensson MA (2011) Secondary insults following traumatic brain injury enhance complement activation in the human brain and release of the tissue damage marker S100B. Acta Neurochir (Wien) 153:90–100

Bohmer AE, Oses JP, Schmidt AP, Peron CS, Krebs CL, Oppitz PP, D'Avila TT, Souza DO, Portela LV,

Stefani MA (2011) Neuron-specific enolase, S100B, and glial fibrillary acidic protein levels as outcome predictors in patients with severe traumatic brain injury. Neurosurgery 68:1624–1631

da Rocha AB, Schneider RF, de Freitas GR, Andre C, Grivicich I, Zanoni C, Fossa A, Gehrke JT, Pereira Jotz G, Kaufmann M, Simon D, Regner A (2006) Role of serum S100B as a predictive marker of fatal outcome following isolated severe head injury or multitrauma in males. Clin Chem Lab Med 44: 1234–1242

Dauberschmidt R, Marangos PJ, Zinsmeyer J, Bender V, Klages G, Gross J (1983) Severe head trauma and the changes of concentration of neuron-specific enolase in plasma and in cerebrospinal fluid. Clin Chim Acta 131:165–170

Dimopoulou I, Korfias S, Dafni U, Anthi A, Psachoulia C, Jullien G, Sakas DE, Roussos C (2003) Protein S-100b serum levels in trauma-induced brain death. Neurology 60:947–951

Donato R (2003) Intracellular and extracellular roles of S100 proteins. Microsc Res Tech 60:540–551

Eng LF (1985) Glial fibrillary acidic protein (GFAP): the major protein of glial intermediate filaments in differentiated astrocytes. J Neuroimmunol 8:203–214

Eng LF, Ghirnikar RS, Lee YL (2000) Glial fibrillary acidic protein: GFAP-thirty-one years (1969–2000). Neurochem Res 25:1439–1451

Gerbitz KD, Summer J, Schumacher I, Arnold H, Kraft A, Mross K (1986) Enolase isoenzymes as tumour markers. J Clin Chem Clin Biochem 24:1009–1016

Guzel A, Er U, Tatli M, Aluclu U, Ozkan U, Duzenli Y, Satici O, Guzel E, Kemaloglu S, Ceviz A, Kaplan A (2008) Serum neuron-specific enolase as a predictor of short-term outcome and its correlation with Glasgow Coma Scale in traumatic brain injury. Neurosurg Rev 31:439–444; discussion 444–435

Herrmann M, Vos P, Wunderlich MT, de Bruijn CH, Lamers KJ (2000) Release of glial tissue-specific proteins after acute stroke: a comparative analysis of serum concentrations of protein S-100B and glial fibrillary acidic protein. Stroke 31:2670–2677

Ingebrigtsen T, Waterloo K, Jacobsen EA, Langbakk B, Romner B (1999) Traumatic brain damage in minor head injury: relation of serum S-100 protein measurements to magnetic resonance imaging and neurobehavioral outcome. Neurosurgery 45:468–475; discussion 475–466

Ishiguro Y, Kato K, Ito T, Nagaya M (1983) Determination of three enolase isozymes and S-100 protein in various tumors in children. Cancer Res 43:6080–6084

Johnsson P, Lundqvist C, Lindgren A, Ferencz I, Alling C, Stahl E (1995) Cerebral complications after cardiac surgery assessed by S-100 and NSE levels in blood. J Cardiothorac Vasc Anesth 9:694–699

Johnsson P, Blomquist S, Luhrs C, Malmkvist G, Alling C, Solem JO, Stahl E (2000) Neuron-specific enolase increases in plasma during and immediately after extracorporeal circulation. Ann Thorac Surg 69: 750–754

Jonsson H, Johnsson P, Hoglund P, Alling C, Blomquist S (2000) Elimination of S100B and renal function after cardiac surgery. J Cardiothorac Vasc Anesth 14: 698–701

Lumpkins KM, Bochicchio GV, Keledjian K, Simard JM, McCunn M, Scalea T (2008) Glial fibrillary acidic protein is highly correlated with brain injury. J Trauma 65:778–782; discussion 782–774

Marangos PJ, Schmechel DE (1987) Neuron specific enolase, a clinically useful marker for neurons and neuroendocrine cells. Annu Rev Neurosci 10:269–295

Meric E, Gunduz A, Turedi S, Cakir E, Yandi M (2010) The prognostic value of neuron-specific enolase in head trauma patients. J Emerg Med 38:297–301

Missler U, Wiesmann M, Wittmann G, Magerkurth O, Hagenstrom H (1999) Measurement of glial fibrillary acidic protein in human blood: analytical method and preliminary clinical results. Clin Chem 45:138–141

Moritz S, Warnat J, Bele S, Graf BM, Woertgen C (2010) The prognostic value of NSE and S100B from serum and cerebrospinal fluid in patients with spontaneous subarachnoid hemorrhage. J Neurosurg Anesthesiol 22:21–31

Mussack T, Biberthaler P, Kanz KG, Wiedemann E, Gippner-Steppert C, Mutschler W, Jochum M (2002) Serum S-100B and interleukin-8 as predictive markers for comparative neurologic outcome analysis of patients after cardiac arrest and severe traumatic brain injury. Crit Care Med 30:2669–2674

Naeimi ZS, Weinhofer A, Sarahrudi K, Heinz T, Vecsei V (2006) Predictive value of S-100B protein and neuron specific-enolase as markers of traumatic brain damage in clinical use. Brain Inj 20:463–468

Nylen K, Ost M, Csajbok LZ, Nilsson I, Blennow K, Nellgard B, Rosengren L (2006) Increased serum-GFAP in patients with severe traumatic brain injury is related to outcome. J Neurol Sci 240:85–91

Nylen K, Ost M, Csajbok LZ, Nilsson I, Hall C, Blennow K, Nellgard B, Rosengren L (2008) Serum levels of S100B, S100A1B and S100BB are all related to outcome after severe traumatic brain injury. Acta Neurochir (Wien) 150:221–227; discussion 227

Olivecrona M, Rodling-Wahlstrom M, Naredi S, Koskinen LO (2009) S-100B and neuron specific enolase are poor outcome predictors in severe traumatic brain injury treated by an intracranial pressure targeted therapy. J Neurol Neurosurg Psychiatry 80:1241–1247

Pelinka LE, Toegel E, Mauritz W, Redl H (2003) Serum S 100 B: a marker of brain damage in traumatic brain injury with and without multiple trauma. Shock 19:195–200

Pelinka LE, Kroepfl A, Leixnering M, Buchinger W, Raabe A, Redl H (2004) GFAP versus S100B in serum after traumatic brain injury: relationship to brain damage and outcome. J Neurotrauma 21:1553–1561

Petzold A, Green AJ, Keir G, Fairley S, Kitchen N, Smith M, Thompson EJ (2002) Role of serum S100B as an early predictor of high intracranial pressure and mortality in brain injury: a pilot study. Crit Care Med 30: 2705–2710

Raabe A, Seifert V (1999) Fatal secondary increase in serum S-100B protein after severe head injury. Report of three cases. J Neurosurg 91:875–877

Raabe A, Grolms C, Seifert V (1999a) Serum markers of brain damage and outcome prediction in patients after severe head injury. Br J Neurosurg 13:56–59

Raabe A, Grolms C, Sorge O, Zimmermann M, Seifert V (1999b) Serum S-100B protein in severe head injury. Neurosurgery 45:477–483

Ross SA, Cunningham RT, Johnston CF, Rowlands BJ (1996) Neuron-specific enolase as an aid to outcome prediction in head injury. Br J Neurosurg 10:471–476

Unden J, Bellner J, Eneroth M, Alling C, Ingebrigtsen T, Romner B (2005) Raised serum S100B levels after acute bone fractures without cerebral injury. J Trauma 58:59–61

Unden J, Astrand R, Waterloo K, Ingebrigtsen T, Bellner J, Reinstrup P, Andsberg G, Romner B (2007) Clinical significance of serum S100B levels in neurointensive care. Neurocrit Care 6:94–99

van Geel WJ, de Reus HP, Nijzing H, Verbeek MM, Vos PE, Lamers KJ (2002) Measurement of glial fibrillary acidic protein in blood: an analytical method. Clin Chim Acta 326:151–154

Velasco ME, Ghobrial MW, Ross ER (1985) Neuron-specific enolase and neurofilament protein as markers of differentiation in medulloblastoma. Surg Neurol 23:177–182

Vos PE, Lamers KJ, Hendriks JC, van Haaren M, Beems T, Zimmerman C, van Geel W, de Reus H, Biert J, Verbeek MM (2004) Glial and neuronal proteins in serum predict outcome after severe traumatic brain injury. Neurology 62:1303–1310

Vos PE, Jacobs B, Andriessen TM, Lamers KJ, Borm GF, Beems T, Edwards M, Rosmalen CF, Vissers JL (2010) GFAP and S100B are biomarkers of traumatic brain injury: an observational cohort study. Neurology 75:1786–1793

Wiesmann M, Missler U, Gottmann D, Gehring S (1998) Plasma S-100b protein concentration in healthy adults is age- and sex-independent. Clin Chem 44:1056–1058

Wiesmann M, Steinmeier E, Magerkurth O, Linn J, Gottmann D, Missler U (2010) Outcome prediction in traumatic brain injury: comparison of neurological status, CT findings, and blood levels of S100B and GFAP. Acta Neurol Scand 121:178–185

Woertgen C, Rothoerl RD, Metz C, Brawanski A (1999) Comparison of clinical, radiologic, and serum marker as prognostic factors after severe head injury. J Trauma 47:1126–1130

Cardiovascular Monitoring 42

Karen-Lise Welling

Recommendations

Level I

There is insufficient data to support a Level I recommendation for this topic.

Level II

Arterial blood pressure should be continuously monitored in patients with severe head trauma. Hypotension (systolic pressure <90 mmHg) must be avoided.

Level III

Central venous pressure does not predict preload or blood volume status.

42.1 Overview

Most patients with severe TBI are young with no pre-existing cardiac problems. Other TBI patients may suffer from associated multiple trauma or pre-existing cardiac disease. The intensivist is challenged by the overall goal of obtaining cardiovascular stability in order to prevent development of cerebral ischaemia and secondary injury. The aim of haemodynamic monitoring is to alert the team to crisis before it occurs and to diagnose, treat and monitor response of the cardiovascular system to treatment.

In order to avoid secondary brain injury by correcting hypotension and hypoxia, the question is whether hypotension is caused by hypovolaemia and how do we predict fluid responsiveness (Benjelid and Romand 2003; Michard and Teboul 2002; Rex et al. 2004). Unfortunately, advanced cardiovascular monitoring is not well validated in this patient population, but much information can be gained from basic haemodynamic monitoring. However, even when the TBI patient appears haemodynamically stable, there is no guarantee that perfusion in the cerebral microcirculation is sufficient nor that cerebral oxygenation is adequate (see Chap. 31).

Tips, Tricks, and Pitfalls

- Cardiovascular monitoring serves to alert about a crisis before it occurs and to monitor response to treatment.
- Assess cardiovascular function by performing a physical examination, measurement of HR, blood pressure and urinary output.

K.-L. Welling
Department of Neurointensive Care,
Copenhagen University Hospital (Rigshospitalet),
Blegdamsvej 9, Copenhagen DK-2100,
Denmark
e-mail: karen-lise.welling@rh.regionh.dk

T. Sundstrøm et al. (eds.), *Management of Severe Traumatic Brain Injury*,
DOI 10.1007/978-3-642-28126-6_42, © Springer-Verlag Berlin Heidelberg 2012

- CVP should not be used to make clinical decisions regarding fluid management.
- CO is a global haemodynamic parameter and can be measured invasively, minimal invasively or non-invasively; however, almost no evidence is available on the benefit of monitoring cardiac output in head trauma patients.
- Arterial blood gas analysis provides information on aerobic or anaerobic metabolism as well as oxygenation.
- Central venous saturation, ScvO2, provides information on the global oxidative balance.
- The zero point of the arterial transducer is of great importance; it should be at the level of the ear (see Chap. 30) and not at heart level in patients with severe head injury.

42.2 Background

There is evidence that cardiovascular deterioration in the patient with severe TBI results in secondary brain damage. Thus, detecting signs of deterioration allowing for timely intervention and haemodynamic optimization is one of the crucial goals of management of the patient with severe TBI.

Most patients suffering from TBI are younger, previously healthy people. In the multiple trauma patient, associated injury may result in bleeding complications or damage of other organs, resulting in cardiovascular instability and a need for extended cardiovascular monitoring. Finally, elderly trauma patients may have pre-existing cardiac disease, usually coronary artery disease or hypertension resulting in a diminished cardiovascular capacity rendering them even more vulnerable to hypovolaemia or hypoxia.

In clinical practice, monitoring is often context specific: requirements in the NICU are often different from those in the trauma centre or the rehabilitation facility. Virtually no cardiovascular research is performed on patients suffering from severe head trauma, and extrapolation of studies from other patient groups is difficult and may lead to faulty conclusions. Thus, in general, cardiovascular monitoring in the NICU is limited to basic critical care monitoring and there is no evidence that use of sophisticated monitoring devices necessarily is 'better' for the patient with severe TBI (Boldt 2009). Sophisticated monitoring can be expensive and time consuming, and a wrongly applied monitoring goal or interpreted result can be of great risk to the patient.

One goal of cardiovascular monitoring is to alert the team caring for the TBI patient to impending cardiovascular crisis before it occurs, another is to obtain specific information about a disease, thus facilitating diagnosis, treatment and response to treatment (Pinsky and Payen 2005). In monitoring the patient with TBI, arterial blood pressure and evaluation of volume status is of primary importance. However, adequate perfusion not only relies on sufficient perfusion pressure but also on systemic blood flow, i.e. CO, to deliver oxygen and substrates to the brain and to eliminate metabolic by-products (Boldt 2009). The NICU doctor therefore desires to obtain information on pressure, volume and cardiac output as well as metabolism, and there are several means available to obtain this information. However, a prerequisite for using any monitoring device is a basic physiological understanding of the cardiovascular system.

42.2.1 Physiological Considerations: Preload, Contractility and Afterload

The Frank-Starling law describes the relationship between cardiac preload and left ventricular stroke volume or CO. CO refers to the volume of blood ejected from the heart over a period of time. It can be calculated by multiplying the stroke volume, SV (SV is the blood pumped by the ventricle in one contraction), by the heart rate, HR. Cardiac function is determined by four factors: preload, contractility, afterload and HR. CO is dependent upon adequate preload, and optimization of preload is one of the major targets of haemodynamic management (Schober et al. 2009). It must be noted that the most common reason for arterial hypotension is intravascular hypovolaemia.

Afterload is determined by aortic compliance and the resistance in the peripheral arteries. Finally, HR is of great importance because tachycardia results in diminished filling time and a fall in CO. Ideally, each of the four factors that determine CO should be monitored; however, apart from HR, current methods available for measurement of preload, CO and afterload all use surrogate parameters or have relatively low accuracy (Hadian et al. 2010).

42.2.2 Basic Monitoring of the Patient with TBI

Any evaluation of the haemodynamic status of a TBI patient starts with a basic clinical examination. Is the skin warm and dry or does the patient have a cold and clammy hand? Are the peripheral veins visible? Does auscultation reveal a heart murmur? Is there jugular vein distension? Pulmonary wheezing or rattling? Peripheral oedema? If possible, obtain the patient's history of pre-existing cardiac problems and medications.

42.2.3 Heart Rate and Rhythm

No TBI patients should be without continuous ECG monitoring because of the increased risk of significant disturbances in HR or rhythm. Despite continuous monitoring, more than 75% of arrhythmias and ischaemic episodes are reported to be undetected. Ischaemia can be detected by a standard 12-lead ECG. It is usually defined as ST segment depression of more than 0.1 mV. More important is that ischaemic episodes most commonly occur without significant changes in haemodynamic variables. However, hypertension or tachycardia is known to elicit ischaemia, and continuous ECG monitoring is mainly useful in detecting brady- or tachycardia, resulting in significant changes in blood pressure.

42.2.4 Arterial Blood Pressure

Every patient with severe TBI should be monitored with an indwelling arterial line to obtain continuous blood pressure. Arterial pressure provides information on systolic and diastolic pressure as well as arterial waveform but provides little information on flow and oxygen supply. However, arterial blood pressure, usually expressed as the mean, MAP (MAP = DBP + (SBP - DBP)/3), is used as a surrogate parameter for organ flow.

Hypotension increases morbidity and mortality in TBI (Chestnut et al. 1993). The threshold of blood pressure is not known, but current guidelines recommend that a SBP less than 90 mmHg must be avoided or corrected as quickly as possible (www.braintrauma.org). The threshold of hypotension in the patient with TBI is probably dependent on age and pre-existing disease, e.g. hypertension. MAP is used to calculate CPP (MAP−ICP=CPP), and a CPP more than 60 mmHg is recommended for adults (see Chap. 30). If the patient is hypotensive, the main interest is whether the patient is hypovolaemic and responds with an increase in MAP with fluid administration (fluid responsiveness) or alternatively if vasopressors or inotropics are needed. Blood pressure should only be increased with vasopressors after volume loading.

When the patient is stable, the arterial cannula should be removed due to the risk of thrombosis and embolization. NIBP is used after the patient has reached definite stabilization or is in the rehabilitation period.

42.2.5 Urinary Output

Sufficient urinary output is a simple parameter indicating adequate organ perfusion and volume status. Hourly urinary output should be monitored in all TBI patients. However, attention must be paid to osmotic diuresis caused by mannitol, which may lead to severe hypovolaemia. Also, urinary output cannot be used to monitor organ perfusion or volume status if diuretics are administered. Most cases of low urinary output are caused by hypovolaemia.

42.2.6 Pulse Oximetry

Pulse oximetry is used to diagnose hypoxaemia and is a mainstay in NICU monitoring. It is usually applied to a finger or a toe, but any site allowing proper orientation of the light can be used. If the finger or toe is cold or not well perfused, the registered oxygen saturation (SpO_2) may be false. It is non-invasive, requires no calibration and is usually available within seconds. Onset or worsening of conditions resulting in hypoxia is immediately identified. In the TBI patient, who is otherwise stable, procedures such as suctioning and positioning may cause desaturation. SpO_2 monitoring identifies that and allows the team to treat and prevent these potentially dangerous episodes of hypoxia. The pulse oximeter also acts as a blood pressure and perfusion monitor and displays HR. The accuracy of pulse oximeters is typically within 2% in the area of SpO_2 100–90 and less accurate below 90. However, the clinical relevant observation is a saturation below 90 (corresponding to a PaO_2 of 60 mmHg or 8 kPa), which definitely is a threshold for intervention (www.braintrauma.org).

42.2.7 Central Venous Pressure

For years, CVP has been used almost universally to guide fluid therapy in critically ill patients. However, there is little relationship between CVP and blood volume. Furthermore, CVP is a poor predictor of the haemodynamic response to a fluid challenge and CVP should not be used to make clinical decisions regarding fluid management (Marik et al. 2008; Osman et al. 2007; Kumar et al. 2004).

42.2.8 Venous Saturation

Central venous saturation ($ScvO_2$) is determined by cardiac output, haemoglobin concentration, arterial oxygen content and oxygen consumption. A change in $ScvO_2$ indicates that a change in oxygen transport and demand has occurred. An absolute value of 0.68–0.77 is considered normal (Reinhart et al. 2004); however, a change in $ScvO_2$ is more important that the absolute value, and assuming that haemoglobin, arterial oxygen content and oxygen consumption are constant, $ScvO_2$ reflects cardiac output. A decrease in $ScvO_2$ is easier to interpret than an increase in $ScvO_2$, and in systemic inflammatory response syndrome or sepsis, peripheral blood flow may impair oxygen uptake, so that $ScvO_2$ remains high (Boldt 2009). The interpretation of $ScvO_2$ thus requires consistent and intact vasoregulation, and because the determinants of $ScvO_2$ are multifactorial, the degree of compensation for changes in one variable cannot be predicted. Changes in $ScvO_2$ should alert the NICU doctor for further evaluation of the individual factors influencing oxygen balance, and a low $ScvO_2$ has been associated with increased mortality (Reinhart et al. 2004). A general guideline is that a $ScvO_2$value greater then 0.66 represents adequate reserve, 0.50–0.65 represents limited reserve and less than 0.50 probably reflects inadequate tissue oxygenation.

42.2.9 Lactate

Arterial blood gas analysis provides information on aerobic or anaerobic metabolism as well as oxygenation. Inadequate availability of O_2 at the mitochondrial level results in anaerobic metabolism and lactic acid production. The most common cause of anaerobic metabolism is cellular hypoperfusion (Pinsky and Payen 2005). While the presence of increased blood lactate indicates anaerobic metabolism, the absence of increased blood lactate does not guarantee adequate cellular oxygen supply. Metabolic acidosis in a TBI patient with poor perfusion, hypoxaemia or both must be assumed to be lactic acidosis until proven otherwise.

42.2.10 Cardiac Output

Several methods are currently used to measure CO in patients. These methods include methods using the Fick principle (thermodilution, dye dilution, lithium dilution) and pulse contour methods as well as ultrasonic methods (trans-oesophageal echocardiography, oesophageal Doppler monitoring). Electrical bioimpedance is another technique currently evolving (Button et al. 2007; Berkenstadt et al. 2001; Deflandre et al. 2008; Hofer et al. 2005).

For more than two decades, haemodynamic monitoring in anaesthesia and intensive care was based on the highly invasive and risk-associated PAC, with no proven benefit on outcome. Almost no reports on the use of PAC in TBI patients are available (Powner et al. 2005). Today, however, *less invasive* methods for estimating CO are available, e.g. methods using a pulse contour analysis system or ultrasonic methods (Marik et al. 2009; Berkenstadt et al. 2001; Hofer et al. 2005). With PAC as the gold standard, few studies have compared the systems (Hadian et al. 2010). Estimating CO is of particular interest in situations where cardiac dysfunction is suspected, or the patient does not respond to fluid, and there is a therapeutic dilemma between the choice of vasopressors versus inotropics. Most investigations dealing with individualized goal-directed therapy and protocolled optimization of haemodynamics by means of measurements of CO and derived parameters have been performed in patients having cardiac or other major surgery (Rex et al. 2004; Srinivasa et al. 2011), while there are few, if any, reports on monitoring of CO and outcome on patients with severe head trauma.

42.2.11 Echocardiography and Doppler Techniques

Echocardiography is widely used for evaluating left and right ventricular function, either by the non-invasive trans-thoracal (TTE) or semi-invasive trans-oesophageal (TEE) approach. With the Doppler technique, pressures and blood flow velocities can be measured (Renner et al. 2007). The method requires expensive equipment and a trained specialist.

Oesophageal Doppler facilitates a rapid estimation of CO with no major adverse events but is not validated as a tool to replace invasive determination of CO at present (Hofer et al. 2005; Srinivasa et al. 2011).

42.2.12 Pulse Contour Analysis of Arterial Pressure Curve

Analysis of the arterial pressure curve has gained popularity in estimating cardiac output and fluid responsiveness. Analysis of the arterial pressure curve, either invasively or by skin applied devices, can be used to calculate CO based on HR, MAP and the arterial waveform. Preload can be evaluated by cyclic respiratory variations in the arterial pressure (Deflandre et al. 2008), and a number of commercially available techniques use derived preload parameters such as pulse pressure variation and stroke volume variation to estimate fluid responsiveness (Reuter et al. 2002). Recent studies suggest that these indices are the most reliable predictors of fluid responsiveness in different populations (Marik et al. 2009).

42.2.13 Goal-Directed Therapy in Severe TBI – Which Direction?

In the majority of Scandinavian hospitals, the protocolled management of TBI is based on the American or/and European guidelines. There is good evidence that both protocolized and specialized neuro-critical care improve outcome (Clayton et al. 2004; Elf et al. 2002). However, different principles are used in the 'Lund concept', which is a protocol aimed at non-surgical reduction of increased ICP (Nordström 2007). A second aim in the Lund concept is to improve brain perfusion and oxygenation around contusions by antagonizing vasoconstriction through minimizing sympathetic discharge and refraining from vasoconstrictors (Grände 2006). As previously stated, the threshold of blood pressure that the treating team should aim for in severe TBI is not known and may be individual. However, normalization of blood pressure, blood volume and plasma oncotic pressure as well as general supportive intensive care is also an integrated part of the Lund treatment.

42.2.14 Outside the NICU

When the patient is considered stable with respect to vital organ functions, i.e. the cardiorespiratory and renal system, discharge from the NICU to a neurosurgical ward or a rehabilitation facility takes place. A basic level of clinical evaluation and physical examination is, at this point, how the patient is judged concerning the status of the cardiovascular system. Solitary haemodynamic values are then useful as threshold monitors, e.g. hypotension is always pathological, as is a low urine output. Defining threshold values and coupling to protocolized care can improve care at this time (Pinsky and Payen 2005).

42.3 Specific Paediatric Concerns

Only 20% of children who die from TBI have isolated cerebral injuries, while 80% have associated injuries due to the associated high energy transmission into a small body, e.g. trauma of the thorax. Thus, alertness to deterioration in cardiovascular status is of paramount importance.

HR and blood pressure are related to age, and there are many nomograms available. In general, children are much more dependent upon an appropriate HR than adults. Also, CO can be up to 200 ml/kg which is 2–3 times more than in adults, and that explains the fast rate of deterioration in children developing circulatory collapse. The only method currently validated for evaluation of CO is really ultrasonic evaluation of preload and contractility. The NICU doctor should be alerted if a child less than 1 year has an HR less than 80 or more than 180, or if a child of more than 1 year has an HR less than 60 or more than 180. A helpful guide for calculating target minimum systolic blood pressure in children is 70 mmHg + 2 × age, i.e. a 5-year-old should have a SBP of 90 mmHg. Estimating volume load in children also combines HR, BP, urinary output and capillary filling. Neck vein distension and liver size is useful mostly in volume overload, but in TBI, the challenge is often to detect hypovolaemia. There is no doubt that echocardiography and Doppler techniques are upfront tools in evaluating volume status in children.

References

Benjelid K, Romand JA (2003) Fluid responsiveness in mechanically ventilated patients: a review of indices used in intensive care. Intensive Care Med 29:352–360

Berkenstadt H, Margalit N, Hadani M et al (2001) Stroke volume variation as a predictor of fluid responsiveness in patients undergoing brain surgery. Anesth Analg 92:984–989

Boldt J (2009) Hemodynamic monitoring. Uni-Med verlag AG, Bremen

Button D, Weibel L, Reuthebuch O et al (2007) Clinical evaluation of the FloTrac/Vigileo system and two established continuous cardiac output monitoring devices in patients undergoing cardiac surgery. Br J Anaesth 99:329–336

Chestnut RM, Marshall LF, Klauber MR et al (1993) The role of secondary brain injury in determining outcome from severe brain injury. J Trauma 34:216–222

Clayton TJ, Nelson RJ, Manara AR (2004) Reduction in mortality from severe head injury following introduction of a protocol for intensive care management. Br J Anaesth 93:761–767

Deflandre E, Bonhomme V, Hans P (2008) Delta down compared with delta pulse pressure as an indicator of volaemia during intracranial surgery. Br J Anaesth 100:245–250

Elf K, Nilsson P, Enblad P (2002) Outcome after traumatic brain injury improved by an organized secondary insult program and standardized neurointensive care. Crit Care Med 30:2129–2134

Grände PE (2006) The "Lund concept" for the treatment of severe head trauma – physiological principles and clinical application. Intensive Care Med 32:1475–1484

Hadian M, Kim HK, Severyn DA et al (2010) Cross-comparison of cardiac output trending accuracy of LiDCO, PiCCO, FloTrac and pulmonary artery catheters. Crit Care 14:R212

Hofer CK, Furrer I, Matter-Ensner S et al (2005) Volumetric preload measurement by thermodilution: a comparison with transoesophageal echocardiography. Br J Anaesth 94:650–654

Kumar A, Anel R, Bunnell E et al (2004) Pulmonary artery occlusion pressure and central venous pressure fail to predict ventricular filling volume, cardiac performance, or the response to volume infusion in normal subjects. Crit Care Med 32:691–699

Marik PE, Baram M, Vahid B (2008) Does central venous pressure predict fluid resposiveness? A systematic review of the leterature and the tale of seven mares. Chest 134:172–178

Marik PE, Cavallazzi R, Vasu T et al (2009) Dynamic changes in arterial waveform derived variables and fluid responsiveness in mechanically ventilated patients: a systematic review of the literature. Crit Care Med 37(9):2642–2647

Michard F, Teboul JL (2002) Predicting fluid responsiveness in ICU patients. A critical analysis of evidence. Chest 121:2000–2008

Nordström CJ (2007) The "Lund concept": what it is and what it isn't. Intensive Care Med 33:558

Osman D, Ridel C, Ray P et al (2007) Cardiac filling pressures are not appropriate to predict hemodynamic response to volume challenge. Crit Care Med 35:4–68

Pinsky MR, Payen D (2005) Functional hemodynamic monitoring. Crit Care 9:566–572

Powner DJ, Miller ER, Levine RL (2005) CVP and PaoP measurements are discordant during fluid therapy after traumatic brain injury. J Intensive Care Med 20: 28–33

Reinhart K, Kuhn HJ, Hartog C et al (2004) Continuous central venous and pulmonary artery oxygen saturation monitoring in the critically ill. Intensive Care Med 30:152–1578

Renner J, Gruenewald M, Brand P et al (2007) Global end-diastolic volume as a variable of fluid responsiveness during acute changing loading conditions. J Cardiothorac Vasc Anesth 21:650–654

Reuter DA, Felbinger TW, Schmidt C et al (2002) Stroke volume variations for assessment of cardiac responsiveness to volume loading in mechanically ventilated patients after cardiac surgery. Intensive Care Med 28:392–398

Rex S, Brose MS et al (2004) Prediction of fluid responsiveness in patients during cardiac surgery. Br J Anaesth 93:782–788

Schober P, Loer SA, Schwarte LA (2009) Perioperative hemodynamic monitoring with transesophageal Doppler technology. Anesth Analg 109:340–453

Srinivasa S, Taylor MHG, Sammour T et al (2011) Oesophageal doppler-guided fluid administration in colorectal surgery: critical appraisal of published clinical trials. Acta Anaesthesiol Scand 55:4–13

Pulmonary Monitoring

43

Jacob Koefoed-Nielsen

Recommendations

Level I

There are insufficient data to support a Level I recommendation for this topic.

Level II

There are insufficient data to support a Level II recommendation for this topic.

Level III

Pulse oximetry and capnography monitoring in all endotracheally intubated ICU patients is recommended.

43.1 Overview

Pulmonary monitoring is used in every patient in the ICU. It can be divided into:

- Non-invasive monitoring of the patient
  - Pulse oximetry
- Invasive monitoring of the patient
  - Capnography
  - Arterial blood analysis
- Additional monitoring of the patient during mechanical ventilation
  - Compliance of the respiratory system

Tips, Tricks, and Pitfalls

- Pulse oximetry
  - Methaemoglobin and carboxyhaemoglobin give erroneously high values.
  - Poor peripheral perfusion due to hypothermia, low cardiac output or drugs results in inaccurate values. This appears more commonly with a finger probe compared with an ear probe.
  - Tricuspid regurgitation and patients with arteriovenous shunts for haemodialysis may produce significant venous pulsation and thereby false low values.
  - Movement (e.g. shivering) may cause inaccurate values.
- The capnography curve provides information about:
  - The inspiratory CO_2 level, e.g. rebreathing of exhaled gas
  - Respiratory rate
  - Indication of correct placement of an endotracheal tube in the trachea
  - Airway obstruction (e.g. bronchospasm)

J. Koefoed-Nielsen
Department of Neuro ICU,
Aarhus University Hospital,
Aarhus, Denmark
e-mail: koefoedjacob@dadlnet.dk

T. Sundstrøm et al. (eds.), *Management of Severe Traumatic Brain Injury*,
DOI 10.1007/978-3-642-28126-6_43, © Springer-Verlag Berlin Heidelberg 2012

- End-tidal CO_2
  - End-tidal CO_2 is approximately 0.5–1.0 kPa below arterial PCO_2 during anaesthesia in patients with normal lung function. In patients with poor perfusion of the lungs or intra-pulmonary shunting, lower values may be seen. Use of end-tidal CO_2 as a monitor of absolute arterial PCO_2 is therefore not possible in most ICU patients, but the assessment remains useful for following changes in the patient.
  - A progressive rise may indicate hypoventilation, increased metabolic rate or airway obstruction.
  - A sudden decrease at a fixed level of ventilation indicates a reduction in cardiac output (shock or a pulmonary embolus) while a fall to zero indicates an accidental extubation of the patient or cardiac arrest.
- Arterial blood analysis
  - Delay in analysing a sample (longer than 20 min) may cause a reduction in PO_2 and pH and a significant elevation in PCO_2 due to cellular metabolism. It can be overcome by placing the blood sample in ice after it is obtained.
  - Air bubbles in the sample can elevate PO_2.
- Compliance
  - Lung compliance is related to changes in lung volume and pressures and is affected by pulmonary pathology, e.g. pneumonia or acute lung injury (ALI)/acute respiratory distress syndrome (ARDS), which will cause a decrease in lung compliance.
  - Compliance of the chest wall (ribcage and diaphragm) is affected by body posture, muscle tonus and intra-abdominal hypertension which results in decreased compliance.

43.2 Background

43.2.1 Non-invasive Monitoring of the Patient

43.2.1.1 Pulse Oximetry

Continuous non-invasive monitoring of arterial oxygen saturation using a probe placed on a finger or earlobe is a part of standard monitoring in ICU. Pulse oximetry is a spectrophotometrical in vivo analysis of the Hb molecule emitting red and near infrared light (wavelengths 660 and 940 nm). The accuracy of the method is within 2% above 75% saturation. The result of the analysis is given by digits (normal interval is 92–100%) and as a curve on the monitor (Miller 2009; Singer and Webb 2003). Pulse oximetry approximates arterial blood saturation, but minor difference may be seen. Besides information of the saturation, pulse oximetry can be use to provide information of the circulation using the shape of the curve. The method is unaffected by foetal Hb, pigmentation of the skin, jaundice and anaemia unless very profound.

43.2.2 Invasive Monitoring of the Patient

43.2.2.1 Capnography

Continuous monitoring of exhaled carbon dioxide (CO_2) in endotracheally intubated patients is part of standard monitoring in ICU. Capnography is a spectrophotometrical in vivo analysis of CO_2 using infrared light with a wavelength of 450 nm. The exhaled gas is sampled by mainstream or side stream sampling. The major difference between these sampling methods is the location of the sensor. In mainstream capnometry, the sensor is incorporated very close to the endotracheal tube and the response time is faster than side stream capnometry (Miller 2009; Lumb 2000). The result of the analysis is given by digits (end-tidal CO_2 (=CO_2 concentration in alveoli)) and as a curve on the monitor.

43.2.2.2 Arterial Blood Analysis

A heparinised arterial blood sample analysed in a blood gas machine is a standard in vitro monitoring in ICU (Miller 2009). Arterial blood is used to identify arterial hypoxaemia/hyperoxaemia (low respectively high PO_2) and hypocapnia/hypercapnia (low respectively high PCO_2), followed by the possibility to adjust the ventilator settings in endotracheally intubated patients or to monitor signs of respiratory failure in the non-intubated patient. pH and base deficit values can be reviewed for acidosis and alkalosis, the origin (respiratory or metabolic) and whether any compensation has occurred (pH will be in normal range if compensation has occurred but base deficit values will be out of normal range).

43.2.3 Compliance

Compliance can be determined from the ventilator in the endotracheally intubated patient. The total compliance (elasticity) of the respiratory system is a product of the lung compliance and the compliance of the chest wall (Miller 2009; Lumb 2000). In standard ventilators, it is not possible to monitor the lung compliance and chest wall compliance separate from each other.

43.3 Specific Paediatric Concerns

There are no specific paediatric concerns for this topic.

References

Lumb AB (2000) Nunn's applied respiratory physiology, 5th edn. Butterworth-Heinemann, Edinburgh

Miller R (2009) Miller's anesthesia, 7th edn. Churchill Livingstone, Philadelphia

Singer M, Webb A (2003) Oxford handbook of critical care, 7th edn. Oxford University Press, Oxford

44 Renal Monitoring

Jens Aage Kølsen-Petersen

Recommendations

Level I

There are insufficient data to support a Level I recommendation for this topic.

Level II

There are insufficient data to support a Level II recommendation for this topic.

Level III

Urinary output, plasma concentrations of creatinine and urea, and creatinine clearance may be used as surrogate parameters for kidney function.

J.A. Kølsen-Petersen
Department of Anaesthesia and Intensive Care,
Aarhus University Hospital,
Brendstrupgaardsvej 100,
8200 Skejby, Aarhus, Denmark
e-mail: jaakp@dadlnet.dk

44.1 Overview

The glomerular filtration rate (GFR) is widely accepted as the single best estimate of the overall kidney function (Johnson 2005). In critically ill patients, renal function can be monitored by surrogate parameters such as urinary output, plasma concentrations of creatinine and urea, and creatinine clearance calculated as

$$\text{Creatinine clearance} = \frac{U_{\text{Creatinine}} \times V_{\text{urine}}}{P_{\text{creatinine}}}$$

$U_{\text{Creatinine}}$ and $P_{\text{creatinine}}$ is the concentration of creatinine in urine and plasma, respectively, and V_{urine} is the volume of urine.

Tips, Tricks, and Pitfalls

- Monitor urinary output and plasma concentrations of creatinine and urea daily. If renal function deteriorates, add creatinine clearance calculated from 2- or 24-h urine samples.
- Creatinine [μmol/L] urea [mmol/L] ratio below ten indicates prerenal cause (hypovolaemia) (Baum et al. 1975).

T. Sundstrøm et al. (eds.), *Management of Severe Traumatic Brain Injury*,
DOI 10.1007/978-3-642-28126-6_44, © Springer-Verlag Berlin Heidelberg 2012

44.2 Background

Acute kidney injury is a common complication and adversely affects outcome in critically ill trauma patients (Bagshaw et al. 2008). Nevertheless, there are no randomised clinical trials addressing the effect of renal monitoring on outcome in critically ill patients (Johnson 2005). The kidneys regulate intravascular volume, osmolality, acid-base and electrolyte balance, and excrete the end products of metabolism and drugs. Most of these functions depend on the kidneys ability to filtrate water. The glomerular filtration rate (GFR) is thus widely accepted as the best marker for the overall kidney function (Johnson 2005). The GFR can be measured directly, e.g. by inulin clearance (Johnson 2005) which is however expensive and time consuming. The clearance of creatinine, a product of muscle metabolism, closely approximates the GFR (Baum et al. 1975). Creatinine is secreted at a relatively constant speed depending on the muscle mass. It is filtered in the glomeruli and to a minor extent (7–10%) secreted by the tubules in the normal kidney. When kidney function declines and GFR decreases, the creatinine secretion is much greater than the filtered load leading to an overestimation of the GFR (Bellomo et al. 2004). For clinical purposes, however, it is important to determine whether renal function is stable or getting worse or better. This can usually be determined by measuring plasma creatinine alone (Bellomo et al. 2004). Plasma urea and urine output are non-specific markers of renal function (Bellomo et al. 2004). Urea is formed in the liver as a major end product of the metabolism of the nitrogen-containing substances. It is filtered in the glomerulus but undergoes extensive tubular reabsorption depending on the urine flow (Baum et al. 1975). Apart from the kidney function, the plasma urea concentration depends on the clinical situation, e.g. degree of catabolism, gastro-intestinal bleeding, infection, administration of steroids, dietary protein, liver function, and hydration. Urine output may be normal or high despite severe renal failure (non-oliguric). The combination of urine output, plasma creatinine, and creatinine clearance provides the basis for the RIFLE classification of acute renal failure (Bellomo et al. 2004).

Estimated GFR (eGFR) calculated from equations that take into account plasma creatinine and certain patient variables (age, gender, and body size) has been shown to be clinically useful for evaluating kidney function in a broad range of clinical settings but has not been sufficiently validated in non-steady state situations with acute changes in renal function (Johnson 2005). An automated calculator using the best available equation, the abbreviated Modification of Diet in Renal Disease (MDRD) formula (Johnson 2005), can be accessed on the Internet at http://kidney.org.au.

44.3 Specific Paediatric Concerns

The principles outlined above also apply for children. However, the reference values for the glomerular filtration rate and plasma creatinine change as the child grows. The GFR is 15–30% of normal adult values at birth, reaches 50% on the fifth to tenth day and gradually attains adult values in the second year of life. The normal plasma creatinine increases as the muscle mass increases and reaches adult values in puberty (Schwartz et al. 1976).

The plasma concentration of urea is normally 3–6 mmol/L throughout childhood and increases in the same situations as mentioned above.

References

Bagshaw SM et al (2008) A multi-center evaluation of early acute kidney injury in critically ill trauma patients. Ren Fail 30:581–589

Baum N et al (1975) Blood urea nitrogen and serum creatinine. Physiology and interpretations. Urology 5:583–588

Bellomo R et al (2004) Acute renal failure - definition, outcome measures, animal models, fluid therapy and information technology needs: the Second International Consensus Conference of the Acute Dialysis Quality Initiative (ADQI) Group. Crit Care 8:R204–R212

Johnson D (2005) The CARI guidelines. Evaluation of renal function. Nephrology (Carlton) 10 Suppl 4:S133–S176

Schwartz GJ et al (1976) A simple estimate of glomerular filtration rate in children derived from body length and plasma creatinine. Pediatrics 58:259–263

Neuroendocrine Monitoring 45

Marianne Klose and Ulla Feldt-Rasmussen

Recommendations

Level I

There are insufficient data to support a Level I recommendation for this topic.

Level II

Routine testing for pituitary insufficiency in the acute phase is not recommended.

Testing for pituitary insufficiency, especially hypoadrenalism, is recommended if clinically indicated.

Level III

Testing for pituitary insufficiency is recommended after severe TBI.

Testing for pituitary insufficiency is not recommended in all TBI patients.

If pituitary insufficiency is discovered and treated within the first year after TBI, it is recommended to retest the patient after 1 year or more.

45.1 Overview

Severe TBI may impact the hypothalamic-pituitary-peripheral hormone system during the acute phase but may also lead to long-term consequences in terms of persistent posttraumatic hypopituitarism. Many factors have been shown to influence the normal adaptive hypothalamo-pituitary response to acute critical illness including mechanisms affecting e.g. metabolism, hormone binding, and production. In TBI, there is an additional risk of structural damage causing direct interruption of the normal hypothalamic-pituitary function, with the risk of persistent damage. In the acute phase after TBI, it is particularly difficult to distinguish the two components.

Anterior pituitary hormone alterations are frequently encountered in the acute phase after TBI. The relevance and therapeutic implications of such endocrine changes are still debated. Acute-phase assessment of the growth hormone, thyroid, and gonadal axis is not recommended, as there is currently no evidence of a clinical benefit. Untreated adrenal insufficiency can be life threatening, and biochemical assessment is difficult in the acute phase. To avoid overlooking the condition, the diagnosis should mainly be based on the clinical picture, and immediate treatment instituted on suspicion.

M. Klose (✉)
Medicinsk Endokrinologisk Klinik PE-2131,
Rigshospitalet, Blegdamsvej 9,
2100 København Ø, Denmark
e-mail: klose@rh.dk

U. Feldt-Rasmussen
Medicinsk Endokrinologisk Klinik PE-2132,
Rigshospitalet, Blegdamsvej 9,
2100 København Ø, Denmark
e-mail: ufeldt@rh.dk

T. Sundstrøm et al. (eds.), *Management of Severe Traumatic Brain Injury*,
DOI 10.1007/978-3-642-28126-6_45, © Springer-Verlag Berlin Heidelberg 2012

The temporal relationship between TBI and hypopituitarism is poorly understood. Longitudinal studies examining TBI patients at variable time points from the acute phase to years after the trauma have reported transient, permanent, and de novo deficiencies all through the time span (Agha et al. 2005; Kleindienst et al. 2009; Klose et al. 2007b; Tanriverdi et al. 2006). Part of this variation may be ascribed to diagnostic difficulties, including those caused by the stress of severe illness, but may also in some cases be related to medication effects.

Over the last years, long-term anterior pituitary hormone deficiency has been reported with a prevalence of 15–83% in selected cohorts, suggesting that long-term posttraumatic hypopituitarism might be a more common complication in TBI than previously believed (Table 45.1). Although some studies have failed to show such high frequency (van der Eerden et al. 2010), this has raised concerns whether undiagnosed and thus untreated hypopituitarism may contribute to the mortality and severe morbidity seen in TBI. The magnitude of this contribution has not yet been defined, and although some outcome studies have indicated that posttraumatic hypopituitarism is of clinical significance, with important impacts on health-related quality of life and lipid status (Kelly et al. 2006; Klose et al. 2007c), the findings have not been consistent (Pavlovic et al. 2010). However, current status is that expert panels have proposed recommendations for hormone assessment of pituitary insufficiency and consequent appropriate replacement after TBI (Ghigo et al. 2005; Ho 2007). Unfortunately, the area lacks valid clinical, biochemical, or other predictors, and it has not yet been clarified which part of the TBI population that should be tested (Klose and Feldt-Rasmussen 2008). Finally, data are still awaited to document the effect of hormone replacement therapy in this patient category, and until such data are available, one should be cautious to introduce uncritical routine anterior pituitary testing and replacement therapy. Meanwhile, more pragmatic recommendations have to be given, e.g. neuroendocrine evaluation should be considered at any stage when clinically indicated in a patient who has suffered TBI. Certain categories of patients may be at a greater risk, including those with increased ICP, CT abnormalities, diffuse axonal injury, and those with basal skull fractures and should be regarded with a higher priority for pituitary assessment.

Tips, Tricks, and Pitfalls

- Involvement of a specialised medical endocrinologist is mandatory for proper choice of hypothalamic-pituitary tests as well as their interpretation.
- Normal plasma sodium does not exclude presence of severe life-threatening hypoadrenalism.
- If reduced or lacking response to vasopressors, secondary hypoadrenalism should be suspected.
- Diabetes insipidus is a strong indicator for hypothalamo-pituitary damage.
- Patients with high ICP, CT abnormalities, and basal skull fractures are at greater risk for hypothalamo-pituitary damage.

45.2 Background

45.2.1 Anterior Pituitary Hormone Deficiency Following TBI – Aetiology

The aetiology of posttraumatic hypopituitarism remains incompletely understood, but current evidence indicates the role of both primary mechanical injury and secondary injury from hypotension, hypoxia, anaemia, and brain swelling causing restriction of flow in the hypophyseal portal vessels. Support of this pathophysiologic concept comes from autopsy studies from fatally head-injured patients in which up to one third sustained anterior pituitary gland necrosis (Ceballos 1966; Crompton 1971; Kornblum and Fisher 1969). It is however unclear whether these data from fatal cases can be generalised to explain long-term hypopituitarism in TBI survivors. Two recent MR studies may support the hypothesis. An observational case–control study including 41 patients with non-lethal head trauma demonstrated acute changes in terms of pituitary

Table 45.1 Recent publications on the prevalence of long-term posttraumatic anterior pituitary dysfunction

				Anterior pituitary function (%)							
Authors	Time from injury (months)	*n*	GCS <13	Total	Multiple hypopituitarism	GH deficiency[a]	ACTH deficiency	LH/FSH deficiency	TSH deficiency	↑ PRL	Predictors
Kelly et al. (2000)	Median 26	22	–	36	23	18	5	23	5	0	Diffuse brain swelling, GCS
Lieberman et al. (2001)	Median 13	70	–	69	18	15	46	1	22	10	None
Agha et al. (2004)	Median 17	102	100%	29	6	11 (8)	13	12	1	12	None
Bondanelli et al. (2004)	Range 12–64	50	86%	54	12	28 (20)	0	14	10	8	GCS score
Popovic et al. (2004)	Median 44	67	100%	34	10	15 (8)	7	9	4	4	None
Aimaretti et al. (2005)	12	70	45%	23	10	20	7	11	6	6	None
Leal-Cerro et al. (2005)	>12	170[b]	100%	25	16	6	6	17	6	–	None
Schneider et al. (2006)	12	70	78%	36	4	10	9	20	3	14	None
Tanriverdi et al. (2006)	12	52	40%	51	10	33	19	8	6	8	None
Herrmann et al. (2006)	Range 5–47	76	100%	24	7	8	2	17	2	–	None
Klose et al. (2007a)	Median 13	104	58%	15	6	15	5	2	2	10	Increased ICP, low GCS
Wachter et al. (2009)		53	24%	25	2	2	4	1	6	–	None
Kleindienst et al. (2009)	>24	23	78%	83	30	39	0	48	0	5	Low GH first week post-TBI
van der Eerden et al. (2010)	3–30	107	28%	<1	0	0	<1	0	0	–	ND

GCS Glasgow Coma Scale score
[a]Given as severe GHD (partial GHD)
[b]Only 99 patients were tested

enlargement, pituitary haemorrhages, infarctions, signal abnormalities, and/or partial stalk transection in about 30% of adult TBI patients (Maiya et al. 2007). Secondly, other observational data have suggested that patients with long-term post-TBI hypopituitarism have a higher frequency of loss of pituitary volume or empty sella, abnormal pituitary gland signal heterogeneity, perfusion deficits, and/or lack of posterior pituitary signal as compared to TBI patients with normal pituitary function (Schneider et al. 2007). Likewise, Bavisetty et al. (2008) reported the degree of injury as defined by acute CT to be the strongest predictor for long-term deficiencies; Klose et al. (2007a) reported that a normal CT excluded development of long-term deficiencies, whereas indirect indicators of increased trauma severity including increased ICP were predictive of long-term deficiency in their cohort of 104 patients; and Schneider et al. found other indicators of more severe TBI such as diffuse axonal injury and basal skull fractures to be predictive (Schneider et al. 2008). Most studies however failed to show a relationship between injury-related factors and the development of long-term hypopituitarism (Klose and Feldt-Rasmussen 2008), and the role of acute CT was recently contradicted by Kleindienst et al. (2009) who did not find any relationship between acute or late CT findings and development of hypopituitarism.

Furthermore, the effects of transient stress from critical illness and medication are mechanisms to be considered in the acute phase. Adrenal cortisol synthesis can be impaired by the use of the anaesthetic agent etomidate and the antifungal agent ketoconazole; exogenous corticosteroid therapy may suppress the HPA axis and induce adrenal atrophy that may persist months after cessation, and hepatic metabolism of cortisol may be enhanced by drugs such as phenytoin.

45.2.2 Acute-Phase Anterior Pituitary Hormone Deficiency

Presence of hypothalamic-anterior pituitary-peripheral hormone alterations is a very common phenomenon in the acute phase after TBI and may resemble the biochemical picture of central hypogonadism or hypothyroidism (Van den Berghe et al. 1998), whereas secretion of stress hormones, such as prolactin, growth hormone (GH), adrenocorticotrophin (ACTH), cortisol (Annane et al. 2000; Beishuizen et al. 2001; Hamrahian et al. 2004), and vasopressin (AVP) (Jochberger et al. 2006), is increased. The degree of such alterations is typically related to disease severity and associated with higher morbidity and mortality (Barton et al. 1987; De Groot 2006; Span et al. 1992). The changes are not disease specific but a hallmark in acute and critical illness as such and appear to be part of important adaptive mechanisms regulating the inflammatory response, caused by cytokine activation among other factors. Acute illness per se can also result in variable changes of metabolism in all the hormone-binding proteins, and a number of drugs used for life support in intensive care units affect the binding of the hormones to their binding proteins. The interpretation of biochemical findings thus entails plenty of problems, independent on whether total or free hormone measurements is used, and currently there are no reliable diagnostic cut-offs for anterior pituitary hormone deficiency in critically ill patients.

The hypothalamic-pituitary-adrenal (HPA) axis deserves special interest, as untreated hypoadrenalism may have a major impact for the patient's outcome. During critical illness, profound and variable changes occur in the HPA axis, including HPA activation (Annane et al. 2000; Hamrahian et al. 2004; Vanhorebeek et al. 2006), decreased cortisol-binding globulin (CBG) the first week after admission (Beishuizen et al. 2001; Hamrahian et al. 2004) leading to increased circulating free cortisol, and increased tissue sensitivity to glucocorticoids (Molijn et al. 1995). All these changes complicate assessment as the usual biochemical definitions of hypoadrenalism cannot be used (Annane et al. 2000; Cooper and Stewart 2003; Hamrahian et al. 2004). Therefore, the threshold that best describes the patients at need for acute or chronic glucocorticoid replacement is still to be defined.

A number of studies have assessed the acute neuroendocrine changes following TBI, in order to investigate the correlation to trauma severity, metabolic derangement, and variables that may predict outcome (Cernak et al. 1999; Cohan et al. 2005; Della et al. 1998; Feibel et al. 1983; Hackl et al. 1991). The clinical implications of these finding however remain unclear. Four longitudinal studies have been designed to evaluate the relation between acute and long-term pituitary hormone status after TBI. Agha et al. (2005) found secondary gonadotropin, growth hormone (GH), corticotrophin (ACTH), and thyrotropin (TSH) deficiency in 80%, 18%, 16%, and 2%, respectively, of 56 patients with moderate or severe TBI. At 1-year follow-up, hormonal abnormalities had recovered in most patients, whereas others had developed de novo deficiencies, and although persistent GH and ACTH deficiency was associated with more severe acute-phase growth hormone and cortisol hyposecretion, the authors were unable to identify biochemical predictors of persistent hypopituitarism. Tanriverdi et al. (2006) reported pituitary hormone deficiency to affect 50% of 52 evaluated patients, primarily affecting the gonadotroph axis. However, individual data showed no obvious relationship between early and late pituitary dysfunctions. Klose et al. (2007b) described acute hormone alterations in 76% of 46 patients, with patients suffering the most severe TBI exhibiting the highest prevalence of alterations mimicking hypogonadotropic hypogonadism and central hypothyroidism, hyperprolactinaemia, and increased HPA activity. They were unable to identify biochemical predictors of persistent hypopituitarism but reported that no de novo deficiencies were recorded from 3 to 12 months post-TBI, whereas late recovery was observed in 1 out of 7 patients being hypopituitary at 3 months. Kleindienst et al. (2009) described hormone alterations in 83% of 71 patients, recovering in most within 2 years of follow-up. They reported that initial low GH levels predicted persistent deficiency 2 years post-TBI. The existing data rely on rather small cohorts only allowing for case description, and therefore clear conclusions and recommendations on this issue are difficult.

Case reports have provided clinical data to justify an increased attention towards the potential presence of secondary hypoadrenalism occurring from the acute phase in TBI patients. In order to illustrate the potential pitfall in diagnosing the causes of hyponatraemia in TBI patients, Agha et al. (2007) reported data from three patients with severe TBI, who were initially misdiagnosed as SIADH. In two cases, hypoadrenalism was suspected due to the combination of hyponatraemia, hypoglycaemia, and hypotension, and in the third case because plasma sodium did not correct with fluid restriction. All three patients had extremely low baseline cortisol of 33–110 nmol/L and undetectable ACTH levels. The condition ameliorated in all upon glucocorticoid replacement. Patients may however present with more subtle signs and symptoms.

45.2.3 Long-Term Anterior Pituitary Hormone Deficiency

Anterior pituitary hormone deficiency following TBI has traditionally been considered very rare and mainly reported as single cases or case series. Over the last decade, using more refined evaluation procedures, including dynamic testing for GH deficiency, long-term anterior pituitary hormone deficiency, has been reported with a prevalence of 15–83% in selected cohorts (Table 45.1). The diversity in the reported prevalence is likely to be explained by different study populations, study designs, and diagnostic procedures used. The high prevalence reported has recently lead expert panels to include TBI in endocrine guidelines regarding whom and when to test for GH deficiency, and several screening programs have been proposed (Behan et al. 2008; Ghigo et al. 2005; Ho 2007). Screening has recently been challenged by the study by van der Eerden et al. (2010) including an emergency-department-based cohort. Partial hypocortisolism was reported in 1 out of 107 patients, indicating that routine pituitary screening in unselected patients after TBI is unlikely to be cost-effective. However, it must still be remembered that no good predictors have yet been identified, although direct and indirect markers of increased trauma severity seem indicative (Table 45.1).

Very few data exist on the possible clinical implication of anterior pituitary hormone deficiency in TBI patients, and again data are conflicting. Kelly et al. (2006) described higher rates of at least one marker of depression and reduced health-related quality of life (HRQoL) in GH-deficient patients. Klose at al. (2007c) found that when adjusted for confounders such as age, trauma severity, and body mass index, posttraumatic hypopituitarism was an independent predictor of the classical phenotypic features of hypopituitarism, including an unfavourable lipid and body-composition profile, as well as worsened HRQoL. Bondanelli et al. (2007) found that peak GH was an independent predictor of poorer outcome as measured by rehabilitation scales evaluating cognition, disability, and functional dependency, whereas Pavlovic et al. (2010) found no correlation between neuropsychological variables and stimulated peak GH or insulin-like growth factor-I (IGF-I) levels.

45.3 Specific Paediatric Concerns

There are no specific paediatric concerns. The diagnostic set-up should follow the general guidelines for neuroendocrine assessment whatever the cause.

References

Agha A, Rogers B, Sherlock M, O'Kelly P, Tormey W, Phillips J, Thompson CJ (2004) Anterior pituitary dysfunction in survivors of traumatic brain injury. J Clin Endocrinol Metab 89:4929–4936

Agha A, Phillips J, O'Kelly P, Tormey W, Thompson CJ (2005) The natural history of post-traumatic hypopituitarism: implications for assessment and treatment. Am J Med 118:1416

Agha A, Walker D, Perry L, Drake WM, Chew SL, Jenkins PJ, Grossman AB, Monson JP (2007) Unmasking of central hypothyroidism following growth hormone replacement in adult hypopituitary patients. Clin Endocrinol (Oxf) 66:72–77

Aimaretti G, Ambrosio MR, Di Somma C, Gasperi M, Cannavo S, Scaroni C, Fusco A, Del Monte P, De Menis E, Faustini-Fustini M, Grimaldi F, Logoluso F, Razzore P, Rovere S, Benvenga S, Uberti EC, De Marinis L, Lombardi G, Mantero F, Martino E, Giordano G, Ghigo E (2005) Residual pituitary function after brain injury-induced hypopituitarism: a prospective 12-month study. J Clin Endocrinol Metab 90(11):6085–6092

Annane D, Sebille V, Troche G, Raphael JC, Gajdos P, Bellissant E (2000) A 3-level prognostic classification in septic shock based on cortisol levels and cortisol response to corticotropin. J Am Med Assoc 283:1038–1045

Barton RN, Stoner HB, Watson SM (1987) Relationships among plasma cortisol, adrenocorticotrophin, and severity of injury in recently injured patients. J Trauma 27:384–392

Bavisetty S, Bavisetty S, McArthur DL, Dusick JR, Wang C, Cohan P, Boscardin WJ, Swerdloff R, Levin H, Chang DJ, Muizelaar JP, Kelly DF (2008) Chronic hypopituitarism after traumatic brain injury: risk assessment and relationship to outcome. Neurosurgery 62:1080–1093

Behan LA, Phillips J, Thompson CJ, Agha A (2008) Neuroendocrine disorders after traumatic brain injury. J Neurol Neurosurg Psychiatry 79:753–759

Beishuizen A, Thijs LG, Vermes I (2001) Patterns of corticosteroid-binding globulin and the free cortisol index during septic shock and multitrauma. Intensive Care Med 27:1584–1591

Bondanelli M, De Marinis L, Ambrosio MR, Monesi M, Valle D, Zatelli MC, Fusco A, Bianchi A, Farneti M, Degli ECI (2004) Occurrence of pituitary dysfunction following traumatic brain injury. J Neurotrauma 21:685–696

Bondanelli M, Ambrosio MR, Cavazzini L, Bertocchi A, Zatelli MC, Carli A, Valle D, Basaglia N, Uberti EC (2007) Anterior pituitary function may predict functional and cognitive outcome in patients with traumatic brain injury undergoing rehabilitation. J Neurotrauma 24:1687–1697

Ceballos R (1966) Pituitary changes in head trauma (analysis of 102 consecutive cases of head injury). Ala J Med Sci 3:185–198

Cernak I, Savic VJ, Lazarov A, Joksimovic M, Markovic S (1999) Neuroendocrine responses following graded traumatic brain injury in male adults. Brain Inj 13:1005–1015

Cohan P, Wang C, McArthur DL, Cook SW, Dusick JR, Armin B, Swerdloff R, Vespa P, Muizelaar JP, Cryer HG, Christenson PD, Kelly DF (2005) Acute secondary adrenal insufficiency after traumatic brain injury: a prospective study. Crit Care Med 33:2358–2366

Cooper MS, Stewart PM (2003) Corticosteroid insufficiency in acutely ill patients. N Engl J Med 348:727–734

Crompton MR (1971) Hypothalamic lesions following closed head injury. Brain 94:165–172

De Groot LJ (2006) Non-thyroidal illness syndrome is a manifestation of hypothalamic-pituitary dysfunction, and in view of current evidence, should be treated with appropriate replacement therapies. Crit Care Clin 22:57–86, vi

Della CF, Mancini A, Valle D, Gallizzi F, Carducci P, Mignani V, De ML (1998) Provocative hypothalamopituitary axis tests in severe head injury: correlations with severity and prognosis. Crit Care Med 26:1419–1426

Feibel J, Kelly M, Lee L, Woolf P (1983) Loss of adrenocortical suppression after acute brain injury: role of increased intracranial pressure and brain stem function. J Clin Endocrinol Metab 57:1245–1250

Ghigo E, Masel B, Aimaretti G, Leon-Carrion J, Casanueva FF, Dominguez-Morales MR, Elovic E, Perrone K, Stalla G, Thompson C, Urban R (2005) Consensus guidelines on screening for hypopituitarism following traumatic brain injury. Brain Inj 19:711–724

Hackl JM, Gottardis M, Wieser C, Rumpl E, Stadler C, Schwarz S, Monkayo R (1991) Endocrine abnormalities in severe traumatic brain injury–a cue to prognosis in severe craniocerebral trauma? Intensive Care Med 17:25–29

Hamrahian AH, Oseni TS, Arafah BM (2004) Measurements of serum free cortisol in critically ill patients. N Engl J Med 350:1629–1638

Herrmann BL, Rehder J, Kahlke S, Wiedemayer H, Doerfler A, Ischebeck W, Laumer R, Forsting M, Stolke D, Mann K (2006) Hypopituitarism following severe traumatic brain injury. Exp Clin Endocrinol Diabetes 114:316–321

Ho KK (2007) Consensus guidelines for the diagnosis and treatment of adults with GH deficiency II: a statement of the GH Research Society in association with the European Society for Pediatric Endocrinology, Lawson Wilkins Society, European Society of Endocrinology, Japan Endocrine Society, and Endocrine Society of Australia. Eur J Endocrinol 157:695–700

Jochberger S, Morgenthaler NG, Mayr VD, Luckner G, Wenzel V, Ulmer H, Schwarz S, Hasibeder WR, Friesenecker BE, Dunser MW (2006) Copeptin and arginine vasopressin concentrations in critically ill patients. J Clin Endocrinol Metab 91:4381–4386

Kelly DF, Gonzalo IT, Cohan P, Berman N, Swerdloff R, Wang C (2000) Hypopituitarism following traumatic brain injury and aneurysmal subarachnoid hemorrhage: a preliminary report. J Neurosurg 93:743–752

Kelly DF, McArthur DL, Levin H, Swimmer S, Dusick JR, Cohan P, Wang C, Swerdloff R (2006) Neurobehavioral and quality of life changes associated with growth hormone insufficiency after complicated mild, moderate, or severe traumatic brain injury. J Neurotrauma 23:928–942

Kleindienst A, Brabant G, Bock C, Maser-Gluth C, Buchfelder M (2009) Neuroendocrine function following traumatic brain injury and subsequent intensive care treatment: a prospective longitudinal evaluation. J Neurotrauma 26:1435–1446

Klose M, Feldt-Rasmussen U (2008) Does the type and severity of brain injury predict hypothalamo-pituitary dysfunction? Does post-traumatic hypopituitarism predict worse outcome? Pituitary 11:255–261

Klose M, Juul A, Poulsgaard L, Kosteljanetz M, Brennum J, Feldt-Rasmussen U (2007a) Prevalence and predictive factors of post-traumatic hypopituitarism. Clin Endocrinol (Oxf) 67:193–201

Klose M, Juul A, Struck J, Morgenthaler NG, Kosteljanetz M, Feldt-Rasmussen U (2007b) Acute and long-term pituitary insufficiency in traumatic brain injury: a prospective single-centre study. Clin Endocrinol (Oxf) 67:598–606

Klose M, Watt T, Brennum J, Feldt-Rasmussen U (2007c) Posttraumatic hypopituitarism is associated with an unfavorable body composition and lipid profile, and decreased quality of life 12 months after injury. J Clin Endocrinol Metab 92:3861–3868

Kornblum RN, Fisher RS (1969) Pituitary lesions in craniocerebral injuries. Arch Pathol 88:242–248

Leal-Cerro A, Flores JM, Rincon M, Murillo F, Pujol M, Garcia-Pesquera F, Dieguez C, Casanueva FF (2005) Prevalence of hypopituitarism and growth hormone deficiency in adults long-term after severe traumatic brain injury. Clin Endocrinol (Oxf) 62:525–532

Lieberman SA, Oberoi AL, Gilkison CR, Masel BE, Urban RJ (2001) Prevalence of neuroendocrine dysfunction in patients recovering from traumatic brain injury. J Clin Endocrinol Metab 86:2752–2756

Maiya B, Newcombe V, Nortje J, Bradley P, Bernard F, Chatfield D, Outtrim J, Hutchinson P, Matta B, Antoun N, Menon D (2007) Magnetic resonance imaging changes in the pituitary gland following acute traumatic brain injury. Intensive Care Med 34(3):468–475

Molijn GJ, Spek JJ, van Uffelen JC, de Jong FH, Brinkmann AO, Bruining HA, Lamberts SW, Koper JW (1995) Differential adaptation of glucocorticoid sensitivity of peripheral blood mononuclear leukocytes in patients with sepsis or septic shock. J Clin Endocrinol Metab 80:1799–1803

Pavlovic D, Pekic S, Stojanovic M, Zivkovic V, Djurovic B, Jovanovic V, Miljic N, Medic-Stojanoska M, Doknic M, Miljic D, Djurovic M, Casanueva F, Popovic V (2010) Chronic cognitive sequelae after traumatic brain injury are not related to growth hormone deficiency in adults. Eur J Neurol 17:696–702

Popovic V, Pekic S, Pavlovic D, Maric N, Jasovic-Gasic M, Djurovic B, Medic SM, Zivkovic V, Stojanovic M, Doknic M, Milic N, Djurovic M, Dieguez C, Casanueva FF (2004) Hypopituitarism as a consequence of traumatic brain injury (TBI) and its possible relation with cognitive disabilities and mental distress. J Endocrinol Invest 27:1048–1054

Schneider HJ, Schneider M, Saller B, Petersenn S, Uhr M, Husemann B, von Rosen F, Stalla GK (2006) Prevalence of anterior pituitary insufficiency 3 and 12 months after traumatic brain injury. Eur J Endocrinol 154:259–265

Schneider HJ, Samann PG, Schneider M, Croce CG, Corneli G, Sievers C, Ghigo E, Stalla GK, Aimaretti G (2007) Pituitary imaging abnormalities in patients with and without hypopituitarism after traumatic brain injury. J Endocrinol Invest 30:RC9–RC12

Schneider M, Schneider HJ, Yassouridis A, Saller B, von Rosen F, Stalla GK (2008) Predictors of anterior pituitary insufficiency after traumatic brain injury. Clin Endocrinol (Oxf) 68:206–212

Span LF, Hermus AR, Bartelink AK, Hoitsma AJ, Gimbrere JS, Smals AG, Kloppenborg PW (1992) Adrenocortical function: an indicator of severity of disease and survival in chronic critically ill patients. Intensive Care Med 18:93–96

Tanriverdi F, Senyurek H, Unluhizarci K, Selcuklu A, Casanueva FF, Kelestimur F (2006) High risk of hypopituitarism after traumatic brain injury: a prospective investigation of anterior pituitary function in the acute phase and 12 months after trauma. J Clin Endocrinol Metab 91:2105–2111

Van den Berghe G, de Zegher F, Bouillon R (1998) Clinical review 95: acute and prolonged critical illness as different neuroendocrine paradigms. J Clin Endocrinol Metab 83:1827–1834

van der Eerden AW, Twickler MT, Sweep FC, Beems T, Hendricks HT, Hermus AR, Vos PE (2010) Should anterior pituitary function be tested during follow-up of all patients presenting at the emergency department because of traumatic brain injury? Eur J Endocrinol 162:19–28

Vanhorebeek I, Peeters RP, Vander PS, Jans I, Wouters PJ, Skogstrand K, Hansen TK, Bouillon R, Van den Berghe G (2006) Cortisol response to critical illness: effect of intensive insulin therapy. J Clin Endocrinol Metab 91:3803–3813

Wachter D, Gundling K, Oertel MF, Stracke H, Boker DK (2009) Pituitary insufficiency after traumatic brain injury. J Clin Neurosci 16:202–208

46 Microbiological Surveillance

Mikala Wang and Jens Kjølseth Møller

Recommendations

Level I

There is insufficient data to support a Level I recommendation for this topic.

Level II

There is insufficient data to support a Level II recommendation for this topic.

Level III

Routine CSF surveillance sampling is not recommended.

46.1 Overview

Routine surveillance of CSF from patients with EVDs is not recommended due to reports suggesting that routine sampling of CSF does not expedite detection of infection, may increase risk of iatrogenic infection, and leads to antimicrobial therapy of contaminants. It is recommended that CSF samples should only be obtained on clinical indication.

Tips, Tricks, and Pitfalls
- Obtain CSF sample on clinical indication.
- Avoid unnecessary handling of EVD.

46.2 Background

Routine surveillance of CSF from patients with EVDs is common practice in many institutions in order to detect infection sooner, thereby hopefully minimizing complications of ventriculitis. However, this premise has been drawn into question by a recent prospective study of 230 patients where daily routine analysis of CSF (Gram's stain, culture, glucose, protein, leucocytes) had no significant predictive value in the diagnosis of EVD-related ventriculitis (Schade et al. 2006). This finding concurs with the results of a retrospective study of 157 children with EVD where daily routine cultures of CSF failed to decrease the time to detection of VRI. The latter study concludes that CSF culture should be performed on clinical signs of infection such as new fever (>38.5) or peripheral leucocytosis, neurological deterioration, or change in CSF appearance in order to detect infection in a

M. Wang, (✉)
Department of Clinical Microbiology,
Aarhus University Hospital,
8200, Skejby, Aarhus, Denmark
e-mail: mikala.wang@skejby.rm.dk

J.K. Møller
Department of Clinical Microbiology, Vejle Hospital,
Vejile, Demark
e-mail: jkm@dadlnet.dk

T. Sundstrøm et al. (eds.), *Management of Severe Traumatic Brain Injury*,
DOI 10.1007/978-3-642-28126-6_46, © Springer-Verlag Berlin Heidelberg 2012

timely fashion (Hader and Steinbok 2000). These reports suggest that routine sampling of CSF does not help detect infection sooner.

Furthermore, frequent CSF sampling and thereby more frequent handling of ventricular drains may increase risk of iatrogenic infection. Korinek et al. recently reported a 50% decrease in infection after the implementation of a strict institutional protocol for EVD care (Korinek et al. 2005). In this study, the major risk factors for EVD-related infection identified were CSF leaks and protocol violations such as CSF sampling without appropriate indication. Protocol violations were four times higher in the patients that subsequently incurred a CSF infection (Hoefnagel et al. 2008). Other recent reports likewise show significant reduction in CSF infection rate by implementing a strict protocol for EVD management including no routine sampling (Dasic et al. 2006; Hoefnagel et al. 2008; Leverstein-van Hall et al. 2010).

Finally, the increased frequency of CSF culture will invariably lead to the increased detection of contaminants. The finding of contaminants in CSF samples often leads to uncertainty in the clinical setting and has been reported to result in unnecessary treatment or procedures being instituted (Hader and Steinbok 2000).

On the basis of these reports suggesting that routine sampling of CSF does not expedite detection of infection, may increase risk of iatrogenic infection, and leads to antimicrobial therapy of contaminants, we do not recommend routine surveillance of CSF but find that CSF samples should only be obtained on clinical indication.

46.3 Specific Paediatric Concerns

There are no specific concerns for the paediatric patient population for this topic.

References

Dasic D, Hanna SJ, Bojanic S, Kerr RS (2006) External ventricular drain infection: the effect of a strict protocol on infection rates and a review of the literature. Br J Neurosurg 20(5):296–300

Hader WJ, Steinbok P (2000) The value of routine cultures of the cerebrospinal fluid in patients with external ventricular drains. Neurosurgery 46(5):1149–1153

Hoefnagel D, Dammers R, Laak-Poort MP, Avezaat CJ (2008) Risk factors for infections related to external ventricular drainage. Acta Neurochir (Wien) 150(3): 209–214

Korinek AM, Reina M, Boch AL, Rivera AO, De Bels D, Puybasset L (2005) Prevention of external ventricular drain-related ventriculitis. Acta Neurochir (Wien) 147(1):39–45

Leverstein-van Hall MA, Hopmans TE, van der Sprenkel JW, Blok HE, van der Mark WA, Hanlo PW et al (2010) A bundle approach to reduce the incidence of external ventricular and lumbar drain-related infections. J Neurosurg 112(2):345–353

Schade RP, Schinkel J, Roelandse FW, Geskus RB, Visser LG, Van Dijk JM et al (2006) Lack of value of routine analysis of cerebrospinal fluid for prediction and diagnosis of external drainage-related bacterial meningitis. J Neurosurg 104(1):101–108

Part VIII

Treatment in Neurointensive Care

Guidelines for Treatment of Patients with Severe Traumatic Brain Injury: Treatment Algorithms

47

Niels Juul

Recommendations

Level I

There are insufficient data to support a Level I recommendation of a single-treatment algorithm for TBI patients.

Level II

There are insufficient data to support a Level II recommendation of a single-treatment algorithm for TBI patients.

Level III

There is Level III evidence supporting care of TBI patients in a specialized neurointensive care unit.

There is Level III evidence supporting appointment of neurointensivists in a neurointensive care unit.

There is Level I, II, and III evidence supporting single parts of the treatment algorithm presented in this chapter. The evidence will be presented in the subchapters concerning the treatment modalities.

N. Juul
Department of anaesthesia, Aarhus University Hospital, Noerrebrogade 44, 8000 Aarhus C, Denmark
e-mail: nielsjuul@privat.dk

47.1 Overview

No single-treatment algorithm of TBI patients has been shown to be superior to another in a clinical randomized study. Clinical guidelines have been developed by ABIC (Bullock et al. 1996) with several updates, the last in 2007 (Brain Trauma Foundation et al. 2007) and EBIC (Maas et al. 1997) and the Lund therapy (Grände 2006). In addition, national guidelines such as the Danish (Welling et al. 2010) and single centre guidelines, such as the one from Addenbrooke's Hospital (Menon 1999), have been published.

None of the published guidelines have been tested in randomized controlled studies. Numerous investigations with historical controls have been published, including single centre reports (Grände 2006) and multicentre trials of single interventions (Yurkewicz 2005).

Level III evidence supports that patients with TBI should be admitted to the nearest neurosurgical department with a specialized neurointensive care unit. The protocol-driven therapy, guided by specialists, will ensure adequate observation and management, especially for patients with intracranial hypertension (Patel et al. 2002). Even patients with injuries that do not necessitate neurosurgical intervention have been shown to have a better outcome in these facilities. Level III evidence suggests that appointment of a neurointensivist to a neurosurgical intensive care unit not only decreased length of stay by 17% but also lead to a relative reduction in mortality of 21% (Varelas et al. 2004).

T. Sundstrøm et al. (eds.), *Management of Severe Traumatic Brain Injury*,
DOI 10.1007/978-3-642-28126-6_47, © Springer-Verlag Berlin Heidelberg 2012

Level III evidence supports that protocol-driven therapy yields a better outcome on mortality and morbidity than treatment initiated at the attending surgeons discretion (Elf et al. 2002). Parts of the guidelines presented in this chapter are supported by Level I evidence (avoidance of steroids in large doses (Edwards et al. 2005)) or Level II evidence (detrimental effect of prophylactic hyperventilation (Muizellar et al. 1991)) or Level III evidence (use of craniectomy as treatment option (Cooper et al. 2011)) to name a few. Evidence supporting the interventions in the algorithm is presented in the following chapters.

Neurointensive care has evolved tremendously over the last decades, with an overwhelming amount of scientific data on display. Guidelines will never be completely up to date, and caution must be taken not to adhere to closely to an outdated part of a guideline.

Tips, Tricks, and Pitfalls

- Start brain protective treatment as soon as the patient is in the emergency room.
- Initiate treatment according to the algorithm without delay.
- Remember that most interventions have side effects; consider changing to another option if side effects are significant.
- Re-evaluate the treatment plan frequently, at least twice a day.
- Ineffective treatment should be stopped.

47.2 Background

The algorithm presented in Fig. 47.1 is developed by the Danish Neurotrauma Committee (Welling et al. 2010), based on the ABIC and EBIC guidelines.

Patients with severe head injury should be received in a trauma centre with neurosurgical capacity, preferably initially, but if not, transferred to a neurosurgical unit as soon as possible.

The patients should be intubated and receive up-to-date intensive care treatment with focus on prevention of secondary brain injuries. Special caution should be focused on avoidance of hypotension or hypoxia, hyperglycaemia or hypoglycaemia, and hyperthermia or hypothermia. In fact, all *hyper* and *hypo* should be avoided and the intensive care concentrated on ensuring *normo* in most areas of the field.

No specific drug has been shown to be superior to others concerning sedation of neurotrauma patients. Sedation should be sufficient to ameliorate the stress response, but allowing for intermittent test of motor response. Wake-up tests, as used in general intensive care, should be used with caution.

ICP should be monitored with the most accurate methods available. CPP monitoring: Zero point of arterial line by meatus acusticus externus. The CPP goal is not supported by Level I or II evidence. The trend in most guidelines has been to reduce the CPP aim from 70 to 60 mmHg in the past decade. Most clinical and experimental investigations have failed to show beneficial effects of increasing CPP above 60, but the detrimental effects of a CPP below 50 seem clear. In children, the CPP should be according to age and related normal BP in the age group.

Patients should be positioned with a slightly elevated head rest, and caution should be taken not to restrict blood flow in the jugular veins and thus increase cerebral blood volume. Bringing oxygen to the suffering brain is of paramount importance in neurointensive therapy. The PaO_2 is to be kept above 12 kPa; PEEP can be applied and blood may be given a little more readily than in the normal trauma patient to ensure the oxygen-bearing capacity of the circulating blood. Patients should be normoventilated; the brain is very vulnerable to hypocapnia, especially during the first 24 h after injury. If light hyperventilation is indicated, advanced neuromonitoring must be ensured.

Both hyper- and hypoglycaemia is linked to increased morbidity and mortality. The Danish guideline recommends blood glucose to be kept at 5–8 mmol/l, thus minimizing the risk of hypoglycaemia. Enteral feeding should be initiated as soon as possible, and 100% enteral nutrition is the goal during the first week after injury.

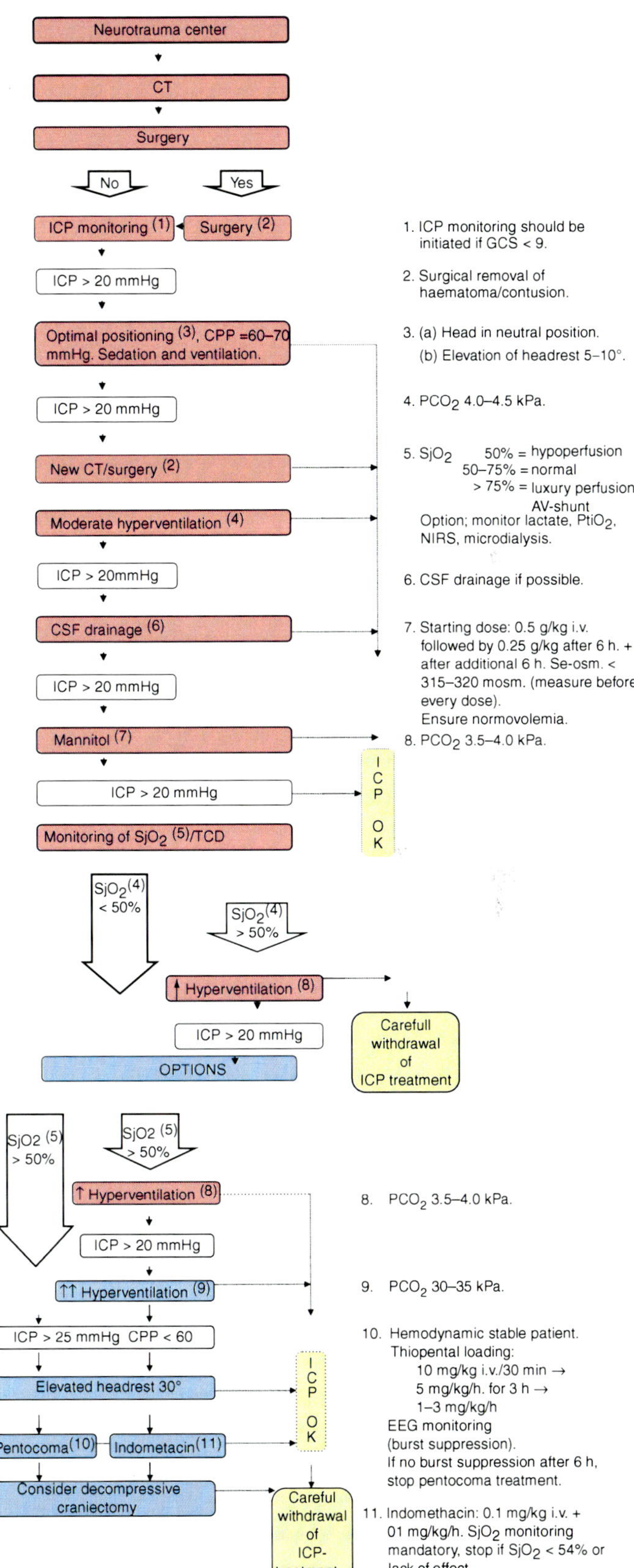

Fig. 47.1 Treatment algorithm for patients with severe brain injury developed by the Danish Neurotrauma Committee (Welling et al. 2010), based on the ABIC and EBIC guidelines (Welling et al. 2010)

It is still to be proven that hypothermia after severe TBI leads to a better outcome, but there is agreement about aggressive treatment of hyperthermia.

47.3 Specific Paediatric Concerns

Recommendations

Level I and II

There are insufficient data to support a Level I or II recommendation of a single-treatment algorithm for paediatric TBI patients.

Level III

There is Level III evidence supporting care of paediatric TBI patients in a paediatric trauma centre with additional neurosurgical expertise.

There has been published one treatment guideline for the paediatric neurotrauma population (Adelson et al. 2003). Compared to the literature for adult TBI patients, the evidence for treatment of the paediatric population is even more scarce. Creating guidelines for children is more difficult than for adults due to the development phases across age groups. In a retrospective study from Pennsylvania, it was shown that children with TBI had a better outcome if they were treated in a paediatric trauma centre (Potoka et al. 2000).

The most difficult question is which blood pressure and CPP to aim for in children with TBI. The goal for MAP and CPP must be in accordance with the normal pressure for the injured child and thus set at a lower level than for adults. In a retrospective cohort study of 118 children (age 7.4 ± 4.6 years), it was found that no children with a mean CPP<40 mmHg survived, but there was no relationship between survival and increments of CPP>40 mmHg (Downard et al. 2000). Parallel to studies in adults, mortality increases dramatically when children are hypotensive or hypoxic on arrival to hospital (Pigula et al. 1993).

Special paediatric considerations will be discussed in the relevant sections of the following chapters.

References

Adelson PD, Bratton SL, Carney NA, Chesnut RM, du Coudray HE, Goldstein B, Kochanek PM, Miller HC, Partington MD, Selden NR, Warden CR, Wright DW, American Association for Surgery of Trauma; Child Neurology Society; International Society for Pediatric Neurosurgery; International Trauma Anesthesia and Critical Care Society; Society of Critical Care Medicine; World Federation of Pediatric Intensive and Critical Care Societies (2003) Guidelines for the acute medical management of severe traumatic brain injury in infants, children, and adolescents. Chapter 19. The role of anti-seizure prophylaxis following severe pediatric traumatic brain injury. Pediatr Crit Care Med 4(3 Suppl):S2–S76

Bullock R, Chesnut RM, Clifton G, Ghajar J, Marion DW, Narayan RK, Newell DW, Pitts LH, Rosner MJ, Wilberger JW (1996) Brain Trauma Foundation, American Association of Neurological Surgeons, Joint Section on Neurotrauma and Critical Care: guidelines for the management of severe head injury. Updates in US trauma foundation/guidelines. J Neurotrauma 13:641–734

Cooper DJ, Rosenfeld JV, Murray L, Arabi YM, Davies AR, D'Urso P, Kossmann T, Ponsford J, Seppelt I, Reilly P, Wolfe R, the DECRA Trial Investigators and the Australian and New Zealand Intensive Care Society Clinical Trials Group (2011) Decompressive craniectomy in diffuse traumatic brain injury. N Engl J Med 364:1493–1502

Downard C, Hulka F, Mullins RJ, Piatt J, Chesnut R, Quint P, Mann NC (2000) Relationship of cerebral perfusion pressure and survival in pediatric brain-injured patients. J Trauma 49:654–659

Edwards P, Arango M, Balica L, Cottingham R, El-Sayed H, Farrell B, Fernandes J, Gogichaisvili T, Golden N, Hartzenberg B, Husain M, Ulloa MI, Jerbi Z, Khamis H, Komolafe E, Laloë V, Lomas G, Ludwig S, Mazairac G, Muñoz Sanchéz Mde L, Nasi L, Olldashi F, Plunkett P, Roberts I, Sandercock P, Shakur H, Soler C, Stocker R, Svoboda P, Trenkler S, Venkataramana NK, Wasserberg J, Yates D, Yutthakasemsunt S, CRASH trial collaborators (2005) Final results of MRC CRASH, a randomised placebo-controlled trial of intravenous corticosteroid in adults with head injury- outcomes at 6 months. Lancet 4–10:1957–1959

Elf K, Nilsson P, Enblad P (2002) Outcome after traumatic brain injury improved by an organized secondary insult program and standardized neurointensive care. Crit Care Med 30(9):2129–2134

Grände PO (2006) The "Lund concept" for the treatment of severe head trauma – physiological principles and clinical application. Intensive Care Med 32:1475–1484

Maas AI, Dearden M, Teasdale GM, Braakman R, Cohadon F, Iannotti F, Karimi A, Lapierre F, Murray G, Ohman J, Persson L, Servadei F, Stocchetti N, Unterberg A (1997) EBIC Guidelines for management of severe head injury in adults. European Brain Injury Consortium. Acta Neurochir (Wien) 139:286–294

Menon DK (1999) Cerebral protection in severe brain injury: physiological determinants of outcome and their optimisation. Br Med Bull 55:226–258

Muizellar JP, Marmerou A, Ward JD, Kontos HA, Choi SC, Becker DP, Young HF (1991) Adverse effects of prolonged hyperventilation in patients with severe head injury; a randomized clinical trial. J Neurosurg 75(5):731–739

Patel HC, Menon DK, Tebbs S, Hawker R, Hutchinson PJ, Kirkpatrick PJ (2002) Specialist neurocritical care and outcome from head injury. Intensive Care Med 28:547–553

Pigula FA, Wald SL, Shackford SR, Vane DW (1993) The effect of hypotension and hypoxia on children with severe head injuries. J Pediatr Surg 28:310–316

Potoka DA, Schall LC, Gardener MJ, Stafford PW, Peitzman AB, Ford HR (2000) Impact of pediatric trauma centers on mortality in a statewide system. J Trauma 49:237–245

The Brain Trauma Foundation; The American Association of Neurological Surgeons; Congress of Neurological Surgeons (2007) Guidelines for the management of severe traumatic brain injury. J Neurotrauma 24(Suppl 1):S1–S106

Varelas PN, Conti MM, Spanaki MV, Potts E, Bradford D, Sunstrom C, Fedder W, Hacein Bey L, Jaradeh S, Genarelli TA (2004) The impact of a neurointensivist-led team on a semiclosed neurosciences intensive care unit. Crit Care Med 32:2919–2928

Welling KL, Eskesen V, Romner B, The Danish Neurotrauma Committee (2010) Neurointensive care of severe traumatic brain injury. Ugeskr Laeger 172:2091–2094 (Danish)

Yurkewicz L, Weaver J, Bullock MR, Marshall LF (2005) The effect of the selective NMDA receptor antagonist traxoprodil in the treatment of traumatic brain injury. J neurotrauma dec; 22(12):1428–1443

The Lund Therapy for Severe Head Trauma

48

Per-Olof Grände and Peter Reinstrup

Recommendations

Level I

There have been no Level I studies performed to evaluate the Lund therapy relative to more conventional treatments.

Level II

There are no Level II studies supporting the Lund therapy.

Level III

There have been several Level III studies that support the Lund therapy.

P.-O. Grände (✉) • P. Reinstrup
Department of Anaesthesia and Intensive Care, Lund University and Lund University Hospital, SE-22185 Lund, Sweden
e-mail: per-olof.grande@med.lu.se; peter.reinstrup@med.lu.se

48.1 Overview of the Lund Guidelines

1. Normalization of the normally raised arterial blood pressure (providing normovolemia) by anti-hypertensive therapy in terms of β_1 antagonist (e.g. metoprolol 1 mg/mL, 1–2 mL/h or 50 mg × 1–2 per os for an adult), α_2 agonist (clonidine diluted to 15 μg/mL, 0.5–1 mL/h or 150 μg × 1–3 per os for an adult) and angiotensin II antagonist (e.g. losartan 50 mg × 1–2 per os for an adult). If necessary, head elevation (max 15°) can be used to reduce cerebral perfusion pressure. In children and adolescents, the doses should be adapted to their age.
2. An arterial blood pressure resulting in too low a CPP (CPP below 50–55 mmHg in adults and below 40 mmHg in small children) may be an indication of a concealed hypovolemia and can be treated with extra fluid substitution (see (4) below). If CPP is still too low, the anti-hypertensive treatment can be reduced. If possible, refrain from using vasoconstrictors and inotropic support. The therapy may be guided by a microdialysis catheter placed in the penumbra zone.
3. Normalization of the plasma oncotic pressure with a colloid solution, preferably 20% albumin solutions up to a plasma albumin concentration of 33–38 g/L.
4. A blood volume expanding therapy aimed at preservation of normovolemia by infusion of

T. Sundstrøm et al. (eds.), *Management of Severe Traumatic Brain Injury*,
DOI 10.1007/978-3-642-28126-6_48, © Springer-Verlag Berlin Heidelberg 2012

albumin (preferably 20% solutions) to normal albumin concentrations (33–38 g/L) and by maintenance of a haemoglobin concentration above 120 g/L (leukocyte-depleted blood). A crystalloid (e.g. normal saline or 5% glucose solution with electrolytes at 1.0–1.5 L/day for an adult, and correspondingly lower volumes for children), can be given to obtain an adequate general fluid balance and urine production. The blood pressure response from additional volumes of blood and albumin or passive leg elevation will show if a low blood pressure can be explained by hypovolemia. The volemic state can also be checked with PPV (PPV > 10 may indicate hypovolemia). The need for vasopressors is small when following this therapy. Diuretics can be used (not mannitol).

5. Anti-stress therapy in terms of midazolam 5 mg/mL (0–3 mL/h for the adult), fentanyl 0.05 mg/mL (0–3 mL/h for the adult), α_2 agonist and $\beta_1$antagonist (see under (1) above) to reduce catecholamine concentration in plasma. Catecholamine concentration in plasma should also be kept low by avoiding noradrenalin and by not using active cooling. Wake-up tests should not be used until start of the weaning procedure, and do not extubate until ICP has stabilized at a normal level.
6. If there are problems with high ICP (above 20–25 mmHg), the following measures can be taken: (1) surgical removal of available haematomas and contusions, (2) start of thiopental (pentothal, 50 mg/mL) initiated by treatment in bolus doses of 1–3 mL followed by a continuous infusion of 1–3 mg/kg/h for the adult for at most 2 days (be aware of the risk with respiratory insufficiency with long term use of this drug) (3) or decompressive craniotomy.
7. Use low-energy nutrition (15–20 kcal/kg/day for an adult, but relatively more energy for small children), if possible by enteral nutrition. Keep blood glucose in the range of 5–8 mmol/L, and electrolytes should be normal.
8. Mechanical ventilation (preferably volume-controlled), keeping a normal PaO_2 and a normal $PaCO_2$. PEEP (6–8 cm H_2O) is mandatory to prevent atelectasis.
9. Drainage of CSF can be used via a ventricular catheter (not by lumbar puncture) and should be performed from a relatively high pressure level to reduce the risk of ventricular collapse, which may result in brainstem herniation.

Tips, Tricks, and Pitfalls

- Use the therapy within the framework of the guidelines.
- Start the therapy early after arrival at the hospital to counteract the development of brain oedema and an increase in ICP.
- A relatively normal haemoglobin concentration helps to avoid hypovolemia and optimize oxygenation.
- Osmotherapy should be avoided except in an acute situation to prevent acute brainstem herniation e.g. during transportation.
- Decompressive craniotomy can be used to prevent brainstem herniation.

48.2 Background

The Lund concept for treatment of severe head injury was initially a theoretical concept based on basal haemodynamic physiological principles for regulation of brain volume and perfusion in the injured brain. These principles have later on found strong support in experimental and clinical studies, including clinical outcome studies involving adults and children. Recent updates of the US guidelines have moved closer to the Lund concept. In its main principles, the Lund concept has not changed since its introduction.

The Lund therapy is a physiology-based therapy for severe traumatic head injury, which combines two main goals, namely, halting or treating the development of a vasogenic brain oedema (the ‘ICP goal’) and a simultaneous, intensified support of the perfusion of the penumbra zone (the 'perfusion goal'). The purpose of the therapy is to improve outcome by preventing brainstem herniation and by reducing cell death of the vulnerable penumbra zone. The principle behind the Lund therapy is normalization of essential haemodynamic and biochemical parameters. For an overview of its theoretical background and therapeutic guidelines, see Grände 2006. The Lund therapy is applicable to all ages. Outcome studies with the Lund therapy have so far been promising (Eker et al. 1998; Wahlström et al. 2005). No Level I or II studies have been performed regarding either the components of the traditional guidelines such as the US guideline and the European guideline in their original versions (Bullock et al. 1996; Maas et al. 1997) or in their updated versions (The Brain Trauma Foundation et al. 2007), or regarding the Lund concept (Grände 2006). A recent study showed about half the mortality rate with the Lund concept (Liu et al. 2010).

The 'ICP goal' of the therapy is mainly based on the hypothesis that an imbalance between the transcapillary hydrostatic and the oncotic pressures creating filtration will result in a vasogenic brain oedema provided the blood–brain barrier (BBB) is passively permeable to small solutes. Such a situation can exist in meningitis and after a head trauma. In head trauma patients, disruption of BBB may occur, especially around cerebral contusions. According to this hypothesis, the brain oedema can be counteracted or prevented by reducing a raised hydrostatic capillary pressure and normalization of a lowered plasma oncotic pressure.

The 'perfusion goal' is based on the hypothesis that there is better perfusion and oxygenation of the penumbra zone if the plasma concentration of catecholamines is kept low by preventing hypovolemia (counteracting baroreceptor reflex activation), by avoiding infusion of vasoconstrictors, by avoiding stress, by not using active cooling and by avoiding low haemoglobin concentrations and hyperventilation (the patient should be normocapnic). The normal haemoglobin concentration will help to give a better oxygenation of the brain and to preserve a normovolemic state. An ICP measuring device should be installed. Our present knowledge of the risk with hyperventilation has been discussed in more detail in a special chapter of this book, as have recommendations regarding fluid therapy. The use of albumin as plasma volume expander is justified due to the relatively small volumes of albumin needed to maintain normovolemia when following the principles of the Lund therapy. See the chapter on fluid therapy in this book. Enteral nutrition is preferable and over-nutrition should be avoided, especially when using parenteral nutrition. Low-dose prostacyclin is an option to improve microcirculation of the penumbra zone (Grände et al. 2000).

A CT scan should be performed as soon as possible after arrival at the hospital. We also recommend that the therapy should be started early, which may help to prevent the development of an increase in ICP. If possible, extensive intracerebral bleedings and available contusions should be surgically evacuated. The Lund therapy is applicable to all ages if doses and physiological parameters are adapted to the patient's age (Eker et al. 1998; Naredi et al. 1998; Wahlström et al. 2005). The therapy can be used independently of the prevailing autoregulatory capacity.

48.3 Specific Paediatric Concerns

The principles of the Lund concept are applicable to all ages if doses of pharmacological substances are adapted to the age. While a lowest CPP of 50 mmHg can be accepted in the adult, providing an optimal fluid therapy maintaining normovolemia, relatively lower values can be accepted in children and down to 38–40 mmHg in the smallest children but also providing an optimal fluid therapy.

References

Bullock R, Chesnut RM, Clifton G, Ghajar J, Marion DW, Narayan RK, Newell DW, Pitts LH, Rosner MJ, Wilberger JW (1996) Guidelines for the management of severe head injury. Brain Trauma Foundation. Eur J Emerg Med 3(2):109–127

Eker C, Asgeirsson B, Grände PO, Schalén W, Nordström CH (1998) Improved outcome after severe head injury with a new therapy based on principles for brain volume regulation and preserved microcirculation. Crit Care Med 26(11):1881–1886

Grände PO (2006) The "Lund concept" for the treatment of severe head trauma–physiological principles and clinical application. Intensive Care Med 32(10):1475–1484

Grände PO, Möller AD, Nordström CH, Ungerstedt U (2000) Low-dose prostacyclin in treatment of severe brain trauma evaluated with microdialysis and jugular bulb oxygen measurements. Acta Anaesthesiol Scand 44(7):886–894

Liu CW, Zheng YK, Lu J, Yu WH, Wang B, Hu W, Zhu KY, Zhu Y, Hu WH, Wang JR, Ma JP (2010) Application of Lund concept in treating brain edema after severe head injury. Zhongguo Wei Zhong Bing Ji Jiu Yi Xue 22(10): 610–613

Maas AI, Dearden M, Teasdale GM, Braakman R, Cohadon F, Iannotti F, Karimi A, Lapierre F, Murray G, Ohman J, Persson L, Servadei F, Stocchetti N, Unterberg A (1997) EBIC-guidelines for management of severe head injury in adults. European Brain Injury Consortium. Acta Neurochir (Wien) 139(4):286–294

Naredi S, Edén E, Zäll S, Stephensen H, Rydenhag B (1998) A standardized neurosurgical neurointensive therapy directed toward vasogenic edema after severe traumatic brain injury: clinical results. Intensive Care Med 24(5):446–451

The Brain Trauma Foundation; The American Association of Neurological Surgeons; Congress of Neurological Surgeons (2007) Guidelines for the management of severe traumatic brain injury. J Neurotrauma 24(Suppl 1):S1–S106

Wahlström MR, Olivecrona M, Koskinen LO, Rydenhag B, Naredi S (2005) Severe traumatic brain injury in pediatric patients: treatment and outcome using an intracranial pressure targeted therapy–the Lund concept. Intensive Care Med 31(6):832–839

49 Comparative Analysis of Various Guidelines for Treatment of Severe TBI

Per-Olof Grände and Niels Juul

Recommendations

Level I

There is no Level I evidence supporting the hypothesis that one of the described guidelines is superior to another.

Level II

There is no Level II evidence supporting the hypothesis that one of the described guidelines is superior to another.

Level III

There is no Level III evidence supporting the hypothesis that one of the described guidelines is superior to another.

P.-O. Grände (✉)
Department of Anaesthesia and Intensive Care,
Lund University and Lund University Hospital,
SE-22185 Lund, Sweden
e-mail: per-olof.grande@med.lu.se

N. Juul
Department of Anaesthesia, Aarhus University
Hospital, Noerrebrogade 44,
DK-8000 Aarhus C, Denmark
e-mail: nielsjuul@privat.dk

T. Sundstrøm et al. (eds.), *Management of Severe Traumatic Brain Injury*,
DOI 10.1007/978-3-642-28126-6_49, © Springer-Verlag Berlin Heidelberg 2012

49.1 Overview of Guidelines

49.1.1 Comparing Guidelines for the Adult

	US guideline, 2007 updated version	European guidelines (EBIC)	Addenbrooke guidelines	Rosner protocol	Lund concept
CPP, blood pressure	CPP 50–70 mmHg	CPP>60–70 mmHg MAP>90 mmHg	CPP>70 mmHg	CPP > 70 mmHg	Optimal CPP 60–70 mmHg and min 50 mmHg, during normovolemia. Min MAP 65–70 mmHg. Blood pressure reducing therapy an option
Ventilation	Volume-controlled normoventilation Moderate hyperventilation at raised ICP	Volume-controlled hyperventilation to 4.0–4.5 kPa in PCO_2. May be intensified at a high ICP	Volume-controlled hyperventilation at a raised ICP to 3.5–4.0 kPa in PCO_2 if $SjO_2>55\%$	Hyperventilation accepted	Volume-controlled normoventilation
Oxygenation	$PO_2>8$ kPa	PO_2 12–13 kPa	Not specified	Not specified	PO_2 12–13 kPa
Analgesics, sedatives	Not specified Barbiturate and propofol at high ICP	Yes. Not specified	Propofol, midazolam, fentanyl	Not specified	Deep sedation (midazolam, fentanyl). No wake-up tests. Propofol only in the weaning phase
ICP monitoring	If abnormal CT scan and unconscious	If considered desirable	All patients with severe TBI	All patients with severe TBI	All patients with severe TBI
ICP treatment initiated	ICP>20 mmHg	ICP>20–25 mmHg	ICP > 20–25 mmHg	Not specified	Early independent of ICP
High-dose barbiturates	To control a high ICP if hemodynamically stable	To control a refractory high ICP	Burst supression pattern to control a refractory high ICP	Not used	Not used. Low doses (1–3 mg/kg/h) for at most 2 days can be used at refractory raised ICP
Hyperosmolar therapy	Mannitol to control a raised ICP, 0.25–1 g/kg	Mannitol to control a raised ICP, S-Osm<315 mosm	Mannitol to control a raised ICP, S-Osm<320 mosm	Mannitol to control a raised ICP if CPP<70 mmHg	Not used except to prevent acute brainstem herniation during transportation
CSF drainage	Not specified	Can be used	An option	Can be used to control CPP	With caution from a relatively high level via ventricular drainage. CT control of ventricular size

(continued)

	US guideline, 2007 updated version	European guidelines (EBIC)	Addenbrooke guidelines	Rosner protocol	Lund concept
Fluids/fluid balance, erythrocyte transfusion	Normovolemia. Fluids not specified	Normovolemia. Fluids not specified. Hb > 110 g/L recommended	Normovolemia. Fluids and optimal Hb values not discussed	Normovolemia to moderate hypervolemia, Hct 30–35%	Normovolemia with albumin 20% (s-alb 35–40 g/L) and erythrocytes (leukocyte depleted) to Hb > 120 g/L (Hct 35%). Crystalloids up to 1–1.5L/day
Vasopressors/ inotropy	Can be used to maintain CPP	Recommended to maintain CPP	Recommended to maintain CPP	Recommended to maintain a high CPP	Should be avoided. If still used, in lowest possible doses
Nutrition	Enteral or parenteral nutrition, full replacement after 1 week	Early enteral feeding	Early enteral feeding	Not specified	Enteral feeding. Full replacement (15–20 kcal/kg/d) day 2–3
Anti-seizure prophylaxis	Not recommended	Not recommended	Can be used	Not discussed	Not used
Surgical therapy		Evacuation of epidural/subdural hematomas. Craniotomy in exceptional cases			Evacuation of hematomas Decompressive craniotomy when indicated to prevent brainstem herniation
Temp control	Active cooling an option	Not discussed	Active cooling to 33°C if CPP < 70 mmHg and ICP > 25 mmHg	Not discussed	Normothermia. High fever treated pharmacologically. No active cooling

Comparison between various guidelines for treatment of a severe TBI in adults in terms of the latest updated version of US guidelines from 2007 (The Brain Trauma Foundation et al. 2007), the European Brain Injury Consortium's (EPIC) guidelines (Maas et al. 1997), the Addenbrooke guidelines from Cambridge (Menon 1999), the Rosner protocol (Rosner et al. 1995) and the Lund concept (Grände 2006)

49.1.2 The Brain Trauma Foundation Guidelines and the Lund Concept for Treatment of the Pediatric Population

Blood pressure, CPP, and oxygenation

US guidelines: CPP > 40 mmHg. Min SBP 70 mmHg + (2 × age)^2, up to 1 year, min systolic blood pressure (SBP) 90 mmHg + (2 × age)^2 above 1 year. Pa O_2 > 8 kPa.

Lund concept: CPP > 38–50 mmHg depending on age from new born up to 18 years of age. These values provide a normovolemic condition. SBP not discussed. Pa O2 12–13 kPa.

Initiation of ICP treatment

US guidelines: At an ICP > 20 mmHg.

Lund concept: Early independent of ICP to counteract the increase in ICP.

Use of hyperventilation

US guidelines: Mild hyperventilation 4.0–4.6 kPa at a raised ICP.

Lund concept: Normoventilation preferably volume controlled.

CSF drainage

US guidelines: An option at a refractory intracranial hypertension.

Lund concept: Intermittently with caution at a high ICP from a relatively high level via ventricular drainage. CT control to detect and prevent ventricular collapse.

Hyperosmolar therapy

US guidelines: Options for mannitol 0.25–1 g/kg to serum osmol < 320 mosm/L and for hypertonic saline to serum osmol < 360 mosm/L.

Lund concept: Not recommended. Exceptionally, it can be used for prevention of acute brain stem herniation under transportation and to offer space during brain operation.

Fluid/fluid balance and erythrocyte therapy

US guidelines: Normovolemia. Type of fluids and how to verify normovolemia is not specified.

Lund concept: Normovolemia. Moderate crystalloid infusions combined with albumin (preferably 20% solutions) as the main plasma volume expander resulting in an albumin concentration of 32–40 g/L. The infusions should be given slowly. Erythrocyte transfusion (leukocyte-depleted blood) to maintain a haemoglobin concentration of about 120 g/L.

Vasopressors

US guidelines: Vasopressors can be used to increase CPP and SPB.

Lund concept: vasopressors should be avoided.

Sedation, analgesics and musculorelaxation

US guidelines: Sedation, analgesics, and muscle relaxation not specified and left to the treating physician. No propofol.

Lund concept: Midazolam, fentanyl in doses adapted to the age and individually preventing stress and pain. No neuromuscular blockade and no propofol.

High-dose barbiturates

US guidelines: Can be used at a refractory high ICP.

Lund concept: Not used. Lower doses <2–3 mg/kg/h for at most 2 days can be used at a refractory raised ICP.

Steroids

US guidelines: Not used.

Lund concept: Not used. One moderate bolus dose of methylprednisolone can be accepted to reduce a significantly high fever.

Temperature control

US guidelines: Active cooling may be used at refractory high ICP.

Lund concept: Active cooling should not be used. High fever is treated pharmacologically.

Anti-seizure prophylaxis

US guidelines: May be used in patients with a high risk of seizure.

Lund concept: Not used.

Surgical

US guidelines: Decompressive craniotomy an option to control a refractory high ICP. Surgical evacuation of hematomas and contusions not discussed.

Lund concept: Evacuation of large hematomas and surgical available contusions. Decompressive craniotomy can be used as a last resort when indicated to counteract a refractory high ICP.

> **Tips, Tricks, and Pitfalls**
> All guidelines for treatment of severe head injury should be looked upon with humbleness, and there must be an individual evaluation of the treatment to choose.

49.2 Background

49.2.1 Guidelines for the Adult

Various guidelines have been presented during the last 20 years for treatment of severe traumatic brain injury in the adult. The Rosner protocol (Rosner et al. 1995) and the Lund concept

(Asgeirsson et al. 1994) were presented in 1992–1995. The US guideline was presented in 1996 (Bullock et al. 1996), the European guideline in 1997 (Maas et al. 1997) and the Addenbrooke guideline from Cambridge, England, in 1999 (Menon 1999). An elucidatory version of the Lund Concept was published in 2006 (Grände 2006) and the last updated version of the US guideline in 2007 (The Brain Trauma Foundation et al. 2007). All guidelines except the Lund concept can be characterized as cerebral perfusion pressure (CPP)-targeted guidelines, and especially, the US guidelines are based on meta-analytic surveys. The Lund concept instead is based on basal physiological principles for brain volume and brain perfusion regulation and can be characterized as an intracranial pressure (ICP) and perfusion-targeted therapy. While US guidelines are based only on clinical studies, the Lund concept also finds support from experimental studies.

The Lund concept has not changed since its introduction except the use of the vasoconstrictor substance dihydroergotamine. This drug is not recommended any more due to the potential side effects inherent in this type of vasoconstrictor substances and that it has been replaced by other measures to reduce a significantly raised ICP, such as decompressive craniotomy (Grände 2006).

All guidelines recommend continuous measurement of arterial pressure and ICP as well as the use of artificial ventilation. No guideline recommends treatment with steroids, except that the Lund concept accepts one bolus dose of Solu-Medrol (0.5–1 g) to reduce a critically raised body temperature. Active cooling is an option in some conventional guidelines but not in the Lund concept (see Chap. 61). Normal potassium and sodium concentrations are generally recommended. A shift in the treatment paradigm has emerged recently in many 'non-Lund centres' by accepting a lower CPP, indicating that the guidelines have approached in some respect, even though the means to reach the goal are different (see Sect. 49.1 for details).

49.3 Guidelines for the Pediatric Population

Little substantial research has been performed specifically for the pediatric population, defined as <18 years of age, and the pediatric brain injury remains poorly investigated. Treatment of children and adolescents therefore is mainly based on deductions from guidelines developed for adults. Important differences from the adult are lower blood pressure and lower peripheral resistance in the whole body including the brain. This means that perfusion of various organs and the brain is maintained at blood and CPP pressures lower than those recommended for the adult. Specific recommendations for children and adolescents are presented by Brain Trauma Foundation (2010) and for the Lund concept (Wahlström et al. 2005; Grände 2006), while the other guidelines do not specifically address the pediatric population. Like for the adult, the US pediatric guidelines are based on meta-analytic surveys of clinical studies and are a CPP-targeted therapy, and the Lund therapy is based on physiological principles for brain volume and brain perfusion regulation and is more of an ICP and perfusion-targeted therapy. The Lund concept also considers results from experimental studies.

References

Asgeirsson B, Grände PO, Nordström CH (1994) A new therapy of post-trauma brain oedema based on haemodynamic principles for brain volume regulation. Intensive Care Med 20(4):260–267

Bullock R, Chesnut RM, Clifton G, Ghajar J, Marion DW, Narayan RK, Newell DW, Pitts LH, Rosner MJ, Wilberger JW (1996) Guidelines for the management of severe head injury. Brain Trauma Foundation. Eur J Emerg Med 3(2):109–127

Grände PO (2006) The "Lund concept" for the treatment of severe head trauma – physiological principles and clinical application. Intensive Care Med 32(10):1475–1484

Maas AI, Dearden M, Teasdale GM, Braakman R, Cohadon F, Iannotti F, Karimi A, Lapierre F, Murray G, Ohman J, Persson L, Servadei F, Stocchetti N, Unterberg A (1997) EBIC-guidelines for management of severe head injury in adults. European Brain Injury Consortium. Acta Neurochir (Wien) 139(4):286–294

Menon DK (1999) Cerebral protection in severe brain injury: physiological determinants of outcome and their optimisation. Br Med Bull 55(1):226–258

Rosner MJ, Rosner SD, Johnson AH (1995) Cerebral perfusion pressure: management protocol and clinical results. J Neurosurg 83(6):949–962

The Brain Trauma Foundation; Pediatric Guidelines (2010) https://www.braintrauma.org/coma-guidelines

Wahlström MR, Olivecrona M, Koskinen LO, Rydenhag B, Naredi S (2005) Severe traumatic brain injury in pediatric patients: treatment and outcome using an intracranial pressure targeted therapy – the Lund concept. Intensive Care Med 31(6):832–839

Pharmacological Neuroprotection in Severe Traumatic Brain Injury

50

Niklas Marklund

Recommendations

Level I

There is no Level I evidence suggesting that any pharmacological treatment option can improve the outcome of TBI patients.

Level II

There are no data supporting a Level II recommendation for this topic.

Level III

There are numerous studies at evidence Level III. These studies are currently not sufficient to recommend or suggest a pharmacological compound to be administered to TBI patients.

50.1 Overview

The basic pathophysiology of TBI consists of an initial, primary injury including rapid deformation of brain tissue with destruction of brain parenchyma and blood vessels and acute loss of neuronal and glial cells. A key concept in the management of TBI is that not all cell death occurs at the time of primary injury; instead, a cascade of molecular and neurochemical secondary events occur during the initial hours and days with a complex temporal profile. Ultimately, this secondary injury cascade markedly exacerbates the primary injury. Pharmacological attenuation of this secondary injury cascade with the aim of neuroprotection using, e.g. reactive oxygen species scavengers, glutamate receptor modulator, endocannabinoids, hypothermia or magnesium sulphate, has received much attention over several decades in numerous preclinical publications. To date, more than 20 phase III clinical trials have been conducted, and several trials are ongoing (Maas et al. 2010, www.clinicaltrials.gov). Unfortunately, these trials all failed to demonstrate clinical efficacy, and there is no neuroprotective compound currently available for TBI patients. So is neuroprotection for TBI a dead concept not to be pursued clinically or experimentally? Arguably, no. There are likely numerous reasons for the failure of neuroprotective compounds used in clinical trials for TBI, including heterogeneous patient samples and differences in general neurointensive care management. With few exceptions, the pharmacological and hypothermia TBI trials conducted to date have been rather small and have been frequently criticised in terms of study design, route of administration, time window and patient selection (e.g. Marklund and Hillered 2011; Maas et al. 2010).

N. Marklund
Department of Neurosurgery,
Uppsala University Hospital,
751 85, Uppsala, Sweden
e-mail: niklas.marklund@neuro.uu.se

T. Sundstrøm et al. (eds.), *Management of Severe Traumatic Brain Injury*,
DOI 10.1007/978-3-642-28126-6_50, © Springer-Verlag Berlin Heidelberg 2012

It should be emphasised that TBI is not *one* disease; instead, all the different subtypes of TBI may require markedly different treatments. Lack of early mechanistic or established surrogate endpoints and the insensitivity of the rather global outcome measures are specific problems in clinical TBI research. It is also obvious that numerous mistakes have been made in the past when attempting to translate preclinical information into the complex human situation. Such shortcomings of preclinical studies include the use of rodent TBI models reaching at most a moderate level of injury, and additionally, only rarely are pharmacological compounds administered beyond the first post-injury hours. Important lessons for future trials include improved patient classification, knowledge of brain penetration and action of the evaluated compound and more carefully defined and detailed outcome measures. Likely, future pharmacological management of TBI patients needs to combine neuroprotective drugs with compounds enhancing regeneration. Until such pharmacological treatment options are developed, neuroprotection for patients suffering from severe TBI is best provided by improved neurointensive care management with the avoidance, detection and treatment of avoidable factors such as seizures, fever, hypotension, hypoxemia, hyper- and hypoglycaemia, low CPP and high ICP. The present chapter reviews important aspects of pharmacological neuroprotection in severe traumatic brain injury. Hypothermia-induced neuroprotection is discussed in another chapter of this book (Chap. 61).

Tips, Tricks, and Pitfalls

- If you see oedema surrounding a traumatic haematoma and consider using corticosteroids, do not do it. Corticosteroids, perhaps the most evaluated drug candidate for TBI, have never been shown to benefit TBI patients; instead, this treatment was shown to impair the outcome of TBI patients in large clinical trials.
- Nimodipine is effective for aneurysmal subarachnoid haemorrhage although, when evaluated for traumatic subarachnoid haemorrhage, no positive effects were demonstrated in clinical trials.
- Numerous small clinical trials evaluating putative neuroprotective compounds exist, and several of these studies demonstrate some positive effects on the clinical outcome following severe TBI. It is recommended that these compounds, to date, should only be used in the context of clinical trials.
- Hopefully, ongoing clinical trials using e.g. cyclospoin A, erythropoietin, progesterone or citicoline, will provide a pharmacological treatment option for the treatment of TBI.
- Likely, the strict avoidance, detection and treatment of avoidable factors (seizures, fever, hypotension, hypoxemia, hyper- and hypoglycaemia, low CPP, high ICP, etc.) is the best currently available therapy to provide neuroprotection for patients suffering from severe TBI.

50.2 Background

Pharmacological attenuation of the secondary injury cascade (Fig. 50.1) has received much attention over several decades in numerous preclinical publications and clinical trial. Although a detailed description of the secondary injury cascade and all neuroprotective mechanisms is beyond the scope of this chapter (for overview see Marklund and Hillered 2011), key pharmacological compounds evaluated in clinical trials for severe TBI are highlighted below. The use of fluid management, hypertonic saline, mannitol, and various sedative compounds is covered in other chapters of this book.

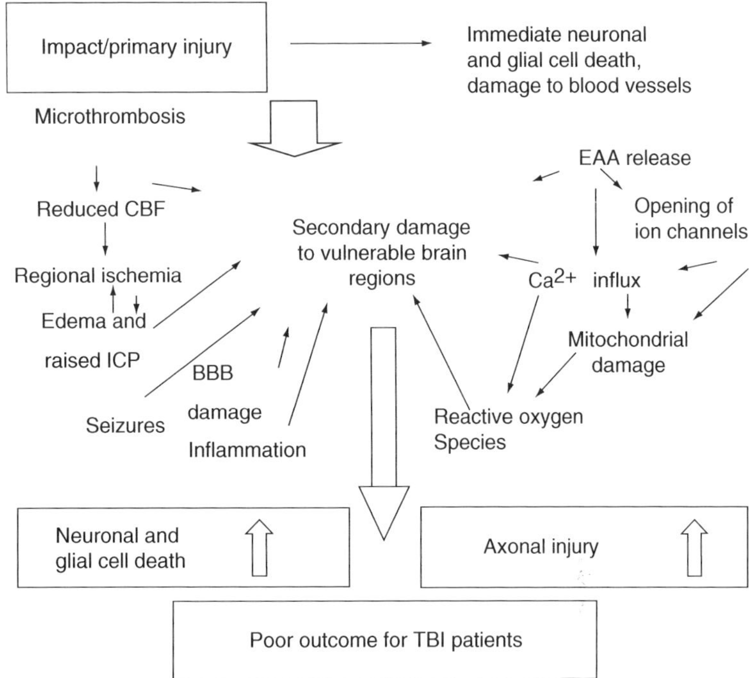

Fig. 50.1 Markedly simplified cartoon of secondary injury events following TBI. *Ca^{2+}* calcium, *rCBF* regional cerebral blood flow, *EAA* excitatory amino acids, *BBB* blood brain barrier

50.2.1 Secondary Injury Cascade

Immediately following the primary injury, there is a profound disturbance of the cellular ion homeostasis across neuronal cell membranes initiated by a marked release of the excitatory amino acid neurotransmitters glutamate and aspartate resulting in an activation of glutamate receptors (a process known as excitotoxicity). As a consequence of this release of glutamate, cellular influx of Na^{+} and Ca^{2+} and efflux of K^{+} is observed and referred to as traumatic depolarization (Faden et al. 1989; Nilsson et al. 1990, 1993). A resulting cerebral oedema with an associated increase in intracranial pressure may be detrimental and negatively influence e.g. cerebral blood flow.

The rapid influx of calcium leads to mitochondrial damage, axonal injury, an increase in free radical production and activation of calcium-dependent destructive proteases (such as caspases and calpains) resulting in cytoskeletal damage (Marklund et al. 2001; Singleton et al. 2001; Israelsson et al. 2008). Mitochondrial dysfunction post-TBI (Verweij et al. 2000; Lifshitz et al. 2004) is an additional unfortunate event since it occurs at the time of increased energy demand due to activation of energy-consuming ion transport systems and cell repair enzymes. The high demand for glucose, demonstrated by an increased local cerebral metabolic rate of glucose, occurs at a time of reduced regional cerebral blood flow, and this uncoupling of blood flow-cerebral metabolism negatively influences the injured brain (Chen et al. 2004). Damaged mitochondria are also a potential source for increased oxidative stress following TBI. Oxidative stress with the increased production of reactive oxygen/nitrogen species (ROS/RNS) and decreased antioxidant defence occurs following TBI and induces damage to cellular membranes and organelles by lipid peroxidation, protein oxidation and nucleotide breakdown (Lewen et al. 2000). Inflammation may be a double-edged sword following TBI. Although some inflammatory pathways may be important for regenerative responses and repair (Lenzlinger et al. 2001; Whitney et al. 2009), numerous experimental studies suggest that part of immune response is exacerbating the primary injury. The acute inflammatory response following TBI includes infiltration of peripheral immune cells, local activation of microglia and astrocytes, release of cytokines and oedema formation resulting from breakdown of the blood-brain barrier (BBB) (Schmidt et al. 2005; Clausen et al. 2009; Ziebell and Morganti-Kossmann 2010).

50.2.2 Neuronal Death and Axonal Damage

Neuronal injury is widespread following TBI and may occur even remote from the site of impact, and there are two major types of cell death occur following TBI: necrosis and apoptosis (Saatman et al. 2006). Damaged mitochondria may contribute to post-injury apoptotic cell death via an opening of the mitochondrial permeability transition pore resulting in release and activation of pro-apoptotic factors including soluble cytochrome c (Lifshitz et al. 2004; Mazzeo et al. 2009). Importantly, TBI-induced cell death continues for months after the injury both in human and experimental TBI (Shiozaki et al. 2001; Bramlett and Dietrich 2002).

For obvious reasons, neuronal cell death has received much attention in TBI research although the presence of traumatic axonal injury is increasingly recognised. Except in those patients with severe TBI dead at the scene of the injury, acute axonal disconnection is rarely observed in survivors of TBI. Rather, axonal disconnection results from complex axolemmal or cytoskeletal changes with impairment of axoplasmic transport (Ferrand-Drake et al. 2003; Buki and Povlishock 2006). Importantly, diffuse axonal injury (DAI) is a dominant contributor to the functional deficits observed in TBI patients and is observed with high frequency in those patients remaining in a persistent vegetative state (Graham et al. 2005). A major limitation to the recovery of TBI patients is that CNS axons do not spontaneously regrow following injury. The reasons for the inability of CNS axons to regenerate are likely multifactorial. The myelin-associated inhibitors of axonal growth may be the most important, and they include the myelin-associated glycoprotein (MAG), oligodendrocyte-myelin glycoprotein (OMgp) and Nogo-A all binding to the neuronal Nogo-66 receptor (NgR1; Sandvig et al. 2004; Walmsley and Mir 2007; Gonzenbach and Schwab 2008). Although damaged axons fail to regenerate and damaged neurons cannot be replaced, patients frequently show a degree of spontaneous improvement (that is often incomplete and unsatisfactory) over the initial months after the injury. This spontaneous behavioural improvement suggests neurophysiological and neuroanatomical adaptive changes of uninjured brain regions that could theoretically be enhanced in order to improve recovery.

50.2.3 Previous Clinical Trials Aiming at Neuroprotection

Clinical trials initiated in the late 1970s and early 1980s began evaluating the corticosteroid dexamethasone and found to be ineffective in improving outcome in cohorts of severely brain-injured patients. Later, the Head Injury Trials (HIT) evaluating nimodipine were published (see Vergouwen et al. 2006). Although the overall results were disappointing, a subgroup analysis suggested a beneficial effect for patients with traumatic subarachnoid haemorrhage, and the HIT3 and HIT4 trials focused on this patient category. Although the HIT 3 study showed a small but significant beneficial effect, the larger HIT 4 trial showed a significant *increase* in poor outcome in nimodipine-treated patients, and nimodipine cannot currently be recommended for TBI patients. In subsequent years, several additional trials were conducted targeting glutamate excitotoxicity and reactive oxygen species, both identified as important targets in animal models of TBI (Marklund and Hillered 2011, Fig. 1). However, neither the ROS scavenging agents tirilazad and PEG-SOD nor the glutamate receptor modulators aptiganel, SNX-111, D-CPP-ene, Selfotel and eliprodil were effective. Based on solid preclinical efficacy, there were great expectations for both the endocannabinoid dexanabinol and magnesium sulphate. In contrast to experimental findings, both compounds failed to demonstrate clinical efficacy, and there were clear indications, at least in the high-dose group, that magnesium sulphate *impaired* the outcome of severe TBI patients (Maas et al. 2006; Temkin et al. 2007).

With few exceptions, most TBI trials to date have been rather small and only infrequently enrolling more than 1,000 patients. The exception is the multicenter randomised MRC-CRASH trial, which evaluated high-dose methylprednisolone for TBI patients, enrolling more than 10,000 patients in the by far largest TBI trial to date. The study included patients with a GCS of 14 and less, which means that the study included the whole range of disability from less injured to more severely injured patients. The results showed a significant *increase* in death and severe disability emphasising that corticosteroids should not be routinely administered to TBI patients (Roberts et al. 2004).

The hormone progesterone has repeatedly shown neuroprotective effects in several animal TBI models, attenuating cerebral oedema and neuronal death and improving behavioural outcome. When progesterone was administered to patients with severe TBI within 8 h following the injury, an improved 3- and 6-month outcome was observed (Xiao et al. 2008) emphasising the need for a larger phase III randomised trial which is currently ongoing (ProTECT trial, Wright et al. 2007). Although the initial trials are promising, larger-scale trials are required before the use of progesterone is recommended for routine use in TBI.

50.2.4 Final Comments

In this chapter, previous and some current trials aiming to achieve neuroprotection for patients with severe TBI have been reviewed. Unfortunately, the pharmacologic concept of neuroprotection for severe human TBI has not been clinically successful so far. In general terms, current pharmacological approaches may be roughly categorised into neuroprotection, inflammatory modulation and enhancement of regeneration. Vast numbers of rodent TBI studies have evaluated calcium channel antagonists, glutamate antagonists, ROS scavengers and anti-inflammatory compounds and repeatedly shown to attenuate behavioural and histological deficit post-TBI. As presented in previous sections, these promising preclinical trials have failed when attempting to translate into the clinical setting. Importantly, injury mechanisms, genetic background, gender, age, type and severity of injury, metabolic state of the brain and other conditions (e.g. other diseases, medication) associated with TBI may clearly influence the TBI and are insufficiently evaluated in preclinical models. Also, much detailed pathophysiological knowledge from experimental TBI has not been confirmed in injured human brain, and the brain penetration of potentially neuroprotective compounds is frequently unknown. Finally, careful selection of patients in terms of injury type and severity based on detailed neuroradiology, age and additional injuries combined with improved secondary outcome measures is likely crucial in the future development of neuroprotective compounds for human TBI.

50.3 Specific Paediatric Concerns

Children are not small adults; instead, the pathophysiology of TBI is frequently different from that of adults. Diffuse injury, in particular diffuse brain swelling, and subdural haematomas are more common than focal TBI in infants and young children compared to adults (see Huh and Raghupathi 2009). To date, no neuroprotective compound has specifically been evaluated in paediatric TBI patients.

References

Bramlett HM, Dietrich WD (2002) Quantitative structural changes in white and gray matter 1 year following traumatic brain injury in rats. Acta Neuropathol 103(6):607–614

Buki A, Povlishock JT (2006) All roads lead to disconnection? – Traumatic axonal injury revisited. Acta Neurochir (Wien) 148:181–193; discussion 193–194

Chen SF, Richards HK, Smielewski P, Johnström P, Salvador R, Pickard JD, Harris NG (2004) Relationship between flow-metabolism uncoupling and evolving axonal injury after experimental traumatic brain injury. J Cereb Blood Flow Metab 24:1025–1036

Clausen F, Hånell A, Björk M, Hillered L, Mir AK, Gram H, Marklund N (2009) Neutralization of interleukin-1beta modifies the inflammatory response and improves histological and cognitive outcome following traumatic brain injury in mice. Eur J Neurosci 30:385–396

Faden AI, Demediuk P, Panter SS, Vink R (1989) The role of excitatory amino acids and NMDA receptors in traumatic brain injury. Science 244:798–800

Ferrand-Drake M, Zhu C, Gidö G, Hansen AJ, Karlsson JO, Bahr BA, Zamzami N, Kroemer G, Chan PH, Wieloch T, Blomgren K (2003) Cyclosporin A prevents calpain activation despite increased intracellular calcium concentrations, as well as translocation of apoptosis-inducing factor, cytochrome c and caspase-3 activation in neurons exposed to transient hypoglycemia. J Neurochem 85: 1431–1442

Gonzenbach RR, Schwab ME (2008) Disinhibition of neurite growth to repair the injured adult CNS: focusing on Nogo. Cell Mol Life Sci 65:161–176

Graham DI, Adams JH, Murray LS, Jennett B (2005) Neuropathology of the vegetative state after head injury. Neuropsychol Rehabil 15:198–213

Huh JW, Raghupathi R (2009) New concepts in treatment of pediatric brain injury. Anesthesiol Clin 27(2): 213–240

Israelsson C, Bengtsson H, Kylberg A, Kullander K, Lewen A, Hillered L, Ebendal T (2008) Distinct cellular patterns of upregulated chemokine expression supporting a prominent inflammatory role in traumatic brain injury. J Neurotrauma 25:959–974

Lenzlinger PM, Morganti-Kossmann MC, Laurer HL, McIntosh TK (2001) The duality of the inflammatory response to traumatic brain injury. Mol Neurobiol 24:169–181

Lewen A, Matz P, Chan PH (2000) Free radical pathways in CNS injury. J Neurotrauma 17:871–890

Lifshitz J, Sullivan PG, Hovda DA, Wieloch T, McIntosh TK (2004) Mitochondrial damage and dysfunction in traumatic brain injury. Mitochondrion 4:705–713

Maas AI, Murray G, Henney H 3rd, Kassem N, Legrand V, Mangelus M, Muizelaar JP, Stocchetti N, Knoller N, Pharmos TBI Investigators (2006) Efficacy and safety of dexanabinol in severe traumatic brain injury: results of a phase III randomised, placebo-controlled, clinical trial. Lancet Neurol 5:38–45

Maas AI, Roozenbeek B, Manley GT (2010) Clinical trials in traumatic brain injury: past experience and current developments. Neurotherapeutics 7:115–126

Marklund N, Hillered L (2011) Animal modeling of traumatic brain injury in pre-clinical drug development – where do we go from here? Br J Pharmacol 164(4): 1207–1229

Marklund N, Lewander T, Clausen F, Hillered L (2001) Effects of the nitrone radical scavengers PBN and S-PBN on in vivo trapping of reactive oxygen species after traumatic brain injury in rats. J Cereb Blood Flow Metab 21:1259–1267

Mazzeo AT, Beat A, Singh A, Bullock MR (2009) The role of mitochondrial transition pore, and its modulation, in traumatic brain injury and delayed neurodegeneration after TBI. Exp Neurol 218:363–370

Nilsson P, Hillered L, Ponten U, Ungerstedt U (1990) Changes in cortical extracellular levels of energy-related metabolites and amino acids following concussive brain injury in rats. J Cereb Blood Flow Metab 10:631–637

Nilsson P, Hillered L, Olsson Y, Sheardown MJ, Hansen AJ (1993) Regional changes in interstitial K+ and Ca2+ levels following cortical compression contusion trauma in rats. J Cereb Blood Flow Metab 13:183–192

Roberts I, Yates D, Sandercock P, Farrell B, Wasserberg J, Lomas G, Cottingham R, Svoboda P, Brayley N, Mazairac G, Laloë V, Muñoz-Sánchez A, Arango M, Hartzenberg B, Khamis H, Yutthakasemsunt S, Komolafe E, Olldashi F, Yadav Y, Murillo-Cabezas F, Shakur H, Edwards P, CRASH trial collaborators (2004) Effect of intravenous corticosteroids on death within 14 days in 10008 adults with clinically significant head injury (MRC CRASH trial): randomised placebo-controlled trial. Lancet 364: 1321–1328

Saatman KE, Feeko KJ, Pape RL, Raghupathi R (2006) Differential behavioral and histopathological responses to graded cortical impact injury in mice. J Neurotrauma 23(8):1241–1253

Sandvig A, Berry M, Barrett LB, Butt A, Logan A (2004) Myelin-, reactive glia-, and scar-derived CNS axon growth inhibitors: expression, receptor signaling, and correlation with axon regeneration. Glia 46:225–251

Schmidt OI, Heyde CE, Ertel W, Stahel PF (2005) Closed head injury – an inflammatory disease? Brain Res Brain Res Rev 48:388–399

Shiozaki T, Akai H, Taneda M, Hayakata T, Aoki M, Oda J, Tanaka H, Hiraide A, Shimazu T, Sugimoto H (2001) Delayed hemispheric neuronal loss in severely head-injured patients. J Neurotrauma 18:665–674

Singleton RH, Stone JR, Okonkwo DO, Pellicane AJ, Povlishock JT (2001) The immunophilin ligand FK506 attenuates axonal injury in an impact-acceleration model of traumatic brain injury. J Neurotrauma 18: 607–614

Temkin NR, Anderson GD, Winn HR, Ellenbogen RG, Britz GW, Schuster J, Lucas T, Newell DW, Mansfield PN, Machamer JE, Barber J, Dikmen SS (2007) Magnesium sulfate for neuroprotection after traumatic brain injury: a randomised controlled trial. Lancet Neurol 6:29–38

Vergouwen MD, Vermeulen M, Roos YB (2006) Effect of nimodipine on outcome in patients with traumatic subarachnoid haemorrhage: a systematic review. Lancet Neurol 5:1029–1032

Verweij BH, Muizelaar JP, Vinas FC, Peterson PL, Xiong Y, Lee CP (2000) Impaired cerebral mitochondrial function after traumatic brain injury in humans. J Neurosurg 93:815–820

Walmsley AR, Mir AK (2007) Targeting the Nogo-A signalling pathway to promote recovery following acute CNS injury. Curr Pharm Des 13:2470–2484

Whitney NP, Eidem TM, Peng H, Huang Y, Zheng JC (2009) Inflammation mediates varying effects in neurogenesis: relevance to the pathogenesis of brain injury and neurodegenerative disorders. J Neurochem 108:1343–1359

Wright DW, Kellermann AL, Hertzberg VS, Clark PL, Frankel M, Goldstein FC, Salomone JP, Dent LL, Harris OA, Ander DS, Lowery DW, Patel MM, Denson DD, Gordon AB, Wald MM, Gupta S, Hoffman SW, Stein DG (2007) ProTECT: a randomized clinical trial of progesterone for acute traumatic brain injury. Ann Emerg Med 49:391–402, 402:391–392

Xiao G, Wei J, Yan W et al (2008) Improved outcomes from the administration of progesterone for patients with acute severe traumatic brain injury: a randomized controlled trial. Crit Care 12:R61

Ziebell JM, Morganti-Kossmann MC (2010) Involvement of pro- and anti-inflammatory cytokines and chemokines in the pathophysiology of traumatic brain injury. Neurotherapeutics 7:22–30

Subacute Surgery in Neurointensive Care

51

Terje Sundstrøm and Knut Wester

Recommendations

Level I

There are insufficient data to support a Level I recommendation for this topic.

Level II

Early, low-threshold decompressive craniectomy in adults with increased intracranial pressure is associated with a poorer outcome compared to conservative treatment.

Bitemporal craniectomy may be preferable at an early stage in children with traumatic brain injury and refractory high intracranial pressure.

Level III

Decompressive procedures (such as bifrontal craniectomy) should always be considered in adults with intractable intracranial hypertension.

Postoperative complications can be avoided by meticulous surgical technique and adequate choice of procedure.

T. Sundstrøm, (✉)
Department of Neurosurgery,
Haukeland University Hospital,
Jonas Lies Vei 65, 5021 Bergen, Norway

Department of Surgical Sciences and
Department of Biomedicine, University of Bergen,
Jonas Lies Vei 91, 5020 Bergen, Norway
e-mail: terje.sundstrom@gmail.com

K. Wester
Department of Surgical Sciences,
University of Bergen,
Jonas Lies Vei 65, 5021 Bergen, Norway

Department of Neurosurgery,
Haukeland University Hospital,
Jonas Lies Vei 65, 5021 Bergen, Norway
e-mail: knut.gustav.wester@helse-bergen.no

51.1 Overview

The possibility of hydrocephalus, brain oedema, or a new or recurrent intracranial haematoma must be investigated by repeated computed tomography (CT) scans in case of neurological deterioration or intractable intracranial hypertension in a head injured patient. Subacute surgery (secondary surgical intervention) should then be considered.

The relevant surgical procedures and their respective indications are described in Part 5 in this book on acute surgical treatment; these principles also apply to subacute surgery. Drainage of cerebrospinal fluid is moreover discussed in the following section. In general, the monitoring and treatment strategies described elsewhere in Part 7 and 8 should be consulted for detailed information on timing, thresholds, and complementary interventions.

T. Sundstrøm et al. (eds.), *Management of Severe Traumatic Brain Injury*,
DOI 10.1007/978-3-642-28126-6_51, © Springer-Verlag Berlin Heidelberg 2012

Tips, Tricks, and Pitfalls

- Continuously re-evaluate the level of treatment according to new developments.
- 'Do not treat the patient with a new CT scan'.
- Prophylactic craniectomy is an unwarranted procedure.
- Always look at the patient and think about possible technical malfunctions and the reliability of the monitoring equipment.
- When doubt exists and consciousness is depressed, intracranial pressure should always be monitored and significant mass lesions removed.
- The first 48 h are most critical in a surgical perspective, but intracranial haematomas can occur at any point in time during neurointensive care.

51.2 Background

There is only Level III evidence for the topics dealt with in this chapter, except two studies with Level II evidence concerning decompressive craniectomy in children (Taylor et al. 2001) and adults (Cooper et al. 2011).

The effectiveness of decompressive craniectomy in adults remains uncertain, and the clinical context has yet to be defined. Nonetheless, clinical experience and results from non-randomized trials and controlled trials with historical controls suggest that craniectomy may be the intervention of choice in selected patients (Sahuquillo and Arikan 2006).

The recently published, randomized controlled Decra study concluded with an increased risk of a poor outcome for patients with refractory high intracranial pressure (ICP) undergoing bifrontotemporoparietal craniectomy as compared to those receiving conservative medical treatment (Cooper et al. 2011). The craniectomy was performed early (within 72 h) in patients with a moderately increased intracranial pressure (20 mmHg) for a short period of time (15 min) and with diffuse brain injuries without mass lesions. Twenty-three percent of the patients assigned to conservative treatment nevertheless underwent a late craniectomy as a life-saving intervention, and these patients were included in the final analyses demonstrating a poorer outcome with craniectomy. This aggressive approach in a subgroup of patients does not really bring clarification to the major problems. Early, prophylactic craniectomy most likely does not have any other effect but preventing a later craniectomy if the ICP cannot be controlled. The ongoing RescueICP trial (www.rescueicp.com) will hopefully allow further conclusions on the efficacy of craniectomy in the adult population.

The Brain Trauma Foundation recommends the use of bifrontal decompressive craniectomy within 48 h of injury for patients with diffuse intractable cerebral oedema and resultant intracranial hypertension (Bullock et al. 2006). Subtemporal decompression, temporal lobectomy, and hemispheric decompressive craniectomy are other options for patients with clinical and radiographic evidence for impending transtentorial herniation.

Intracranial haematomas or contusions diagnosed by the initial CT scan can evolve with enlargement of bleeding and/or perifocal oedema, thereby requiring surgery at a later stage. An intracranial haematoma may also arise after an initial, normal CT scan. It is especially important to be observant with patients undergoing an early CT scan (within a few hours) after the trauma and patients on anticoagulant treatment or with other coagulopathies. Delayed traumatic intracerebral haematomas (DTICHs) is an uncommon phenomenon. DTICHs are haematomas appearing in brain areas described as normal in otherwise abnormal initial CT scans. These usually become clinically apparent within 48 h of injury (Gentleman et al. 1989).

Carotid dissection and cerebral vasospasms are other conditions to be aware of. Both conditions can cause neurological deterioration in a subacute manner. Carotid dissection is often associated with neck trauma (e.g. seat belt injury) and may be followed by development of a hemiparesis without corresponding findings on initial

CT scans. Traumatic arterial spasms are not that uncommon and have a similar time course to that seen with aneurysmal subarachnoid haemorrhage. The clinical significance of vasospasms in traumatic brain injury is still uncertain (Armin et al. 2008).

New or recurrent haematomas are not infrequent after acute surgery for head injuries (Seifman et al. 2011). The vasculature can be injured and the clotting mechanisms can be compromised. Rebleeding at the operative site requiring reoperation has been reported in up to 7% of patients undergoing craniotomy and evacuation of traumatic intracranial haematomas (Bullock et al. 1990). The use of correct surgical techniques and adequate choice of procedures are therefore essential to avoid postoperative complications (see Part 5 on acute surgical treatment).

51.3 Specific Paediatric Concerns

One small prospective, randomized study has investigated the use of early bitemporal craniectomy without duraplasty in children (Taylor et al. 2001). The children had a median age of 120.9 months. Thirteen children were randomized to craniectomy and 14 children to conservative management; the median GCS score was 6 and 5, respectively. The craniectomy was performed at a median of 19.2 h (range 7.3–29.3 h) after the accident. Children who had sustained intracranial hypertension during the first day after admission (ICP 20–24 mmHg for 30 min, 25–29 mmHg for 10 min, 30 mmHg or more for 1 min) or had evidence of herniation (unilaterally dilated pupil or bradycardia) were eligible for randomization. A trend was shown towards greater improvement in intracranial pressure, less time required in the intensive care unit, and improved clinical outcome by adding decompressive craniectomy to conventional medical treatment. Based on this study, a recent Cochrane review concluded that decompressive craniectomy might be justified in patients below the age of 18 years when full medical treatment is unable to control the intracranial pressure (Sahuquillo and Arikan 2006).

References

Armin SS, Colohan AR, Zhang JH (2008) Vasospasm in traumatic brain injury. Acta Neurochir Suppl 104:421–425

Bullock R, Hanemann CO, Murray L, Teasdale GM (1990) Recurrent hematomas following craniotomy for traumatic intracranial mass. J Neurosurg 72:9–14

Bullock MR, Chesnut R, Ghajar J, Gordon D, Hartl R, Newell DW, Servadei F, Walters BC, Wilberger JE, Surgical Management of Traumatic Brain Injury Author Group (2006) Surgical management of traumatic brain injury. Neurosurgery 58:S2-1–S2-62

Cooper DJ, Rosenfeld JV, Murray L, Arabi YM, Davies AR, D'Urso P, Kossmann T, Ponsford J, Seppelt I, Reilly P, Wolfe R, DECRA Trial Investigators; Australian and New Zealand Intensive Care Society Clinical Trials Group (2011) Decompressive craniectomy in diffuse traumatic brain injury. N Engl J Med 364:1493–1502

Gentleman D, Nath F, Macpherson P (1989) Diagnosis and management of delayed traumatic intracerebral haematomas. Br J Neurosurg 3:367–372

Sahuquillo J, Arikan F (2006) Decompressive craniectomy for the treatment of refractory high intracranial pressure in traumatic brain injury. Cochrane Database Syst Rev 1:CD003983. doi:10.1002/14651858.CD003983.pub2

Seifman MA, Lewis PM, Rosenfeld JV, Hwang PY (2011) Postoperative intracranial haemorrhage: a review. Neurosurg Rev 34(4):393–407

Taylor A, Butt W, Rosenfeld J, Shann F, Ditchfield M, Lewis E, Klug G, Wallace D, Henning R, Tibballs J (2001) A randomized trial of very early decompressive craniectomy in children with traumatic brain injury and sustained intracranial hypertension. Childs Nerv Syst 17:154–162

CSF Drainage

52

Lars-Owe D. Koskinen

Recommendations

Level I

There are insufficient data to support a Level I recommendation for this topic.

Level II

There are insufficient data to support a Level II recommendation for this topic.

Level III

Continuous or intermittent CSF drainage is recommended in situations with increased ICP (>20 mmHg) when other measures have failed such as surgical removal of space occupying haematomas and contusions, optimizing of ventilation and sedation.

52.1 Overview

In an early retrospective study in 39 patients, intermittent or continuous CSF drainage was applied, and it was concluded that early drainage was of little use in influencing ICP while later CSF removal had a more pronounced effect (Papo et al. 1981). In a prospective study on 31 patients, it was shown that various volumes of CSF intermittent drainage significantly decreased the ICP with a few mmHg, but in only 6/31 subjects, the decrease was more than 3 mmHg and lasting for more than 10 min (Kerr et al. 2000). A prospective study in 24 subjects, with sustained elevated ICP after other ICP decreasing measures, showed that in about 50% of the cases, the ICP was brought under control after continuous drainage (Timofeev et al. 2008). In a prospective study of 45 patients with sTBI and 55 patients with SAH and presenting refractory ICP elevation, a combination of ventriculostomy and lumbar drainage was shown to reduce the ICP but not to affect outcome (Tuettenberg et al. 2009). In that same study, 12% presented with cerebral herniation and 6% died due to herniation. Some studies have shown an improved outcome after using CSF drainage (Timofeev et al. 2008; Ghajar et al. 1993).

The decrease in ICP after CSF drainage cannot be expected to be long lasting and may not be effective in all subjects as the loss of CSF by time will be replaced by brain oedema. It is discussed whether removal of constitutes of the CSF might have a negative effect on cerebral function and repair. In cases with very narrow ventricles, free-hand ventriculostomy can be difficult. The method maybe complicated by CSF leakage and infections.

L.-O.D. Koskinen
Department of Neurosurgery, Umeå University,
Umeå 901 85, Sweden
e-mail: lars-owe.koskinen@neuro.umu.se

T. Sundstrøm et al. (eds.), *Management of Severe Traumatic Brain Injury*,
DOI 10.1007/978-3-642-28126-6_52, © Springer-Verlag Berlin Heidelberg 2012

Tips, Tricks, and Pitfalls

- CSF drainage can be used when other measures have failed.
- An intermittent drainage is often preferred over continuous.
- The drainage should be against a pressure of about 15–20 mmHg in order to avoid slits ventricles.
- If the drain stops functioning, this can be due to blood, debris, mechanical tubing problems, stopcocks or empty ventricles. Empty ventricles are a serious complication to CSF drainage due to increased risk of brainstem herniation.
- Some drainage systems are sensitive to wrong position of the drainage reservoir resulting in non-functioning airing valves.
- If empty ventricles, close the drain for 20 min and check the function again.
- Beware of a dislocation of the ventricular catheter and the relative high risk of infection.
- If lumbar drainage is used: be aware of the risk of cerebral herniation.

52.2 Background

High ICP is generally considered as one of the main factors influencing the final clinical outcome after TBI (Miller et al. 1977; Narayan et al. 1982; Eisenberg et al. 1988; Jiang et al. 2002; Schreiber et al. 2002; Olivecrona et al. 2010; Marmarou et al. 1991). It has also been reported that those who respond to a given ICP-reducing therapy have a reduced risk of mortality (Farahvar et al. 2011). Several causes of raised ICP can be identified including haematomas, contusions, oedema, disturbance in CSF outflow and resorption. The rationale for removing CSF is based on the Monro-Kellie doctrine (Monro 1783; Kelly 1824) giving space for, e.g. diffuse cerebral oedema. CSF drainage is thus applied in patients with or without signs of acute hydrocephalus. Lundberg (1960) presented some evidence that CSF drainage decreases elevated ICP. It is well understood that drainage of CSF can be effective in reducing ICP in the emergency situation. It is also commonly referred to in textbooks that CSF diversion is an effective treatment of elevated ICP. However, the scientific evidence is spare.

52.3 Specific Paediatric Concerns

The age of the paediatric patient must be considered in deciding the optimal and critical ICP level (Jones et al. 2003). Furthermore, the lower CSF volume in children must be taken into account when deciding the volume to be drained. In 22 paediatric patients, the ICP decreased after CSF drainage (Shapiro and Marmarou 1982). A study reporting on the use of a combination of CSF drainage by ventriculostomy and lumbar drainage in 16 patients showed that ICP was unaffected in two patients who died; in the remaining 14 patients, an abrupt and lasting decrease in ICP was observed (Levy et al. 1995). Continuous drainage of CSF appears more effective in reducing the ICP than intermittent drainage (Shore et al. 2004). In a multicentre study of 41 paediatric patients, it was shown that the mean ICP was significantly higher (43 ± 26 mmHg, $n = 3$) in the deceased group as compared to the survivors (13 ± 4 mmHg, $n = 38$) (Wahlström et al. 2005).

References

Eisenberg HM, Frankowski RF, Contant CF, Marshall LF, Walker MD (1988) High-dose barbiturate control of elevated intracranial pressure in patients with severe head injury. J Neurosurg 69:15–23 [Clinical Trial Randomized Controlled Trial Research Support, U.S. Gov't, P.H.S.]

Farahvar A, Gerber LM, Chiu YL, Hartl R, Carney N, Ghajar J (2011) Response to intracranial hypertension treatment as a predictor of death in patients with severe traumatic brain injury. J Neurosurg 114:1471–1478

Ghajar JBG, Hariri RJ, Patterson RH (1993) Improved outcome from traumatic coma using only ventricular cerebrospinal fluid drainage for intracranial pressure control. Adv Neurosurg 21:5

Jiang JY, Gao GY, Li WP, Yu MK, Zhu C (2002) Early indicators of prognosis in 846 cases of severe traumatic brain injury. J Neurotrauma 19:869–874

Jones PA, Andrews PJ, Easton VJ, Minns RA (2003) Traumatic brain injury in childhood: intensive care time series data and outcome. Br J Neurosurg 17:29–39 [Research Support, Non-U.S. Gov't]

Kelly G (1824) Appearances observed in the dissection of two individuals; death from cold and congestion of the brain. Trans Med Chir Sci Edinb 1:85

Kerr EM, Marion D, Sereika MS, Weber BB, Orndoff AP, Henker R et al (2000) The effect of cerebrospinal fluid drainage on cerebral perfusion in traumatic brain injured adults. J Neurosurg Anesthesiol 12:324–333 [Research Support, Non-U.S. Gov't Research Support, U.S. Gov't, P.H.S.]

Levy DI, Rekate HL, Cherny WB, Manwaring K, Moss SD, Baldwin HZ (1995) Controlled lumbar drainage in pediatric head injury. J Neurosurg 83:453–460 [Case Reports]

Lundberg N (1960) Continuous recording and control of ventricular fluid pressure in neurosurgical practice. Acta Psychiatr Scand Suppl 36:1–193

Marmarou A, Anderson RL, Ward JD, Choi SC, Young HF, Eisenberg HM et al (1991) Impact of ICP instability and hypotension on outcome in patients with severe head trauma. J Neurosurg 75:59–66

Miller JD, Becker DP, Ward JD, Sullivan HG, Adams WE, Rosner MJ (1977) Significance of intracranial hypertension in severe head injury. J Neurosurg 47:503–516 [Research Support, U.S. Gov't, P.H.S.]

Monro A (1783) Observations on the structure and function of the nervous system. Creech & Johnson, Edinburgh

Narayan RK, Kishore PR, Becker DP, Ward JD, Enas GG, Greenberg RP et al (1982) Intracranial pressure: to monitor or not to monitor? A review of our experience with severe head injury. J Neurosurg 56:650–659 [Research Support, U.S. Gov't, P.H.S.]

Olivecrona M, Wildemyr Z, Koskinen LO (2010) The apolipoprotein E epsilon4 allele and outcome in severe traumatic brain injury treated by an intracranial pressure-targeted therapy. J Neurosurg 112:1113–1119 [Randomized Controlled Trial Research Support, Non-U.S. Gov't]

Papo I, Caruselli G, Luongo A (1981) CSF withdrawal for the treatment of intracranial hypertension in acute head injuries. Acta Neurochir 56:191–199

Schreiber MA, Aoki N, Scott BG, Beck JR (2002) Determinants of mortality in patients with severe blunt head injury. Arch Surg 137:285–290

Shapiro K, Marmarou A (1982) Clinical applications of the pressure-volume index in treatment of pediatric head injuries. J Neurosurg 56:819–825 [Research Support, U.S. Gov't, P.H.S.]

Shore PM, Thomas NJ, Clark RS, Adelson PD, Wisniewski SR, Janesko KL et al (2004) Continuous versus intermittent cerebrospinal fluid drainage after severe traumatic brain injury in children: effect on biochemical markers. J Neurotrauma 21:1113–1122 [Comparative Study (Multicenter Study Research Support, Non-U.S. Gov't Research Support, U.S. Gov't, P.H.S.]

Timofeev I, Dahyot-Fizelier C, Keong N, Nortje J, Al-Rawi PG, Czosnyka M et al (2008) Ventriculostomy for control of raised ICP in acute traumatic brain injury. Acta Neurochir Suppl 102:99–104 [Clinical Trial Research Support, Non-U.S. Gov't]

Tuettenberg J, Czabanka M, Horn P, Woitzik J, Barth M, Thome C et al (2009) Clinical evaluation of the safety and efficacy of lumbar cerebrospinal fluid drainage for the treatment of refractory increased intracranial pressure. J Neurosurg 110:1200–1208

Wahlström MR, Olivecrona M, Koskinen LO, Rydenhag B, Naredi S (2005) Severe traumatic brain injury in pediatric patients: treatment and outcome using an intracranial pressure targeted therapy – the Lund concept. Intensive Care Med 31:832–839 [Multicenter Study Research Support, Non-U.S. Gov't]

Hyperventilation

53

Niels Juul

Recommendations

Level I

There are insufficient data to support a Level I recommendation for this topic.

Level II

Prophylactic hyperventilation ($PaCO_2$ of 3.3 kPa or less) is not recommended.

Level III

Hyperventilation is recommended as a temporising measure for the reduction of ICP.

Hyperventilation should be avoided during the first 24 h after injury when CBF often is critically reduced.

If hyperventilation is used, it is recommended to monitor brain oxygen delivery by either SjO_2, $PtiO_2$ measurements, or other means of continuous brain oxygen monitoring.

N. Juul
Department of anaesthesia, Aarhus University Hospital, Noerrebrogade 44, 8000 Aarhus C, Denmark
e-mail: nieljuul@rm.dk

53.1 Overview

Aggressive hyperventilation (arterial $PaCO_2 \leq$ 3.3 kPa) has been a cornerstone in the management of severe traumatic brain injury for more than 20 years because it can cause a rapid reduction of ICP. Brain swelling and elevated ICP develop in 40% of patients with severe TBI (Miller et al. 1977), and high or uncontrolled ICP is one of the most common causes of death and neurologic disability after TBI (Becker et al. 1977). Hyperventilation reduces ICP by causing cerebral vasoconstriction and a subsequent reduction in CBF (Raichle and Plum 1972). Therefore, the assumption has been made that hyperventilation benefits all patients with severe TBI. In a survey from 1995, Ghajar et al. found that hyperventilation was used by 83% of US trauma centres (Ghajar et al. 1995). This number has declined over the years, but as recent as in 2008, the Brain IT group made a survey in European centres showing that early prophylactic hyperventilation was used in more than 50% of cases (Neumann et al. 2008). Research conducted over the past 20 years clearly demonstrates that CBF during the first day after injury is less than half that of normal individuals (Bouma et al. 1992; Muizelaar et al. 1989; Robertson et al. 1988) and that there is a risk of causing cerebral ischemia with aggressive hyperventilation. Histological evidence of cerebral ischemia has been found in most victims of severe TBI who die (Graham and Adams 1971; Ross et al. 1993). A randomised study found significantly poorer outcomes at 3 and 6 months

T. Sundstrøm et al. (eds.), *Management of Severe Traumatic Brain Injury*,
DOI 10.1007/978-3-642-28126-6_53, © Springer-Verlag Berlin Heidelberg 2012

when prophylactic hyperventilation was used, as compared with when it was not (Muizelaar et al. 1991). Thus, limiting the use of hyperventilation following severe TBI may help improve neurologic recovery following injury, or at least avoid iatrogenic cerebral ischemia.

Tips, Tricks, and Pitfalls

- If the ICP is stable and below 20 mmHg, keep the $PaCO_2$ above 4.5 kPa.
- If the patient is monitored with $ETCO_2$ and the pulmonary condition is stable, compare $ETCO_2$ with $PaCO_2$ on a regular basis (once or twice a day). This will diminish the need for arterial blood gas monitoring since the difference between $PaCO_2$ and $ETCO_2$ will, for all good measures, be approximately the same if the pulmonary condition is stable.
- If the ventilator is on pressure control and you want to decrease $PaCO_2$, increase the frequency of ventilations rather than tidal volume, because this will not alter the difference between $ETCO_2$ and $PaCO_2$.
- If the ventilator is on volume control and you increase the minute volume, keep an eye on the peak pressures to decrease the risk of overextension of the lung.
- It is easier to control the hyperventilation if the ventilator setting is on volume control.

53.2 Background

53.2.1 CBF Following TBI

Three studies provide class III evidence that CBF can be dangerously low soon after severe TBI (Bouma et al. 1992; Marion et al. 1991; Sioutos et al. 1995). Two measured CBF were performed with xenon-CT/CBF method during the first 5 days following severe TBI in a total of 67 patients. In one, CBF measurements obtained during the first 24 h after injury were less than 18 mL/100 g/min in 31.4% of patients (Bouma et al. 1992). In the second, the mean CBF during the first few hours after injury was 27 mL/100 g/min (Marion et al. 1991). The third study measured CBF with a thermodiffusion blood flow probe, also during the first 5 days post-injury, in 37 severe TBI patients (Sioutos et al. 1995). Twelve patients had a CBF less than 18 mL/100 g/min up to 48-h post-injury.

53.2.2 $PaCO_2$/CBF Reactivity and Cerebral Oxygen Utilisation

Three class III studies provide the evidence base for this topic (Imberti et al. 2002; Oertel et al. 2002; Sheinberg et al. 1992). Results associating hyperventilation with SjO_2 and $PtiO_2$ values in a total of 102 patients are equivocal. One study showed no consistent positive or negative change in SjO_2 or $PtiO_2$ values (Imberti et al. 2002). A second study associated hyperventilation with a reduction of $PaCO_2$ and subsequent decrease in SjO_2 from 73% to 67%, but the SjO_2 values never dropped below 55% (Oertel et al. 2002). The third study reported hyperventilation to be the second most common identifiable cause of jugular venous oxygen desaturation in a sample of 33 patients (Sheinberg et al. 1992). Studies on regional CBF show significant variation in reduction in CBF following TBI. Two studies indicated lowest flows in brain tissue surrounding contusions or underlying subdural hematomas and in patients with severe diffuse injuries (Marion et al. 1991; Salvant and Muizelaar 1993). Similarly, a third found that CO_2 vasoreactivity was most abnormal in contusions and around subdural hematomas (McLaughlin and Marion 1996). Considering that CO_2 vasoreactivity could range from almost absent to three times normal in these patients, there could be a dangerous reduction in CBF to brain tissue surrounding contusions or underlying subdural clots following hyperventilation. Only one of these three studies (Marion et al. 1991) had adequate design and adequate sample to be included. Two studies associated hyperventilation-induced reduction in CBF with a significant increase in oxygen extraction fraction, but they did not find a significant relationship between hyperventilation and change in the $CMRO_2$ (Diringer et al. 2002; Hutchinson et al. 2002).

53.2.3 Effect of Hyperventilation on Outcome

One class III study involving 890 patients intubated prehospitally showed adverse outcome for both hypo- and hypercapnic patients; those intubated patients arriving at the trauma centre with an $PaCO_2$ between 4.0 and 6.5 kPa had a better survival than those who had been hypo- or hyperventilated, after adjustment for confounding factors (adjusted OR 2.17) (Davis et al. 2006).

One class II RCT of 113 patients used a stratified, randomised design to compare outcomes of severe TBI patients provided normal ventilation ($PaCO_2$ 4.66 ± 0.25 kPa; $n = 41$; control group), hyperventilation ($PaCO_2$ 3.33 ± 0.25 kPa; $n = 36$), or hyperventilation with tromethamine ($n = 36$) (Muizelaar et al. 1991). One benefit of hyperventilation is considered to be minimization of cerebrospinal fluid acidosis. However, the effect on CSF pH may not be sustained due to a loss of HCO_3^- buffer. Tromethamine buffer (THAM) treatment was introduced to test the hypothesis that it would reverse the effects of the loss of buffer. Patients were stratified based on the motor component of the GCS score (1–3 vs. 4–5). The GOS score was used to assess patient outcomes at 3, 6, and 12 months. For patients with a motor GCS of 4–5, the 3- and 6-month GOS scores were significantly lower in the hyperventilated patients than in the control or THAM groups. However, the effect was not sustained at 12 months. Also, the effect was not observed in patients with the lower motor GCS, minimising the sample size for the control, hyperventilation, and THAM groups to 21, 17, and 21, respectively. The absence of a power analysis renders uncertainty about the adequacy of the sample size. The recommendation today is that hyperventilation should be avoided.

53.3 Specific Paediatric Concerns

There are no specific paediatric concerns; children should be treated in accordance with the adult guidelines.

References

Becker DP, Miller JD, Ward JD, Greenberg RP, Young HF, Sakalas R (1977) The outcome from severe head injury with early diagnosis and intensive management. J Neurosurg 47:491–502

Bouma GJ, Muizelaar JP, Stringer WA, Choi SC, Fatouros P, Young HF (1992) Ultra-early evaluation of regional cerebral blood flow in severely head-injured patients using xenon-enhanced computerized tomography. J Neurosurg 77:360–368

Davis DP, Idris AH, Sise MJ, Kennedy F, Eastman AB, Velky T, Vilke GM, Hoyt DB (2006) Early ventilation and outcome in patients with moderate to severe traumatic brain injury. Crit Care Med 34:1202–1208

Diringer MN, Videen TO, Yundt K, Zazulia AR, Aiyagari V, Dacey RG Jr, Grubb RL, Powers WJ (2002) Regional cerebrovascular and metabolic effects of hyperventilation after severe traumatic brain injury. J Neurosurg 96:103–108

Ghajar J, Hariri RJ, Narayan RK, Iacono LA, Firlik K, Patterson RH (1995) Survey of critical care management of comatose, head-injured patients in the United States. Crit Care Med 23:560–567

Graham DI, Adams JH (1971) Ischaemic brain damage in fatal head injuries. Lancet 1:265–266

Hutchinson PJ, Gupta AK, Fryer TF, Al-Rawi PG, Chatfield DA, Coles JP, O'Connell MT, Kett-White R, Minhas PS, Aigbirhio FI, Clark JC, Kirkpatrick PJ, Menon DK, Pickard JD (2002) Correlation between cerebral blood flow, substrate delivery, and metabolism in head injury: a combined microdialysis and triple oxygen positron emission tomography study. J Cereb Blood Flow Metab 22:735–745

Imberti R, Bellinzona G, Langer M (2002) Cerebral tissue PO_2 and $SjvO_2$ changes during moderate hyperventilation in patients with severe traumatic brain injury. J Neurosurg 96:97–102

Marion DW, Darby J, Yonas H (1991) Acute regional cerebral blood flow changes caused by severe head injuries. J Neurosurg 74:407–414

McLaughlin MR, Marion DW (1996) Cerebral blood flow and vasoresponsivity within and around cerebral contusions. J Neurosurg 85:871–876

Miller JD, Becker DP, Ward JD, Sullivan HG, Adams WE, Rosner MJ (1977) Significance of intracranial hypertension in severe head injury. J Neurosurg 47:503–510

Muizelaar JP, Marmarou A, DeSalles AA, Ward JD, Zimmerman RS, Li Z, Choi SC, Young HF (1989) Cerebral blood flow and metabolism in severely head-injured children. Part 1: relationship with GCS score, outcome, ICP, and PVI. J Neurosurg 71:63–71

Muizelaar JP, Marmarou A, Ward JD, Kontos HA, Choi SC, Becker DP, Gruemer H, Young HF (1991) Adverse effects of prolonged hyperventilation in patients with severe head injury: a randomized clinical trial. J Neurosurg 75:731–739

Neumann JO, Chambers IR, Citerio G, Enblad P, Gregson BA, Howells T, Mattern J, Nilsson P, Piper I, Ragauskas A, Sahuquillo J, Yau YH, Kiening K, BrainIT Group (2008) The use of hyperventilation therapy after traumatic brain injury in Europe: an analysis of the Brain IT Group. Intensive Care Med 34:1676–1682

Oertel M, Kelly DF, Lee JH, McArthur DL, Glenn TC, Vespa P, Boscardin WJ, Hovda DA, Martin NA (2002) Efficacy of hyperventilation, blood pressure elevation, and metabolic suppression therapy in controlling intracranial pressure after head injury. J Neurosurg 97:1045–1053

Raichle ME, Plum F (1972) Hyperventilation and cerebral blood flow. Stroke 3:566–575

Robertson CS, Clifton GL, Grossman RG, Ou CN, Goodman JC, Borum P, Bejot S, Barrodale P (1988) Alterations in cerebral availability of metabolic substrates after severe head injury. J Trauma 28:1523–1532

Ross DT, Graham DI, Adams JH (1993) Selective loss of neurons from the thalamic reticular nucleus following severe human head injury. J Neurotrauma 10:151–165

Salvant JB Jr, Muizelaar JP (1993) Changes in cerebral blood flow and metabolism related to the presence of subdural hematoma. Neurosurgery 33:387–393

Sheinberg M, Kanter MJ, Robertson CS, Contant CF, Narayan RK, Grossman RG (1992) Continuous monitoring of jugular venous oxygen saturation in head-injured patients. J Neurosurg 76:212–217

Sioutos PJ, Orozco JA, Carter LP, Weinand ME, Hamilton AJ, Williams FC (1995) Continuous regional cerebral cortical blood flow monitoring in head-injured patients. Neurosurgery 36:943–949

54 Osmotherapy

Jens Aage Kølsen-Petersen

Recommendations

Level I

There are insufficient data to support a Level I recommendation on this topic.

Level II

Mannitol is effective for control of raised intracranial pressure (ICP) at doses of 0.25–1 g/kg body weight. Arterial systolic blood pressure <90 mmHg should be avoided.

Level III

Restrict mannitol use prior to ICP monitoring to patients with signs of transtentorial herniation or progressive neurological deterioration not attributable to extracranial causes.

Hypertonic saline (HTS) is effective for control of increased ICP. HTS can be infused intravenously with or without added colloid as a bolus or continuous infusion in concentrations of 1.6–30%. Electrolytes should be monitored and plasma sodium maintained below 155 mmol/l.

The choice of mannitol or hypertonic saline as a first-line hyperosmolar agent should be left to the treating physician.

54.1 Overview

Reducing the volume of the intracranial content, decreasing ICP, and increasing CPP by drawing water out of the brain into the vascular compartment along an osmotic gradient is a cornerstone in the medical treatment of elevated ICP. Solutions of mannitol and hypertonic saline are effective and used frequently in clinical practice (White et al. 2006; Bhardwaj 2007). Both solutions exert an early effect on ICP due to optimising of rheological properties of the blood resulting in decreased blood viscosity and haematocrit, increasing cerebral blood flow (CBF) and oxygen delivery, and resulting in reflex autoregulatory vasoconstriction of cerebral arterioles that reduces CBV and ICP. This is followed by an osmotic shrinkage of brain cells that peaks after 15–30 min (Ziai et al. 2007).

In absence of definitive evidence regarding administration regimens related to different kinds of brain injury and side effects (e.g. kidney failure, rebound cerebral oedema), the clinician must weigh the value of long-standing clinical acceptance and safety (mannitol) against a newer, potentially more effective therapy with a limited clinical record (hypertonic saline).

J.A. Kølsen-Petersen
Department of Anaesthesia and Intensive Care,
Aarhus University Hospital,
Brendstrupgaardsvej 100,
Skejby, Aarhus N 8200, Denmark
e-mail: jaakp@dadlnet.dk

T. Sundstrøm et al. (eds.), *Management of Severe Traumatic Brain Injury*,
DOI 10.1007/978-3-642-28126-6_54, © Springer-Verlag Berlin Heidelberg 2012

Tips, Tricks, and Pitfalls

- When osmotherapy is required for intracranial hypertension, administer a bolus of 20% mannitol 0.25–1.0 g/kg or 250 ml 3% NaCl over 10–20 min. Alternatively, use a continuous IV infusion of 3% NaCl 1–2 ml/kg/h.
- Maintain Na between 145 and 155 mmol/l.
- Monitor sodium and potassium every 4 h. Allow Na to normalise gradually after ICP has been stabilised.

54.2 Background

The effect of circulating osmotic agents on the brain was first described by Weed and McKibben in 1919 using intravenous infusion of 30% NaCl solutions in doses from 2.2 to 8.8 ml/kg in cats (Weed and McKippen 1919). Later, hyperosmolar solutions of urea, glycerol, and sorbitol were used in the treatment of elevated ICP (Knapp 2005). These agents were largely replaced by mannitol in the 1960s (Knapp 2005). Within the last two decades, concentrated saline solutions have received renewed attention (Ogden et al. 2005). In this chapter, only mannitol and hypertonic saline will be discussed since they are the main substances used in current clinical practice (Bratton et al. 2007).

54.2.1 Mannitol

54.2.1.1 Mechanism of Action

The exact mechanism behind the ICP lowering effect of mannitol in the injured brain is still controversial (Bratton et al. 2007). It is generally proposed to be biphasic with an immediate effect on blood rheology followed by an osmotic effect on brain water (Diringer and Zazulia 2004; Knapp 2005; Ogden et al. 2005; Bratton et al. 2007). Infusion immediately lowers ICP because of cerebral autoregulatory vasoconstriction in response to (1) increased cerebral perfusion pressure and oxygenation due to osmotically induced plasma volume expansion and increased cardiac output (Rosner and Coley 1987; White et al. 2006) and/or (2) increased microcirculation due to shrinkage of erythrocytes and endothelial cells and decreased haematocrit and blood viscosity (Burke et al. 1981; Ogden et al. 2005). After 15–30 min, an osmotic gradient is established over the blood–brain barrier that draws water from the brain into the intravascular space (Paczynski 1997; Diringer and Zazulia 2004; Bratton et al. 2007). The water efflux depends on (1) the osmotic gradient created, (2) the osmotic reflection coefficient of the membrane for that solute (ranging from 0 to 1, where 1 is impermeable), and (3) the hydraulic conductivity of the membrane (Diringer and Zazulia 2004). Mannitol has a reflection coefficient of 0.9 over the intact blood–brain barrier.

Infusion of mannitol to normal rabbits and monkeys in clinical doses (Diringer and Zazulia 2004) and to brain injured rats in supra-clinical doses (Todd et al. 2006) reduces brain water by approximately 2%. The rather modest decrease in brain water may explain why the initial ICP seems to be important for the ICP lowering effect of mannitol since the intracranial compliance curve is steeper at a higher pressure. In a recent meta-analysis of 18 clinical studies, it was found that the ICP decrease was significantly greater when initial ICP was higher than 30 mmHg compared to when it was lower. The dose of mannitol seemed of less importance (Sorani and Manley 2008).

A longer-lasting effect on ICP, though never satisfactorily documented, has been attributed to accelerated absorption of cerebrospinal fluid brought about by the plasma hyperosmolarity (Paczynski 1997; White et al. 2006).

54.2.1.2 Dose and Pharmacokinetics

The recommended dose of mannitol for control of elevated ICP after traumatic brain injury is 0.25–1.0 g/kg body weight (Bratton et al. 2007). The peak ICP lowering effect is seen 15–30 min after infusion and last about 60 min (Sorani and Manley 2008), although a duration of 6 h or more can be seen (Bratton et al. 2007).

There are insufficient data to support a standard treatment (Bratton et al. 2007). Intermittent boluses may be as good as continuous infusion.

Mannitol is not metabolised in mammalian tissues and is excreted unchanged in the urine with an elimination half-life of 0.5–2.5 h (Paczynski 1997). In the presence of intact renal function, accumulation within tissues is unlikely to occur (Paczynski 1997).

54.2.1.3 Side Effects

Infusion of mannitol may cause hypotension that challenges the cerebral perfusion through two different mechanisms. First, rapid infusions may cause a decrease in systemic vascular resistance and hypotension especially in the hypovolemic patient (Paczynski 1997). However, it is rarely a clinical problem during infusions of 0.5–1.5 g/kg over 15–30 min (Paczynski 1997). Second, mannitol is a strong osmotic diuretic that may cause a diuresis five times the infused volume (Paczynski 1997). Hence, a reduction in intravascular volume often accompanies infusion rendering the patient at risk for hypovolaemia (Knapp 2005). Consequently, appropriate fluid replacement is important, e.g. with 0.9% sodium chloride. A Foley catheter is recommended.

Mannitol is excreted unchanged in the urine, and a serum osmolality >320 mOsm/l has been associated with acute tubular necrosis and renal failure (Knapp 2005). However, the data supporting this are limited and come from studies with hypovolemic patients (Diringer and Zazulia 2004; Knapp 2005).

Infusion of hyperosmolar solutions leads to plasma dilution and acute hyponatremia followed by osmotic diuresis with a loss of 'free water' that results in hypernatremia (Paczynski 1997). Potassium, phosphate, and magnesium are lost in the urine putting the patient at risk for electrolyte disturbances (Paczynski 1997). Hyperkalemia has also been reported after infusion of mannitol in clinical doses (Hassan et al. 2007), even complicated with ventricular tachycardia (Seto et al. 2000). Measuring electrolytes and serum osmolality every 2–6 h has been proposed (Knapp 2005).

Continuous or repeated administration of mannitol may lead to osmotic equilibration between the intra- and extracellular compartments through accumulation of intracellular osmolytes in the brain and risk of rebound cerebral oedema when the hyperosmolar infusion is stopped (Diringer and Zazulia 2004). Furthermore, mannitol may cross even the intact (reflection coefficient 0.9) and especially the injured BBB and cause water movement back into the brain (Diringer and Zazulia 2004). There may be a risk of midline shift in the presence of a unilateral lesion (Diringer and Zazulia 2004). However, mannitol is not metabolically trapped in the brain, and there is no reason not to expect that it would exit the way it entered, down its concentration gradient (Diringer and Zazulia 2004). The matter of rebound cerebral oedema after mannitol administration is controversial (Paczynski 1997; Diringer and Zazulia 2004).

54.2.1.4 Clinical Studies

In a recent Cochrane review on mannitol for traumatic brain injury (Wakai et al. 2007), only four randomised controlled clinical studies were found (Schwartz et al. 1984; Smith et al. 1986; Sayre et al. 1996; Vialet et al. 2003). The authors of the Cochrane review concluded that there is insufficient reliable evidence to make recommendations on the use of mannitol in the management of patients with traumatic brain injury (Wakai et al. 2007). The latest guidelines from the Brain Trauma Foundation states that mannitol is effective for control of raised intracranial pressure (level II evidence) and that use of mannitol prior to ICP monitoring should be restricted to patients with signs of transtentorial herniation or progressive neurological deterioration not attributable to extracranial causes (level III evidence) (Bratton et al. 2007).

In a Cochrane review on mannitol for acute ischaemic stroke or non-traumatic intracerebral haemorrhage (Bereczki et al. 2007), three randomised controlled trials were found involving a total of 226 patients (Santambrogio et al. 1978; Kalita et al. 2004; Misra et al. 2005). Based on this review, there is not enough evidence to decide if mannitol improves survival or prevents disability after stoke. The routine use of mannitol in all patients with acute stroke is not recommended (Bereczki et al. 2007).

Mannitol has been used to treat cerebral oedema of other causes, such as acute liver failure (Stravitz et al. 2007; Wendon and Lee 2008), subarachnoid haemorrhage (Jafar et al. 1986; Heuer et al. 2004), and tumour, though corticosteroids are the mainstay therapy for the latter (Kaal and Vecht 2004).

Although mannitol is a time-honoured means of treating intracranial hypertension, hypertonic saline is emerging as an alternative. Hypertonic saline (HTS) is efficacious in the treatment of cerebral oedema and elevations in ICP even in cases refractory to mannitol (Ogden et al. 2005; White et al. 2006; Bhardwaj 2007; Tyagi et al. 2007; Ziai et al. 2007)

54.2.2 Hypertonic Saline

54.2.2.1 Mechanism of Action

The principal ICP-lowering effect of hypertonic saline (HTS) infusion is possibly due to osmotic mobilisation of water from the brain to the intravascular space (Ogden et al. 2005; Bratton et al. 2007; Tyagi et al. 2007). Sodium chloride has a reflection coefficient of 1.0 over the intact blood–brain barrier making it, theoretically, more efficient than mannitol (reflection coefficient 0.9) (Bhardwaj 2007; Himmelseher 2007). It appears from animal studies that the integrity of the BBB is important for the effect of hypertonic saline (White et al. 2006). Thus, hypertonic crystalloid infusions (3–6.5%) primarily dehydrated the uninjured parts of the brain while the water content in the injured parts were unaffected by fluid tonicity (Wisner et al. 1990; Shackford et al. 1992). Similar results come from MRI scans of a patient with traumatic brain injury after infusion of 18% HTS (Saltarini et al. 2002).

Infusion of hypertonic saline has several other consequences that may benefit the brain. Plasma volume increases due to almost instantaneous mobilisation of water from the intracellular compartment of mainly erythrocytes and endothelial cells into the vascular fluid spaces along the osmotic gradient (Tølløfsrud et al. 1998). The MAP and hence the CPP is better preserved or even augmented compared to mannitol (Berger et al. 1994; Qureshi et al. 1999). A typical dose in trauma of 250 ml 7.5% NaCl expands plasma volume by about two to three times the infused volume (Vassar and Holcroft 1992; Kramer 2003; Järvelä et al. 2003).

In addition to increased preload, HTS infusion decreases both right (Kien et al. 1991) and left ventricular afterload through hyperosmotic-induced arteriolar vasodilation (Read et al. 1960; Gazitùa et al. 1971; Goertz et al. 1995). Despite reports of short-lived hyperosmotic-induced impairment of cardiac contractility (Gazitùa et al. 1971), overall cardiac performance increases because of augmented preload and decreased afterload (Goertz et al. 1995). In a porcine model of haemorrhagic shock and brain injury, HTS resuscitation was found to decrease ICP and increase cerebral perfusion pressure, pial arteriolar diameter, cerebral blood flow, and cerebral oxygen delivery compared to resuscitation with Ringer's lactate (Schmoker et al. 1991; Shackford et al. 1994).

In addition to these salutary effects, HTS infusion improves the microcirculation through shrinkage of erythrocytes and ischaemic swollen endothelial cells (Mazzoni et al. 1989, 1990; Corso et al. 1998). Thus, enhanced microcirculation was demonstrated in animal visceral organs after resuscitation from haemorrhagic (Maningas 1987; Kreimeier et al. 1988, 1990; Behrman et al. 1991; Bauer et al. 1993; Vollmar et al. 1994; Corso et al. 1998) and endotoxic (Oi et al. 2000) shock compared to LR infusion (Pascual et al. 2003). Reduction of endothelial-leukocyte interaction decreases capillary plugging by activated sticking leukocytes which further augments nutritional flow (Nolte et al. 1992; Bauer et al. 1993; Vollmar et al. 1994; Härtl et al. 1997; Pascual et al. 2002). Recovery of the microcirculation may explain why both the resting membrane potential and cell volume changed towards pre-shock values after infusion of hypertonic saline compared to isotonic saline with equal amounts of Na and Cl in bled rats (Nakayama et al. 1985) and also why oxygen consumption (VO_2) returned to above baseline after resuscitation with HTS in haemorrhaged larger animals (Kramer et al. 1986; Kreimeier et al. 1990).

Finally, recent studies found hypertonicity to affect immune responses in animals and in human blood cell cultures. It was shown that hypertonicity attenuated neutrophil cytotoxicity (Hampton et al. 1994; Rosengren et al. 1994; Rizoli et al. 1998; Ciesla et al. 2000; Pascual et al. 2002) and at the same time up-regulated immunologic protection furnished by lymphocytes (Junger et al. 1997; Loomis et al. 2001, 2003). The few clinical studies, conducted to date, specifically addressing the immune effect of hypertonic saline infusion, showed little, if any, effect on markers of immune function, and large clinical trials did not convincingly demonstrate benefit in terms of morbidity or mortality (Kolsen-Petersen 2004). Whether the observed immunomodulatory properties of hypertonic saline infusion translate into a clinical significant effect is thus still an open question.

54.2.2.2 Dose and Pharmacokinetics

There is no evidence, yet, to support one concentration of sodium chloride or administration protocol over another for the control of elevated ICP (Bratton et al. 2007; Tyagi et al. 2007). HTS as both bolus and continuous infusions lowers ICP (Tyagi et al. 2007). Concentrations between 1.6% and 30% have been used successfully (Himmelseher 2007; Tyagi et al. 2007). Many studies used 200–300 ml of 3% NaCl since it is equi-osmolar with a 'standard' 20% mannitol regimen (White et al. 2006). The goal is ICP control with a sodium level between 145 and 155 mmol/l either through continuous infusion of 3% HTS solution 1–2 ml/kg/h (Bhardwaj 2007) or through repeated doses of 250 ml (White et al. 2006). Studies with hypotensive trauma patients including those with brain injury often use 250 ml 7.5% NaCl with or without added colloid (Wade et al. 1997a, b; Cooper et al. 2004) based on animal experiments (Dubick et al. 1995).

The pharmacokinetics were studied in healthy men after infusion of 7.5% NaCl 5 ml/kg over 30 min (Drobin and Hahn 2002). Plasma volume was increased by approximately 25% at the end of infusion and decreased over the next 240 min with a half-life about 60 min. The efficacy of ICP reduction and the exact duration of the ICP-lowering effect are difficult to predict in general. Most studies show that ICP remain decreased 1–2 h after infusion (Himmelseher 2007).

54.2.2.3 Side Effects

Infusion of hypertonic saline increases the plasma concentrations of sodium and chloride. The increase in Cl induces a hyperchloremic acidosis (Kolsen-Petersen et al. 2005) that is unlikely to be clinically relevant, except in the most severe cases (Gunnerson et al. 2006). The increase in Na depends on the dose, concentration, and speed of administration of the HTS solution (Kolsen-Petersen 2004). In trauma patients, Na generally reached 150–155 mM measured 30–60 min after infusion of 250 ml NaCl 7.5% with or without colloids over 1–5 min (Maningas et al. 1989; Vassar et al. 1991, 1993a, b; Mattox et al. 1991; Younes et al. 1992). Plasma Na exceeded 155 mM in one-tenth of trauma patients receiving a 250-ml bolus of HSD (Mattox et al. 1991; Younes et al. 1992). Sodium levels below 160 mEq/l are generally well tolerated without worsened outcome in the neurologic intensive care unit (Aiyagari et al. 2006). Thus, as long as plasma sodium is kept in the recommended range (145–155 mmol/l), the hypernatremia possibly benefits ICP and is unlikely to adversely affect outcome (White et al. 2006; Bhardwaj 2007; Himmelseher 2007).

A rapid increase in plasma Na in patients with chronic hyponatremia carries the risk of central pontine myelinolysis. Consequently, pre-existing chronic hyponatremia should be excluded before administration of hypertonic saline, especially in malnourished and alcoholics (Bratton et al. 2007). No human studies with HTS have demonstrated central pontine myelinolysis (Tyagi et al. 2007). Even a mean peak sodium concentration of 171 mmol/l after continuous infusion of 3% NaCl in a paediatric intensive care unit caused no signs on myelinolysis on MRI or post-mortem (Khanna et al. 2000; Peterson et al. 2000).

Highly concentrated sodium chloride infusions, albeit effective in reducing ICP, may impair the BBB and lead to increased water accumulation in the injured brain (Himmelseher 2007). Thus, infusion of 40 ml of 20% NaCl over 20 min 1–5 days after traumatic brain injury decreased the volume of the non-contused hemisphere whereas it increased the volume of the contused hemisphere based on quantitative assessments of CT scans (Lescot et al. 2006). The exact clinical relevance of this observation remains to be determined (Himmelseher 2007). As with mannitol, continuous osmotherapy with HTS may lead to accumulation of intracellular osmolytes and rebound oedema when serum sodium returns towards normal (Ogden et al. 2005; White et al. 2006).

Potassium has been reported to decrease by some authors because of dilution and urinary loss in exchange for sodium (Qureshi and Suarez 2000; Kolsen-Petersen et al. 2005). In other studies, however, a transient increase was found of about 0.5 mM after infusion of 7.5% NaCl 4 ml/kg (Kolsen-Petersen et al. 2005).

In a single study of resuscitation of burn patients, HTS was associated with a fourfold increase in acute renal failure compared with a historical control group receiving Ringer's lactate (Huang et al. 1995). However, no correlation was found between serum sodium and biochemical markers of kidney function in retrospective chart studies in kids with traumatic brain injury (Peterson et al. 2000) or adults with elevated ICP (Froelich et al. 2009) treated with continuous 3% HTS infusion. Nevertheless, patients with Na >155 mmol/l had a higher risk of developing blood urea nitrogen >8.9 mmol/l or creatinine >132.6 μmol/l (Froelich et al. 2009).

Dilution of normal human plasma with hypertonic saline significantly increased prothrombin (PT) and activated partial thromboplastin times (APTT) and decreased platelet aggregation when 10% or more of the plasma was replaced by 7.5% HTS raising concerns of potentially coagulopathy after HTS infusion (Reed et al. 1991). In a later experiments on euvolaemic and haemorrhaged swine, no coagulopathy was found after infusion of 4 ml/kg 7.5% NaCl with 6% dextran (Dubick et al. 1993). None of the clinical trials involving patients with active haemorrhage from penetrating or other non-tamponaded blunt injuries produced evidence that these solutions increase blood loss or mortality (Vassar and Holcroft 1992).

54.2.2.4 Clinical Studies

HTS solutions have been studied for resuscitation of patients with traumatic brain injury. Subgroup analysis in randomised prospective clinical trials with hypotensive trauma patients showed that infusion of 250 ml 7.5% NaCl with 6% dextran 70 (HSD) in addition to standard of care increased survival to discharge compared to Ringer's lactate alone (Vassar et al. 1991) and that the effect was caused by HSD (Vassar et al. 1993a). Subsequent analysis of individual patient data from trials comparing HSD with isotonic crystalloid solution included 223 hypotensive trauma patients with head injury and concluded that patients treated with HSD solutions are twice as likely to survive until discharge (Wade et al. 1997b). However, the only prospective randomised double-blinded trial of hypotensive patients with GCS<9 that compared prehospital infusion of 250 ml 7.5% NaCl and Ringer's lactate found no significant difference in mortality or neurologic outcome (Cooper et al. 2004). The study has been criticised partly on the grounds that the ICP-lowering effect of a single dose of HTS is temporary and that further doses or infusion may be needed in order to show benefit (White et al. 2006).

Control of ICP by repeated doses or infusion of HTS has been investigated in several small, mainly observational, or retrospective studies in both children and adults with traumatic brain injury (White et al. 2006; Bhardwaj 2007). From these studies, it appears that HTS solutions are efficacious in ameliorating cerebral oedema and reducing ICP after brain injury and surgery. However, definitive human trials using hard endpoints are lacking (White et al. 2006; Bhardwaj 2007).

HTS may also be effective in reducing non-trauma-related intracranial hypertension due to ischaemic stroke, tumour, subarachnoid haemorrhage, and acute liver failure (Ogden et al. 2005; White et al. 2006). The results, however, are based on small clinical or animal studies, and the effect on outcome is unknown.

54.2.3 Sugar or Salt?

Mannitol and HTS for treatment of elevated ICP have been compared in few studies using equi-osmolar regimens (White et al. 2006). Based on these animal experiments and small human trials, it appears that HTS may be more effective than mannitol in reducing ICP and has a longer duration of action (White et al. 2006; Ziai et al. 2007). HTS may even reduce ICP refractory to mannitol

Table 54.1 Comparison of mannitol and hypertonic saline

	Mannitol	Hypertonic saline
Dose	Bolus 0.25–1.0 g/kg = 1.25–5 ml/kg 20% mannitol	Infusion or bolus 250 ml 3% NaCl. Target [Na^+] 145–155 mmol/l
Effectiveness	Reflection coefficient 0.9. Effect may decrease with repeated administration	Reflection coefficient 1.0. Potentially greater and more prolonged effect. May work when mannitol refractory
Effect on mortality	Unknown	Unknown
Rheologic effect	Yes	Yes
Diuretic effect	Osmotic diuresis up to five times infused volume	Diuresis up to twice infused volume via increased ANP
Haemodynamic effect	Diuresis may compromise intravascular volume causing hypovolaemia and hypotension	Augments intravascular volume and maintains MAP, CVP, and CO. Increased microcirculation
Other effects	Antioxidant via free radical scavenging	Restores resting membrane potential and cell volume. Immunomodulatory
Maximum serum osmolality (mOsm/l)	320	360
Potential for rebound oedema	Yes	Yes
Half-life	2–4 h	Unknown
Known and potential adverse effects	Hypotension, rebound elevation in ICP, hypokalaemia, haemolysis, and renal failure	Rebound elevation in ICP, hypo- and hyperkalaemia, congestive heart failure, haemolysis, coagulopathy, and central pontine myelinolysis

Adapted after (Ziai et al. 2007) and (Knapp 2005)
ANP atrial natriuretic peptide, *MAP* mean arterial pressure, *CVP* central venous pressure, *CO* cardiac output

administration (Ziai et al. 2007). Whether this leads to decreased mortality is unknown.

The two regimens are compared in Table 54.1.

54.3 Specific Paediatric Concerns

Due to the paucity of class I and II studies focused on the paediatric age group (Adelson et al. 2003; Morrow and Pearson 2010), the recommendations in this chapter are mainly extrapolated from adult studies. This calls for further investigations in children aimed at identifying the best hyperosmolar agent, the optimal treatment regimen and evaluating the long-term neurology outcome.

References

Adelson PD, Bratton SL, Carney NA, Chesnut RM, du Coudray HE, Goldstein B, Kochanek PM, Miller HC, Partington MD, Selden NR, Warden CR, Wright DW (2003) Guidelines for the acute medical management of severe traumatic brain injury in infants, children, and adolescents. Chapter 11. Use of hyperosmolar therapy in the management of severe pediatric traumatic brain injury. Pediatr Crit Care Med 4:S40–S44

Aiyagari V, Deibert E, Diringer MN (2006) Hypernatremia in the neurologic intensive care unit: how high is too high? J Crit Care 21:163–172

Bauer M, Marzi I, Ziegenfuss T, Seeck G, Bühren V, Larsen R (1993) Comparative effects of crystalloid and small volume hypertonic hyperoncotic fluid resuscitation on hepatic microcirculation after hemorrhagic shock. Circ Shock 40:187–193

Behrman SW, Fabian TC, Kudsk KA, Proctor KG (1991) Microcirculatory flow changes after initial resuscitation of hemorrhagic shock with 7.5% hypertonic saline/6% dextran 70. J Trauma 31:589–598; discussion 599–596

Bereczki D, Fekete I, Prado GF, Liu M (2007) Mannitol for acute stroke. Cochrane Database Syst Rev (3):CD001153

Berger S, Schürer L, Härtl R, Deisböck T, Dautermann C, Murr R, Messmer K, Baethmann A (1994) 7.2% NaCl/10% dextran 60 versus 20% mannitol for treatment of intracranial hypertension. Acta Neurochir Suppl (Wien) 60:494–498

Bhardwaj A (2007) Osmotherapy in neurocritical care. Curr Neurol Neurosci Rep 7:513–521

Bratton SL, Chestnut RM, Ghajar J, McConnell Hammond FF, Harris OA, Hartl R, Manley GT, Nemecek A,

Newell DW, Rosenthal G, Schouten J, Shutter L, Timmons SD, Ullman JS, Videtta W, Wilberger JE, Wright DW (2007) Guidelines for the management of severe traumatic brain injury. II. Hyperosmolar therapy. J Neurotrauma 24(Suppl 1):S14–S20

Burke AM, Quest DO, Chien S, Cerri C (1981) The effects of mannitol on blood viscosity. J Neurosurg 55:550–553

Ciesla DJ, Moore EE, Zallen G, Biffl WL, Silliman CC (2000) Hypertonic saline attenuation of polymorphonuclear neutrophil cytotoxicity: timing is everything. J Trauma 48:388–395

Cooper DJ, Myles PS, McDermott FT, Murray LJ, Laidlaw J, Cooper G, Tremayne AB, Bernard SS, Ponsford J, HTS Study Investigators (2004) Prehospital hypertonic saline resuscitation of patients with hypotension and severe traumatic brain injury: a randomized controlled trial. JAMA 291:1350–1357

Corso CO, Okamoto S, Leiderer R, Messmer K (1998) Resuscitation with hypertonic saline dextran reduces endothelial cell swelling and improves hepatic microvascular perfusion and function after hemorrhagic shock. J Surg Res 80:210–220

Diringer MN, Zazulia AR (2004) Osmotic therapy: fact and fiction. Neurocrit Care 1:219–233

Drobin D, Hahn RG (2002) Kinetics of isotonic and hypertonic plasma volume expanders. Anesthesiology 96:1371–1380

Dubick MA, Davis JM, Myers T, Wade CE, Kramer GC (1995) Dose response effects of hypertonic saline and dextran on cardiovascular responses and plasma volume expansion in sheep. Shock 3:137–144

Dubick MA, Kilani AF, Summary JJ, Greene JY, Wade CE (1993) Further evaluation of the effects of 7.5% sodium chloride/6% Dextran-70 (HSD) administration on coagulation and platelet aggregation in hemorrhaged and euvolemic swine. Circ Shock 40:200–205

Froelich M, Ni Q, Wess C, Ougorets I, Härtl R (2009) Continuous hypertonic saline therapy and the occurrence of complications in neurocritically ill patients. Crit Care Med 37:1433–1441

Gazitùa S, Scott JB, Swindall B, Haddy FJ (1971) Resistance responses to local changes in plasma osmolality in three vascular beds. Am J Physiol 220:384–391

Goertz AW, Mehl T, Lindner KH, Rockemann MG, Schirmer U, Schwilk B, Georgieff M (1995) Effect of 7.2% hypertonic saline/6% hetastarch on left ventricular contractility in anesthetized humans. Anesthesiology 82:1389–1395

Gunnerson KJ, Saul M, He S, Kellum JA (2006) Lactate versus non-lactate metabolic acidosis: a retrospective outcome evaluation of critically ill patients. Crit Care 10:R22

Hampton MB, Chambers ST, Vissers MC, Winterbourn CC (1994) Bacterial killing by neutrophils in hypertonic environments. J Infect Dis 169:839–846

Härtl R, Medary MB, Ruge M, Arfors KE, Ghahremani F, Ghajar J (1997) Hypertonic/hyperoncotic saline attenuates microcirculatory disturbances after traumatic brain injury. J Trauma 42:S41–S47

Hassan ZU, Kruer JJ, Fuhrman TM (2007) Electrolyte changes during craniotomy caused by administration of hypertonic mannitol. J Clin Anesth 19:307–309

Heuer GG, Smith MJ, Elliott JP, Winn HR, LeRoux PD (2004) Relationship between intracranial pressure and other clinical variables in patients with aneurysmal subarachnoid hemorrhage. J Neurosurg 101:408–416

Himmelseher S (2007) Hypertonic saline solutions for treatment of intracranial hypertension. Curr Opin Anaesthesiol 20:414–426

Huang PP, Stucky FS, Dimick AR, Treat RC, Bessey PQ, Rue LW (1995) Hypertonic sodium resuscitation is associated with renal failure and death. Ann Surg 221:543–554; discussion 554–557

Jafar JJ, Johns LM, Mullan SF (1986) The effect of mannitol on cerebral blood flow. J Neurosurg 64:754–759

Järvelä K, Koskinen M, Kööbi T (2003) Effects of hypertonic saline (7.5%) on extracellular fluid volumes in healthy volunteers. Anaesthesia 58:878–881

Junger WG, Coimbra R, Liu FC, Herdon-Remelius C, Junger W, Junger H, Loomis W, Hoyt DB, Altman A (1997) Hypertonic saline resuscitation: a tool to modulate immune function in trauma patients? Shock 8:235–241

Kaal EC, Vecht CJ (2004) The management of brain edema in brain tumors. Curr Opin Oncol 16:593–600

Kalita J, Misra UK, Ranjan P, Pradhan PK, Das BK (2004) Effect of mannitol on regional cerebral blood flow in patients with intracerebral hemorrhage. J Neurol Sci 224:19–22

Khanna S, Davis D, Peterson B, Fisher B, Tung H, O'Quigley J, Deutsch R (2000) Use of hypertonic saline in the treatment of severe refractory posttraumatic intracranial hypertension in pediatric traumatic brain injury. Crit Care Med 28:1144–1151

Kien ND, Kramer GC, White DA (1991) Acute hypotension caused by rapid hypertonic saline infusion in anesthetized dogs. Anesth Analg 73:597–602

Knapp JM (2005) Hyperosmolar therapy in the treatment of severe head injury in children: mannitol and hypertonic saline. AACN Clin Issues 16:199–211

Kolsen-Petersen JA (2004) Immune effect of hypertonic saline: fact or fiction? Acta Anaesthesiol Scand 48:667–678

Kolsen-Petersen JA, Nielsen JO, Tonnesen E (2005) Acid base and electrolyte changes after hypertonic saline (7.5%) infusion: a randomized controlled clinical trial. Scand J Clin Lab Invest 65:13–22

Kramer GC (2003) Hypertonic resuscitation: physiologic mechanisms and recommendations for trauma care. J Trauma 54:S89–S99

Kramer GC, Perron PR, Lindsey DC, Ho HS, Gunther RA, Boyle WA, Holcroft JW (1986) Small-volume resuscitation with hypertonic saline dextran solution. Surgery 100:239–247

Kreimeier U, Brückner UB, Messmer K (1988) Improvement of nutritional blood flow using hypertonic- hyperoncotic solutions for primary treatment of hemorrhagic hypotension. Eur Surg Res 20:277–279

Kreimeier U, Brueckner UB, Schmidt J, Messmer K (1990) Instantaneous restoration of regional organ blood flow after severe hemorrhage: effect of small-volume resuscitation with hypertonic- hyperoncotic solutions. J Surg Res 49:493–503

Lescot T, Degos V, Zouaoui A, Preteux F, Coriat P, Puybasset L (2006) Opposed effects of hypertonic saline on contusions and noncontused brain tissue in patients with severe traumatic brain injury. Crit Care Med 34(12): 3029–3033

Loomis WH, Namiki S, Hoyt DB, Junger WG (2001) Hypertonicity rescues T cells from suppression by trauma-induced anti- inflammatory mediators. Am J Physiol Cell Physiol 281:C840–C848

Loomis WH, Namiki S, Ostrom RS, Insel PA, Junger WG (2003) Hypertonic stress increases T cell interleukin-2 expression through a mechanism that involves ATP release, P2 receptor, and p38 MAPK activation. J Biol Chem 278:4590–4596

Maningas PA (1987) Resuscitation with 7.5% NaCl in 6% dextran-70 during hemorrhagic shock in swine: effects on organ blood flow. Crit Care Med 15:1121–1126

Maningas PA, Mattox KL, Pepe PE, Jones RL, Feliciano DV, Burch JM (1989) Hypertonic saline-dextran solutions for the prehospital management of traumatic hypotension. Am J Surg 157:528–533; discussion 533–534

Mattox KL, Maningas PA, Moore EE, Mateer JR, Marx JA, Aprahamian C, Burch JM, Pepe PE (1991) Prehospital hypertonic saline/dextran infusion for post-traumatic hypotension. The U.S.A. Multicenter Trial. Ann Surg 213:482–491

Mazzoni MC et al (1989) Lumenal narrowing and endothelial cell swelling in skeletal muscle capillaries during hemorrhagic shock. Circ Shock 29:27–39

Mazzoni MC, Borgström P, Intaglietta M, Arfors KE (1990) Capillary narrowing in hemorrhagic shock is rectified by hyperosmotic saline-dextran reinfusion. Circ Shock 31:407–418

Misra UK, Kalita J, Ranjan P, Mandal SK (2005) Mannitol in intracerebral hemorrhage: a randomized controlled study. J Neurol Sci 234:41–45

Morrow SE, Pearson M (2010) Management strategies for severe closed head injuries in children. Semin Pediatr Surg 19:279–285

Nakayama S, Kramer GC, Carlsen RC, Holcroft JW (1985) Infusion of very hypertonic saline to bled rats: membrane potentials and fluid shifts. J Surg Res 38:180–186

Nolte D, Bayer M, Lehr HA, Becker M, Krombach F, Kreimeier U, Messmer K (1992) Attenuation of postischemic microvascular disturbances in striated muscle by hyperosmolar saline dextran. Am J Physiol 263:H1411–H1416

Ogden AT, Mayer SA, Connolly ESJ (2005) Hyperosmolar agents in neurosurgical practice: the evolving role of hypertonic saline. Neurosurgery 57:207–215

Oi Y, Aneman A, Svensson M, Ewert S, Dahlqvist M, Haljamäe H (2000) Hypertonic saline-dextran improves intestinal perfusion and survival in porcine endotoxin shock. Crit Care Med 28:2843–2850

Paczynski RP (1997) Osmotherapy. Basic concepts and controversies. Crit Care Clin 13:105–129

Pascual JL, Ferri LE, Seely AJ, Campisi G, Chaudhury P, Giannias B, Evans DC, Razek T, Michel RP, Christou NV (2002) Hypertonic saline resuscitation of hemorrhagic shock diminishes neutrophil rolling and adherence to endothelium and reduces in vivo vascular leakage. Ann Surg 236:634–642

Pascual JL, Khwaja KA, Chaudhury P, Christou NV (2003) Hypertonic saline and the microcirculation. J Trauma 54:S133–S140

Peterson B, Khanna S, Fisher B, Marshall L (2000) Prolonged hypernatremia controls elevated intracranial pressure in head-injured pediatric patients. Crit Care Med 28:1136–1143

Qureshi AI, Suarez JI (2000) Use of hypertonic saline solutions in treatment of cerebral edema and intracranial hypertension. Crit Care Med 28:3301–3313

Qureshi AI, Wilson DA, Traystman RJ (1999) Treatment of elevated intracranial pressure in experimental intracerebral hemorrhage: comparison between mannitol and hypertonic saline. Neurosurgery 44:1055–1063

Read RC, Johnson JA, Vick JA, Meyer MW (1960) Vascular effects of hypertonic solutions. Circ Res 8: 538–548

Reed RL 2nd, Johnston TD, Chen Y, Fischer RP (1991) Hypertonic saline alters plasma clotting times and platelet aggregation. J Trauma 31:8–14

Rizoli SB, Kapus A, Fan J, Li YH, Marshall JC, Rotstein OD (1998) Immunomodulatory effects of hypertonic resuscitation on the development of lung inflammation following hemorrhagic shock. J Immunol 161: 6288–6296

Rosengren S, Henson PM, Worthen GS (1994) Migration-associated volume changes in neutrophils facilitate the migratory process in vitro. Am J Physiol 267: C1623–C1632

Rosner MJ, Coley I (1987) Cerebral perfusion pressure: a hemodynamic mechanism of mannitol and the post-mannitol hemogram. Neurosurgery 21:147–156

Saltarini M, Massarutti D, Baldassarre M, Nardi G, De Colle C, Fabris G (2002) Determination of cerebral water content by magnetic resonance imaging after small volume infusion of 18% hypertonic saline solution in a patient with refractory intracranial hypertension. Eur J Emerg Med 9:262–265

Santambrogio S, Martinotti R, Sardella F, Porro F, Randazzo A (1978) Is there a real treatment for stroke? Clinical and statistical comparison of different treatments in 300 patients. Stroke 9:130–132

Sayre MR, Daily SW, Stern SA, Storer DL, van Loveren HR, Hurst JM (1996) Out-of-hospital administration of mannitol to head-injured patients does not change systolic blood pressure. Acad Emerg Med 3:840–848

Schmoker JD, Zhuang J, Shackford SR (1991) Hypertonic fluid resuscitation improves cerebral oxygen delivery and reduces intracranial pressure after hemorrhagic shock. J Trauma 31:1607–1613

Schwartz ML, Tator CH, Rowed DW, Reid SR, Meguro K, Andrews DF (1984) The University of Toronto head injury treatment study: a prospective, randomized comparison of pentobarbital and mannitol. Can J Neurol Sci 11:434–440

Seto A, Murakami M, Fukuyama H, Niijima K, Aoyama K, Takenaka I, Kadoya T (2000) Ventricular tachycardia caused by hyperkalemia after administration of hypertonic mannitol. Anesthesiology 93:1359–1361

Shackford SR, Schmoker JD, Zhuang J (1994) The effect of hypertonic resuscitation on pial arteriolar tone after brain injury and shock. J Trauma 37:899–908

Shackford SR, Zhuang J, Schmoker J (1992) Intravenous fluid tonicity: effect on intracranial pressure, cerebral blood flow, and cerebral oxygen delivery in focal brain injury. J Neurosurg 76:91–98

Smith HP, Kelly DL Jr, McWhorter JM, Armstrong D, Johnson R, Transou C, Howard G (1986) Comparison of mannitol regimens in patients with severe head injury undergoing intracranial monitoring. J Neurosurg 65:820–824

Sorani MD, Manley GT (2008) Dose–response relationship of mannitol and intracranial pressure: a meta-analysis. J Neurosurg 108:80–87

Stravitz RT, Kramer AH, Davern T, Shaikh AO, Caldwell SH, Mehta RL, Blei AT, Fontana RJ, McGuire BM, Rossaro L, Smith AD, Lee WM, Acute Liver Failure Study Group (2007) Intensive care of patients with acute liver failure: recommendations of the U.S. Acute Liver Failure Study Group. Crit Care Med 35:2498–2508

Todd MM, Cutkomp J, Brian JE (2006) Influence of mannitol and furosemide, alone and in combination, on brain water content after fluid percussion injury. Anesthesiology 105:1176–1181

Tølløfsrud S, Tønnessen T, Skraastad O, Noddeland H (1998) Hypertonic saline and dextran in normovolaemic and hypovolaemic healthy volunteers increases interstitial and intravascular fluid volumes. Acta Anaesthesiol Scand 42:145–153

Tyagi R, Donaldson K, Loftus CM, Jallo J (2007) Hypertonic saline: a clinical review. Neurosurg Rev 30:277–289

Vassar MJ, Fischer RP, O'Brien PE, Bachulis BL, Chambers JA, Hoyt DB, Holcroft JW (1993a) A multicenter trial for resuscitation of injured patients with 7.5% sodium chloride. The effect of added dextran 70. The Multicenter Group for the study of hypertonic saline in trauma patients. Arch Surg 128:1003–1011

Vassar MJ, Holcroft JW (1992) Use of hypertonic-hyperoncotic fluids for resuscitation of trauma patients. J Int Care Med 7:189–198

Vassar MJ, Perry CA, Gannaway WL, Holcroft JW (1991) 7.5% sodium chloride/dextran for resuscitation of trauma patients undergoing helicopter transport. Arch Surg 126:1065–1072

Vassar MJ, Perry CA, Holcroft JW (1993b) Prehospital resuscitation of hypotensive trauma patients with 7.5% NaCl versus 7.5% NaCl with added dextran: a controlled trial. J Trauma 34:622–632; discussion 632–633

Vialet R, Albanèse J, Thomachot L, Antonini F, Bourgouin A, Alliez B, Martin C (2003) Isovolume hypertonic solutes (sodium chloride or mannitol) in the treatment of refractory posttraumatic intracranial hypertension: 2 mL/kg 7.5% saline is more effective than 2 mL/kg 20% mannitol. Crit Care Med 31:1683–1687

Vollmar B, Lang G, Menger MD, Messmer K (1994) Hypertonic hydroxyethyl starch restores hepatic microvascular perfusion in hemorrhagic shock. Am J Physiol 266:H1927–H1934

Wade CE, Kramer GC, Grady JJ, Fabian TC, Younes RN (1997a) Efficacy of hypertonic saline dextran (HSD) in patients with traumatic hypotension: meta-analysis of individual patient data. Acta Anaesthesiol Scand Suppl 110:77–79

Wade CE, Grady JJ, Kramer GC, Younes RN, Gehlsen K, Holcroft JW (1997b) Individual patient cohort analysis of the efficacy of hypertonic saline/dextran in patients with traumatic brain injury and hypotension. J Trauma 42:S61–S65

Wakai A, Roberts I, Schierhout G (2007) Mannitol for acute traumatic brain injury. Cochrane Database Syst Rev (1):CD001049

Weed LH, McKippen PS (1919) Experimental alteration of brain bulk. Am J Physiol 48:531–555

Wendon J, Lee W (2008) Encephalopathy and cerebral edema in the setting of acute liver failure: pathogenesis and management. Neurocrit Care 9:97–102

White H, Cook D, Venkatesh B (2006) The use of hypertonic saline for treating intracranial hypertension after traumatic brain injury. Anesth Analg 102:1836–1846

Wisner DH, Schuster L, Quinn C (1990) Hypertonic saline resuscitation of head injury: effects on cerebral water content. J Trauma 30:75–78

Younes RN, Aun F, Accioly CQ, Casale LP, Szajnbok I, Birolini D (1992) Hypertonic solutions in the treatment of hypovolemic shock: a prospective, randomized study in patients admitted to the emergency room. Surgery 111:380–385

Ziai WC, Toung TJ, Bhardwaj A (2007) Hypertonic saline: first-line therapy for cerebral edema? J Neurol Sci 261:157–166

Barbiturates for ICP Management 55

Mads Rasmussen

Recommendations

Level I

There are insufficient data to support a Level I recommendation for this topic.

Level II

Prophylactic administration of barbiturates to induce burst suppression EEG is not recommended.

High-dose barbiturate administration is recommended to control elevated ICP refractory to maximum standard medical and surgical treatment. Hemodynamic stability is essential before and during barbiturate therapy.

Level III

No barbiturate regimen has been shown to be superior to another.

M. Rasmussen
Department of Anaesthesia, Section of Neuroanaesthesia, Aarhus University Hospital,
Nørrebrogade 44, 8000 Aarhus C, Denmark
e-mail: mads.rasmussen@vest.rm.dk, mads.rasmussen@ki.au.dk

55.1 Overview

The ICP-lowering and cerebral protective effects of barbiturates are believed to be due to the coupling of cerebral blood flow to regional cerebral metabolic demand. By suppression of cerebral metabolic demand, barbiturates reduce cerebral metabolism and thereby lowers cerebral blood flow and cerebral blood volume and thus ICP. Other effects of barbiturates include alterations in vascular tone and resistance and inhibition of excitotoxicity (Shapro 1985).

During the last six decades, barbiturates have been used to manage high ICP (Horsley 1937).

Currently, high dosages of barbiturates are used in patients with severe head injury and high ICP refractory to standard medical and surgical treatment. This practice is recommended by the Brain Trauma Foundation Guidelines because this is the only second-level measure for which there is level II evidence to reduce intracranial pressure (Brain Trauma Foundation Guidelines 2007).

A systematic review conducted by the Cochrane injuries group concluded that there is no evidence that barbiturate therapy in patients with severe head injury improves outcome. Barbiturate therapy results in a fall in blood pressure in one of four patients. This hypotensive effect may offset any ICP-lowering effect on cerebral perfusion pressure (Roberts and Sydenham 2009).

A number of different therapeutic regimens using thiopental have been applied. No documentation

T. Sundstrøm et al. (eds.), *Management of Severe Traumatic Brain Injury*,
DOI 10.1007/978-3-642-28126-6_55, © Springer-Verlag Berlin Heidelberg 2012

has been presented, however, that one regimen is superior to another. I suggest the following protocol:

Use a loading dose of 10 mg/kg over 30 min followed by infusion of 5 mg/kg/h for 3 h and a subsequent infusion of 1–3 mg/kg/h thereafter. If the effect is absent after the initial 30 min, it is unlikely that barbiturate therapy will work and you should discontinue further thiopentone infusion. The need for barbiturate therapy can be re-evaluated. An electroencephalographic monitoring may be used to evaluate the existence of a burst suppression pattern, which implies near maximal reduction in cerebral metabolism.

Tips, Tricks, and Pitfalls

- Only initiate barbiturate therapy in hemodynamically stable patients. Patients may receive vasopressors, but they must not be hypotensive.
- Use barbiturate therapy in patients with ICP greater than 20 mmHg refractory to other standard treatments with appropriate sedation (propofol/midazolam), mannitol, hypertonic saline, ventricular drainage, and moderate hyperventilation (3.6–4.5 kPa)

55.2 Background

55.2.1 Effect of Barbiturate Therapy on Intracranial Pressure

Two studies have examined the effect of barbiturate administration on intracranial pressure. Eisenberg et al. randomly assigned 73 patients with severe head injury, GCS of 4–8, and intractable ICP to either pentobarbital or no pentobarbital (Eisenberg et al. 1988). The results indicated a 2:1 benefit for those treated with pentobarbital with regard to ICP control. A smaller proportion of the patients in the barbiturate group had uncontrolled ICP (68% versus 83%). The relative risk for uncontrolled ICP was 0.81 (95% CI 0.62–1.06).

Ward et al. (1985) allocated 53 patients with severe head injury to receive either pentobarbital or no pentobarbital (Ward et al. 1985). Similar to the Eisenberg study, mean ICP was lower in the barbiturate-treated patients. There was no difference in 1-year mortality. Hypotension (systolic blood pressure <80 mmHg) occurred in 54% of the patients in the pentobarbital group and in 7% of the patients in the control group.

55.2.2 Barbiturate Therapy Versus Mannitol: Effect on Intracranial Pressure

Schwartz et al. compared prophylactic pentobarbital and mannitol for ICP control in 59 patients with severe head injury. Pentobarbital was less effective than mannitol for control of elevated ICP, and there was no difference in mortality between the two drugs (RR = 1.21; 95% CI 0.75–1.94) (Schwartz et al. 1984).

55.2.3 Penthobarbital Versus Thiopental for ICP Control

Pérez-Bárcena et al. randomized 44 patients suffering from severe head injury to either pentobarbital or thiopental. Inclusion criteria were GCS < 8 after resuscitation or neurological deterioration during the first week after trauma and with an ICP > 20 mmHg refractory to first tier measures as defined by the Brain Trauma Foundation. Fewer patients had uncontrollable ICP with thiopental. There was no significant difference with regard to neurological outcome. Incidence of hypotension was equal in the two groups (Pérez-Bárcena et al. 2008).

55.2.4 Systematic Review of Barbiturate-Randomized Controlled Trials

In 1999 and 2009, the Cochrane injuries group completed a systematic review of barbiturates for acute traumatic brain injury. They included data from six trials. The pooled risk ratio for death (barbiturate vs. no barbiturate) was 1.09 (95% CI 0.81–1.47). Two randomized studies examined the effect of barbiturates on ICP. In one study, the results indicated that ICP was better controlled with barbiturate treatment. In another study, however, there was no effect on ICP with prophylactic barbiturate treatment. Barbiturate therapy is associated with increased incidence of hypotension (RR = 1.80; 95% CI 1.19–2.70) (Roberts and Sydenham 2009).

55.3 Specific Pediatric Concerns

There is only limited information on the use of barbiturates in pediatric head injury. Similar to the adult recommendations, the recent guidelines for the management of pediatric severe traumatic brain injury suggest that barbiturates may be effective in lowering high ICP refractory to medical and surgical therapy. They suggested the therapeutic regime as mentioned in Sect. 55.1 (Adelson et al. 2003).

References

Adelson PD, Bratton SL, Carney NA, Chesnut RM, du Coudray HE, Goldstein B, Kochanek PM, Miller HC, Partington MD, Selden NR, Warden CR, Wright DW, American Association for Surgery of Trauma, Child Neurology Society, International Society for Pediatric Neurosurgery, International Trauma Anesthesia and Critical Care Society, Society of Critical Care Medicine, World Federation of Pediatric Intensive and Critical Care Societies (2003) Guidelines for the management of severe traumatic head injury in infants, children and adolescents. Chapter 13. The use of barbiturates in the control of intracranial hypertension in severe pediatric brain injury. Pediatr Crit Care Med 4(3 suppl):S49–S52

Eisenberg HM, Frankowski RF, Contant CF, Marshall LF, Walker MD (1988) High-dose barbiturate control of elevated intracranial pressure in patients with severe head injury. J Neurosurg 69:15–23

Horsley JS (1937) The intracranial pressure during barbital narcosis. Lancet 1:141–143

Pérez-Bárcena J, Llompart-Pou JA, Homar J, Abadal JM, Raurich JM, Frontera G, Brell M, Ibáñez J, Ibáñez J (2008) Pentobarbital versus thiopental in the treatment of refractory intracranial hypertension in patients with traumatic brain injury: a randomized controlled trial. Crit Care 12(4):R112

Roberts I, Sydenham E (2009) Barbiturates for acute traumatic brain injury. Cochrane Database Syst Rev (4):CD 000033. doi 10.1002/14651858

Schwartz ML, Tator CH, Rowed DW, Reid SR, Meguro K, Andrews DF (1984) The University of Toronto head injury treatment study: a prospective, randomized comparison of pentobarbital and mannitol. Can J Neurol Sci 11:434–440

Shapro HM (1985) Barbiturates in brain ischemia. Br J Anaesth 57:82–95

The Brain Trauma Foundation: The American Association of Neurological Surgeons (2007) The Joint Section on Neurotrauma and Critical Care. Anesthetics, analgetics and sedatives. J Neurotrauma 24(suppl 1):71–76

Ward JD, Becker DP, Miller JD, Choi SC, Marmarou A, Wood C, Newlon PG, Keenan R (1985) Failure of prophylactic barbiturate coma in the treatment of severe head injury. J Neurosurg 62:383–388

Fluid Haemodynamics in Patients with Severe TBI

56

Per-Olof Grände and Niels Juul

Recommendations

Level I

There are insufficient data to support a Level I recommendation for a specific fluid therapy in TBI patients.

Level II

There has been one Level II study (the SAFE-TBI study) supporting the use of normal saline rather than 4% albumin in TBI patients.

Level III

There have been Level III studies supporting the use of albumin in TBI patients.

There are insufficient data to support the use of synthetic colloids in severe TBI.

P.-O. Grände (✉)
Department of Anaesthesia and Intensive Care, Lund University and Lund University Hospital, SE-22185 Lund, Sweden
e-mail: per-olof.grande@med.lu.se

N. Juul
Department of Anaesthesia, Aarhus University Hospital Noerrebrogade 44, DK-8000 Aarhus C, Denmark
e-mail: nielsjuul@privat.dk

56.1 Overview

The support for saline or other *crystalloid* solutions as the main plasma volume expanders in TBI patients is supported by the results of the SAFE-TBI study. This fluid regimen is cheaper than other fluid regimens using albumin or synthetic colloids. A crystalloid solution is distributed throughout the whole of the extracellular space of the body, which means that only 20–25% of the volume infused will stay intravascularly and the rest will be relatively quickly distributed to the interstitial space of the body. The maintenance of normovolemia with saline or other crystalloids therefore means the need for large volumes, resulting in interstitial oedema with potential side effects in terms of increased lung water, greater diffusion distances, and an increased risk of compartment syndrome. What may be more important in the TBI patient is that distribution of crystalloids will occur also to the brain interstitium, provided the blood–brain barrier (BBB) has become permeable for small solutes. There is apparently a risk that the use of saline will trigger the development of tissue oedema not only in organs away from the brain but also in the brain itself in TBI patients (Grände 2006; Jungner et al. 2010). Large volumes of saline may also induce adverse hyperchloraemic acidosis.

Albumin has a molecular weight of 69 kDa and is the most essential natural plasma protein. In contrast to synthetic colloids, all the molecules are of the same size, are negatively charged, and

T. Sundstrøm et al. (eds.), *Management of Severe Traumatic Brain Injury*,
DOI 10.1007/978-3-642-28126-6_56, © Springer-Verlag Berlin Heidelberg 2012

are not degraded to smaller molecules. As will be discussed below, the fact that albumin is not degraded may be an advantage by exerting a more sustained plasma volume expansion, but it may also be a disadvantage if albumin accumulates in the interstitium. Allergic reactions with albumin are rare. The protein concentration in plasma is reduced after a TBI, reflecting increased leakage of plasma proteins to the interstitium—being beyond the recirculation capacity of the lymphatic system. According to the 2-pore theory of transvascular fluid exchange (Rippe and Haraldsson 1994), plasma proteins are transferred to the interstitium through the relatively few large pores at the end of the capillary network and in venules, following the fluid stream mainly through convection. In the large pores, the hydrostatic pressure is the dominating force, as the transcapillary oncotic absorbing force is significantly reduced across the pores. This means that even in the normal state, there is a continuous leakage of plasma and plasma proteins from the intravascular space to the extravascular space across these pores, but the capacity of the recirculating lymphatic system is large enough to prevent hypovolaemia and tissue oedema. The loss of plasma fluid is dependent on the number of large pores and on the magnitude of the force of the hydrostatic pressure. This means that there is a risk that the more albumin infused to compensate for hypovolaemia, the more leakage of plasma fluid there will be. Thus, the use of albumin as plasma volume expander should include measures that reduce the transcapillary leakage to volumes below the capacity of the lymphatic system. According to physiological principles of transcapillary fluid exchange as described by the 2-pore theory, leakage of plasma fluid to the interstitium can be reduced by maintaining the hydrostatic capillary pressure low. This can be accomplished by avoiding high arterial pressures. The leakage can also be reduced using low infusion rates and higher concentrations of the albumin solution. Physiotherapy may also reduce the need for albumin by stimulating the lymphatic drainage system. As discussed below, avoidance of low haemoglobin concentrations may also reduce the need for albumin infusions.

By increasing the plasma oncotic pressure, albumin may induce absorption of fluid from the brain, provided BBB is permeable to small solutes (Tomita et al. 1994; Grände 2006; Jungner et al. 2010). This regime may be questioned if the BBB is disrupted to a large extent, resulting in leakage of albumin to the brain. However, considering the low protein concentration in cerebrospinal fluid of about 2 g/L at most after a severe head injury, most likely reflecting approximately the same concentrations in the brain interstitium, these concentrations are very low compared to the normal plasma protein concentration of approximately 60 g/L. Protein leakage cannot therefore have any significant influence on the transcapillary oncotic absorbing force in the brain. The plasma oncotic effect may help to maintain ICP at an adequate level or to reduce a raised ICP. There are insufficient data to give a general support for the use of synthetic colloids to severe TBI patients.

56.1.1 Erythrocyte Transfusion

No studies have been performed to date that can be used for guidance in the treatment with erythrocyte transfusion in patients with severe TBI. One study from Canada (Hébert et al. 1999) could not show any beneficial effects of erythrocyte transfusion in a general intensive care material, but no TBI patients were included and leukocyte-depleted blood was not used. A more recent study, on the other hand, showed that higher haemoglobin concentrations are associated with improved outcome after subarachnoid haemorrhage (Naidech et al. 2007), and another study showed improved oxygenation of red blood cell transfusion regardless of baseline haemoglobin concentration (Zygun et al. 2009). Due to the uncertainty regarding optimal haemoglobin concentration, very low haemoglobin concentrations down to 70 g/L (4.3 mmol/L) have been accepted in many neurointensive care units, while other units more or less normalize the haemoglobin concentration as recommended in the Lund concept (see Chap. 48).

Low haemoglobin concentrations mean larger plasma volume to maintain normovolemia. This means a greater need for plasma volume expanders to reach normovolemia from a hypovolemic state, which also means more transcapillary leakage of plasma and more tissue oedema according to the 2-pore theory. It has also been shown in the dog that plasma leakage to the interstitium is higher with a low haemoglobin concentration than with a more normal one (Valeri et al. 1986). These considerations indicate that haemoglobin concentration is of importance in the fluid therapy of TBI patients and a relatively normal haemoglobin level may be optimal. Normalization of a low haemoglobin value also improves oxygenation of the injured brain (Smith et al. 2005; Dhar et al. 2009), which is of added importance in TBI patients since avoidance of brain ischaemia is a most important issue in neurointensive care.

Blood transfusion does have side effects, however, especially proinflammatory effects when using non-leukocyte-depleted blood and when using blood stored for longer periods of time. Side effects of erythrocyte transfusion can be reduced by using leukocyte-depleted blood and fresher blood products, and the blood volume expanding effect and oxygenation effect of blood transfusion in TBI patients may override any potentially adverse effects.

56.1.2 How to Confirm the Status of the Volumetric State

A relatively normal protein and haemoglobin concentration may help to maintain an adequate intravascular volume. The use of Swan-Ganz catheters, PICCO catheters, and other advanced vascular-monitoring devices are rarely indicated in the treatment of TBI patients. The arterial blood pressure response on a bolus dose of a plasma volume expander or erythrocytes, the arterial blood pressure response following leg tilting, and the PPV index of the arterial curve may be tools by which to evaluate the volumetric state of the patient.

56.1.3 Guidance on Fluid Treatment with Crystalloids and Albumin

The use of crystalloids as plasma volume expander means that relatively large volumes must be infused to maintain normovolemia, and there is often a need for vasopressors to keep an adequate cerebral perfusion pressure. Be aware of the fact that this fluid therapy means general tissue oedema and that there is a potential risk of hyperchloraemic acidosis when using large volumes of saline.

Albumin should be used up to relatively normal albumin concentrations (33–38 g/L). Even though 20% albumin is to be preferred, also lower concentrations can be used. Avoid over-transfusion with albumin. In addition, a crystalloid solution should be used (e.g. 1–1.5 L/day for an adult) to maintain an adequate fluid balance and urine production.

The need for albumin as a plasma volume expander can be restricted by: (1) giving albumin at a low infusion rate (e.g. 100 mL of 20% albumin over 4 h), (2) avoiding high arterial pressures by avoiding vasopressors and sometimes using antihypertensive treatment, and (3) keeping the haemoglobin concentration at a relatively normal level (>120 g/L) (leukocyte-depleted and very recently stored erythrocytes should preferably be used).

56.1.4 Electrolytes

As with other patients in the intensive care setting, preservation of normal concentrations of electrolytes such as sodium, potassium, and chloride ions is important in patients with a severe head injury. The infusion of potassium should be adapted to maintain its concentration within normal limits of 3.6–4.4 mmol/L. High values of chloride ions should be avoided to avoid hyperchloraemic acidosis. It is especially emphasized that low concentrations of sodium may have severe adverse effects in head-injured patients as hyponatraemia can be associated with the development of brain oedema. If not adequately treated, hyponatraemia is quite common in these patients.

In the literature, hyponatraemia after a head injury has been classified by mainly two different syndromes, the cerebral salt-wasting syndrome (CSWS) and the syndrome of inappropriate secretion of antidiuretic hormone (SIADH). In CSWS, there is an elevation of brain natriuretic peptide (BNP) levels, which results in reduction in the efficacy of aldosterone and hence reduction in the ability to reabsorb sodium in the kidneys, resulting in excretion of salt in the urine. The SIADH is more common in neurological patients and results from an excessive secretion of antidiuretic hormone; water is retained with risk of hypervolaemia and reduced plasma sodium and should be treated with sodium substitution in combination with diuretics. CSWS is a rarer cause of hyponatraemia, but it may be diagnosed as hyponatraemia in combination with excessive production of slightly hypertonic urine. It should be treated with sodium substitution in combination with fluid substitution in volumes related to the amount of urine production. If the polyuria is extensive, the patient may be treated with low doses of ADH analogue. Adrenal gland failure may occur early after a traumatic brain injury and can be diagnosed from analysis of pituitary and adrenal hormones. If it results in severe hypoglycaemia, hypotension, and hyponatraemia, treatment with adrenocorticotrophin hormones can be considered.

56.1.5 Vasopressors

Previously, all traditional guidelines recommended the use of vasopressors to maintain a CPP of above 70 mmHg, and both inotropic support and vasoconstrictors such as phenylephrine and noradrenaline were used. By the change in the recommendations of CPP from a minimal value of 70 mmHg down to 50–60 mmHg in the most recent update of the US guidelines, the need for vasopressors has been reduced, if this guideline is followed.

With the Lund therapy, more or less complete avoidance of vasopressors is recommended. Still, CPP stays in the range of 60–70 mmHg in most patients using this guideline, due to a more strict avoidance of hypovolaemia by albumin infusions towards normal albumin concentration in plasma and by giving erythrocyte transfusion up to a relatively normal haemoglobin concentration. According to the principles behind the Lund therapy, the avoidance of vasopressors may reduce the increase in ICP, reduce the need for plasma volume expanders to maintain normovolemia, and result in a less compromised microcirculation and better oxygenation of hypoxic areas of the brain and in the rest of the body (see Chap. 48).

Tips, Tricks, and Pitfalls

If using a crystalloid as the main plasma volume expander, be aware that:

- Relatively large volumes are needed to maintain normovolaemia.
- Crystalloids are associated with general tissue oedema, including the injured brain.
- Saline is associated with hyperchloraemic acidosis.

If using albumin as main plasma volume expander, the need for albumin may be reduced by:

- Using high-concentration solutions
- Using low infusion rates
- Avoiding high blood pressures and vasopressors
- Avoiding low haemoglobin concentrations
- Frequent physiotherapy to activate the lymphatic recirculation system

56.2 Background

As in other trauma patients, the TBI patient suffers from a general increase in microvascular permeability resulting in an increase in transcapillary leakage of plasma fluid to the interstitium. This leakage results in hypovolaemia if the transcapillary escape rate (TER) (normally 5–6% of total plasma volume per hour) is increased above the capacity of the lymphatic recirculation system (Haskell et al. 1997). If not adequately treated, most patients with severe TBI suffer from hypovolaemia, resulting in activation of the baroreceptor reflex with increased sympathetic discharge and catecholamine release. Avoidance of hypovolaemia is essential in patients with severe TBI for maintenance of perfusion and oxygenation of the injured brain—and especially of the most injured parts of the brain (Rise et al. 1998). This means that there is a need for transfusion with blood volume expanders to restore blood volume to a normovolemic condition. Traditional guidelines for treatment of severe TBI give no recommendations on how to treat these patients regarding the type and strategy of fluid therapy. In principle, we lack generally accepted clinical studies that would be used for guidance on fluid treatment in these patients. Saline and albumin are the most common plasma volume expanders used in clinical practice today for TBI patients. The only randomized study regarding fluid therapy in TBI patients during ICU treatment to be published so far (The SAFE Study Investigators 2007) showed better outcome with normal saline than with 4% albumin, while other smaller studies have indicated beneficial effects with albumin (Tomita et al. 1994; Bernard et al. 2008; Rodling Wahlström et al. 2009; Jungner et al. 2010). The SAFE-TBI study has resulted in more frequent use of normal saline and other crystalloids and less frequent use of albumin during the last few years in many neurointensive care units all over the world. Neither the American Guidelines nor the European Brain Injury Consortium guidelines—in their original or updated versions for treatment of TBI—suggest any strategies for fluid management (Bullock et al. 1996; Maas et al. 1997; Stocchetti et al. 2001; The Brain Trauma Foundation 2007). Thus, no consensus about the type of fluid substitution, which volumes and infusion rates to use, or which concentration of albumin solution to use for an optimal fluid treatment has been developed. We also lack studies and recommendations about the optimal haemoglobin concentration in patients with severe TBI, an issue also of importance in maintaining an adequate blood volume, as erythrocytes comprise a large proportion of the blood volume. This is of added importance at a time where restraints, due to the risk of transfusion with contaminated blood, give rise to strict local criteria for blood transfusion. The two main blood volume expanding alternatives used today, crystalloids and albumin, in combination with their most important physiological features have been described above.

The unexpected results from the SAFE-TBI study may indicate that normal saline is a better choice than 4% albumin as plasma volume expander in TBI patients. The SAFE-TBI study can be criticized, however, for several reasons. As it represents a subgroup from a larger study, it can be criticized from a statistical point of view. Norepinephrine was used in high doses in that study, to reach a CPP of above 70 mmHg, and it has been documented both experimentally and in patients that norepinephrine induces a significant loss of plasma proteins to the interstitium (Dubniks et al. 2007; Nygren et al. 2010). Especially for the albumin group, this may have resulted in extracranial complications in terms of general tissue oedema and ARDS (Contant et al. 2001; Grände 2008). This conclusion finds support in the fact that the worse outcome with albumin in the SAFE-TBI study was not an effect of a higher ICP and therefore can most likely be attributed to extracranial events. Thus, even though the SAFE-TBI study has been the only randomized study published so far regarding fluid therapy in TBI patients and formally fulfils the demand for a level I–II study, after a critical evaluation, the results cannot be used for a general recommendation of avoiding albumin and using only normal saline or other crystalloids as plasma volume expander (Grände 2008).

With the lack of recommendations in conventional guidelines on how to treat patients with severe TBI regarding plasma volume substitution, this chapter has described the two main alternatives used in clinical practice today: (1) a fluid regime using mainly crystalloids as recommended through the SAFE-TBI study and (2) an alternative regimen based on physiological and pathophysiological principles for transcapillary fluid exchange using mainly albumin combined with crystalloids. In principle, the later regimen agrees with that suggested in the Lund concept for treatment of severe TBI patients (Grände 2006), which is described in another chapter of this book (Chap. 48). Synthetic colloids such as HES solutions and gelatin have been given as plasma volume expanders in TBI patients in Europe, but no human trials have been published that focus especially on TBI patients. It must be assumed, however, that the physiological effect of colloids on TBI patients in regions of the body other than the brain is the same as in non-brain-injured patients; thus, it seems reasonable to use synthetic colloids in situations where plasma expansion is indicated and blood products or albumin are not indicated.

References

Bernard F, Al-Tamimi YZ, Chatfield D, Lynch AG, Matta BF, Menon DK (2008) Serum albumin level as a predictor of outcome in traumatic brain injury: potential for treatment. J Trauma 64(4):872–875

Bullock R, Chesnut RM, Clifton G, Ghajar J, Marion DW, Narayan RK, Newell DW, Pitts LH, Rosner MJ, Wilberger JW (1996) Guidelines for the management of severe head injury. Brain Trauma Foundation. Eur J Emerg Med 3(2):109–127

Contant CF, Valadka AB, Gopinath SP, Hannay HJ, Robertson CS (2001) Adult respiratory distress syndrome: a complication of induced hypertension after severe head injury. J Neurosurg 95(4):560–568

Dhar R, Zazulia AR, Videen TO, Zipfel GJ, Derdeyn CP, Diringer MN (2009) Red blood cell transfusion increases cerebral oxygen delivery in anemic patients with subarachnoid hemorrhage. Stroke 40(9):3039–3044

Dubniks M, Persson J, Grände PO (2007) Effect of blood pressure on plasma volume loss in the rat under increased permeability. Intensive Care Med 33(12):2192–2198

Grände PO (2006) The "Lund Concept" for the treatment of severe head trauma – physiological principles and clinical application. Intensive Care Med 32(10):1475–1484

Grände PO (2008) Time out for albumin or a valuable therapeutic component in severe head injury? Acta Anaesthesiol Scand 52(6):738–741

Haskell A, Nadel ER, Stachenfeld NS, Nagashima K, Mack GW (1997) Transcapillary escape rate of albumin in humans during exercise-induced hypervolemia. J Appl Physiol 83(2):407–413

Hébert PC, Wells G, Blajchman MA, Marshall J, Martin C, Pagliarello G, Tweeddale M, Schweitzer I, Yetisir E (1999) A multicenter, randomized, controlled clinical trial of transfusion requirements in critical care. Transfusion Requirements in Critical Care Investigators, Canadian Critical Care Trials Group. N Engl J Med 340(6):409–417

Jungner M, Grände PO, Mattiasson G, Bentzer P (2010) Effects on brain edema of crystalloid and albumin fluid resuscitation after brain trauma and hemorrhage in the rat. Anesthesiology 112(5):1194–1203

Maas AI, Dearden M, Teasdale GM, Braakman R, Cohadon F, Iannotti F, Karimi A, Lapierre F, Murray G, Ohman J, Persson L, Servadei F, Stocchetti N, Unterberg A (1997) EBIC-guidelines for management of severe head injury in adults. European Brain Injury Consortium. Acta Neurochir (Wien) 139(4):286–294

Naidech AM, Jovanovic B, Wartenberg KE, Parra A, Ostapkovich N, Connolly ES, Mayer SA, Commichau C (2007) Higher hemoglobin is associated with improved outcome after subarachnoid hemorrhage. Crit Care Med 35(10):2383–2389

Nygren A, Redfors B, Thorén A, Ricksten SE (2010) Norepinephrine causes a pressure-dependent plasma volume decrease in clinical vasodilatory shock. Acta Anaesthesiol Scand 54(7):814–820

Rippe B, Haraldsson B (1994) Transport of macromolecules across microvascular walls: the two-pore theory. Physiol Rev 74(1):163–219

Rise IR, Risöe C, Kirkeby O (1998) Cerebrovascular effects of high intracranial pressure after moderate hemorrhage. J Neurosurg Anesthesiol 10(4):224–230

Rodling Wahlström M, Olivecrona M, Nyström F, Koskinen LO, Naredi S (2009) Fluid therapy and the use of albumin in the treatment of severe traumatic brain injury. Acta Anaesthesiol Scand 53(1):18–25

Smith MJ, Stiefel MF, Magge S, Frangos S, Bloom S, Gracias V, Le Roux PD (2005) Packed red blood cell transfusion increases local cerebral oxygenation. Crit Care Med 33(5):1104–1108

Stocchetti N, Penny KI, Dearden M, Braakman R, Cohadon F, Iannotti F, Lapierre F, Karimi A, Maas A Jr, Murray GD, Ohman J, Persson L, Servadei F, Teasdale GM, Trojanowski T, Unterberg A, European Brain Injury Consortium (2001) Intensive care management of head-injured patients in Europe: a survey from the European brain injury consortium. Intensive Care Med 27(2):400–406

The Brain Trauma Foundation, The American Association of Neurological Surgeons, Congress of Neurological Surgeons (2007) Guidelines for the management of severe traumatic brain injury. J Neurotrauma 24(Suppl 1):S1–S106

The SAFE Study Investigators (2007) Saline or albumin for fluid resuscitation in patients with traumatic brain injury. N Engl J Med 357:874–884

Tomita H, Ito U, Tone O, Masaoka H, Tominaga B (1994) High colloid oncotic therapy for contusional brain edema. Acta Neurochir Suppl (Wien) 60:547–549

Valeri CR, Donahue K, Feingold HM, Cassidy GP, Altschule MD (1986) Increase in plasma volume after the transfusion of washed erythrocytes. Surg Gynecol Obstet 162(1):30–36

Zygun DA, Nortje J, Hutchinson PJ, Timofeev I, Menon DK, Gupta AK (2009) The effect of red blood cell transfusion on cerebral oxygenation and metabolism after severe traumatic brain injury. Crit Care Med 37:1074–1078

Sedation: Including Pain Treatment and Withdrawal Symptoms

57

Silvana Naredi

Recommendations

Level I

There are insufficient data to support a Level I recommendation for sedation and analgesia.

Level II

Prophylactic use of barbiturates to the level of burst suppression on EEG is not recommended.

Barbiturate administration to control elevated ICP is recommended, but careful control of haemodynamic stability is essential during barbiturate therapy.

Propofol is also recommended for the control of ICP, but high-dose propofol can be associated with significant morbidity.

Level III

When barbiturates and propofol are used, normovolemia must be maintained in order to avoid hypotension.

To minimize the risk for the propofol infusion syndrome, the maximum dose of propofol administered should be 4 mg/kg/h and caution must be taken when propofol infusion exceeds 48 h, especially in children.

S. Naredi
Department of Anesthesiology and Intensive Care, Umeå University Hospital, S90185 Umeå, Sweden
e-mail: silvana.naredi@anestesi.umu.se

57.1 Overview

Several different sedative and analgesic agents have been used for sedation and analgesia in severe TBI (Table 57.1). Barbiturates have been used for treatment of TBI for decades. Treatment of pain and avoidance of stress and agitation with the help of sedatives and analgesics could theoretically help to keep ICP within acceptable levels. Sedation and analgesia may thus be beneficial. However, sedation makes it impossible to perform repeated neurological exams, and all sedative agents have adverse haemodynamic effects. The scientific evidence for the effect of sedation and analgesia in patients with severe TBI has been lacking. In the first two editions of the guidelines from the Brain Trauma Foundation, little scientific information was provided regarding the use of sedation and analgesia in patients with TBI. In the last edition from 2007, a chapter on "Anaesthetics, Analgesics, and Sedatives" have been added (Bratton et al. 2007).

Tips, Tricks, and Pitfalls

- A strategy to reduce the incidence of withdrawal symptoms is to gradually reduce drug doses.
- In trauma emergency situations, ketamine is probably safe to use.

T. Sundstrøm et al. (eds.), *Management of Severe Traumatic Brain Injury*,
DOI 10.1007/978-3-642-28126-6_57, © Springer-Verlag Berlin Heidelberg 2012

Table 57.1 Effects of commonly employed anaesthetics/analgesics in patients with severe traumatic brain injury

Anaesthetic/ analgesic agent	Cerebral metabolism	ICP	Adverse effects	Comments
Barbiturates	⇓	⇓	Hypotension	Maintain normovolemia Monitor with EEG
Propofol	⇓	⇔ (⇓)	Hypotension Propofol infusion syndrome	Maintain normovolemia <4 mg/kg/h
Midazolam	⇓	⇔		Long duration
Ketamine	⇔	⇔		Haemodynamic stability Limited data available in severe TBI
Opioids	⇔	⇔ (⇑)	Hypotension	Maintain normovolemia Continuous infusion

57.2 Background

Administration of sedatives and analgesics is necessary for stress reduction in the treatment of severe TBI. The scientific evidence regarding which drugs to use are scarce, and all available drugs used have their pros and cons. Specific concern should be taken when using propofol for longer periods of time and in high doses, due to the propofol infusion syndrome.

57.2.1 Barbiturates

Barbiturates are believed to decrease ICP by the coupling of decreased cerebral metabolic demands to reduced cerebral blood flow, thus reducing cerebral blood volume and intracranial pressure.

The Cochrane Injuries Group published a systematic review in 1999, updated in 2009 with the same conclusion, on the effects of barbiturates in patients with acute traumatic brain injury. Data from six trials were included in the review, and the overall conclusion was that there is no evidence supporting improved outcome with barbiturate therapy in patients with severe TBI. This lack of effect could be due to that barbiturates induce hypotension, especially in hypovolemic patients. When barbiturates are used, extreme caution must therefore be taken to maintenance of normovolemia in order to avoid hypotension. Barbiturate therapy should also preferably be monitored by continuous electroencephalography in order to titrate the lowest possible dose (Roberts and Sydenham 1999; Bratton et al. 2007).

57.2.2 Propofol

Propofol is extensively used for sedation in critically ill patients, including patients with severe TBI. Propofol has a short duration, which makes it possible to examine a patient neurologically briefly after termination of propofol administration. In experimental studies, propofol has been shown to reduce cerebral metabolism. In clinical studies, propofol has maintained or decreased ICP. Propofol can cause hypotension, and careful titration of propofol is therefore needed in haemodynamically unstable or hypovolemic patients (McKeage and Perry 2003; Bratton et al. 2007).

Although propofol has been administered safely in millions of patients during the last two decades, an increasing number of reports have described fatal complications, both in children and adults, after prolonged infusion of the drug. The adverse fatal effects include myocardial failure, lactic acidosis, hyperkalemia, rhabdomyolysis, lipemia, and acute renal failure, and have taken together, been defined as the propofol infusion syndrome. Young age, acute neurological injury, and catecholamine infusions are described as risk factors for the propofol infusion syndrome. A maximum rate of 4 mg/kg/h should be used in patients with severe TBI, and caution must be taken when propofol infusion exceeds 48 h. If lactic acidosis develops or the need for inotropic support increases, in the absence of obvious reasons, propofol should be discontinued (McKeage and Perry 2003; Bratton et al. 2007; Kam and Cardone 2007; Kotani et al. 2008; Otterspoor et al. 2008).

57.2.3 Midazolam

Midazolam is commonly used for sedation in neurosurgical intensive care units. Midazolam given as a continuous infusion for a prolonged period of time will accumulate in the body, which causes substantially prolonged duration and difficulties in assessment of patients after termination of the drug. Midazolam has minimal cardiovascular effect, at least in a normovolemic patient.

Midazolam reduces cerebral metabolism and cerebral blood flow in a dose-related fashion. The reduction in cerebral blood flow is linked to the reduction in cerebral metabolism. Midazolam has no obvious significant effect on ICP (Papazian et al. 1993; Albanese et al. 2004; Bratton et al. 2007).

57.2.4 Ketamine

The possible beneficial effects of the *N*-methyl-D-aspartate (NMDA) receptor antagonist ketamine in patients with severe TBI remain essentially unknown because of the persisting view that the drug should be avoided in patients with a cerebral injury. Ketamine is associated with haemodynamic stability, decreasing the need for vasopressors. The possibility to use ketamine in patients with a cerebral injury has received increasing interest during the last years. Increased glutamate concentrations have been found after brain injury, which has stimulated the idea to use NMDA receptor antagonists in the treatment of a cerebral injury (Himmelseher and Durieux 2005).

In clinical studies of patients with severe TBI, the combination ketamine/midazolam was as effective as the combination midazolam/sufentanil in controlling ICP and CPP (Bourgoin et al. 2003, 2005). In trauma emergency situations, ketamine can probably be used safely. Still, no robust evidence exists of a neuroprotective effect of ketamine in humans.

57.2.5 Analgesics

The most commonly used analgesics in patients with severe TBI have been opioid agonists, and among those, morphine is the most extensively used. The opioid agonists fentanyl, sufentanil, and alfentanil have become increasingly popular because of their short duration. Studies have shown an increase in ICP and a decrease in MAP after bolus doses of opioid agonists. The underlying mechanism of opioid effects on ICP is not evaluated in detail. Opioids may induce histamine release, inducing a decrease in cerebral vascular resistance and a fall in systemic blood pressure. Elevation of ICP by opioid agonists could also be caused by a compensatory autoregulatory cerebral vasodilation following a decrease in MAP. To avoid a reduction in MAP and in order to use opioid agonists safely, patients with a severe TBI should always be kept normovolemic, and it may be better to administer analgesics in continuous infusion instead of giving bolus injections (Albanese et al. 1999; Bratton et al. 2007).

57.2.6 $\alpha 2$ Agonists

Stress reduction in patients with severe TBI can be obtained by combining sedatives (midazolam, propofol, and thiopental) and analgesics with $\alpha 2$ agonists. This therapeutic approach is used in the 'Lund concept', where clonidine is used for two purposes: reduction of systolic blood pressure and reduction of stress response (Grande 2006). The use of $\alpha 2$ agonists (clonidine, dexmedetomidine) for sedation in patients with severe TBI has not been evaluated in randomized studies.

57.2.7 Withdrawal

Opioid and benzodiazepine administration for a longer period of time (>5–7 days) increases the risk for abstinence symptoms after termination of the drugs. The risk for withdrawal abstinence increases with abrupt termination or rapid tapering. Prevention and management of withdrawal symptoms is important in that it can aggravate patient distress. One strategy to reduce the incidence of withdrawal symptoms has been to slowly reduce doses of the drugs and utilization of α2 agonists (clonidine, dexmedetomidine).

The scientific evidence supporting the use of α2 agonists for avoidance of withdrawal symptoms is sparse and limited to case reports and small retrospective studies. Consensus regarding the best strategy to avoid drug withdrawal symptoms in critically ill patients is lacking (Honey et al. 2009).

57.3 Specific Paediatric Concerns

Children seem to be overrepresented among the reported cases of propofol infusion syndrome. This could be due to their lower glycogen stores and higher dependency on fat metabolism (Bratton et al. 2007; Kam and Cardone 2007; Kotani et al. 2008; Otterspoor et al. 2008). Administration of benzodiazepines and/or opioids for sedation in critically ill children may induce withdrawal symptoms after termination of the drugs. To reduce the incidence of withdrawal symptoms, the total doses of benzodiazepines and/or opioids administered should be kept as low as possible to control ICP. A daily tapering rate of 10–20% has been recommended in several studies; however, this strategy did not result in total absence of withdrawal symptoms (Ista et al. 2007).

References

Albanese J, Garnier F et al (2004) The agents used for sedation in neurointensive care unit. Ann Fr Anesth Reanim 23(5):528–534

Albanese J, Viviand X et al (1999) Sufentanil, fentanyl, and alfentanil in head trauma patients: a study on cerebral hemodynamics. Crit Care Med 27(2):407–411

Bourgoin A, Albanese J et al (2003) Safety of sedation with ketamine in severe head injury patients: comparison with sufentanil. Crit Care Med 31(3):711–717

Bourgoin A, Albanese J et al (2005) Effects of sufentanil or ketamine administered in target-controlled infusion on the cerebral hemodynamics of severely brain-injured patients. Crit Care Med 33(5):1109–1113

Bratton SL, Chestnut RM et al (2007) Guidelines for the management of severe traumatic brain injury. XI. Anesthetics, analgesics, and sedatives. J Neurotrauma 24(Suppl 1):S71–S76

Grande PO (2006) The "Lund Concept" for the treatment of severe head trauma – physiological principles and clinical application. Intensive Care Med 32(10): 1475–1484

Himmelseher S, Durieux ME (2005) Revising a dogma: ketamine for patients with neurological injury? Anesth Analg 101(2):524–534, table of contents

Honey BL, Benefield RJ et al (2009) Alpha2-receptor agonists for treatment and prevention of iatrogenic opioid abstinence syndrome in critically ill patients. Ann Pharmacother 43(9):1506–1511

Ista E, van Dijk M et al (2007) Withdrawal symptoms in children after long-term administration of sedatives and/or analgesics: a literature review. "Assessment remains troublesome". Intensive Care Med 33(8): 1396–1406

Kam PC, Cardone D (2007) Propofol infusion syndrome. Anaesthesia 62(7):690–701

Kotani Y, Shimazawa M et al (2008) The experimental and clinical pharmacology of propofol, an anesthetic agent with neuroprotective properties. CNS Neurosci Ther 14(2):95–106

McKeage K, Perry CM (2003) Propofol: a review of its use in intensive care sedation of adults. CNS Drugs 17(4):235–272

Otterspoor LC, Kalkman CJ et al (2008) Update on the propofol infusion syndrome in ICU management of patients with head injury. Curr Opin Anaesthesiol 21(5):544–551

Papazian L, Albanese J et al (1993) Effect of bolus doses of midazolam on intracranial pressure and cerebral perfusion pressure in patients with severe head injury. Br J Anaesth 71(2):267–271

Roberts I, Sydenham E (1999) Barbiturates for acute traumatic brain injury. Cochrane Database Syst Rev (3):CD000033

Nutrition

58

Anne Berit Guttormsen, Bram de Hoog, and Jennie Hernæs

Recommendations

Level I

Additional parenteral nutrition (PN) should be avoided in patients that tolerate enteral nutrition (EN) to target energy intake.

There are insufficient data to support Level I recommendation for when to start artificial nutrition, the preferable route of feeding (enteral (EN) or parenteral (PN)), energy and protein requirements and the level of blood sugar in patients with severe traumatic brain injury (TBI).

Level II

There is Level II evidence supporting that starting tailored nutrition within 72 h improves outcome in intensive care patients. Both hypocaloric and hypercaloric nutrition seems harmful.

A.B. Guttormsen (✉)
Department of Anaesthesia and Intensive Care, Haukeland University Hospital, Bergen, Norway

Department of Surgical Sciences, Section of Anaesthesiology, University of Bergen, Bergen, Norway
e-mail: anne.guttormsen@helse-bergen.no

B. de Hoog
Department of Anaesthesia and Intensive Care, Haukeland University Hospital, Bergen, Norway
e-mail: bram.johan.de.hoog@helse-bergen.no

J. Hernæs
Department of Clinical Nutrition, Haukeland University Hospital, Bergen, Norway
e-mail: jennie.hernaes@helse-bergen.no

Level III

An evaluation of patient nutritional status, i.e. bodyweight, height, weight loss and food intake, the last week before admission is recommended.

Continuous infusion of insulin is feasible to control blood sugar in the intensive care setting. Both hypo- and hyperglycaemia are deleterious in patients with TBI. The suggested target range for blood sugar is 6–9 mmol/l.

58.1 Overview

Individual nutritional support is an important component in all patient care and might contribute to better outcome and optimal rehabilitation (Singer et al. 2011). Hyperglycaemia is associated with worse outcome, and serum glucose of 6–9 mmol/l seems optimal (Bechir et al. 2010; Meierhans et al. 2010; Kansagara et al. 2011).

In the acute phase, nutrition has third priority after stabilization of vital functions (ventilation, hemodynamics) and intracranial pressure. Enteral nutrition (EN) is preferred and should be initiated within 24–48 h after the injury. EN should be supplied through a soft tube through the mouth (only if the patient is on a ventilator) or nasal cavity to the stomach. In the rehabilitation phase, percutaneous enteral gastrostomy (PEG) may be the preferable route. The technique is debatable and has complications (Kurien et al. 2010). If less than 1,500 kcal (1,500 ml) is administered, EN needs to be supplemented with vitamins and micronutrients

T. Sundstrøm et al. (eds.), *Management of Severe Traumatic Brain Injury*,
DOI 10.1007/978-3-642-28126-6_58, © Springer-Verlag Berlin Heidelberg 2012

Table 58.1 Nutrition guideline

TBI patients that cannot eat should start artificial nutrition
If there is no contraindications for EN, insert a gastric feeding tube and start EN as soon as possible, within 24–48 h
Measure (indirect calorimetry) or estimate EE (25–50 kcal/kg, dependant on days after injury). Repeat at regular intervals, preferably every week in stable patients
Use a feeding protocol to increase and monitor EN
Start supplemental PN if energy demands are not reached within 72 h
Increase PN to caloric target over 2–3 days to prevent metabolic derangement, especially in unstable patients
Use small bowel feeding when gastric fluid retention prevents full EN
Assess protein requirement and loss once to twice weekly in intensive care until nitrogen balance is achieved
Stable patients who can feed themselves are assessed regularly for malnutrition with a screening tool (Kondrup et al 2003). Fortify ordinary food and give ONS or EN and PN if needed

ONS oral nutritional supplements in the form of liquid sip feeds, bars, puddings and powders, *EN* enteral nutrition, *PN* parenteral nutrition

to cover basal requirements. To increase energy intake, a concentrated EN formula may be used, i.e. 1.5 kcal/ml. Consider using EN-containing fibre to normalize bowel function, especially in the rehabilitation phase. There are possible interactions between continuous EN and peroral medications. Be aware that concomitant administration of EN might diminish or delay absorption of phenytoin (Cook et al. 2008).

Parenteral nutrition (PN) is added if nutritional needs are not gained within 72 h (Singer et al. 2009). However, recently the EPaNIC study (Casaer et al. 2011), comparing early (24-48 h) and late (8 days) PN in critically ill patients, has questioned early initiation of PN if EN fails. In the intensive care phase, most of the TBI patients have a multi-lumen central venous catheter. One of the lumens should be dedicated to i.v. nutrition if PN is needed. PN with lower osmolality can be supplied via a peripheral line for a shorter period of time, i.e. 2–3 days. The line should be inspected at least once a day, and the peripheral line should be changed once every second day to avoid phlebitis.

PN is most conveniently administered from 3-chamber bags comprising glucose, fat and amino acids. These solutions contain 1 kcal/ml solution; the content of glucose, fat and amino acids differs between manufacturers. Bags for peripheral administration contain <1 kcal/ml, i.e. administered volume must be higher to reach energy target.

Energy supply should be tailored. Stress metabolism is unpredictable, and therefore energy demand is best measured with indirect calorimetry (Cook et al. 2008). Although recommended, very few departments use indirect calorimetry because the equipment is expensive and the technique is cumbersome. Overfeeding is harmful (Griffiths 2007; Turner 2010) due to increased metabolism, excessive CO_2, and heat production. These metabolic changes elevate ICP (dilatation of brain arteries), especially in patients that are not on a ventilator (Table 58.1).

The following basal needs can be used when calculating energy and nutrient requirements, but individual adaptations must be considered.

Catabolic state (early)	25 kcal/kg/24 h
Anabolic state (late)	30–50[a] kcal/kg/24 h
Glucose requirements	
Glucose	2–3 g/kg/24 h
Lipid requirements	
Lipid	0.5–2 g/kg/24 h
Protein requirements	
Protein (nitrogen)	1–1.5 g/kg/24 t (~0.16–0.24 g N/kg/24 h)
Electrolyte requirements	
Sodium	1–1.4 mmol/kg/24 h (might be considerably higher in salt loosing conditions)
Potassium	0.7–0.9 mmol/kg/24 h
Phosphate	0.15–0.30 mmol/kg/24 h
Magnesium	0.04 mmol/kg/24 h
Calcium	0.11 mmol/kg/24 h

[a]The highest energy supply during rehabilitation. In the rehabilitation phase body weight should guide energy supply

Fluid Requirements

The supplement of fluid is an integrated part of nutritional support. The basal requirement of fluid is approximately 30 ml/kg/24 h, and the administered volume has to be adjusted according to the clinical situation.

Tips, Tricks and Pitfalls

- *Ordinary food and oral nutritional supplements*
  - If the patient is able to drink and/or eat, he/she should be encouraged to do so. Do measure intake.
- *Enteral nutrition*
  - Start EN with 20 ml/h of a standard solution (1.0 kcal/ml). Increase with 10–20 ml every 8th hour while monitoring gastric retention. Modest increase in delivery may prevent diarrhoea.
  - In patients with gastric retention, a motility agent can be added like erythromycin (200 mg × 2–3/day) over a period of maximal 3 days.
  - In case of gastrointestinal paresis due to opioids, use peripherally functioning antagonists: naloxone 3–6 mg × 3 orally or give parenteral methylnaltrexon.
  - In failed enteral nutrition, also treat constipation.
  - If motility agents do not solve the gastric retention problem, the feeding tube can be positioned in the small bowel with the help of gastroscopy.
  - If need for EN for more than 2–4 weeks, PEG should be the preferred route.
- *Parenteral nutrition*
  - During administration of PN, a central venous access is preferable.
  - Daily requirements should be administered as three chamber bags. Trace elements and micronutrients (water-soluble and fat-soluble vitamins) must be added.
- *Amount of energy*
  - In the rehabilitation phase, body weight should be measured one to two times a week.
  - Stable bodyweight, or slowly increased body weight, hints that energy supply is sufficient. Be aware that oedema will also increase body weight.

58.2 Background

After TBI, swallow problems are common, leading to malnutrition, dehydration and aspiration pneumonia. As during other critical illness, TBI induces a hypermetabolic response mediated by cytokines, other inflammatory mediators, hormones (norepinephrine, epinephrine, ACTH and cortisol, growth hormone, prolactin and vasopressin) and endorphins (Cook et al. 2008). Concomitant production of glucose coupled with insulin resistance leads to hyperglycaemia.

Due to the hypermetabolic response, resting energy expenditure (REE) might be considerably increased compared with estimates done according to the Harris-Benedict formula (Frankenfield et al. 2007). There is an inverse relationship between Glasgow Coma Scale score and REE. Energy requirement is difficult to predict because many other factors influence metabolism. Muscle relaxants, mechanical ventilation, opioids and sedation all reduce REE to a variable degree. Agitation, seizures, increased body temperature and catecholamines increase metabolism (http://www.lll-nutrition.com).

Early EN-containing glutamine is associated with fewer infections in trauma patients. Glutamine might also have favourable effects in TBI patients (Yang and Xu 2007). EN is preferred if tolerated (Lochs et al. 2006; Singer et al. 2009).

Failed enteral feeding because of high gastric residual volume is a common problem in critically ill patients (Fraser and Bryant 2010). Using prokinetic drugs can enhance gastric motility. Metoclopramide 10 mg q 3–4/day is generally used in general intensive care patients, but may not be effective in TBI patients. Erythromycin is a motilin agonist. Its use as a prokinetic to achieve nutritional goals may be equivalent to small bowel feeding in the short term (Boivin and Levy 2001). There are resistance issues since erythromycin is an antibiotic, and it is not efficient with prolonged use (Nguyen et al. 2007). Combining both agents has better results with prolonged feeding (Fraser and Bryant 2010). Small bowel feeding is recommended if gastric feeding is still unsuccessful despite motility agents. It may also reduce the incidence of ventilator-associated pneumonia in patients at risk (Heyland et al. 2003).

PN is indicated in heavily sedated patients (barbiturate coma) due to gastric retention and GI paralyses, or if EN does not reach nutritional requirements. Close monitoring of electrolytes (sodium, potassium and phosphate), acid–base balance, blood glucose and liver status and triglycerides is important during the critical care phase of injury.

In TBI patients, standard equations for estimating energy demand, like Harris Benedict, Mifflin-St-Jeor and Iretons-Jones (Frankenfield et al. 2007), are inaccurate and indirect calorimetry should be used if available. Patients with severe TBI can lose 10–15% of lean body mass in 1 week and 30% of body weight in 2–3 weeks if nutritional intervention is not started. Tailored caloric intake probably improve outcome (Singer et al. 2011)

During intensive care, patients with TBI might have problems with fluid and electrolyte (primarily sodium) balance. It is therefore mandatory to closely monitor fluid balance, serum sodium and excretion of sodium in the urine to avoid hyponatremia and hypovolaemia. Stress metabolism induces a catabolic state with gluconeogenesis and breakdown of skeletal muscle. Loss of nitrogen and muscle is high (>20 gN/24 h or >600 g of muscle tissue/24 h) and aggravated by steroids. Restoration of nitrogen balance is often not achieved until 2–3 weeks after the injury. Protein requirements are a matter of debate in critically ill patients (Wolfe et al. 1983; Larsson et al. 1990; Ishibashi et al. 1998; Seron Arbeloa et al. 1999). There is no evidence supporting that amino acid infusion of more than 1.5 g/kg/day leads to a better nitrogen balance. It may instead lead to an augmented urea production. Correcting nitrogen balance will not reverse the catabolic state (Clifton et al. 1986; Streat and Hill 1987; Young et al. 1987), but will lead to a positive nitrogen balance earlier (Twyman et al. 1985). Overall nitrogen loss will decrease. Supplementation of amino acids is necessary to maintain protein syntheses. It is possible to calculate nitrogen balance in patients with normal renal function. To do so, 24-h urine is collected to measure urea excretion. Nitrogen supply=(protein intake (g))/6.25, and nitrogen loss=urine urea (mmol) times 0.028+4 g (correcting for non-urinary loss) (Sabotka 2004). In critically ill patients, nitrogen loss is higher than nitrogen supply.

Studies on cerebral glucose level using microdialysis suggest that a blood glucose level between 6 and 9 mmol/l results in optimal cerebral glucose concentration in TBI patients. Insulin therapy started at blood glucose levels above 7 mmol/l had positive effect on cerebral metabolism (Bechir et al. 2010; Meierhans et al. 2010). Kansagara and collaborators (Kansagara et al. 2011) have performed a systematic review summarizing available data from 1950 to 2010. They conclude that tight blood glucose control often causes hypoglycaemia, and that there is no consistent evidence that tight blood glucose control is better than a less strict glycaemic control. ESPEN guidelines advocate a serum glucose level below 10 mmol/l (Singer et al. 2009). During intensive care, blood glucose is controlled with continuous infusion of insulin.

In TBI patients, serum zinc concentration decline due to sequestration in the liver and increased secretion in the urine. Zinc is a cofactor for substrate metabolism and is important for immune and NMDA receptor function (Cook et al. 2008). One study indicates that zinc supplementation in the immediate period after head injury is favourable, as the study group had improved neurologic recovery. Further, serum pre-albumin concentrations were significantly higher in the zinc-supplemented group 3 weeks after injury, which might indicate better nutritional status (Young et al. 1996). Decreased food intake and/or insufficient nutritional support aggravates malnutrition and effect outcome. Despite this, it is important not to feed too much energy, eventually causing obesity, which has negative effects for the daily care of the patient. Support with artificial nutrition should decrease in line with increase in oral food intake, always making sure energy demands are met.

58.3 Specific Paediatric Concerns

There are not enough data to support a level I recommendation for how to perform nutritional support in paediatric patients with TBI. As in adults, energy and protein requirement are increased, and guidelines recommend supplementation of 130–160% of measured or calculated basal energy expenditure. There are few studies on the optimal route or timing of nutrition. However, one study found that hyperglycaemia was an independent predictor for death and poor cerebral outcome in children (Cochran et al. 2003).

References

Bechir M, Meierhans R, Brandi G, Sommerfeld J, Fasshauer M, Cottini SR, Stocker R, Stover JF (2010) Insulin differentially influences brain glucose and lactate in traumatic brain injured patients. Minerva Anestesiol 76:896–904

Boivin MA, Levy H (2001) Gastric feeding with erythromycin is equivalent to transpyloric feeding in the critically ill. Crit Care Med 29:1916–1919

Casaer MP, Mesotten D, Hermans G, Wouters PJ, Schetz M, Meyfroidt G, Van Cromphaut S, Ingels C, Meersseman P, Muller J, Vlasselaers D, Debaveye Y, Desmet L, Dubois J, Van Assche A, Vanderheyden S, Wilmer A, Van den Berghe GN (2011) Early versus late parenteral nutrition in critically ill adults. Engl J Med. 365(6):506–17. Epub 2011 Jun 29

Clifton GL, Robertson CS, Choi SC (1986) Assessment of nutritional requirements of head-injured patients. J Neurosurg 64:895–901

Cochran A, Scaife ER, Hansen KW, Downey EC (2003) Hyperglycemia and outcomes from pediatric traumatic brain injury. J Trauma 55:1035–1038

Cook AM, Peppard A, Magnuson B (2008) Nutrition considerations in traumatic brain injury. Nutr Clin Pract 23:608–620

Frankenfield D, Hise M, Malone A, Russell M, Gradwell E, Compher C (2007) Prediction of resting metabolic rate in critically ill adult patients: results of a systematic review of the evidence. J Am Diet Assoc 107:1552–1561

Fraser RJ, Bryant L (2010) Current and future therapeutic prokinetic therapy to improve enteral feed intolerance in the ICU patient. Nutr Clin Pract 25:26–31

Griffiths RD (2007) Too much of a good thing: the curse of overfeeding. Crit Care 11:176

Heyland DK, Dhaliwal R, Drover JW, Gramlich L, Dodek P (2003) Canadian clinical practice guidelines for nutrition support in mechanically ventilated, critically ill adult patients. JPEN J Parenter Enteral Nutr 27:355–373

Ishibashi N, Plank LD, Sando K, Hill GL (1998) Optimal protein requirements during the first 2 weeks after the onset of critical illness. Crit Care Med 26:1529–1535

Kansagara D, Fu R, Freeman M, Wolf F, Helfand M (2011) Intensive insulin therapy in hospitalized patients: a systematic review. Ann Intern Med 154:268–282

Kondrup J, Rasmussen HH, Hamberg O, Stanga Z (2003) Nutritional risk screening (NRS2002): a new method based on an analyses of controlled clinical trials. Clin Nutr. 22:321–336

Kurien M, McAlindon ME, Westaby D, Sanders DS (2010) Percutaneous endoscopic gastrostomy (PEG) feeding. BMJ 340:c2414

Larsson J, Lennmarken C, Martensson J, Sandstedt S, Vinnars E (1990) Nitrogen requirements in severely injured patients. Br J Surg 77:413–416

Lochs H, Allison SP, Meier R, Pirlich M, Kondrup J, Schneider S, van den Berghe G, Pichard C (2006) Introductory to the ESPEN guidelines on enteral nutrition: terminology, definitions and general topics. Clin Nutr 25:180–186

Meierhans R, Bechir M, Ludwig S, Sommerfeld J, Brandi G, Haberthur C, Stocker R, Stover JF (2010) Brain metabolism is significantly impaired at blood glucose below 6 mM and brain glucose below 1 mM in patients with severe traumatic brain injury. Crit Care 14:R13

Nguyen NQ, Chapman MJ, Fraser RJ, Bryant LK, Holloway RH (2007) Erythromycin is more effective than metoclopramide in the treatment of feed intolerance in critical illness. Crit Care Med 35:483–489

Sabotka L (2004) Basics in clinical nutrition. Publishing House Galen, Prague

Seron Arbeloa C, Avellanas Chavala M, Homs Gimeno C, Larraz Vileta A, Laplaza Marin J, Puzo Foncillas J (1999) Evaluation of a high protein diet in critical care patients. Nutr Hosp 14:203–209

Singer P, Anbar R, Cohen J, Shapiro H, Shalita-Chesner M, Lev S, Grozovski E, Theilla M, Frishman S, Madar Z (2011) The tight calorie control study (TICACOS): a prospective, randomized, controlled pilot study of nutritional support in critically ill patients. Intensive Care Med 37:601–609

Singer P, Berger MM, Van den Berghe G, Biolo G, Calder P, Forbes A, Griffiths R, Kreyman G, Leverve X, Pichard C, ESPEN (2009) ESPEN guidelines on parenteral nutrition: intensive care. Clin Nutr 28:387–400

Streat SJ, Hill GL (1987) Nutritional support in the management of critically ill patients in surgical intensive care. World J Surg 11:194–201

Turner P (2010) Providing optimal nutritional support on the intensive care unit: key challenges and practical solutions. Proc Nutr Soc 69:574–581

Twyman D, Young AB, Ott L, Norton JA, Bivins BA (1985) High protein enteral feedings: a means of achieving positive nitrogen balance in head injured patients. JPEN J Parenter Enteral Nutr 9:679–684

Wolfe RR, Goodenough RD, Burke JF, Wolfe MH (1983) Response of protein and urea kinetics in burn patients to different levels of protein intake. Ann Surg 197:163–171

Yang DL, Xu JF (2007) Effect of dipeptide of glutamine and alanine on severe traumatic brain injury. Chin J Traumatol 10:145–149

Young B, Ott L, Twyman D, Norton J, Rapp R, Tibbs P, Haack D, Brivins B, Dempsey R (1987) The effect of nutritional support on outcome from severe head injury. J Neurosurg 67:668–676

Young B, Ott L, Kasarskis E, Rapp R, Moles K, Dempsey RJ, Tibbs PA, Kryscio R, McClain C (1996) Zinc supplementation is associated with improved neurologic recovery rate and visceral protein levels of patients with severe closed head injury. J Neurotrauma 13:25–34

59 Management of External Drain-Related CNS Infection

Mikala Wang and Jens Kjølseth Møller

Recommendations

Level I

There are insufficient data to support a Level I recommendation for this topic.

Level II

There are insufficient data to support a Level II recommendation for this topic.

Level III

Prophylactic catheter exchange, irrigation of catheters, or prophylactic antibiotic therapy for patients with an EVD is not recommended.

Strict adherence to a sterile protocol for insertion and maintenance of a closed system is advised. The EVD should be removed on a timely fashion. There is insufficient evidence to support a recommendation of antimicrobial-impregnated catheters.

Antimicrobial therapy should only be initiated in suspected VRI, VRI, or ventriculitis. As empirical therapy in head trauma patients with CNS infection, we recommend administration of a broad-spectrum cephalosporin, e.g. ceftriaxone. In patients with clinical signs of VRI, we recommend systemic administration of cefuroxime and vancomycin intrathecally as empirical therapy, in the event of a Gram-positive isolate. As empirical therapy in the event of a Gram-negative isolate, we recommend administration of ceftriaxone i.v. In fulminant ventriculitis, we recommend intrathecal gentamicin. We recommend suspension of treatment when the patient has shown clinical resolution and three consecutive sterile CSF cultures have been obtained.

59.1 Overview

Central nervous system (CNS) infection is a common complication to external drainage of cerebrospinal fluid (CSF) leading to extended duration of hospitalization, neurological sequelae, or even death.

In the following, ventriculostomy-related infections are defined by the presence of clinical symptoms of CNS infection such as new fever, nuchal rigidity, decreased mental status, and neurological deterioration. Supporting the clinical diagnosis are laboratory parameters indicating a deterioration of the biochemical profile of the CSF and/or a positive Gram stain/culture from CSF. Deterioration of the CSF biochemical

M. Wang (✉)
Department of Clinical Microbiology,
Aarhus University Hospital, Skejby, Aarhus N
8200, Denmark
e-mail: mikala.wang@skejby.rm.dk

J.K. Møller
Department of Clinical Microbiology,
Vejle Hospital, Vejle, Denmark
e-mail: jkm@dadlnet.dk

T. Sundstrøm et al. (eds.), *Management of Severe Traumatic Brain Injury*,
DOI 10.1007/978-3-642-28126-6_59, © Springer-Verlag Berlin Heidelberg 2012

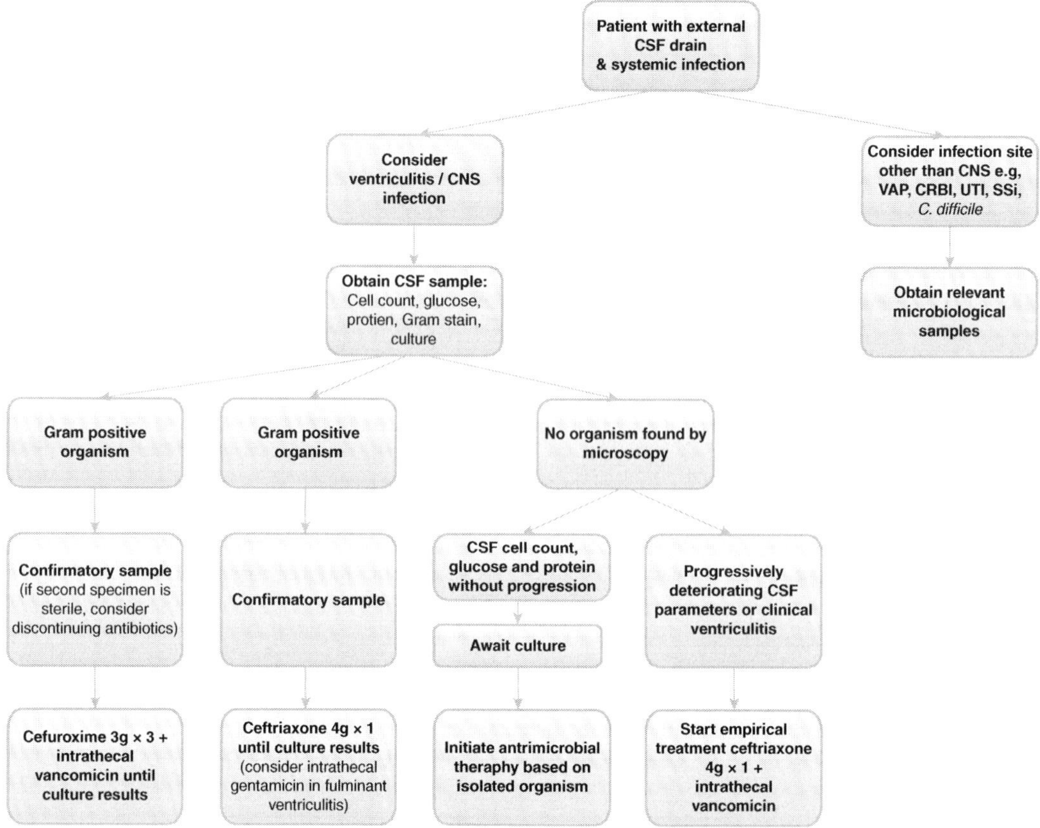

Fig. 59.1 Operational algorithm for the management of ventriculostomy-related infections

profile is defined by progressively advancing CSF pleocytosis, declining CSF glucose, and increasing CSF protein. An operational algorithm for the management of ventriculostomy-related infections is shown in Fig. 59.1.

Risk factors for external CSF drain-related infections are prophylactic catheter exchange, unnecessary manipulation of catheters, neurosurgical procedures, cranial fractures, haemorrhagic CSF, and CSF leaks. The use of antimicrobial-impregnated catheters shows promise in preventing CSF infections; however, further studies are required. Prophylactic antibiotic therapy should not be instituted in patients with external CSF drains as several studies indicate that prophylactic use of systemic antibiotics select for more resistant pathogens leading to increased mortality.

Tips, Tricks, and Pitfalls

- Obtain microbiological samples before initiating antimicrobial therapy.
- Consider other origins of infection: ventilator-associated pneumonia (VAP), catheter-related blood stream infection (CRBSI), urinary tract infection (UTI), *Clostridium difficile* enterocolitis, sinusitis, and surgical site infection (SSI).
- Obtain the following samples from the head trauma patient with an infection of unknown origin:
  1. CSF for Gram stain, culture, cell count, glucose, and protein
  2. Blood cultures × 2 (from CVC and peripheral blood)

3. Sputum for culture/PCR
4. Swabs/aspirates from possible surgical site infection
5. Urine for culture
6. Faeces for *C. difficile* (if the patient has diarrhoea)

- In the event of a positive Gram stain or culture from an EVD, always get a second sample before initiating antimicrobial therapy in order to confirm a positive finding.
- In the event of persistent CSF infection despite appropriate antibiotic therapy, replace the EVD.
- In the event of a CSF infection rate >10% in patients with EVD, an investigation of the institutional procedures for the insertion and care of the EVD should be initiated.

59.2 Background

CNS infection in the TBI patient is primarily caused by the breach of barriers due to trauma or by neurosurgical interventions such as the placement of CNS drains. The following chapter focuses mainly on management of drain-related CNS infections, as these require highly specialized knowledge; however, this chapter also suggests a general empirical treatment strategy for CNS infection in the TBI patient.

59.2.1 Diagnosis

The interpretation of studies on infections related to external ventricular drains (EVD) has been impeded by the lack of a universally agreed upon definition of ventriculostomy-related infection (VRI) which has made a comparison of results exceedingly difficult. Previously, VRI has been defined by a positive cerebrospinal fluid (CSF) culture drawn from an EVD or lumbar puncture (LP) (Mayhall et al. 1984) without taking the CSF biochemical profile or the clinical status of the patient into consideration. This definition has led to an overestimation of the true incidence as the possibility of contamination or colonization was not taken into account. Efforts to establish more stringent diagnostic criteria for VRI have been partly hindered by the fact that both clinical symptoms and laboratory findings can be relatively non-specific. The traditional symptoms of CNS infection – nuchal rigidity, fever, decreased level of consciousness, and neurological deterioration – can be difficult to ascertain in the brain trauma patient with decreased level of consciousness. Furthermore, the less pathogenic organisms that are commonly isolated in VRI, such as coagulase-negative staphylococci, generally cause mild, non-specific symptoms. Moreover, the aseptic CNS inflammation caused by the presence of a foreign body, e.g. an EVD, can create a similar CSF profile as seen in CNS infection with pleocytosis, decreased CSF glucose, and increased CSF protein.

Lozier et al. have proposed new diagnostic criteria for VRI where the abnormal CSF profile is not defined in absolute terms but rather viewed as a progression in comparison to the earlier biochemical profile of the patient. By these criteria, ventriculitis is defined by the presence of clinical symptoms of CNS infection such as fever, nuchal rigidity, decreased mental status, and neurological deterioration in conjunction with progressively advancing CSF pleocytosis, declining CSF glucose, increasing CSF protein, and a positive Gram stain/culture. VRI is defined by the same laboratory findings but no clinical symptoms other than fever. A suspected VRI is defined by abnormal CSF profile, lack of clinical symptoms other than fever, and the absence of a positive Gram stain/culture. A positive Gram stain/culture from a patient with expected CSF profile and no symptoms of infection other than fever is considered a contaminant. If isolated in repeat culture from the same patient with no changes in CSF profile or clinical status, it is deemed colonization of the catheter (Lozier et al. 2002).

59.2.2 Epidemiology

VRI is a frequent complication to the use of EVD with incidence rates ranging between 0% and

22% in the literature. A recent review pooled data from 23 studies showing an average incidence of positive CSF cultures of 8.8% per patient and 8.1% per EVD (Lozier et al. 2002). As previously mentioned, the true incidence of VRI remains elusive due to the varying definitions of drain-related CNS infection. Ventriculostomy-related infections have a reported low mortality from 0% to 2.8%; however, they are associated with increased morbidity.(Bota et al. 2005; Flibotte et al. 2004; Holloway et al. 1996; Schade et al. 2005) The majority of reports show a preponderance of Gram-positive cocci – mainly coagulase-negative staphylococci and some *Staphylococcus aureus* – consistent with normal skin flora comprising up to 75–85% of isolates. Gram-negative rods are also commonly isolated and normally comprise up to 15–20%. Fungi, although occasionally found, are still a rare cause of VRI. The mortality of VRI appears to depend on the causative agent as studies with a large proportion of Gram-negative infections report a far higher mortality rate of up to 58% (Buckwold et al. 1977; Lu et al. 1999; Lyke et al. 2001; Mombelli et al. 1983). Gram-negative CNS infections have been associated with the prophylactic use of antibiotics covering the Gram-positive spectrum thus selecting for Gram-negative organisms, multiresistant bacteria, and fungi (Alleyne et al. 2000; Aucoin et al. 1986; Korinek et al. 2006; Lyke et al. 2001; May et al. 2006; Poon et al. 1998; Stoikes et al. 2008). Furthermore, a long hospital stay and head trauma also predispose for Gram-negative CNS infection (Berk and McCabe 1980; Buckwold et al. 1977; Mombelli et al. 1983).

59.2.3 Risk Factors

A number of risk factors for VRI of relevance to head trauma patients have been identified. Several reports show that hemorrhagic CSF increases the risk of VRI (Aucoin et al. 1986; Holloway et al. 1996; Mayhall et al. 1984; Stenager et al. 1986; Sundbarg et al. 1988). Cranial fractures, both basilar cranial fractures and depressed cranial fractures, have also been demonstrated to have a statistically significant association with VRIs (Aucoin et al. 1986; Holloway et al. 1996; Luerssen et al. 1993; Mayhall et al. 1984). Likewise, neurosurgical procedures such as craniotomy have been reported to increase the incidence of VRIs (Holloway et al. 1996; Luerssen et al. 1993; Mayhall et al. 1984; Sundbarg et al. 1988). Interestingly, it has also been shown that concomitant systemic infection increases the risk of VRI, however, not by the same organism causing the systemic infection, leading to speculation that this increased incidence could be due to relative immunosuppression brought on by systemic infection (Bota et al. 2005; Clark et al. 1989; Holloway et al. 1996).

Regarding risk factors pertaining to the catheter, maintenance of a closed drainage system has been hypothesized to be essential to prevent infection. In line with this theory, irrigation of the EVD has been demonstrated to significantly increase the risk of CNS infection (Aucoin et al. 1986; Mayhall et al. 1984). Likewise, Korinek et al. reported in a recent paper how the implementation of a rigid protocol for insertion and care for the EVD with strict adherence to sterile technique and maintenance of a closed system resulted in a significant reduction in drain-related infections from 12.2% to 5.7%. Protocol violations such as catheter manipulations and inappropriate CSF sampling were major risk factors for infection in this study as the score for protocol violation was four times higher in the infected group than in non-infected patients (Korinek et al. 2005). Another major risk factor for infection identified in this study was CSF leakage around the EVD in concurrence with other reports (Bogdahn et al. 1992; Holloway et al. 1996; Lyke et al. 2001; Rebuck et al. 2000; Schade et al. 2005; Sundbarg et al. 1988). These studies emphasize the importance of maintenance of a closed system and adherence to strict procedures in the insertion and management of the EVD in order to prevent infection.

There is controversy in the literature concerning the significance of the duration of catheterization as pertaining to the risk of infection. A number of studies have found duration of drainage to be a risk factor for VRI with variable data regarding when the infection rate starts increasing. Several of these reports suggest that more than 5 days of catheterization is a risk factor for VRI (Aucoin et al. 1986; Clark et al. 1989; Holloway et al. 1996; Luerssen et al. 1993; Mayhall et al. 1984; Narayan et al. 1982; Paramore and Turner 1994), and one report by Holloway et al. notes a decline in infection after day 10 (Holloway et al. 1996). However, other reports demonstrate increasing infection rates up to day 6 after which infection rates decline (Kanter et al. 1985; Paramore and Turner 1994). Conversely, numerous studies show no relationship between duration of EVD and infection (Korinek et al. 2005; Pfisterer et al. 2003; Smith and Alksne 1976; Stenager et al. 1986; Sundbarg et al. 1988; Winfield et al. 1993). Hoefnagel et al. found duration to be a risk factor in a recent study; however, prolonged duration of catheterization was associated with frequent CSF sampling thus confounding the result (Hoefnagel et al. 2008). As the incidence and mechanism of infection depends on the local practice regarding sterile technique and maintenance of a closed system in the management of external ventricular drains, we believe that a unifying conclusion pertaining to duration of catheterization as a risk factor may not be possible to draw. Reports from studies implementing a strict protocol for EVD management suggest that duration of catheterization is not an independent risk factor for drain-related infection when strict adherence to sterile technique and maintenance of a closed is upheld (Korinek et al. 2005).

59.2.4 Prevention

In order to prevent ventriculostomy-related infections, various interventions such as prophylactic catheter exchange, tunnelling of external ventricular drains, prophylactic antibiotics, and impregnated catheters have been investigated. The results of these interventions will be reviewed in the following section.

Based on the assumption that duration of catheterization is a risk factor for VRI, prophylactic catheter exchange has been proposed as a means to decrease EVD-related infections (Mayhall et al. 1984). Two retrospective studies based on analysis of data from The Traumatic Coma Data Bank and The Medical College of Virginia Neurocore Data Bank were unable to demonstrate any preventive effect of routine exchange of EVD (Holloway et al. 1996; Luerssen et al. 1993). On the contrary, data from The Traumatic Coma Data Bank suggested a higher CSF infection rate in centres with routine revision of EVDs (16.8%) as opposed to those that did not (7.8%), closely approaching statistical significance ($p=0.054$) (Luerssen et al. 1993). Furthermore, a prospective randomized controlled trial to determine the prophylactic effect of routine exchange of catheter every 5 days showed no decrease in infections rates but also suggested a trend towards higher infection rate among those prophylactically changed (Wong et al. 2002). In line with these observations, several studies have reported a correlation between multiple catheters and VRI (Arabi et al. 2005; Clark et al. 1989; Lo et al. 2007; Rebuck et al. 2000; Sundbarg et al. 1988); however, this correlation is being disputed by others who report no association between the two (Alleyne et al. 2000; Holloway et al. 1996; Lyke et al. 2001; Mayhall et al. 1984). Based on these reports, we do not recommend prophylactic change of catheters.

The use of an extended tunnelling technique for EVDs has been proposed to reduce infection rates and was indeed initially reported to result in a zero rate of infection (Friedman and Vries 1980). However, subsequent studies did report drain-related infections despite tunnelling of catheters but reported lower rates of infection than untunnelled catheters (Khanna et al. 1995; Kim et al. 1995; Leung et al. 2007). As no randomized controlled trials have been performed to verify this claim, there is insufficient evidence to recommend the use of tunnelling technique with EVDs. However, tunnelling of EVDs has become common practice amongst neurosurgeons and has been demonstrated to reduce infection rates in the context of central venous catheters (CVC) (Mermel 2000).

Another common practice in order to prevent drain-related infection is the administration of prophylactic antimicrobial therapy, either periprocedural or for the duration of the drainage period. Regarding the use of periprocedural antibiotics for the insertion of EVDs, there are no studies available. Our local practice does not call for periprocedural antibiotics for the insertion of an external drain. However, there are several studies on the effect of giving systemic antibiotics for the duration of the drainage period. One randomized prospective study demonstrated significant reduction in CSF infection in patients receiving prophylactic antibiotics for the duration of the drainage period compared to those did not receive antibiotics; however, this reduction was at the expense of selecting for more resistant pathogens such as MRSA and Candida species (Poon et al. 1998). Other studies have shown no effect on infection rates by the administration of prophylactic antibiotics (Alleyne et al. 2000; Aucoin et al. 1986; May et al. 2006; Mayhall et al. 1984; Rebuck et al. 2000; Rosner and Becker 1976; Stenager et al. 1986; Stoikes et al. 2008) however, a shift towards multi-drug-resistant organisms, fungi, and Gram negatives was likewise observed in several of these studies among patients receiving continuous antibiotic treatment (Aucoin et al. 1986; May et al. 2006; Stoikes et al. 2008). A dominance of Gram-negative CNS infections (82%) was also observed in a prospective study by Lyke and co-workers, and it was hypothesized that this was partly due to selective pressure induced by the antibiotic prophylaxis given for the duration of catheterization. This shift towards more resistant pathogens led to an unusually high mortality rate of 22% and significant morbidity in the infected group (Lyke et al. 2001). This is in striking contrast to reported mortality rates 0–2.8% from patient groups where no prophylactic antibiotics were given (Bota et al. 2005; Flibotte et al. 2004; Holloway et al. 1996; Schade et al. 2005). On the basis of these reports, we do not recommend the administration of prophylactic antibiotics as there is insufficient evidence supporting a reduction in infection incidence. More importantly, several studies using prophylactic antibiotics demonstrate increased mortality and morbidity due to a selection for more resistant microorganisms.

The ability of antimicrobial-impregnated catheters to prevent VRI is in the process of being investigated, and the preliminary results are promising. A multi-centre prospective randomized controlled trial using minocycline-/rifampicin-impregnated catheters showed significant reduction in positive CSF culture rates and colonization rates (Zabramski et al. 2003). In a prospective randomized study, Wong et al. reported comparable infection rates in patients using clindamycin-rifampicin-impregnated catheters as in patients receiving dual prophylactic antibiotic coverage (Wong et al. 2008). Likewise, a recent clinical trial showed significant decrease in positive CSF cultures when using clindamycin-rifampicin-coated catheters (Tamburrini et al. 2008). Although there were no reports of induction of bacterial resistance in these studies, the concern has been expressed, substantiated by in vitro studies demonstrating induced resistance in staphylococci exposed to minocycline-rifampicin catheters (Sampath et al. 2001; Tambe et al. 2001). Moreover, increased rifampicin resistance in coagulase-negative staphylococci associated with use of minocycline-rifampicin-impregnated CVCs has been reported in an intensive care setting (Wright et al. 2001). However, the increased rifampicin resistance of staphylococci in vivo by the use of these catheters has thus far not been corroborated by other clinical trials. Another cause for concern are reports demonstrating significant increase in Candida colonization when using minocycline-rifampicin-coated CVCs (Leon et al. 2004; Sampath et al. 2001).

Catheters impregnated with silver nanoparticles have also been studied for the use in external drainage. In CVCs, the efficacy of silver-coated catheters have thus far to be demonstrated; however, the preliminary results in external drains are more encouraging. In vitro studies have demonstrated their antibacterial effect and shown that silver toxicity is not an issue (Galiano et al. 2008; Roe et al. 2008). A recent pilot study reported significant reduction in positive CSF cultures in patients with silver-impregnated catheters (Lackner et al. 2008), and a larger retrospective study likewise found decreased culture-positive rates in patients with a silver-coated EVD;

however, the difference in this study was not significant (Fichtner et al. 2010). Silver resistance has previously been described in burn units due to use of silver as an antiseptic, and there is concern that the use of silver-coated catheters will select for antibiotic resistance as studies suggest that silver resistance can confer cross-resistance to multiple antibiotics (McHugh et al. 1975; Pirnay et al. 2003). Antimicrobial-impregnated catheters show promise in preventing CSF infection; however, further evidence is required in order to support a recommendation. Moreover, due to the risk of induction of bacterial resistance, we cannot support a general recommendation of these catheters; however, they may have a place in recurrent or persistent infection. The implementation of a strict protocol for insertion and care for the catheter with emphasis on sterile technique and avoidance of unnecessary catheter manipulation remains the best way to prevent drain-related CNS infection.

59.2.5 Treatment

Due to the propensity for Gram-negative meningitis in head trauma patients (Mombelli et al. 1983; Rincon and Badjatia 2006), we suggest an empirical strategy in this patient population of ceftriaxone 4 g×1 on clinical diagnosis of CNS infection. In the event of a Gram-negative Gram stain/culture, intraventricular gentamicin should be considered in the context of fulminant ventriculitis. This approach is not recommended in neonates due to a controlled trial where infants with meningitis/ventriculitis were randomized to receive systemic antibiotics alone or systemic antibiotics in combination with intraventricular gentamicin. This study was terminated early due to the significantly higher mortality rate in the group receiving intraventricular gentamicin (43%) compared to those receiving systemic antibiotics alone (13%) (McCracken et al. 1980).

In the event of a Gram-positive isolate in the presence of clinical CNS infection, we recommend initiation of antimicrobial therapy with cefuroxime 3 g×3 i.v. in combination with vancomycin intrathecally until culture results. If the isolated organism proves to be methicillin resistant, only intrathecal vancomycin therapy is continued. In case of fulminant ventriculitis due to a methicillin-resistant microorganism or if the isolate is a MRSA, we recommend systemic linezolid therapy in combination with intrathecal vancomycin.

With regards to the duration of antimicrobial therapy in drain-related infections, there is little evidence to lean on and recommendations range from less than a week to over 3 weeks (Whitehead and Kestle 2001). Some differentiate based on the isolated pathogen, recommending at least 1 week of antimicrobial therapy in the case of coagulase-negative staphylococci, whereas *S. aureus* and Gram-negative isolates should be treated for a minimum of 10–14 days (Tunkel et al. 2004). However, if the patient's response to antimicrobial therapy is inadequate, longer duration of treatment may be required. In case of insufficient clinical response despite appropriate antibiotic therapy, we recommend replacing the EVD. Our local practice is to suspend treatment when the patient has shown clinical response and had three consecutive sterile CSF cultures.

59.3 Specific Paediatric Concerns

Intraventricularly administered gentamicin is not recommended in neonates.

References

Alleyne CH Jr, Hassan M, Zabramski JM (2000) The efficacy and cost of prophylactic and perioprocedural antibiotics in patients with external ventricular drains. Neurosurgery 47(5):1124–1127

Arabi Y, Memish ZA, Balkhy HH, Francis C, Ferayan A, Al Shimemeri A et al (2005) Ventriculostomy-associated infections: incidence and risk factors. Am J Infect Control 33(3):137–143

Aucoin PJ, Kotilainen HR, Gantz NM, Davidson R, Kellogg P, Stone B (1986) Intracranial pressure monitors. Epidemiologic study of risk factors and infections. Am J Med 80(3):369–376

Berk SL, McCabe WR (1980) Meningitis caused by gram-negative bacilli. Ann Intern Med 93(2):253–260

Bogdahn U, Lau W, Hassel W, Gunreben G, Mertens HG, Brawanski A (1992) Continuous-pressure controlled, external ventricular drainage for treatment of acute hydrocephalus–evaluation of risk factors. Neurosurgery 31(5):898–903

Bota DP, Lefranc F, Vilallobos HR, Brimioulle S, Vincent JL (2005) Ventriculostomy-related infections in critically ill patients: a 6-year experience. J Neurosurg 103(3):468–472

Buckwold FJ, Hand R, Hansebout RR (1977) Hospital-acquired bacterial meningitis in neurosurgical patients. J Neurosurg 46(4):494–500

Clark WC, Muhlbauer MS, Lowrey R, Hartman M, Ray MW, Watridge CB (1989) Complications of intracranial pressure monitoring in trauma patients. Neurosurgery 25(1):20–24

Fichtner J, Guresir E, Seifert V, Raabe A (2010) Efficacy of silver-bearing external ventricular drainage catheters: a retrospective analysis. J Neurosurg 112(4):840–846

Flibotte JJ, Lee KE, Koroshetz WJ, Rosand J, McDonald CT (2004) Continuous antibiotic prophylaxis and cerebral spinal fluid infection in patients with intracranial pressure monitors. Neurocrit Care 1(1):61–68

Friedman WA, Vries JK (1980) Percutaneous tunnel ventriculostomy. Summary of 100 procedures. J Neurosurg 53(5):662–665

Galiano K, Pleifer C, Engelhardt K, Brossner G, Lackner P, Huck C et al (2008) Silver segregation and bacterial growth of intraventricular catheters impregnated with silver nanoparticles in cerebrospinal fluid drainages. Neurol Res 30(3):285–287

Hoefnagel D, Dammers R, Laak-Poort MP, Avezaat CJ (2008) Risk factors for infections related to external ventricular drainage. Acta Neurochir (Wien) 150(3):209–214

Holloway KL, Barnes T, Choi S, Bullock R, Marshall LF, Eisenberg HM et al (1996) Ventriculostomy infections: the effect of monitoring duration and catheter exchange in 584 patients. J Neurosurg 85(3):419–424

Kanter RK, Weiner LB, Patti AM, Robson LK (1985) Infectious complications and duration of intracranial pressure monitoring. Crit Care Med 13(10):837–839

Khanna RK, Rosenblum ML, Rock JP, Malik GM (1995) Prolonged external ventricular drainage with percutaneous long-tunnel ventriculostomies. J Neurosurg 83(5):791–794

Kim DK, Uttley D, Bell BA, Marsh HT, Moore AJ (1995) Comparison of rates of infection of two methods of emergency ventricular drainage. J Neurol Neurosurg Psychiatry 58(4):444–446

Korinek AM, Baugnon T, Golmard JL, van Effenterre R, Coriat P, Puybasset L (2006) Risk factors for adult nosocomial meningitis after craniotomy: role of antibiotic prophylaxis. Neurosurgery 59(1):126–133

Korinek AM, Reina M, Boch AL, Rivera AO, De Bels D, Puybasset L (2005) Prevention of external ventricular drain-related ventriculitis. Acta Neurochir (Wien) 147(1):39–45

Lackner P, Beer R, Broessner G, Helbok R, Galiano K, Pleifer C et al (2008) Efficacy of silver nanoparticles-impregnated external ventricular drain catheters in patients with acute occlusive hydrocephalus. Neurocrit Care 8(3):360–365

Leon C, Ruiz-Santana S, Rello J, de la Torre MV, Valles J, Alvarez-Lerma F et al (2004) Benefits of minocycline and rifampin-impregnated central venous catheters. A prospective, randomized, double-blind, controlled, multicenter trial. Intensive Care Med 30(10):1891–1899

Leung GK, Ng KB, Taw BB, Fan YW (2007) Extended subcutaneous tunnelling technique for external ventricular drainage. Br J Neurosurg 21(4):359–364

Lo CH, Spelman D, Bailey M, Cooper DJ, Rosenfeld JV, Brecknell JE (2007) External ventricular drain infections are independent of drain duration: an argument against elective revision. J Neurosurg 106(3):378–383

Lozier AP, Sciacca RR, Romagnoli MF, Connolly ES Jr (2002) Ventriculostomy-related infections: a critical review of the literature. Neurosurgery 51(1):170–181

Lu CH, Chang WN, Chuang YC, Chang HW (1999) Gram-negative bacillary meningitis in adult post-neurosurgical patients. Surg Neurol 52(5):438–443

Luerssen TG, Chesnut RM, Van Berkum-Clark M, Marshall LF, Klauber MR, Blunt BA (1993) Post traumatic cerebrospinal fluid infections in the Traumatic Coma Data Bank: the influence of the type and management of ICP monitors. In: Intracranial pressure VIII: proceedings of the 8th international symposium on intracranial pressure. Springer, Berlin, pp 42–45

Lyke KE, Obasanjo OO, Williams MA, O'Brien M, Chotani R, Perl TM (2001) Ventriculitis complicating use of intraventricular catheters in adult neurosurgical patients. Clin Infect Dis 33(12):2028–2033

May AK, Fleming SB, Carpenter RO, Diaz JJ, Guillamondegui OD, Deppen SA et al (2006) Influence of broad-spectrum antibiotic prophylaxis on intracranial pressure monitor infections and subsequent infectious complications in head-injured patients. Surg Infect (Larchmt) 7(5):409–417

Mayhall CG, Archer NH, Lamb VA, Spadora AC, Baggett JW, Ward JD et al (1984) Ventriculostomy-related infections. A prospective epidemiologic study. N Engl J Med 310(9):553–559

McCracken GH Jr, Mize SG, Threlkeld N (1980) Intraventricular gentamicin therapy in gram-negative bacillary meningitis of infancy. Report of the Second Neonatal Meningitis Cooperative Study Group. Lancet 1(8172):787–791

McHugh GL, Moellering RC, Hopkins CC, Swartz MN (1975) Salmonella typhimurium resistant to silver nitrate, chloramphenicol, and ampicillin. Lancet 1(7901):235–240

Mermel LA (2000) Prevention of intravascular catheter-related infections. Ann Intern Med 132(5):391–402

Mombelli G, Klastersky J, Coppens L, Daneau D, Nubourgh Y (1983) Gram-negative bacillary meningitis in neurosurgical patients. J Neurosurg 59(4):634–641

Narayan RK, Kishore PR, Becker DP, Ward JD, Enas GG, Greenberg RP et al (1982) Intracranial pressure: to monitor or not to monitor? A review of our experience with severe head injury. J Neurosurg 56(5):650–659

Paramore CG, Turner DA (1994) Relative risks of ventriculostomy infection and morbidity. Acta Neurochir (Wien) 127(1–2):79–84

Pfisterer W, Muhlbauer M, Czech T, Reinprecht A (2003) Early diagnosis of external ventricular drainage infection: results of a prospective study. J Neurol Neurosurg Psychiatry 74(7):929–932

Pirnay JP, De Vos D, Cochez C, Bilocq F, Pirson J, Struelens M et al (2003) Molecular epidemiology of *Pseudomonas aeruginosa* colonization in a burn unit: persistence of a multidrug-resistant clone and a silver sulfadiazine-resistant clone. J Clin Microbiol 41(3): 1192–1202

Poon WS, Ng S, Wai S (1998) CSF antibiotic prophylaxis for neurosurgical patients with ventriculostomy: a randomised study. Acta Neurochir Suppl 71:146–148

Rebuck JA, Murry KR, Rhoney DH, Michael DB, Coplin WM (2000) Infection related to intracranial pressure monitors in adults: analysis of risk factors and antibiotic prophylaxis. J Neurol Neurosurg Psychiatry 69(3):381–384

Rincon F, Badjatia N (2006) Central nervous system infections in the neurointensive care unit. Curr Treat Options Neurol 8(2):135–144

Roe D, Karandikar B, Bonn-Savage N, Gibbins B, Roullet JB (2008) Antimicrobial surface functionalization of plastic catheters by silver nanoparticles. J Antimicrob Chemother 61(4):869–876

Rosner MJ, Becker DP (1976) ICP monitoring: complications and associated factors. Clin Neurosurg 23: 494–519

Sampath LA, Tambe SM, Modak SM (2001) In vitro and in vivo efficacy of catheters impregnated with antiseptics or antibiotics: evaluation of the risk of bacterial resistance to the antimicrobials in the catheters. Infect Control Hosp Epidemiol 22(10):640–646

Schade RP, Schinkel J, Visser LG, Van Dijk JM, Voormolen JH, Kuijper EJ (2005) Bacterial meningitis caused by the use of ventricular or lumbar cerebrospinal fluid catheters. J Neurosurg 102(2):229–234

Smith RW, Alksne JF (1976) Infections complicating the use of external ventriculostomy. J Neurosurg 44(5):567–570

Stenager E, Gerner-Smidt P, Kock-Jensen C (1986) Ventriculostomy-related infections – an epidemiological study. Acta Neurochir (Wien) 83(1–2):20–23

Stoikes NF, Magnotti LJ, Hodges TM, Weinberg JA, Schroeppel TJ, Savage SA et al (2008) Impact of intracranial pressure monitor prophylaxis on central nervous system infections and bacterial multi-drug resistance. Surg Infect (Larchmt) 9(5):503–508

Sundbarg G, Nordstrom CH, Soderstrom S (1988) Complications due to prolonged ventricular fluid pressure recording. Br J Neurosurg 2(4):485–495

Tambe SM, Sampath L, Modak SM (2001) In vitro evaluation of the risk of developing bacterial resistance to antiseptics and antibiotics used in medical devices. J Antimicrob Chemother 47(5):589–598

Tamburrini G, Massimi L, Caldarelli M, Di Rocco C (2008) Antibiotic impregnated external ventricular drainage and third ventriculostomy in the management of hydrocephalus associated with posterior cranial fossa tumours. Acta Neurochir (Wien) 150(10):1049–1055

Tunkel AR, Hartman BJ, Kaplan SL, Kaufman BA, Roos KL, Scheld WM et al (2004) Practice guidelines for the management of bacterial meningitis. Clin Infect Dis 39(9):1267–1284

Whitehead WE, Kestle JR (2001) The treatment of cerebrospinal fluid shunt infections. Results from a practice survey of the American Society of Pediatric Neurosurgeons. Pediatr Neurosurg 35(4):205–210

Winfield JA, Rosenthal P, Kanter RK, Casella G (1993) Duration of intracranial pressure monitoring does not predict daily risk of infectious complications. Neurosurgery 33(3):424–430

Wong GK, Poon WS, Ng SC, Ip M (2008) The impact of ventricular catheter impregnated with antimicrobial agents on infections in patients with ventricular catheter: interim report. Acta Neurochir Suppl 102:53–55

Wong GK, Poon WS, Wai S, Yu LM, Lyon D, Lam JM (2002) Failure of regular external ventricular drain exchange to reduce cerebrospinal fluid infection: result of a randomised controlled trial. J Neurol Neurosurg Psychiatry 73(6):759–761

Wright F, Heyland DK, Drover JW, McDonald S, Zoutman D (2001) Antibiotic-coated central lines: do they work in the critical care setting? Clin Intensive Care 12(1): 21–28

Zabramski JM, Whiting D, Darouiche RO, Horner TG, Olson J, Robertson C et al (2003) Efficacy of antimicrobial-impregnated external ventricular drain catheters: a prospective, randomized, controlled trial. J Neurosurg 98(4):725–730

60 Management of Other Infections

Steinar Skrede

Recommendations

For all the major groups of infections dealt with in this chapter, several Level I recommendations and a large number of Level II and III recommendations exist. Further reading of specific guidelines is recommended.

Level I

To lower risk of ventilator associated pneumonia (VAP) in the general intensive care unit patient population, intubation and reintubation should, whenever possible, be avoided and non-invasive ventilation be used. Body position affects risk of aspiration and VAP during mechanical ventilation. Empiric treatment of patients with hospital-acquired pneumonia (HAP) or VAP requires the use of antibiotics at optimal doses by the intravenous route. Monotherapy with selected agents can be used for patients with severe HAP or VAP in the absence of resistant pathogens. In patients with good clinical response, efforts should be made to shorten the duration of therapy, given that *Pseudomonas* or related bacterial species are not involved. In intravascular catheter-related bloodstream infections, two pairs of blood cultures should be obtained prior to initiation of antibiotic therapy. A definite diagnosis requires that the same microorganism grows from at least one percutaneous blood culture and from a culture of the catheter tip. Peripheral intravenous catheters with associated pain, erythema, or swelling should be removed. In suspected catheter-related urinary tract infection, other possible sources of infection must be ruled out. Catheters should remain closed, and duration of catheterization should be as short as possible. Systemic antimicrobial treatment of asymptomatic catheter associated bacteriuria is generally not recommended. In the initial episode of *Clostridium difficile* infection (CDI) where oral therapy is possible, patients with non-severe infection should be given metronidazole by the oral route.

Level II

In patients with suspected VAP and the presence of a new or progressive radiographic pulmonary infiltrate, accompanied by purulent secretions, fever of 38°C, leucopoenia, or leucocytosis, the use of antibiotics is warranted. Initial empiric therapy can be guided by a Gram stain of a reliable tracheal aspirate. Initial treatment should not be postponed in patients identified to be in need of antibiotic treatment. A negative tracheal aspirate has a strong negative predictive value for VAP in selected patients. Prophylactic administration of systemic antibiotics for 24 h at the time of intubation has demonstrated to reduce the risk of hospital-acquired pneumonia (HAP) in patients with closed brain trauma. Antimicrobial treatment of

S. Skrede
Department of Medicine, Haukeland University Hospital, Jonas Lies vei 65, N – 5021 Bergen, Norway
e-mail: steinar.skrede@helse-bergen.no

T. Sundstrøm et al. (eds.), *Management of Severe Traumatic Brain Injury*,
DOI 10.1007/978-3-642-28126-6_60, © Springer-Verlag Berlin Heidelberg 2012

catheter-related urinary tract infection is recommended only in symptomatic cases. Removing or replacing a catheter that has been in place for more than 7 days is recommended before initiating antimicrobial treatment. Treatment should be adjusted as soon as culture results are available. In cases of suspected CDI, testing for the microbe or its toxin should be performed on diarrheal stool. Toxin testing is most important; however, the sensitivity of the tests may be questionable. Repeated testing in the same episode should not be performed. Any other antimicrobial therapy should be minimized to reduce the risk of CDI according to local antimicrobial stewardship programmes. To lower the risk of recurrence of CDI, the antimicrobial suspected to initiate this infection should be discontinued as soon as possible. In initial episodes of severe CDI, vancomycin is the drug of choice. The antimicrobial treatment of the first recurrence of CDI should usually be the same as for the first episode of CDI. There are several other Level II recommendations. The reader should refer to topic-specific guidelines for further details selected.

Level III

For the major groups of infections dealt with in this chapter, a substantial number of Level III recommendations exist. Further reading of selected guidelines is recommended.

60.1 Overview

Patients in need of neurointensive care are at high risk of acquiring infections during all phases of the hospital stay. In a critical care unit, approximately 50% of patients will undergo infections. Patients with reduced consciousness and neurologic deficits will be at particular risk of acquiring infections, and almost three out of four will receive antimicrobial therapy. In the initial phase, the need for surgery, mechanical ventilatory support, the use of central venous catheters, and urinary catheters contribute to the risk of infection. The most common infections are hospital-acquired pneumonia (HAP), catheter-related bloodstream infection, and urosepsis. Surgical wound infections also occur, as does *Clostridium difficile* infection, and infections associated with ventriculostomy catheters. After treatment in the intensive care unit, patients with reduced consciousness and neurologic deficits will be at particular risk of acquiring infections. This is in part explained by a need for long-lasting hospital stays. Furthermore, the frequent use of broad-spectrum antibiotics during neurointensive care puts the patient at risk for late-appearing infectious complications, such as antibiotic associated diarrhoea. Any medical therapy of these patients may be affected by infections, as altered hemodynamics affects pharmacokinetics, and the risk of drug interactions will increase upon initiation of treatment with selected antimicrobials in severe infections. In this chapter, methods for identifying and treating infections in the adult population in the neurointensive care unit will be dealt with. The reader is provided with a list of recommended literature (Ortiz and Lee 2006; Martin and Yost 2011; Colorado et al. 2007; American Thoracic Society and Infectious Diseases Society of America 2005; Torres and Carlet 2001; Chastre et al. 2003; Sirvent et al. 1997; Mermel et al. 2001, 2009; Tenke et al. 2008; Hooton et al. 2010; Musa et al. 2010; Bauer et al. 2009; Cohen et al. 2010). For further details, please refer to specific guidelines for the groups of infections considered in this chapter.

Tips, Tricks, and Pitfalls

- Patients in neurocritical care units are at high risk of acquiring nosocomial infection.
- Fever and reduced GCS may be early signs; however, initial symptoms are often scarce and unspecific.
- When infection is suspected, clinical examination and relevant microbiological tests must be undertaken rapidly.
- The use of bactericidal broad-spectrum antibiotics administered intravenously is often indicated.

60.2 Background

The incidence of serious infections in the neurointensive care unit is high. Commonly, the initial clinical presentation is unspecific. However, most patients will develop fever. A reduced level of consciousness is frequently observed in any infection, not only in infections involving the CNS. The most likely infection in this patient group is hospital-acquired pneumonia (HAP). Many of these cases are attributable to the use of mechanical ventilator. In these patients, the initial use of broad-spectrum antimicrobials is warranted. Intravascular catheter-related infection is commonly associated with bloodstream infection (BSI) frequently seen in neurointensive care units and is to be suspected in cases without other evident primary source of infection. In BSI, antibiotic treatment should be aiming at covering Gram-positive pathogens. Catheter associated urinary tract infection should be suspected in any intensive care unit patient with signs of systemic inflammatory response syndrome (SIRS). Asymptomatic bacterial colonization may easily be misinterpreted, and efforts should be made to secure the diagnosis of infection before treatment is initiated in symptomatic cases. Many patients in the neurointensive care unit are monitored or treated with indwelling ventriculostomy catheters. If properly established and maintained, the incidence of related infections is low. However, the lethality in these infections is high, and efforts to establish a diagnosis should be made early before treatment starts. Broad-spectrum antimicrobials penetrating the blood–brain barrier should be chosen (see Chap. 59). Finally, the patient population is at risk of acquiring *Clostridium difficile* infection (CDI) during the hospital stay. The earliest symptoms of CDI in these patients may be indistinguishable from any of the other infections considered before symptoms from the gastrointestinal tract are evident. Following basic hygiene rules is of greatest importance to avoid CDI and to limit its spread in institutions when it occurs. Metronidazole administered enterally is the preferred initial treatment. Vancomycin is the primary choice in selected cases. For the patient in the neurointensive care unit, identifying the source of infection and identifying the pathogen causing disease will result in significantly lower mortality risk.

60.2.1 Hospital-Acquired Pneumonia (HAP)

Among the infections occurring in the neuro intensive care unit, pneumonia is the most common. Nosocomial pneumonia is defined at peneumonia presenting later than 48 h after admittance and can be categorized as health care associated pneumonia (HCAP), hospital-acquired pneumonia (HAP), or ventilator associated pneumonia (VAP). In HCAP, risk factors are immobilization, neurologic deficits, aspiration, long-lasting stays, and co-morbidity. Furthermore, the risk for developing VAP is related to the time of mechanical ventilation. The management of patients in these three groups of pneumonia is essentially similar. However, all cases of HCAP are divided into early-onset (within 4 days of admittance) and late-onset pneumonias. The clinical management is different in these subgroups. In early-onset VAP, predominating microbes are *Streptococcus pneumoniae* and *Haemophilus influenzae*. *Staphylococcus aureus* is also seen. In late VAP, Gram-negative intestinal bacilli may be involved. Any VAP may be seen in approximately 10–25% of patients requiring intubation. In VAP, the risk of death is increased, and substantially so if the initial antimicrobial therapy given is inappropriate. Prompt clinical diagnosis, supported by efforts to rapidly identify pathogen, and administration of appropriate antibiotics without further delay are recommended in these patients. Therapeutic options include cephalosporins, piperacillin-tazobactam, carbapenems, aminoglycosides, and quinolones. In pneumococcal disease, penicillin G is also an option. The value of combination therapy is not established. Antibiotic treatment of assumed VAP on the sole basis of radiographic findings and clinical judgement will lead to substantial overuse of antimicrobial agents.

60.2.2 Intravascular Catheter-Related Bloodstream Infection (CRBSI)

Detailed recommendations for diagnosis and management of infections related to short-term and long-term indwelling intravenous catheters are established (2001) and recently updated (2009). CRBSI is a frequent infection in intensive care units, reaching 15% of all nosocomial infections in 2009, carrying a high mortality rate. The most common pathogen in CRBSI is coagulase-negative staphylococci. In cases of *Staphylococcus aureus* and coagulase-negative staphylococci, penicillinase-resistant penicillins are preferred. In case of oxacillin resistance, vancomycin is preferred to daptomycin or linezolid. In enterococcal disease, ampicillin is preferred for susceptible isolates. If the isolate is ampicillin resistant, vancomycin is the first choice. In both cases, aminoglycosides can be considered in combination. Gram-negative intestinal bacilli are treated empirically with third-generation cephalosporins. Depending on identity of the microbe and susceptibility testing, carbapenems, an aminopenicillin plus a penicillinase inhibitor, or fluoroquinolones may be considered as therapeutic agents. In most situations, intravascular catheters are recommended to be removed in established infection. Short-term catheters are preferably removed, as are long-term central venous catheters in patients with disseminated bacterial disease, such as accompanying endocarditis or bone infection. In long-term catheter use, these should be removed in cases caused by *Staphylococcus aureus*, Gram-negative bacilli, or *Candida* species. As soon as the diagnosis is substantiated, the catheters should be removed and antibiotics administered intravenously by a different access.

60.2.3 Catheter-Related Urinary Tract Infection (UTI)

UTI is the most prevalent nosocomial infection, commonly seen in patients who have had urological manipulation or permanent urethral catheterization. In intensive care units, UTI is primarily associated with indwelling catheters. UTIs increase the length of stay but have less effect on risk for mortality compared to VAP and BSI. Indications for the use of urinary catheters are to monitor production of urine, in obstruction, or in the perioperative period. Following established guidelines for catheter care decreases the risk for infection. Short-term catheterization is defined as catheter in place for less than 1 week. Most episodes of bacteriuria in this situation are asymptomatic. In long-term catheterization, the risk of morbidity is higher. Enteric microbes are the most prevalent pathogens encountered, *E. coli* being the commonest. However, ascending infections and bacteraemia are unusual. The most common clinical finding in symptomatic UTI is fever. Some patients will fulfil sepsis criteria (clinical infection accompanied by at least two of four signs of SIRS; temperature >38°C or <36°C, pulse rate >90/min, respiratory rate >20/min, leucocytes in peripheral blood >12 or $<4\times10^9$/L, or $PaCO_2 < 4.3$ kPa in arterial blood gas sample). However, localizing symptoms as tenderness, obstruction, or haematuria must be sought. Generally, treatment of asymptomatic bacteriuria is not recommended in most cases, but highly selected cases may benefit from treatment. Urine cultures from long-term indwelling catheters are always positive. It is therefore difficult to establish a definitive diagnosis of CR-UTI when there are no localizing symptoms. It is recommended that blood cultures and urinary cultures are taken prior to antibiotic therapy. In cases where catheters have been in place more than 2 weeks at the onset of UTI, the catheters should be replaced if its use is still indicated, and urine culture should be obtained from the new catheter to help guide treatment. In absence of evident clinical signs of CR-UTI, other diagnosis must be ruled out. Antibiotic treatment is recommended in symptomatic infection, i.e. BSI, pyelonephritis, prostatitis, and epididymitis. Empirical treatment is given using broad-spectrum antibiotics based on knowledge of local microbiological conditions, but treatment must later be tailored according to culture results. These infections are often monobacterial, and there is an increased risk that the causal microbe will be (multi-) drug resistant.

60.2.4 *Clostridium difficile* Infection (CDI)

Antibiotic associated diarrhoea is, by definition, unexplained diarrhoea occurring in association with administration of antibiotics, used either in prophylaxis or treatment of infection. The majority of cases of colitis associated with antibiotic therapy are caused by *Clostridium difficile*. CDI is an important and emerging cause of nosocomial infection. Although frequent in hospital, CDI is rarely acquired in neurocritical care units according to recent data. The clinical presentation of CDI can be anything from minor diarrhoea to severe, even life-threatening disease. Antibiotics frequently associated with the disease are cephalosporins, clindamycin, aminopenicillins, and quinolones. All antibiotics may, in principle, predispose patients to CDI, and it may appear epidemically in hospitals. Major risk factors for acquiring CDI are advanced age, long hospital stays, and exposure to antibiotics, including those given as prophylaxis before surgery. The most frequently used diagnostic test is detection of *Clostridium difficile* toxins in one stool sample. In up to one-fourth of patients, diarrhoea will resolve upon discontinuation of the ongoing antibiotic therapy. Supportive measures and avoiding antiperistaltic drugs are recommended. Antibiotics are indicated for patients with moderate or severe CDI or for patients with significant co-morbidity. Oral metronidazole and oral vancomycin are the antibiotics used in primary therapy of CDI. Hospitalized patients should be treated in isolate, and hygiene measures must be emphasized and undertaken. Relapses are frequent. Then several treatment options exist. Updated treatment recommendations from the European Society of Clinical Microbiology and Infectious Diseases (ESCMID) (2009) as well as from the Society for Healthcare Epidemiology of America (SHEA)/Infectious Diseases Society of America (IDSA) have recently been published (2010).

60.2.5 Ventricular Catheterization-Related Infection

Management of ventricular catheterization-related infections is dealt with in a separate section (see Chap. 59).

60.3 Specific Paediatric Concerns

There are age-dependent limitations in use of several antibiotics. However, most key antimicrobial agents may be offered to the paediatric patient population in the neurocritical care unit, with dosages based on patient age and/or weight. The use of local guidelines for use of antibiotics in children is recommended.

References

American Thoracic Society, Infectious Diseases Society of America (2005) Guidelines for the management of adults with hospital-acquired, ventilator-associated, and healthcare-associated pneumonia. Am J Respir Crit Care Med 171(4):388–416

Bauer MP, Kuijper EJ, van Dissel JT (2009) European Society of Clinical Microbiology and Infectious Diseases (ESCMID): treatment guidance document for *Clostridium difficile* infection (CDI). Clin Microbiol Infect 15(12):1067–1079

Chastre J, Wolff M, Fagon JY, Chevret S, Thomas F, Wermert D et al (2003) Comparison of 8 vs 15 days of antibiotic therapy for ventilator-associated pneumonia in adults: a randomized trial. JAMA 290(19): 2588–2598

Cohen SH, Gerding DN, Johnson S, Kelly CP, Loo VG, McDonald LC et al (2010) Clinical practice guidelines for *Clostridium difficile* infection in adults: 2010 update by the Society for Healthcare Epidemiology of America (SHEA) and the Infectious Diseases Society of America (IDSA). Infect Control Hosp Epidemiol 31(5):431–455

Colorado L, Vizcaychipi M, Herbert S (2007) Incidence of bacteremia in a neurocritical unit. Crit Care 11(S2): S26–S27

Hooton TM, Bradley SF, Cardenas DD, Colgan R, Geerlings SE, Rice JC et al (2010) Diagnosis, prevention, and treatment of catheter-associated urinary tract infection in adults: 2009 International Clinical Practice Guidelines from the Infectious Diseases Society of America. Clin Infect Dis 50(5):625–663

Martin SJ, Yost RJ (2011) Infectious diseases in the critically ill patients. J Pharm Pract 24(1):35–43

Mermel LA, Farr BM, Sherertz RJ, Raad II, O'Grady N, Harris JS et al (2001) Guidelines for the management of intravascular catheter-related infections. J Intraven Nurs 24(3):180–205

Mermel LA, Allon M, Bouza E, Craven DE, Flynn P, O'Grady NP et al (2009) Clinical practice guidelines for the diagnosis and management of intravascular catheter-related infection: 2009 update by the Infectious Diseases Society of America. Clin Infect Dis 49(1):1–45

Musa SA, Robertshaw H, Thomson SJ, Cowan ML, Rahman TM (2010) *Clostridium difficile*-associated disease acquired in the neurocritical care unit. Neurocrit Care 13(1):87–92

Ortiz R, Lee K (2006) Nosocomial infections in neurocritical care. Curr Neurol Neurosci Rep 6(6):525–530

Sirvent JM, Torres A, El-Ebiary M, Castro P, de Battle J, Bonet A (1997) Protective effect of intravenously administered cefuroxime against nosocomial pneumonia in patients with structural coma. Am J Respir Crit Care Med 155(5):1729–1734

Tenke P, Kovacs B, Bjerklund Johansen TE, Matsumoto T, Tambyah PA, Naber KG (2008) European and Asian guidelines on management and prevention of catheter-associated urinary tract infections. Int J Antimicrob Agents 31(Suppl 1):S68–S78

Torres A, Carlet J (2001) Ventilator-associated pneumonia. European Task Force on ventilator-associated pneumonia. Eur Respir J 17(5):1034–1045

Body Temperature in TBI Patients

61

Per-Olof Grände and Bertil Romner

Recommendations

Level I

Active cooling to subnormal temperature in TBI patients should be avoided.

Level II

There is support for the avoidance of high fever, but no support for active cooling.

Level III

Level III studies support the use of active cooling in TBI patients, a conclusion not supported from Level I or II studies. Paracetamol or methylprednisolone can be used to control fever in TBI patients. Normothermia is the optimal temperature for a TBI patient.

P.-O. Grände (✉)
Department of Anaesthesia and Intensive Care, Lund University and Lund University Hospital, SE-22185 Lund, Sweden
e-mail: per-olof.grande@med.lu.se

B. Romner
Department of Neurosurgery 2092, Rigshospitalet, 2100 Copenhagen, Denmark
e-mail: bertil.romner@rh.regionh.dk

61.1 Overview

Based on experimental and clinical studies, there is a general view that fever is detrimental to TBI patients (Thompson et al. 2003). An important goal in the treatment of these patients has therefore been to prevent or reduce fever. So far, we lack evidence-based consensus regarding how to reduce temperature in TBI patients. Fever can be reduced pharmacologically by affecting the thermostat or by active cooling of the patient. During the last 10–15 years, it has also been suggested that active cooling to subnormal temperatures (32–34°C) should be beneficial due to its well-known neuroprotective effect, as demonstrated in animal studies after brain ischaemia and also in humans after near-drowning and after active cooling following heart resuscitation, and the fact that hypothermia decreases an increased intracranial pressure (Polderman 2008). The mechanisms behind the hypothermia-induced neuroprotection are not clarified, but the reduced neuronal metabolism and the inflammatory response, and the reduction in toxic substances such as glutamate and a scavenging effect may be involved. It was therefore believed that active cooling should be beneficial in TBI patients, but we still lack studies giving support for active cooling in clinical practice. In this chapter, we give recommendations on how and when temperature should be reduced and the goal temperature in TBI patients, based on the results of the most recent studies and current knowledge in this field. It will be concluded that active cooling is associated with

T. Sundstrøm et al. (eds.), *Management of Severe Traumatic Brain Injury*,
DOI 10.1007/978-3-642-28126-6_61, © Springer-Verlag Berlin Heidelberg 2012

side effects and that we lack support for its use in TBI patients, and it can therefore not be recommended.

Tips, Tricks, and Pitfalls

- Avoid active cooling in TBI patients.
- Temperature can be reduced by affecting the thermostat pharmacologically with paracetamol (1 g×2–4 p.o.) and when there is persistent fever above 38.5°C with one bolus dose of methylprednisolone (Solu-Medrol) (0.5–1.0 g i.v.).
- Normothermia is the optimal temperature.

61.2 Background

61.2.1 Active Cooling of the Patient

In spite of the fact that reduction of fever by active cooling to a normal temperature has been used in clinical practice in TBI patients for decades, there have been no studies confirming the effect of this therapeutic measure on outcome. There have been many studies on TBI patients, however, that have analyzed the effect of active cooling to subnormal temperatures on outcome. Several smaller studies have suggested that there is improved outcome with active cooling (Marion et al. 1997; Adelson et al. 2005), but the best trials on children and adults could not confirm any beneficial effects with active cooling (Clifton et al. 2001, 2011; Hutchison et al. 2008). A comprehensive analysis of the best studies supported the view that active cooling to subnormal temperatures has no beneficial effect on outcome in TBI patients; instead, these studies indicated that active cooling may worsen outcome—a conclusion strongly supported by a recent Cochrane analysis (Sydenham et al. 2009). Furthermore, we still lack any support for the view that treatment of fever to a normal or subnormal temperature by active cooling is beneficial. Thus, at this stage, active cooling cannot be recommended as a therapy to reduce temperature in TBI patients.

There are some specific characteristics of the TBI patients that may explain why the well-established neuroprotective effect of active cooling does not result in improved outcome (Grände et al. 2009). Active cooling always means a difference between the body temperature and the temperature stipulated by the thermostat. This difference creates a metabolic stress with the purpose of restoring body temperature to the level before, resulting in an increase in plasma catecholamines, and muscle shivering is a visible component of this stress response. There is a great risk, however, that the increased catecholamine concentration after active cooling will further reduce the already compromised circulation of the penumbra zone. There is also a great risk that ventilatory adjustment to the lower metabolism is not performed, leading to a hyperventilation-induced worse perfusion of the penumbra zone. Hypothermia also means a lower blood pressure, resulting in more frequent use of vasopressors, which may not only reduce perfusion of the penumbra zone but also increase the risk of development of ARDS (Robertson et al. 1999) and loss of plasma volume to the interstitium (Dubniks et al. 2007). Finally, reduction of the body temperature to subnormal values may induce coagulation disturbances and increase the volumes of the contusional bleedings (Rundgren and Engström 2008).

61.2.2 Pharmacological Reduction of Body Temperature

From a physiological point of view, fever should be treated by adjusting the thermostat to normal temperature levels. Several types of new temperature-reducing substances have been tested experimentally, but, so far, none of these drugs can be used clinically due to severe side effects. This means that at the moment, paracetamol and steroids are the only temperature-reducing substances available in clinical practice. Paracetamol has side effects in terms of inhibition of the endogenous production of prostacyclin and has toxic effects on the liver, but in reasonable doses, it can be used to reduce fever. Steroids (methylprednisolone) effectively reduce fever in a bolus dose of 0.5–1 g in man. A specific randomized study analysing the effect of methylprednisolone on TBI, the Crash study (Edwards et al. 2005), showed worse outcome in TBI patients (GCS <14) when using steroids, but steroids were given in a very high dose of more than 20 g for 2 days in that study. The results of the Crash study support the conclusion that corticosteroids should not be used routinely in the treatment of head injury. This does not mean, however, that the fever-reducing effect of one bolus dose of methylprednisolone at the low dose of 0.5–1 g to an adult cannot be used to reduce fever. Such a dose may significantly reduce fever for up to 2 days, and the beneficial fever-reducing effect most likely overrides the potential adverse effects shown by the 20–40 times larger doses in the Crash study. A subsequent increase in blood glucose can be controlled by insulin.

61.3 Specific Paediatric Concerns

The highest quality randomized trials performed for the adult and the paediatric population have not shown any beneficial effects of active hypothermia following TBI (Clifton et al. 2001, 2011). The best paediatric study performed so far (Hutchison et al. 2008) strongly indicated that hypothermia may even worsen outcome. This means that active hypothermia should not be used in the paediatric population.

References

Adelson PD, Ragheb J, Kanev P, Brockmeyer D, Beers SR, Brown SD, Cassidy LD, Chang Y, Levin H (2005) Phase II clinical trial of moderate hypothermia after severe traumatic brain injury in children. Neurosurgery 56(4):740–754

Clifton GL, Miller ER, Choi SC, Levin HS, McCauley S, Smith KR Jr, Muizelaar JP, Wagner FC Jr, Marion DW, Luerssen TG, Chesnut RM, Schwartz M (2001) Lack of effect of induction of hypothermia after acute brain injury. N Engl J Med 344(8):556–563

Clifton GL, Valadka A, Zygun D, Coffey CS, Drever P, Fourwinds S, Janis LS, Wilde E, Taylor P, Harshman K, Conley A, Puccio A, Levin HS, McCauley SR, Bucholz RD, Smith KR, Schmidt JH, Scott JN, Yonas H, Okonkwo DO (2011) Very early hypothermia induction in patients with severe brain injury (the National Acute Brain Injury Study: Hypothermia II): a randomised trial. Lancet Neurol 10(2):131–139

Dubniks M, Persson J, Grände PO (2007) Effect of blood pressure on plasma volume loss in the rat under increased permeability. Intensive Care Med 33(12):2192–2198

Edwards P, Arango M, Balica L, Cottingham R, El-Sayed H, Farrell B, Fernandes J, Gogichaisvili T, Golden N, Hartzenberg B, Husain M, Ulloa MI, Jerbi Z, Khamis H, Komolafe E, Laloë V, Lomas G, Ludwig S, Mazairac G, Muñoz Sanchéz Mde L, Nasi L, Olldashi F, Plunkett P, Roberts I, Sandercock P, Shakur H, Soler C, Stocker R, Svoboda P, Trenkler S, Venkataramana NK, Wasserberg J, Yates D, Yutthakasemsunt S, CRASH trial collaborators (2005) Final results of MRC CRASH, a randomised placebo-controlled trial of intravenous corticosteroid in adults with head injury-outcomes at 6 months. Lancet 365(9475):1957–1959

Grände PO, Reinstrup P, Romner B (2009) Active cooling in traumatic brain-injured patients: a questionable therapy? Acta Anaesthesiol Scand 53(10):1233–1238

Hutchison JS, Ward RE, Lacroix J, Hébert PC, Barnes MA, Bohn DJ, Dirks PB, Doucette S, Fergusson D, Gottesman R, Joffe AR, Kirpalani HM, Meyer PG, Morris KP, Moher D, Singh RN, Skippen PW, Hypothermia Pediatric Head Injury Trial Investigators and the Canadian Critical Care Trials Group (2008) Hypothermia therapy after traumatic brain injury in children. N Engl J Med 358(23):2447–2456

Marion DW, Penrod LE, Kelsey SF, Obrist WD, Kochanek PM, Palmer AM, Wisniewski SR, DeKosky ST (1997) Treatment of traumatic brain injury with moderate hypothermia. N Engl J Med 336(8):540–546

Polderman KH (2008) Induced hypothermia and fever control for prevention and treatment of neurological injuries. Lancet 371:1955–1969, Review

Robertson CS, Valadka AB, Hannay HJ, Contant CF, Gopinath SP, Cormio M, Uzura M, Grossman RG (1999) Prevention of secondary ischemic insults after severe head injury. Crit Care Med 27(10):2086–2095

Rundgren M, Engström M (2008) A thromboelastometric evaluation of the effects of hypothermia on the coagulation system. Anesth Analg 107(5):1465–1468

Sydenham E, Roberts I, Alderson P (2009) Hypothermia for traumatic head injury. Cochrane Database Syst Rev (2):CD001048

Thompson HJ, Tkacs NC, Saatman KE, Raghupathi R, McIntosh TK (2003) Hyperthermia following traumatic brain injury: a critical evaluation. Neurobiol Dis 12(3):163–173

Neuroendocrine Treatment

62

Marianne Klose and Ulla Feldt-Rasmussen

Recommendations

Level I

There are insufficient data to support a Level I recommendation for this topic.

Level II

Immediate treatment of hypoadrenalism is recommended upon clinical suspicion.

Level III

When pituitary insufficiency is discovered and treated within 6 months after TBI, it is recommended to retest the patient after 1 year or more.

62.1 Overview

Presence of pituitary hormone alterations is a very common phenomenon in the acute phase after TBI. However, the diagnosis entails plenty of problems, and currently there are no reliable diagnostic cut-offs for anterior pituitary hormone deficiency in critically ill patients (for details see Chap. 45). Furthermore, no evidence exists to support a clinical benefit from hormonal replacement therapy with growth hormone (GH), thyroid hormone, or reproductive hormones in the critically ill. The diagnosis of adrenal failure and management of this disorder also remains controversial, with poor agreement among the experts. The threshold that best describes the patients at need for acute or chronic glucocorticoid replacement is still to be defined and is likely to depend on the underlying illness. At present time, recommendations will have to be pragmatic and mainly rely on the clinical evaluation of the patient, where a combination of hyponatraemia, hypoglycaemia, and hypotension is highly suggestive (Agha et al. 2005; Cooper and Stewart 2003), but not prerequisite, of secondary hypoadrenalism, and should elicit immediate therapeutic trial of glucocorticoid replacement. The subsequent treatment response should guide further treatment and follow-up.

Long-term anterior pituitary hormone deficits are being described with a higher frequency than previously thought. Although some studies have subsequently failed to show such high frequency (van der Eerden et al. 2010), concerns have been raised whether undiagnosed and thus untreated hypopituitarism may contribute to the mortality and severe morbidity seen in TBI. The magnitude of this contribution has not yet been defined, and although some outcome studies have indicated

M. Klose (✉)
Medicinsk Endokrinologisk Klinik PE-2131,
Rigshospitalet, Blegdamsvej 9,
2100 København, Denmark
e-mail: klose@rh.dk

U. Feldt-Rasmussen
Medicinsk Endokrinologisk Klinik PE-2132,
Rigshospitalet, Blegdamsvej 9,
2100 København, Denmark
e-mail: ufeldt@rh.dk

T. Sundstrøm et al. (eds.), *Management of Severe Traumatic Brain Injury*,
DOI 10.1007/978-3-642-28126-6_62, © Springer-Verlag Berlin Heidelberg 2012

that posttraumatic hypopituitarism is of clinical significance with important impacts on health-related quality of life, lipid status (Kelly et al. 2006; Klose et al. 2007), and rehabilitation (Bondanelli et al. 2007), the findings have not been consistent (Pavlovic et al. 2010). However, current status is that expert panels have proposed recommendations for hormone assessment of pituitary insufficiency and consequent appropriate replacement after TBI (Ghigo et al. 2005; Ho 2007). Which subgroups of patients that should be considered for assessment, and at what time point is still debated, and data are still awaited to document the effect of hormone replacement therapy in this patient category. Until such data are available, one should be cautious to introduce uncritical routine anterior pituitary testing and replacement therapy.

Tips, Tricks, and Pitfalls

- Treatment of hypoadrenalism with replacement dosages of hydrocortisone is recommended upon clinical suspicion. Important diagnostic clues are hemodynamic instability despite adequate fluid resuscitation.
- TBI patients may develop long-term hypopituitarism. Involvement of a specialised medical endocrinologist is mandatory for proper decision of hypothalamo-pituitary tests, their interpretation, and treatment.
- Long-term treatment of anterior pituitary hormone deficits should follow the general guidelines for treatments of these deficiencies whatever the cause.

62.2 Background

62.2.1 Acute Phase Anterior Pituitary Hormone Deficiency

Currently, no evidence exists to suggest introduction of anterior pituitary hormone screening in critical illness, due to both the aforementioned diagnostic difficulties and lack of evidence of the beneficial effects from hormonal substitution. Treatment with pharmacological doses of GH has been shown to increase morbidity and mortality (Takala et al. 1999), whether or not administration of thyroid hormone is beneficial or harmful remains controversial (De Groot 2006; Stathatos et al. 2001), and no conclusive clinical benefit has been demonstrated for androgen treatment in prolonged critical illness (Angele et al. 1998). The evidence of a clinical benefit from glucocorticoid replacement therapy relies on case reports, where initiation of glucocorticoid causes improvement in the patient's condition and clinical symptoms (Agha et al. 2005; Webster and Bell 1997). However, considering the fact that an insufficient glucocorticoid production is lethal, randomised clinical trials will never be performed.

62.2.2 Long-Term Anterior Pituitary Hormone Deficiency

The negative effects of glucocorticoid, thyroid, and gonadal hormone deficiencies are well recognised, as is the beneficial effect from appropriate replacement therapy. Yet randomised clinical trials have never been performed in such classical endocrine deficiencies, and neither are randomised studies available to document such effect in TBI patients. These deficiencies and their treatment, however, have more distinct clinical features, than, e.g., GH deficiency, which is the most frequently reported deficiency in TBI patients. It is associated with impaired linear growth and attainment of normal body composition in children, but in adults the features are less specific with reduced lean body mass, decreased exercise capacity, reduced bone mineral density, unfavourable changes in the lipid profile, and decreased quality of life in adults. There are only few available data on treatment effect in this specific subpopulation of patients with anterior pituitary hormone deficiency. In order to evaluate the effect of human GH replacement therapy as documented in the German Pfizer International Metabolic (KIMS) database, clinical and other outcome variables were compared at baseline and after 1 year of hGH replacement, in 84 TBI patients and 84 patients with deficiency due to a non-functioning pituitary adenoma (NFPA) (Kreitschmann-Andermahr et al. 2008). At 1-year follow-up, IGF-I SDS levels had increased to the normal range, and quality of life (QoL) as measured by the QoL – Assessment of Growth Hormone Deficiency (AGHDA) questionnaire – improved significantly in TBI as in NFPA patients, thus suggesting that TBI patients with GH deficiency benefit from hGH replacement in terms of improved QoL in a similar fashion as do NFPA patients. However, there is still inadequate literature to demonstrate that pituitary replacement therapy improves neuro-cognitive symptoms, psychosocial problems, and work-related activities in TBI patients (High et al. 2010; Maric et al. 2010; Reimunde et al. 2011).

62.3 Specific Paediatric Concerns

Paediatric survivors of severe TBI in particular may develop pituitary dysfunction. Recent studies have reported very discrepant results as concern the prevalence of posttraumatic hypopituitarism in children and adolescents (Einaudi et al. 2006; Khadr et al. 2010; Moon et al. 2010; Niederland et al. 2007; Poomthavorn et al. 2008), and thus no guidelines have yet been proposed. At this level, it is recommended that, as in adults, treatment of long-term posttraumatic hypopituitarism should follow the general guidelines for treatments of the present deficiencies whatever the cause.

References

Agha A, Sherlock M, Thompson CJ (2005) Post-traumatic hyponatraemia due to acute hypopituitarism. QJM 98:463–464

Angele MK, Ayala A, Cioffi WG, Bland KI, Chaudry IH (1998) Testosterone: the culprit for producing splenocyte immune depression after trauma hemorrhage. Am J Physiol 274:C1530–C1536

Bondanelli M, Ambrosio MR, Cavazzini L, Bertocchi A, Zatelli MC, Carli A, Valle D, Basaglia N, Uberti EC (2007) Anterior pituitary function may predict functional and cognitive outcome in patients with traumatic brain injury undergoing rehabilitation. J Neurotrauma 24:1687–1697

Cooper MS, Stewart PM (2003) Corticosteroid insufficiency in acutely ill patients. N Engl J Med 348: 727–734

De Groot LJ (2006) Non-thyroidal illness syndrome is a manifestation of hypothalamic-pituitary dysfunction, and in view of current evidence, should be treated with appropriate replacement therapies. Crit Care Clin 22: 57–86, vi

Einaudi S, Matarazzo P, Peretta P, Grossetti R, Giordano F, Altare F, Bondone C, Andreo M, Ivani G, Genitori L, de Sanctis C (2006) Hypothalamo-hypophysial dysfunction after traumatic brain injury in children and adolescents: a preliminary retrospective and prospective study. J Pediatr Endocrinol Metab 19:691–703

Ghigo E, Masel B, Aimaretti G, Leon-Carrion J, Casanueva FF, Dominguez-Morales MR, Elovic E, Perrone K, Stalla G, Thompson C, Urban R (2005) Consensus guidelines on screening for hypopituitarism following traumatic brain injury. Brain Inj 19:711–724

High WM Jr, Briones-Galang M, Clark JA, Gilkison C, Mossberg KA, Zgaljardic DJ, Masel BE, Urban RJ (2010) Effect of growth hormone replacement therapy on cognition after traumatic brain injury. J Neurotrauma 27:1565–1575

Ho KK (2007) Consensus guidelines for the diagnosis and treatment of adults with GH deficiency II: a statement of the GH Research Society in association with the European Society for Pediatric Endocrinology, Lawson Wilkins Society, European Society of Endocrinology, Japan Endocrine Society, and Endocrine Society of Australia. Eur J Endocrinol 157:695–700

Kelly DF, McArthur DL, Levin H, Swimmer S, Dusick JR, Cohan P, Wang C, Swerdloff R (2006) Neurobehavioral and quality of life changes associated with growth hormone insufficiency after complicated mild, moderate, or severe traumatic brain injury. J Neurotrauma 23:928–942

Khadr SN, Crofton PM, Jones PA, Wardhaugh B, Roach J, Drake AJ, Minns RA, Kelnar CJ (2010) Evaluation of pituitary function after traumatic brain injury in childhood. Clin Endocrinol (Oxf) 73:637–643

Klose M, Watt T, Brennum J, Feldt-Rasmussen U (2007) Posttraumatic hypopituitarism is associated with an unfavorable body composition and lipid profile, and decreased quality of life 12 months after injury. J Clin Endocrinol Metab 92:3861–3868

Kreitschmann-Andermahr I, Poll EM, Reineke A, Gilsbach JM, Brabant G, Buchfelder M, Fassbender W, Faust M, Kann PH, Wallaschofski H (2008) Growth hormone deficient patients after traumatic brain injury–baseline characteristics and benefits after growth hormone replacement–an analysis of the German KIMS database. Growth Horm IGF Res 18:472–478

Maric NP, Doknic M, Pavlovic D, Pekic S, Stojanovic M, Jasovic-Gasic M, Popovic V (2010) Psychiatric and neuropsychological changes in growth hormone-deficient patients after traumatic brain injury in response to growth hormone therapy. J Endocrinol Invest 33:770–775

Moon RJ, Sutton T, Wilson PM, Kirkham FJ, Davies JH (2010) Pituitary function at long-term follow-up of childhood traumatic brain injury. J Neurotrauma 27:1827–1835

Niederland T, Makovi H, Gal V, Andreka B, Abraham CS, Kovacs J (2007) Abnormalities of pituitary function after traumatic brain injury in children. J Neurotrauma 24:119–127

Pavlovic D, Pekic S, Stojanovic M, Zivkovic V, Djurovic B, Jovanovic V, Miljic N, Medic-Stojanoska M, Doknic M, Miljic D, Djurovic M, Casanueva F, Popovic V (2010) Chronic cognitive sequelae after traumatic brain injury are not related to growth hormone deficiency in adults. Eur J Neurol 17:696–702

Poomthavorn P, Maixner W, Zacharin M (2008) Pituitary function in paediatric survivors of severe traumatic brain injury. Arch Dis Child 93:133–137

Reimunde P, Quintana A, Castanon B, Casteleiro N, Vilarnovo Z, Otero A, Devesa A, Otero-Cepeda XL, Devesa J (2011) Effects of growth hormone (GH) replacement and cognitive rehabilitation in patients with cognitive disorders after traumatic brain injury. Brain Inj 25:65–73

Stathatos N, Levetan C, Burman KD, Wartofsky L (2001) The controversy of the treatment of critically ill patients with thyroid hormone. Best Pract Res Clin Endocrinol Metab 15:465–478

Takala J, Ruokonen E, Webster NR, Nielsen MS, Zandstra DF, Vundelinckx G, Hinds CJ (1999) Increased mortality associated with growth hormone treatment in critically ill adults. N Engl J Med 341:785–792

van der Eerden AW, Twickler MT, Sweep FC, Beems T, Hendricks HT, Hermus AR, Vos PE (2010) Should anterior pituitary function be tested during follow-up of all patients presenting at the emergency department because of traumatic brain injury? Eur J Endocrinol 162:19–28

Webster JB, Bell KR (1997) Primary adrenal insufficiency following traumatic brain injury: a case report and review of the literature. Arch Phys Med Rehabil 78:314–318

63 Mechanical Ventilation in NICU

Jacob Koefoed-Nielsen

Recommendations

Level I

Lung-protected ventilation with low tidal volume is recommended in all patients suffering from ALI/ARDS.

Level II

Invasive ventilation is recommended in the neurotrauma patient with respiratory failure if not fully conscious and able to protect the airways.

The presence of ALI/ARDS is found to be an independent predictor of increased mortality and poor neurological outcome.

Level III

PEEP combined with lung recruitment is recommended (open lung concept). The fraction of inspired oxygen in mechanically ventilated patients should be below 0.6 (= 60%)

J. Koefoed-Nielsen
Department of Neuro ICU,
Aarhus University Hospital,
Aarhus, Denmark
e-mail: koefoedjacob@dadlnet.dk

63.1 Overview

The purpose of mechanical ventilation is to improve gas exchange (O_2 and CO_2); mechanical ventilation can however not improve the gas exchange function of the lung but only support/replace the work done by the respiratory muscles. Mechanical ventilation can be managed in two different ways: non-invasive (tight-fitting face mask) and invasive (endotracheal intubation) (Lumb 2000). Invasive ventilation is the gold standard in neurotrauma patients because the patient has to be fully conscious and able to cooperate if non-invasive ventilation shall be successful.

Tips, Tricks, and Pitfalls

- Lung-protected ventilation, 6–8 ml tidal volume/kg ideal body weight, is recommended in all patients.
- The use of high fraction of inspired oxygen during long-time ventilation is not recommended. The aim should be below 0.6 (= 60% oxygen in the inspired air).
- In patients without lung pathology, 5 cm H_2O PEEP is a good setting to use initially.

T. Sundstrøm et al. (eds.), *Management of Severe Traumatic Brain Injury*,
DOI 10.1007/978-3-642-28126-6_63,

63.2 Background

Invasive ventilation is normally achieved by application of controlled intermittent positive pressure ventilation to the airways of the patient. There are two phases of the respiratory cycle: inspiration, during which the pressure is intermittently raised by the ventilator and the inspired gas flow into the lung is in accordance with the resistance and compliance of the respiratory system, followed by expiration, a passive process as a result of falling pressure in the ventilator (Lumb 2000).

A general complication to mechanical ventilation even in healthy lungs is the formation of atelectases. An atelectasis is a part of the lung, which due to collapse does not participate in gas exchange, thereby creating a shunt whereby blood reaches the arterial system without passing through ventilated regions of the lung. To reduce the formation of atelectases, the use of positive end-expiratory pressure (PEEP) is applied. An atelectasis can be reversed by so-called lung recruitment, where collapsed alveoli will reopen when a higher transpulmonary pressure is applied than that at which they collapsed. The lung recruitment will improve the gas exchange. One of the most obvious side effects of mechanical ventilation (and PEEP) is the effect on the hemodynamic system of the patient. It is caused by an elevation of the intra-thoracic pressure, which decreases the venous return to the heart, resulting in a decrease in cardiac output and a reduction in arterial pressure and CPP (Klinger 1996; Pinsky 1990). This effect has been estimated to be a 10% reduction in cardiac output in a group of patients without lung pathology at 0 cm PEEP. If PEEP is applied, the reduction in cardiac output is higher. PEEP also increases the pressure in the sagittal sinus, but the interference with the venous outflow can be reduced if PEEP is lower than ICP and if the patient's head is elevated 30°.

The negative effect on the hemodynamic system can partially be counteracted with fluid replacement or use of cardiovascular agents (Lumb 2000).

Another important side effect of mechanical ventilation is ventilator-associated lung injury (VALI) (Tremblay et al. 2006). Several factors have been proposed to contribute to VALI: pre-existing lung damage (e.g. trauma, pneumonia), high inspired oxygen concentrations, high inspiratory airway pressure (pneumothorax), and cyclical opening and closure of the alveoli during ventilation (atelectrauma). Cyclical opening and closure of the alveoli can be counteracted by sufficient PEEP (Farias et al. 2005). In healthy lungs, the risk of damage to the lung during mechanical ventilation is very low, even after many cycles of breath-by-breath collapse and re-expansion (Taskar et al. 1995).

In 10–25% of patients with isolated brain injury, the condition is complicated by ALI/ARDS. ALI/ARDS are associated with an inflammatory condition in the lung, and the ventilation of the lung is affected by massive atelectases and a reduction of end-expiratory lung volume (Holland et al. 2003). The compliance of the lung is markedly reduced because of increased interstitial fluid and alveolar oedema. The increased weight of the lung will lead to further collapse of the alveoli. There is a potential risk of damage caused by the mechanical ventilation because re-expansion of collapsed alveoli will lead to local shear stress, which may tear epithelial cells from the basal membrane of the alveoli, creating a vicious circle. In the terminal phase of ALI/ARDS, the lungs become massively consolidated. This results in severe hypoxemia, even when the fraction of inspired oxygen is 1.0 (100%) and there is a persisting hypercapnia caused by large dead space/intrapulmonary shunts and ventilation-perfusion mismatch. Not all patients proceed to the terminal stage, and the condition may resolve at any time, but it is difficult to predict the course of the individual patient. ALI/ARDS may be complicated by other organ failures, leading to multi-organ dysfunction syndrome.

There is no diagnostic laboratory test to confirm ALI/ARDS, but four criteria must be present (Bernard et al. 1994):

1. Acute onset of respiratory failure
2. Severe hypoxia with a ratio between PO_2 and fraction of inspired oxygen (FiO_2) of less than 40 kPa (300 mmHg) if ALI and 26.7 kPa (200 mmHg) if ARDS

3. Chest X-ray: New bilateral diffuse infiltrations
4. One to three cannot be explained by left arterial hypertension (pulmonary artery wedge pressure less than 18 mmHg)

The presence of ALI/ARDS in patients suffering from traumatic brain injury is found to be an independent predictor of increased mortality and poor neurological outcome (Holland et al. 2003). The knowledge that mechanical ventilation can lead to lung damage has received major attention in the past years. According to the 2000 guidelines from the ARDS network, the recommendation for ventilator settings in ALI/ARDS is a low tidal volume, also known as protective ventilation (Brower 2000). This is today the only ventilator setting that has proved to reduce the risk of VALI and to improve patient survival.

Although PEEP is also used in the ventilator treatment of ALI/ARDS in order to prevent repeated closure and reopening of alveoli, the optimal PEEP is difficult to estimate because of individual differences in the pulmonary responses to PEEP (Gattinoni et al. 2006). The same consideration is relevant regarding lung recruitment, which would also seem obvious to apply in ventilator treatment together with adequate PEEP, so-called open lung concept (Lachmann 1992). But as in the case with PEEP, the use of lung recruitment in ICU has not proved to reduce mortality (Meade et al. 2008; Grasso et al. 2005; Mercat et al. 2008). Furthermore, lung recruitment also elevates intra-thoracic pressure; consequently, patients suffering from hypovolaemia are at risk of decreased blood pressure. At present, no specific method to perform lung recruitment is better than another. However, lung recruitment using inspiratory airway pressure above 40 cm H_2O must be considered carefully because of the risk of barotraumas (Gattinoni 2008).

Mechanical ventilation with low tidal volume may result in a degree of hypercapnia, which is a challenge in patients with severe brain injury where tight CO_2 control is important.

A review by Mascia concerning ALI in patients with severe brain injury is published in Neurocrit Care (Marcia 2009).

63.3 Specific Paediatric Concerns

There are no specific concerns. In general, apply the same ventilator settings (tidal volume and PEEP), but be very careful if you attempt to recruit the lungs.

References

Bernard GR et al (1994) The American-European Consensus Conference on ARDS. Definitions, mechanisms, relevant outcomes, and clinical trial coordination. Am J Respir Crit Care Med 149(3 Pt 1):818–824

Brower RG (2000) The ARDS Clinical Trials Network. Ventilation with lower tidal volume as compared with traditional tidal volumes for acute lung injury and the acute respiratory distress syndrome. N Engl J Med 342(18):1301–1308

Farias LL et al (2005) Positive end-expiratory pressure prevents lung mechanical stress caused by recruitment/derecruitment. J Appl Physiol 98(1):53–61

Gattinoni L (2008) Refining ventilatory treatment for acute lung injury and acute respiratory distress syndrome. JAMA 299(6):691–693

Gattinoni L et al (2006) Lung recruitment in patients with the acute respiratory distress syndrome. N Engl J Med 354(17):1775–1786

Grasso S et al (2005) Effects of high versus low positive end-expiratory pressure in acute respiratory distress syndrome. Am J Respir Crit Care Med 171(9):1002–1008

Holland MC et al (2003) The development of acute lung injury is associated with worse neurologic outcome in patients with severe traumatic brain injury. J Trauma 55:106–111

Klinger JR (1996) Hemodynamics and positive end-expiratory pressure in critically ill patients. Crit Care Clin 12(4):841–864

Lachmann B (1992) Open up the lung and keep the lung open. Intensive Care Med 18(6):319–321

Lumb AB (2000) Nunn's applied respiratory physiology, 5th edn. Butterworth-Heinemann, Edinburgh

Marcia L (2009) Acute lung injury in patients with severe brain injury: a double hit model. Neurocrit Care 11(3):417–426

Meade MO et al (2008) Ventilation strategy using low tidal volumes, recruitment maneuvers, and high positive end-expiratory pressure for acute lung injury and acute respiratory distress syndrome: a randomized controlled trial. JAMA 299(6):637–645

Mercat A et al (2008) Positive end-expiratory pressure setting in adults with acute lung injury and acute respiratory distress syndrome: a randomized controlled trial. JAMA 299(6):646–655

Pinsky MR (1990) The effects of mechanical ventilation on the cardiovascular system. Crit Care Clin 6(3):663–678

Taskar V et al (1995) Healthy lungs tolerate repetitive collapse and reopening during short periods of mechanical ventilation. Acta Anaesthesiol Scand 39(3): 370–376

Tremblay LN et al (2006) Ventilator-induced lung injury: from the bench to the bedside. Intensive Care Med 32(1):24–33

64 Seizures

Elisabeth Ronne-Engström

Recommendations

Level I

There are insufficient data to support a Level I recommendation regarding either treatment for early posttraumatic seizures (PTS) or anti-seizure prophylaxis after head trauma.

Level II

Early posttraumatic seizures should be treated. Anticonvulsants are indicated to decrease the incidence of early PTS (within 7 days of injury).

Level III

When seizures occur, it is important to re-evaluate the clinical situation with respect to intracranial lesions requiring surgical intervention.

Prophylactic anti-seizure therapy may be considered as a treatment option to prevent early PTS in young paediatric patients and infants at high risk for seizures following head injury.

E. Ronne-Engström
Department of Neurosurgery,
Uppsala University Hospital, Uppsala Sweden
e-mail: elisabeth.ronne.engstrom@akademiska.se

64.1 Overview

There are no randomised, controlled, double-blind studies regarding treatment of early seizures after TBI, but from observational studies in the literature, there are good reasons to believe that seizures should be treated as soon as they occur. The basic idea with neurointensive care of TBI is to identify and treat conditions that compromise the brain's supply and use of oxygen and glucose. Seizure activity in the acute phase impairs this in a number of ways and can therefore worsen the brain trauma. Neuronal firing causes a massive release of the potentially neurotoxic transmitter glutamate (GLU). In order to clear the synaptic space from GLU, there is an efficient glial uptake. However, this is highly energy dependent. Seizures increase the energy demand which can cause an energy failure in the brain into a manifest ischemia due to energy failure. Seizure activity can also cause significant changes in cerebral blood flow, with both increases and decreases observed.

It is debated whether anticonvulsant prophylaxis after head trauma should be used or not. The Brain Trauma Foundation states in its latest review (Bratton et al. 2007) that there is evidence that an adequate treatment with phenytoin reduces the incidence of early seizures but that no effects on outcome were seen. A major confounding factor is that earlier studies base their conclusions on clinically observable seizures. The Brain Trauma Foundation states accordingly that more studies are needed and that such

T. Sundstrøm et al. (eds.), *Management of Severe Traumatic Brain Injury*,
DOI 10.1007/978-3-642-28126-6_64, © Springer-Verlag Berlin Heidelberg 2012

studies should use continuous EEG monitoring to identify seizures.

Once seizures occur, it could either be a result of the original trauma or they could indicate that new intracranial lesions have developed. Treatment of repeated seizures and status epilepticus is a matter for qualified neurointensive care and could need multimodality monitoring and a team approach including neurosurgeons, neurologists, neurophysiologists and neurointensivists.

Tips, Tricks, and Pitfalls

- When seizures occur, exclude development of new intracranial lesions needing surgical intervention.
- Remember possible withdrawal symptoms for alcohol/drug addicts with TBI.
- *Treatment of single seizures*:
  - Intravenous diazepam 10 mg or lorazepam 2–4 mg.
  - Consider prophylaxis with phenytoin.
- *Treatment of repeated seizures*:
  - Start continuous treatment as well as prophylaxis.
  - Monitor vital functions and EEG.
  - Low threshold for intubation and artificial ventilation to enable more intense treatment.
  - Choice should be based on local traditions for sedation of intubated patients.
  - Propofol infusion is commonly used. A bolus dose of 1–3 mg/kg is followed by infusion of 1.0–7.5 mg/kg/h until seizure activity is gone. Midazolam can also be used, together with propofol or as only drug, and starts with a bolus of 0.2 mg/kg i.v. followed by infusion of 0.1–0.5 mg/kg/h.
  - Phenytoin is added as prophylaxis with 15–20 mg FE/kg i.v. followed by 250 FE×3. It is important that adequate serum concentrations are achieved and daily checks are advised.
  - If seizures still are present, lorazepam, levetiracetam, lamotrigine, carbamazepine or valproate could be added.
- *Treatment of status epilepticus if not resolved with the treatment above*:
  - Thiopental infusion. Bolus dose is 100–250 mg and is followed by 50 mg every 2–3 min until EEG is low voltage without seizure activity or burst suppression. This is followed by an infusion of 3–5 mg/kg/h. There should be 12–24 h free from seizures before the treatment stops. Note: the patient has to be on mechanical ventilation with a strict control on electrolytes, temperature and vital organ functions.

64.2 Background

Seizures occurring after traumatic brain injury (TBI) are usually described as early, within first week after trauma or late. These are two different phenomena, probably also to some extent with separate neurobiological backgrounds. The true incidence of early seizures is presently discussed. Based on clinical observations, the incidence was estimated to ~10%. However, continuous EEG monitoring shows that early seizures are more common and are seen in up to 50% of TBI patients that are admitted to neurointensive care. Early seizures were more often seen in older patients and in those with subdural/epidural haematomas alone or in combination with brain contusions (Vespa et al. 1999; Ronne-Engstrom and Winkler 2006).

Late seizures manifest as posttraumatic epilepsy and develop in approximately 5% of TBI. The risk is higher after severe TBI. Posttraumatic epilepsy accounts for 20% of symptomatic epilepsy in the population (see Lowenstein 2009) and is more common after penetrating injury, severe closed injury and focal lesions (Pohlmann-Eden and Bruckmeir 1997; Annegers and Coan 2000).

Early seizures are also believed to be a risk factor for posttraumatic epilepsy. Apparently, there is a time lag and a time window for therapeutic intervention before the traumatic brain scar matures into a chronic epileptic region.

There are two main indications for monitoring and treatment of seizures after head trauma:

- Seizure activity in the acute phase can be deleterious for the injured brain and has repeatedly been shown to be associated with a worse outcome.
- To lower the risk for posttraumatic epilepsy since early seizures are believed to be a risk factor for this.

64.2.1 The Relation of Seizures to the Acute Brain Injury

There are several mechanisms by which seizure activity in the acute phase can exacerbate the brain trauma. Neuronal firing causes a massive release of the potentially neurotoxic transmitter glutamate (GLU). Extracellular glutamate release during seizure activity was demonstrated with intracerebral microdialysis in patients with chronic epilepsy (During and Spencer 1993; Ronne-Engstrom et al. 1992) and in TBI patients (Vespa et al. 1998). Another problem is that the postsynaptic glial uptake of GLU is highly energy dependent (see Magistretti and Pellerin 1999). Seizure activity can thus cause a significant increase in the energy demand. In the acute phase after trauma, with an already strained brain metabolism, an increased energy demand can result in a manifest ischaemia due to energy failure with higher demands than availability (Samuelsson et al. 2007). Seizure activity can also cause significant changes in cerebral blood flow. This has been demonstrated with different techniques, e.g. cortical blood flow measurements using laser Doppler fibre attached to subdural strip electrodes (Ronne-Engstrom et al. 1993). Increased, as well as a decreased, cerebral blood flow was detected during seizures. Both these situations are potentially harmful. Increased CBF could increase ICP by vasodilatation, and a decreased CBF could worsen an energy failure situation. The blood flow changes are probably coupled to the changes in metabolic demands. Vespa showed (Vespa et al. 2007) that patients with TBI and repetitive non-convulsive seizures had both higher mean ICP and higher lactate/pyruvate ratio as measured with intracerebral microdialysis, marking an increased glucose metabolism.

64.2.2 NICU Management

64.2.2.1 Seizure Monitoring

The general idea with the NICU monitoring is to identify and treat conditions that compromise the oxygen and glucose supply to the brain or that increase the metabolic demands, e.g. fever and epileptic seizures. The EEG pattern depends on the integrity of the brain structures as well as on the cerebral blood flow and metabolism. Continuous EEG is therefore theoretically ideal as a monitoring facility. EEG is in fact so far the only available method for online real-time monitoring of the brain's functions. There are still some problems, such as the availability of EEG reading on a 24-h basis. However, since EEG today is done digitally, computerised treatment of the EEG signal can facilitate the EEG reading. An example of this is the use of the trends of the EEG's total power (Vespa 2005). High values can indicate seizure activity, and when this is found, raw EEG during this time period is studied. Another advantage of digital EEG is that it allows for web-based EEG reading.

64.2.2.2 Prophylaxis

It is debated whether anticonvulsant prophylaxis should be used or not. A major confounding factor when reading the literature is that earlier studies base their conclusions on clinically observable seizures. The Brain Trauma Foundation has in their guidelines for treatment of TBI also reviewed the scientific bases for anti-seizure prophylaxis (Bratton et al. 2007). Their conclusion is that there is evidence that an adequate treatment with phenytoin reduces the incidence of early seizures, but not of posttraumatic epilepsy. Furthermore, valproate may have a comparable effect but may also be associated with a higher mortality. They also state that more studies are needed on the effect on outcome by reducing early seizures and that such studies should use continuous EEG monitoring to identify seizures.

Using drugs with anticonvulsant properties, e.g. midazolam in sedating intubated patients could be an alternative anti-seizure prophylaxis. No seizures were monitored in a study were most of the patients were sedated with thiopental and midazolam (Olivecrona et al. 2009).

64.2.2.3 Treatment of Seizures

When seizures occur, it is important to re-evaluate the clinical situation to see if something has changed. This could be the development of a brain contusion, subdural hematoma or a cortical venous thrombosis. One should also keep in mind the possibility of withdrawal symptoms for alcohol/drug addicts with TBI. Early posttraumatic seizures should be treated as soon as they occur, which is easier if the unit has a programmed treatment. The suggested treatments below are from Uppsala University Hospital treatment program for seizures in neurointensive care.

Single seizures could be treated with intravenous diazepam 10 mg i.v. or lorazepam 2–4 mg i.v. Prophylaxis with phenytoin should be considered.

In case of *repeated seizures*, treatment as well as prophylaxis should be started. It is preferred that continuous EEG monitoring is used to ensure that the patient becomes seizure free from the treatment. Respiration and cardiovascular functions should also be monitored, and the threshold for intubation and mechanical ventilation should be low.

The choice of pharmacological substances must be based on local traditions of what is used for sedation of intubated patients. Propofol infusion is often used. A bolus dose of 1–3 mg/kg is given, followed by 1-5 mg/kg/h. Treatment should not extend 48 h. Midazolam infusion is also efficient. Midazolam starts with a bolus of 0.2 mg/kg i.v. followed by 0.1–0.5 mg/kg/h. To this is Pheytoin infusion, 15-20mg FE/kg, followed by intermittent doses of 250mg FE/kg x 3. It is important that adequate serum concentrations are achieved and daily checks are advised.

If seizures still are present, lorazepam, levetiracetam, lamotrigine, carbamazepine or valproate can be added. Anticonvulsant drugs have many side effects including interaction with other drugs, skin reactions, deranged liver function and haematologic disturbances, such as clotting disturbances, which can be especially serious for TBI patients.

Status epilepticus that does not resolve with the treatment above could be treated with thiopental infusion. Bolus dose is 100–250 mg and is followed by 50 mg every 2–3 min until EEG is low voltage without seizure activity or burst suppression. This is followed by an infusion of 3–5 mg/kg/h. There should be at least 12–24 h free from seizures before the treatment stops. The patient with thiopental treatment has to be on mechanical ventilation with a strict control on electrolytes, temperature and vital organ functions.

64.3 Specific Paediatric Concerns

There are only a few studies in the literature regarding children and early posttraumatic seizures. In one study, 7% had immediate seizures (Emanuelson and Uvebrant 2009). This contrasts to a recent study showing that as much as 68% of children with moderate and severe TBI developed early posttraumatic seizures. The two groups probably represent different severities of TBI (Liesemer et al. 2011).

According to the Brain Trauma Foundation, prophylactic use of anti-seizure therapy is not recommended for children with severe traumatic brain injury (TBI) for preventing late posttraumatic seizures (Level II) (Adelson et al. 2003). They state also that prophylactic anti-seizure therapy may be considered as a treatment option to prevent early PTS in young paediatric patients and infants at high risk for seizures following head injury (Level III).

Treatment of seizures and status epilepticus in children should follow similar strategies as in adults. However, the doses and choices of drugs should be carefully considered after the individual circumstances. In Sweden, propofol is only recommended for starting sedation of children >1 month, but not for continuous sedation of children <16 years. Continuous EEG monitoring could be very valuable.

References

Adelson PD, Bratton SL, Carney NA, Chesnut RM, Du Coudray HEM, Goldstein B, Kochanek PM, Miller HC, Partington MD, Selden NR, Warden CR, Wright DW (2003) Guidelines for the acute medical treatment of severe traumatic brain injury in infants, children and adolescents. Chapter 19; The role of anti-seizure prophylaxis following severe traumatic brain injury. Pediatr Crit Care Med 31(6 Suppl):S488–S491

Annegers JF, Coan SP (2000) The risks of epilepsy after traumatic brain injury. Seizure 9(7):453–457

Bratton SL et al (2007) Guidelines for the management of severe traumatic brain injury. XIII. Antiseizure prophylaxis. J Neurotrauma 24 Suppl 1:S83–S86

During MJ, Spencer DD (1993) Extracellular hippocampal glutamate and spontaneous seizure in the conscious human brain. Lancet 341(8861):1607–1610

Emanuelson I, Uvebrant P (2009) Occurrence of epilepsy during the first 10 years after traumatic brain injury acquired in childhood up to the age of 18 years in the south western Swedish population-based series. Brain Inj 23(7):612–616

Liesemer K et al (2011) Early post-traumatic seizures in moderate to severe pediatric traumatic brain injury: rates, risk factors, and clinical features. J Neurotrauma 28(5):755–762

Lowenstein DH (2009) Epilepsy after head injury: an overview. Epilepsia 50(Suppl 2):4–9

Magistretti PJ, Pellerin L (1999) Astrocytes couple synaptic activity to glucose utilization in the brain. News Physiol Sci 14:177–182

Olivecrona M et al (2009) Absence of electroencephalographic seizure activity in patients treated for head injury with an intracranial pressure-targeted therapy. J Neurosurg 110(2):300–305

Pohlmann-Eden B, Bruckmeir J (1997) Predictors and dynamics of posttraumatic epilepsy. Acta Neurol Scand 95(5):257–262

Ronne-Engstrom E, Winkler T (2006) Continuous EEG monitoring in patients with traumatic brain injury reveals a high incidence of epileptiform activity. Acta Neurol Scand 114(1):47–53

Ronne-Engstrom E et al (1992) Intracerebral microdialysis of extracellular amino acids in the human epileptic focus. J Cereb Blood Flow Metab 12(5):873–876

Ronne-Engstrom E, Carlson H, Blom S, Flink R, Gazelius B, Spännare B, Hillered L (1993) Monitoring of cortical blood flow in human epileptic foci using laser doppler flowmetry. J Epilepsy 6:145–151

Samuelsson C et al (2007) Cerebral glutamine and glutamate levels in relation to compromised energy metabolism: a microdialysis study in subarachnoid hemorrhage patients. J Cereb Blood Flow Metab 27(7):1309–1317

Vespa P (2005) Continuous EEG monitoring for the detection of seizures in traumatic brain injury, infarction, and intracerebral hemorrhage: "to detect and protect". J Clin Neurophysiol 22(2):99–106

Vespa P et al (1998) Increase in extracellular glutamate caused by reduced cerebral perfusion pressure and seizures after human traumatic brain injury: a microdialysis study. J Neurosurg 89(6):971–982

Vespa PM et al (1999) Increased incidence and impact of nonconvulsive and convulsive seizures after traumatic brain injury as detected by continuous electroencephalographic monitoring. J Neurosurg 91(5):750–760

Vespa PM et al (2007) Nonconvulsive electrographic seizures after traumatic brain injury result in a delayed, prolonged increase in intracranial pressure and metabolic crisis. Crit Care Med 35(12):2830–2836

65 Autonomic Dysfunction

Christina Rosenlund

Recommendations

Level I

Hyper-metabolism and nitrogen loss follow acute severe cerebral injury, and high protein diet is vital.

Level II

Weight loss following dystonia is causing problems in rehabilitation settings.

Level III

If there are clinical signs of autonomic dysfunction and other explanations for the symptoms are ruled out, it is recommended to try treatment with intrathecal baclofen.

If there is no response to treatment with a lumbar dosage of 200 μg baclofen, further testing is without purpose.

C. Rosenlund
Department of Neurosurgery,
Odense University Hospital,
Sdr. Boulevard 29, 5000 Odense, DK
e-mail: chrisstenrose@gmail.com

65.1 Overview

Autonomic dysfunction is defined by dystonia (paroxystic increase in muscle tone) and at least one of the below following symptoms:

1. Hyperthermia
2. Arterial hypertension
3. Tachypnea
4. Tachycardia
5. Sweating
6. Hyper-salivation/increase in bronchial secretion

Autonomic dysfunction can cause systemic disorders, contractures (joints) and excessive weight loss because of a massive loss of muscle protein. If there are clinical signs of autonomic dysfunction and other explanations for the symptoms are ruled out, it is recommended to try treatment with intrathecal baclofen. The differential diagnoses for these symptoms are:

Other cerebral lesions
Hydrocephalus
Shunt infection
Shunt dysfunction
Systemic infection
Cardiac disorder

When the decision to treat is made, a test dose of baclofen is given to test the response to treatment.

T. Sundstrøm et al. (eds.), *Management of Severe Traumatic Brain Injury*,
DOI 10.1007/978-3-642-28126-6_65, © Springer-Verlag Berlin Heidelberg 2012

The test dose is given through a lumbar puncture; 2 ml CSF is sent to microbiological examination. Give only one dose of baclofen per day.

Dosage adults	Day 1	Day 2	
(Baclofen)	100 μg	200 μg	
Dosage children	Day 1	Day 2	Day 3
<10 kg	25 μg	35 μg	50 μg
10–30 kg	35 μg	50 μg	75 μg
>30 kg	50 μg	75 μg	100 μg

If there is an effect on the symptoms (reduction or disappearance of symptoms) following administration of 100 μg, consider placing a spinal catheter and an external pump. If there is no response to treatment with 200 μg, further testing is without purpose. This is also the recommendation following the third test dosage when treating children (Kock-Jensen 2007).

Placement of a spinal catheter for continuous infusion with baclofen through an external pump (Kock-Jensen 2007):

1. Pre-puncture antibiotics (dicloxacillin 1 g i.v. or cefuroxime 1.5 g i.v.).
2. Use a thin epidural/ spinal catheter.
3. Sterile cover after thorough cleansing.
4. The catheter is placed in the subarachnoid space via puncture at level L3/L4.
5. The catheter is lead approximately 10 cm in cranial direction.
6. Catheter loop at access point. Sterile drape afterwards.
7. The catheter is fastened with a patch along the back and fixated at the level of the clavicle.
8. A catheter filter is mounted.
9. An injection pump is mounted.

Initial dosage is 5–10 μg/h, which gives a daily dose of 120–240 μg. Treatment dosages of up to 800 μg/day can be necessary to have maximal effect on the condition, in a few cases even more than that. With a concentration in the injection pump of 10 μg baclofen/ml, the infusion is programmed to run at a speed of 0.5–1 ml/h.

Dosage baclofen (10 μg/ml):

μg/h	2	5	10	15	20	25	30
ml/h (à 10 μg/ml)	0.2	0.5	1.0	1.5	2.0	2.5	3.0
μg/24 h	48	120	240	360	480	600	720

The dosage can be increased with 10–15% every 6 h until maximal effect is reached (disappearance of symptoms) while observing for effect and/or side effects. The spinal catheter can be used for 3–6 days. The patient must be observed for signs of infection, and daily measurement of CRP and leukocytes is necessary. Sometimes the autonomic dysfunction has disappeared completely within a few days of treatment with baclofen (<1 week). If this is not the case and the treatment cannot be discontinued, the patient needs to get an internal pump implanted. Side effects of the treatment are rare and are in that case related to an overdose (Sidenius 2010; Kock-Jensen 2007):

Urine retention
Muscle hypotonia
Excessive salivation
Confusion, vertigo and somnolence
Nausea, vomiting
Depression of respiration (very seldom)
Coma
Convulsions

Interaction: Antihypertensives and tricyclic antidepressants (Sidenius 2010)

Tips, Tricks, and Pitfalls

- If the patient has an external drain from the ventricular system, you can use this to administrate baclofen. NB! The dosage of baclofen is 1/10 of the dosage given through a lumbar puncture, i.e. test dosage is 10 μg instead of 100 μg baclofen.
- It is possible to give bolus baclofen through the spinal catheter instead of administering continuous baclofen. The maximal dosage is 200 μg (adults), and the bolus interval must be at least 6 h.

65.2 Background

65.2.1 Dystonia

The stretch and bend reflexes are under normal circumstances regulated from the superior centres in the brainstem and the brain through γ-neurons which are balancing the stimulating and inhibitory impulses. Damage to the brain or spinal cord can cause a downregulation of the threshold for synaptic excitation at the level of the segmental anterior horn cell, which causes an abnormal increase in reflex activity. This is the definition of spasticity, clinically seen as resistance of the muscle to stretch until a point of sudden collapse (clasp-knife effect). Dystonia is a variant of spasticity and are clinically characterised as abnormal, involuntary and often painful contractions of muscles with both agonistic and antagonistic function, resulting in a persisting contracture, for example, torticollis and talipes equinus (club foot) (Albright et al. 2001; Blackman et al. 2004).

65.2.2 Autonomic Dysfunction

Autonomic dysfunction typically appears following diffuse and severe cerebral lesions, such as diffuse axonal injury, hypoxia and severe CNS infection and is characterised by tachycardia, tachypnea, arterial hypertension, sweating, hypersalivation, hyper-secretion and dystonia. Autonomic dysfunction ('paroxystic autonomic instability disorder') is paroxystic in nature and can be provoked by minor sensory stimuli (light touch or a sound). The condition is often clinically visible in the period of coma remission, when the patient is out of, or reduced in, sedation from days to a few weeks after the cerebral damage (Baguley et al. 2004; Kock-Jensen 2007). Autonomic dysfunction can result in systemic dysfunction, contractures and a severe weight loss because of loss of muscle protein (Blackman et al. 2004; François et al. 2001). The initiating time for neurorehabilitation is delayed because of a prolonged stay in the intensive care unit. When measured with Glasgow Outcome Score (GOS) and Functional Independence Measure (FIM), the outcome for these patients is worse after rehabilitation than in patients with equally severe trauma but without autonomic dysfunction. The condition can be fatal and can alternatively persist for weeks, months or even years when left untreated, resulting in painful contractures and problems regarding rehabilitation and care. There is no documented treatment for autonomic dysfunction, and often it is chosen to minimise the symptoms with sedation, analgesics and/or beta-antagonists (Baguley et al. 2004; Blackman et al. 2004). Sedation is not a treatment, and the patients are still suffering from autonomic dysfunction. Prolonged sedation increases the risk of complications such as bacteraemia, ventilation-associated pneumonia (VAP), secondary complications to immobility/inactivity and those related to drugs (accumulation, tolerance, withdrawal symptoms, circulatory problems) (Walder and Tramer 2004). Baclofen treatment has been shown to eliminate the autonomic symptoms and dystonia in several case studies (Albright et al. 2001; Becker et al. 2000; Blackman et al. 2004; Brennan and Whittle 2008; Cuny et al. 2001; François et al. 2001; Meythaler et al. 1999; Turner 2003). There are no reported complications to the treatment except for a few with catheter-related infections or ruptures. In some cases, it is sufficient to treat only for a few days (3–4) in the acute phase, which means that the patient does not need further treatment. Becker et al. studied four patients (aged 21, 28, 29 and 34) with autonomic dysfunction following different primary TBI (Becker et al. 2000). One patient had a treated obstructive hydrocephalus and did not respond to lumbar, intrathecal baclofen at 100 μg and died from uncontrollable autonomic dysfunction. The other three patients received intrathecal baclofen through intraspinal or intraventricular catheters without any complications. The optimal dosage was 400–450 μg baclofen/24 h. Baclofen treatment was instituted 1–2 weeks posttraumatically. Only one patient needed an internal pump before he left the intensive care unit. The others did not show signs of autonomic dysfunction after a short period of treatment. Cuny et al. (2001) did also treat four patients (1, 19, 23 and 37 years old) who suffered from autonomic dysfunction following TBI (initial GCS 4–7) with intrathecal baclofen. The treatment was initiated 23–68 days posttraumatically and was continuously infused for a period of 6 days. The optimal dosage was 144–600 μg baclofen/24 h. The autonomic dysfunction disappeared in all four patients through the test period. Three patients needed an internal, programmable baclofen pump. One patient had a ruptured catheter afterwards, which was replaced without complications. There were no other complications to the treatment. This treatment is used in Denmark in some of the neurosurgical departments and is given to patients suffering from autonomic dysfunction following a severe cerebral injury hence diffuse axonal injury (DAI), stroke (e.g. malignant arteria cerebri media infarction), anoxic damage, CNS infection or sequelae from SAH. The treatment at the Department of Neurosurgery in Aarhus and Odense and at the semi-intensive care unit (MOBE) at Hammel Neurorehabilitation Centre has shown very promising results.

65.2.3 Weight Loss

It is well documented in nine class I studies (Brain Trauma Foundation 1995) that hypermetabolism and excessive nitrogen loss follow acute severe cerebral injury. Thus, it is found that a resting patient, in coma and with an isolated TBI, has an energy expenditure of 140% of expected metabolic rate (variability 120–250%). The same patient in relaxation (pancuronium bromide or barbiturate) has an energy use of 100–120% of the expected metabolic rate. This finding suggests that most of the excessive use of energy is related to muscle tone. Less than 10% of the expended calories are from protein resources under normal circumstances (healthy, average men). In a patient with an acute severe cerebral injury, who receives a total coverage of expended energy through the diet including 10 g of nitrogen/day, the catabolism of protein reaches as high as 30% of the energy sources used; this results in a loss of nitrogen of 14–25 g/day. It has been shown that the earliest normalisation of the nitrogen balance begins in the third week posttraumatically and often later than that. It is also shown that there is a tendency for the nitrogen loss to increase in the beginning of the posttraumatic phase with a peak in the second week. Most of the parenteral and enteral dietary products for hyper-metabolic conditions have a maximal content of protein of 20%. Excessive weight loss is still the result because the nitrogen balance will be negative despite the reduced nitrogen loss (Brain Trauma Foundation 1995). Weight loss is a huge problem in patients suffering from autonomic dysfunction (Baguley et al. 2004; Blackman et al. 2004).

65.2.4 Baclofen

Baclofen (4-amino-3-(4-chlorophenylic)-gamma -aminobutyric acid) is a well-known and well-tested product, which has been used as treatment for spinal spasticity for the last 40 years and for dystonia for the latest years as well, also when the dystonia is a part of an autonomic dysfunction (Albright 1996; Sidenius 2010; Kock-Jensen 2007). Baclofen has an agonistic impact on the GABA-B receptors, which binds to and stimulates the pre-synaptic GABA-B receptors in the brainstem and spinal cord. Baclofen inhibits the mono- and poly-synaptic reflexes and GABA metabolism hence spasticity. When administered intrathecally, the dosage needed to treat is much lower compared with orally administered baclofen, especially because of the poor passage of orally administered baclofen across the blood-brain barrier (Sidenius 2010; Meythaler et al. 1999).

65.3 Specific Paediatric Concerns

Children are treated as adults except regarding the dosage (See Sect. 65.1). There are no randomised studies to document the effect of intrathecal treatment with baclofen on autonomic dysfunction. There is on the other hand a convincing amount of cases that show the effectiveness of the treatment. Baclofen itself is a well-known pharmacologic compound with as well as no side effects when administered intrathecally. Autonomic dysfunction is a potentially fatal condition, or at least a condition that complicates and lowers the outcome significantly for the patients.

References

Albright AL (1996) Baclofen in the treatment of cerebral palsy. J Child Neurol 11:77–83

Albright AL et al (2001) Intrathecal baclofen for generalized dystonia. Dev Med Child Neurol 43:652–657

Baguley IJ et al (2004) Pharmacological management of dysautonomia following traumatic brain injury. Brain Inj 18(5):409–417

Becker R et al (2000) Intrathecal baclofen alleviates autonomic dysfunction in severe brain injury. J Clin Neurosci 7:316–319

Blackman JA et al (2004) Paroxysmal autonomic instability with dystonia after brain injury. Arch Neurol 61(6):980

Brain Trauma Foundation (1995) Chapter 14: Nutritional support of brain-injured patients. In: Guidelines for the management of severe head injury. Brain Trauma Foundation, New York

Brennan PM, Whittle IR (2008) Intrathecal baclofen therapy for neurological disorders: a sound knowledge base but many challenges remain. Br J Neurosurg 18:1–12

Cuny E et al (2001) Dysautonomia syndrome in the acute recovery phase after traumatic brain injury: relief with intrathecal baclofen therapy. Brain Inj 15:917–925

François B et al (2001) Intrathecal baclofen after traumatic brain injury: early treatment using a new technique to prevent spasticity. J Trauma 50:158–161

Sidenius P (2010) Medicin.dk. Spasticitet. Infomatum a/s. 34. udgave, 1. oplag 2010; 327

Kock-Jensen C (2007) Intrathecal baclofen through bolus/external pump. Regionshospitalet Hammel Neurocenter. Instruks. Local Publication 1–8

Meythaler JM et al (1999) Long-term continuously infused intrathecal baclofen for spastic-dystonic hypertonia in traumatic brain injury: 1-year experience. Arch Phys Med Rehabil 80:13–19

Turner MS (2003) Early use of intrathecal baclofen in brain injury in pediatric patients. Acta Neurochir Suppl 87:81–83

Walder B, Tramer MR (2004) Analgesia and sedation in critically ill patients. Swiss Med Wkly 134:333–346

66 Prophylaxis Against Venous Thromboembolism in Patients with Traumatic Brain Injury

Morten Zebitz Steiness

Recommendations

Level I

There are insufficient data to support a Level I recommendation for this topic.

Level II

There are insufficient data to support a Level II recommendation for this topic.

Level III

Mechanical prophylaxis with compression stockings or intermittent pneumatic compression is recommended unless lower extremity injuries prevent it and should be continued until full mobilisation.

Pharmacological prophylaxis with a low molecular weight heparin (LMWH) or low dose unfractionated heparin (UFH) should be used in combination with mechanical prophylaxis.

However, there is an increased risk for expansion in existing haematomas, so it is recommended to wait for a 24-h control CT to make sure that there is no progression in existing haematomas or new pathology.

There is insufficient evidence to support recommendations of drug, dose or further timing, but due to the existing risk of progression in haematomas, we recommend the lowest prophylactic dose of the departments preferred LMWH. We recommend LMWH because it is administered once daily and has a lower risk of heparin induced thrombocytopenia.

66.1 Overview

Patients with severe traumatic brain injury (TBI) are at significant risk of developing venous thromboembolic complications. The risk has been estimated to 20% in the absence of any prophylaxis (Knudson et al. 2004). Another review found an estimated risk of pulmonary embolism (PE) of 0.38% among patients with severe TBI (Page et al. 2004). Unfortunately, we only have publications supporting Level III evidence in this high risk population of trauma patients.

Tips, Tricks, and Pitfalls

- Avoid dehydration
- Use compression stockings
- Early mobilisation and physiotherapy
- Keep operation time as short as possible
- Beware of positioning during surgery

M.Z. Steiness
Department of Neurosurgery,
Aaalborg Hospital, Hobrovej 18-22,
9100 Aalborg, Denmark
e-mail: zebitz@yahoo.com

T. Sundstrøm et al. (eds.), *Management of Severe Traumatic Brain Injury*,
DOI 10.1007/978-3-642-28126-6_66, © Springer-Verlag Berlin Heidelberg 2012

66.2 Background

66.2.1 Mechanical Prophylaxis

A number of studies have demonstrated the efficacy and safety of mechanical prophylaxis with either graduated compression stockings or intermittent pneumatic compression. The relative risk of venous thrombosis has been reduced >50% (Skillman et al. 1978; Turpie et al. 1989) without any changes in mean arterial pressure, ICP or central venous pressure as documented by Davidson et al. (1993). However, due to the lack of class II data, the recommendations are made on the basis of Level III evidence.

66.2.2 Pharmacological Prophylaxis

Among *elective* neurosurgical patients, we have Level I evidence regarding pharmacological prophylaxis (Agnelli et al. 1998); however, it is difficult to extrapolate these strong dates into the population of TBI patients without being very careful.

Studies among patients with TBI suggest that LMWH is efficacious in reducing the risk of VTE; however, data show a trend towards an increased risk of intracranial bleeding. Case studies suggest that LMWH prophylaxis should not be initiated pre- or perioperatively and not before a 24-h control CT has been performed, demonstrating no progression in existing haematomas or new intracranial bleedings (Black et al. 1986; Gerlach et al. 2003; Kleindienst et al. 2003; Norwood et al. 2002).

There are no data supporting specific recommendations regarding drug choice or dose.

66.3 Specific Paediatric Concerns

There are no specific paediatric concerns, except that children are less prone to thrombotic complications than adults.

References

Agnelli G, Piovella F, Buoncristiani P et al (1998) Enoxaparin plus compression stocking compared with compression stocking alone in the prevention of venous thromboembolism after elective neurosurgery. N Engl J Med 339:80–85

Black PM, Baker MF, Snook CP (1986) Experience with external pneumatic calf compression in neurology and neurosurgery. Neurosurgery 18:440–444

Davidson JE, Williams DC, Hoffman MS (1993) Effect of intermittent pneumatic leg compression on intracranial pressure in brain-injured patients. Crit Care Med 21:224–227

Gerlach R, Scheuer T, Beck J et al (2003) Risk of postoperative hemorrhage intracranial surgery after early nadroparin administration: results of a prospective study. Neurosurgery 53:1028–1034

Kleindienst A, Harvey HB, Mater E et al (2003) Early antithrombotic prophylaxis with low molecular weight heparin in neurosurgery. Acta Neurochir (Wien) 145:1085–1090

Knudson MM, Ikossi DG, Khaw L et al (2004) Thromboembolism after trauma: an analysis of 1602 episodes from the American college of surgeons national trauma data bank. Ann Surg 240:490–496

Norwood SH, McAuley CE, Berne JD et al (2002) Prospective evaluation of the safety of enoxaparin prophylaxis for venous thromboembolism in patients with intracranial hemorrhagic injuries. Arch Surg 137:696–701

Page RB, Spott MA, Krishnamurthy S et al (2004) Head injury and pulmonary embolism: a retrospective report based on the Pennsylvania Trauma Outcomes study. Neurosurgery 54:143–148

Skillman JJ, Collins RE, Coe NP et al (1978) Prevention of deep vein thrombosis in neurosurgical patients: a controlled, randomized trial of external pneumatic compression boots. Surgery 83:354–358

Turpie AG, Hirsh J, Gent M et al (1989) Prevention of deep vein thrombosis in potential neurosurgical patients. A randomized trial comparing graduated compression stockings alone or graduated compression stockings plus intermittent compression with control. Arch Intern Med 149:679–681

Brain Injury and the Haemostatic System

67

Martin Engström

Recommendations

Level I

There are insufficient data to support a Level I recommendation for this topic.

Level II

There are insufficient data to support a Level II recommendation for this topic.

Level III

Thrombocytopenia as well as signs of impaired humoral coagulation PT has been associated with progressive intracerebral haemorrhage and worse outcome in patients suffering from traumatic brain injury (TBI).

M. Engström
Onkologi-, Thorax- och Medicindivisionen (OTM),
Akademiska Sjukhuset,
751 85 Uppsala, Sweden
e-mail: martin.engstrom@akademiska.se

67.1 Overview

Progressive haemorrhage is a feared complication to different kinds of brain injuries, e.g. traumatic brain injury (TBI), spontaneous intracerebral haemorrhage (ICH) and subarachnoid haemorrhage (SAH). The evidence supporting any treatment option aiming at preventing or stopping progressive haemorrhage is weak. There is low-grade support for correcting abnormalities of the coagulation system, such as prolonged prothrombin time (PT) and thrombocytopenia after TBI and ICH. Other recommendations miss supporting evidence.

Haemorrhage is an important component in several types of brain injuries. Intracranial haemorrhage can be divided into intracerebral and extracerebral haemorrhage. The skull strictly restricts the intracranial volume and any mass occupying intracranial volume may have severe consequences. If intracranial haemorrhage occurs, the blood may occupy intracranial volume and cause the intracranial pressure to increase, a well-known reason for morbidity and mortality in brain-injured patients. Local tissue damage caused by intracerebral haemorrhage is another very important contributor to bad outcome in brain-injured patients. The great risks associated with intracranial haemorrhage of any type may explain why the brain has developed into the organ with the highest amounts of tissue factor (TF). TF is the most important trigger of the coagulation system. It is located subendothelially in blood vessels and is exposed to the blood stream in cases of blood vessel injury.

T. Sundstrøm et al. (eds.), *Management of Severe Traumatic Brain Injury*,
DOI 10.1007/978-3-642-28126-6_67, © Springer-Verlag Berlin Heidelberg 2012

The reason for the injury caused by haemorrhage can be the mass effect as well as direct tissue damage. The mass effect is most prominent in spontaneous intracerebral haemorrhage (ICH) but also traumatic brain injury (TBI) and non-traumatic subarachnoid haemorrhage may be complicated by mass effects caused by haemorrhage. Tissue damage caused by haemorrhage may be prominent in TBI patients where a combination of tissue damage and mass effect due to petechial bleeding and swelling around contusions is not uncommon.

Tips, Tricks, and Pitfalls

- Correct prolonged PT in patients suffering from traumatic brain injury.
- Correct severe thrombocytopenia in patients suffering from traumatic brain injury.
- Consider pros and cons thoroughly before deciding whether to use pharmacologic DVT prophylaxis. Mechanic pneumatic compression may be an alternative.

67.2 Background

67.2.1 The Coagulation System

For haemostasis to occur, several components of the coagulation system must work together in a balanced way. If the balance is altered, either excess bleeding or excess coagulation leading to pathologic thrombosis formation may occur.

The haemostatic process involves cellular elements, the blood vessel wall and circulating coagulation factors. The coagulation has traditionally been viewed as a cascade starting with primary haemostasis, where primary haemostasis is considered as the formation of a platelet plug where a blood vessel has been disrupted. Once a platelet plug was formed, secondary haemostasis was initiated involving the circulating coagulation factors leading to formation of a fibrin mesh armouring the platelet plug, according to this traditional view. The secondary haemostasis was divided into two separate pathways, the intrinsic and the extrinsic pathway.

The traditional view on the coagulation process presented above has today been abandoned in favour of a new model. Haemostasis is today considered to occur in three phases: initiation, amplification and propagation. This model was described some 15 years ago and is today the generally accepted model (Hoffman and Monroe 2001). The new model presumes a close cooperation between cellular and humoral components, where the initiation of the coagulation process takes place when the blood vessel wall is injured and subendothelial tissue is exposed to the blood stream. TF and extravascular matrix proteins are exposed, and at the same time as platelets adhere to the exposed extravascular tissue and become activated, TF interacts with activated coagulation factor VII (FVIIa). The interaction between TF and FVIIa initiates the coagulation process and several of the steps in the coagulation process occur on the surface of the activated platelets. Close interaction between cellular and humoral elements is thus required for haemostasis to occur.

The haemostatic system is affected when the biochemical properties of blood is changed or when homeostasis is changed in different ways. Hypothermia has been proven to impair the activity of the individual coagulation factors resulting in a coagulopathic state at low body temperatures (Johnston et al. 1994; Wolberg et al. 2004). Another important factor affecting the coagulation is the acid-base balance. When pH is lowered, the coagulation system is less effective, resulting in impaired ability to coagulate blood (Meng et al. 2003; Engstrom et al. 2006a, b). This finding has been studied in various settings and may be of importance when we study the pathologic processes caused by brain injury.

The procoagulant system is balanced by an anti-coagulant system inhibiting coagulation and by a fibrinolytic system responsible for the resolution of formed blood clots. Closely linked to the procoagulant system, there is a number of anticoagulant factors as well, where the most important probably are tissue factor pathway inhibitor (TFPI), inhibiting the TF/FVIIa complex, and the proteins C and S, inhibiting coagulation factors Va and VIIIa. Anti-thrombin (AT) is a circulating protein inactivating a number of coagulation factors and the activity of AT is accelerated by the presence of heparin.

Fibrinolysis is important to resolve already formed clots and the fibrinolytic system is activated when tissue-type plasminogen activator (t-PA) converts plasminogen into plasmin, a protease able to degrade fibrin into fibrin degradation products.

Without a finely tuned balance between the procoagulant system, the anti-coagulant system and the fibrinolytic system, bleeding or thrombosis will be the inevitable result.

67.2.2 Traumatic Brain Injury

It is well documented that TBI leads to activation of the coagulation system and a consumptive coagulopathy may develop after brain trauma. A potential explanation for this activation may be that, as the brain is very rich in TF, large amounts of TF is released at the time of injury and that this release results in general activation of the coagulation system, but the mechanisms have not been fully elucidated.

The activation can be documented as increases in prothrombin time (PT), activated partial thromboplastin time (aPTT) and fibrin degradation products (FDP) (Auer and Ott 1979; Hulka et al. 1996; Chiaretti et al. 2001; Keller et al. 2001; Vavilala et al. 2001). It is also well known that activation of the coagulation system, as documented using the mentioned lab tests, is associated with progression of intracranial haemorrhagic complications and to worse outcome. Progression of haemorrhagic complications as such has also been found to be associated to worse outcome (Lobato et al. 1991).

The most commonly progressive haemorrhagic complication after TBI is progression of intracerebral contusions, a common complication after TBI, but a complication which may develop late (Stein et al. 1992; Chiaretti et al. 2001; Oertel et al. 2002; Engstrom et al. 2005).Contusions may be barely identifiable on an initial CT scan, but 24–48 h later, large areas of the brain may be affected by contusions. The brain volume affected by haemorrhagic contusions has been found to be very closely linked to the volume of non-functional brain tissue on long-term follow-up using CT scan (von Oettingen et al. 2002). Studies have shown that thrombocytopenia at admission after TBI is a strong predictor of progressive haemorrhage and increase of the size of intracerebral contusions (Engstrom et al. 2005).

As the contusions grow for a prolonged period of time, it has been hypothesised that there is a window of opportunity for an intervention aimed at stopping the progressive haemorrhage. This view is also supported by the findings that patients taking anti-coagulant medication or anti-platelet drugs have a worse outcome after TBI than patients not taking such medication (Mina et al. 2002). Understanding the reasons for the prolonged bleeding is of importance if measures to stop the bleeding are to be developed. Through microdialysis studies, it has been found that increased levels of lactate often are found in parts of the brain affected by a brain trauma (Reinstrup et al. 2000). The increase in lactate levels is likely to be caused by impaired circulation and inadequate oxygenation of the tissue, but also mitochondrial dysfunction may be a factor. The lactate levels are similar to levels which in blood would correspond to a pH of 6.8, a pH level at which the coagulation system has been found to be severely impaired (Meng et al. 2003; Engstrom et al. 2006a, b).

Therapeutic options are few for intervention after TBI with the aim of decreasing complications caused by progressive haemorrhage, and the evidence supporting the clinical management is weak. Management often includes correction of prolonged PT using, e.g. fresh frozen plasma (FFP) and avoidance of thrombocytopenia when the platelet count falls below 50–100 × 10^9/L using platelet transfusions, even though the scientific support for these measures are weak. Due to the evidence of poor outcome after TBI in patients treated with vitamin K antagonists, it is common to normalise the PT using FFP or coagulation factor concentrates, e.g. prothrombin complex concentrate (PCC) (Hulka et al. 1996; Keller et al. 2001).

The use of thrombosis prophylaxis for TBI patients has been subject for debate, and firm recommendations are difficult to provide. Deep vein thrombosis (DVT) and pulmonary embolism (PE) are well-known and feared complications to immobilisation after neurosurgical procedures and trauma. However, there is also adequate fear of haemorrhagic complications if thrombosis prophylaxis is administered early after TBI.

Clinical studies investigating the potential effect of procoagulant pharmaceutical agents have been discussed, and at least one such has been performed and revealed a non-significant trend towards less progression of the haemorrhage in patients having received rFVIIa early after trauma (Narayan et al. 2008). The scientific support for such treatment is weak, but there are case reports in the literature when recombinant activated factor VIIa (rFVIIa) has been used (Zaaroor et al. 2008). The case reports are positive and use of rFVIIa in selected patients may be considered, especially when profuse bleeding during surgery occurs, despite the weak evidence.

67.3 Specific Paediatric Concerns

There is no support for differentiating the treatment between the paediatric and the adult TBI populations.

References

Auer LM, Ott E (1979) Disturbances of the coagulatory system in patients with severe cerebral trauma II. Platelet function. Acta Neurochir (Wien) 49(3–4): 219–226

Chiaretti A, Pezzotti P, Mestrovic J et al (2001) The influence of hemocoagulative disorders on the outcome of children with head injury. Pediatr Neurosurg 34(3):131–137

Engstrom M, Romner B, Schalen W et al (2005) Thrombocytopenia predicts progressive hemorrhage after head trauma. J Neurotrauma 22(2):291–296

Engstrom M, Schott U, Nordstrom CH et al (2006a) Increased lactate levels impair the coagulation system – a potential contributing factor to progressive hemorrhage after traumatic brain injury. J Neurosurg Anesthesiol 18(3):200–204

Engstrom M, Schott U, Romner B et al (2006b) Acidosis impairs the coagulation: a thromboelastographic study. J Trauma 61(3):624–628

Hoffman M, Monroe DM 3rd (2001) A cell-based model of hemostasis. Thromb Haemost 85(6):958–965

Hulka F, Mullins RJ, Frank EH (1996) Blunt brain injury activates the coagulation process. Arch Surg 131(9): 923–927; discussion 927–928

Johnston TD, Chen Y, Reed RL 2nd (1994) Functional equivalence of hypothermia to specific clotting factor deficiencies. J Trauma 37(3):413–417

Keller MS, Fendya DG, Weber TR (2001) Glasgow Coma Scale predicts coagulopathy in pediatric trauma patients. Semin Pediatr Surg 10(1):12–16

Lobato RD, Rivas JJ, Gomez PA et al (1991) Head-injured patients who talk and deteriorate into coma. Analysis of 211 cases studied with computerized tomography. J Neurosurg 75(2):256–261

Meng ZH, Wolberg AS, Monroe DM 3rd et al (2003) The effect of temperature and pH on the activity of factor VIIa: implications for the efficacy of high-dose factor VIIa in hypothermic and acidotic patients. J Trauma 55(5):886–891

Mina AA, Knipfer JF, Park DY et al (2002) Intracranial complications of preinjury anticoagulation in trauma patients with head injury. J Trauma 53(4):668–672

Narayan RK, Maas AI, Marshall LF et al (2008) Recombinant factor VIIA in traumatic intracerebral hemorrhage: results of a dose-escalation clinical trial. Neurosurgery 62(4):776–786; discussion 786–788

Oertel M, Kelly DF, McArthur D et al (2002) Progressive hemorrhage after head trauma: predictors and consequences of the evolving injury. J Neurosurg 96(1): 109–116

Reinstrup P, Stahl N, Mellergard P et al (2000) Intracerebral microdialysis in clinical practice: baseline values for chemical markers during wakefulness, anesthesia, and neurosurgery. Neurosurgery 47(3):701–709; discussion 709–710

Stein SC, Young GS, Talucci RC et al (1992) Delayed brain injury after head trauma: significance of coagulopathy. Neurosurgery 30(2):160–165

Vavilala MS, Dunbar PJ, Rivara FP et al (2001) Coagulopathy predicts poor outcome following head injury in children less than 16 years of age. J Neurosurg Anesthesiol 13(1):13–18

von Oettingen G, Bergholt B, Gyldensted C et al (2002) Blood flow and ischemia within traumatic cerebral contusions. Neurosurgery 50(4):781–788; discussion 788–790

Wolberg AS, Meng ZH, Monroe DM 3rd et al (2004) A systematic evaluation of the effect of temperature on coagulation enzyme activity and platelet function. J Trauma 56(6):1221–1228

Zaaroor M, Soustiel JF, Brenner B et al (2008) Administration off label of recombinant factor-VIIa (rFVIIa) to patients with blunt or penetrating brain injury without coagulopathy. Acta Neurochir (Wien) 150(7):663–668

Steroids

68

Jens Jakob Riis

Recommendations

Level I

Administration of high-dose corticosteroids to patients with brain trauma is directly harmful with considerable side effects and should therefore not be used routinely.

Level II

Data are insufficient to support Level II recommendations for this subject.

Level III

Data are insufficient to support Level III recommendations for this subject.

68.1 Overview

Corticosteroids to brain trauma patients have for a long time been an important and controversial topic; so far, there has not been consensus regarding the possible benefits or adverse effects of administration of corticosteroids to such patients. High-dose methylprednisolone to patients with trauma-induced spinal transection has been abandoned in many Nordic trauma centres due to (1) lack of evidence for beneficial effect, (2) harmful effect on brain trauma patients with spinal cord injuries, and (3) the significant side effects, e.g. hyperglycaemia, gastric ulcers/bleeding, increased risk of infection, psychosis and impairment of wound healing (Poungvarin 2004).

Trauma-induced brain oedema can be seen alone, in conjunction with contusions or after removal of, e.g. an acute subdural haematoma. Basically, the brain oedema in trauma patients is a mixture of vasogenic and cytotoxic oedema (Papadopoulos et al. 2004). So far, it has not been proven that corticosteroids have the same effect on oedema in trauma patients as it has in brain tumour patients. Administration of corticosteroids in order to decrease traumatically induced oedema, e.g. around cerebral contusions, has not been widespread due to lack of evidence of effect; the knowledge of possible serious side effects is probably another explanation.

The use of corticosteroids in TBI patients has been directed against the brain oedema (Dearden et al. 1986; Giannotti et al. 1984; Grände 2006; Kamano 2000; Rabinstein 2006) and the inflammatory response but has also been directed against hyperpyrexia/fever. Corticosteroids have been used in patients where paracetamol and cooling have proved ineffective in lowering the body temperature, as hyperpyrexia/fever in itself is a negative prognostic factor in brain trauma

J.J. Riis
Department of Neurosurgery,
Aarhus Aaarhus University Hospital,
DK-8000, Aarhus, Denmark
e-mail: jenjakri@rm.dk

T. Sundstrøm et al. (eds.), *Management of Severe Traumatic Brain Injury*,
DOI 10.1007/978-3-642-28126-6_68, © Springer-Verlag Berlin Heidelberg 2012

(Audibert et al. 2009; Ginsbury and Busto 2003; Poldermann 2008; Poldermann and Herold 2009).

Tips, Tricks and Pitfalls

- Avoid using corticosteroids, especially high dose, in all brain trauma patients.

68.2 Background

A systematic review in 1997 in *British Medical Journal* by Alderson and Robertson suggested a reduction in mortality on 1–2% in patients who received steroids (Alderson and Robertson 1997). Two thousand patients were included in this study that encouraged the use of corticosteroids in this setting.

Corticosteroids to patients with brain tumours with peritumoural oedema is a well-established routine, and the effect on tumour, and thereby ultimately oedema-induced symptoms, e.g. paresis, is significant. The oedema of tumours is thought to be secondary to disrupted blood–brain barrier (BBB), and corticosteroids' mechanism of action is supposed to be decreasing the permeability of the tight junctions and thereby stabilising the damaged BBB (Raslan and Bhardwaj 2007; Sinha et al. 2004).

The CRASH study (Roberts et al. 2004) was a cornerstone what use of corticosteroids in brain trauma is concerned. It was supposed to include 20,000 patients, but the inclusion of patients was terminated prematurely because an interim analysis showed that 21% of the patients in the steroid group were dead within 2 weeks of randomisation compared with 18% in the placebo group. The patients received, within 8 h of the head injury, either a bolus dose of 2 g of methylprednisolone and afterwards 0.4 g/h for the next 48 h, or an infusion of placebo. All included patients had a GCS of 14 or less. Ten thousand and eight patients had been included when the study was closed. The relative risk (RR) for death from all causes was 1.18 (95% CI; 1.09–1.27; $p=0.001$). There was no increase in complications (infections, gastric bleeding, etc.) in the group allocated to corticosteroids contrary to the findings in the Cochrane review mentioned earlier (Alderson and Roberts 2005). The reason for the increased mortality has never been elucidated. The weakness of the CRASH study was its inability to rule out the primary cause of death in the corticosteroid group; so far, nobody has been able to explain the higher mortality in the corticosteroid group.

Because of that, corticosteroids are no longer used routinely in brain trauma patients, although some authors (Giannotti et al. 1984; Grände 2006; Kamano 2000) have emphasised that corticosteroids are not ineffective and hazardous in this matter.

Cerebral oedema following brain trauma is supposed to be of both vasogenic and cytotoxic origin (Papadopoulos et al. 2004). No studies has so far proved that administration of corticosteroids has a beneficial effect on these types of oedema as far as brain trauma patients are concerned; the use has been on empirical basis and has been abandoned in many trauma centres.

A Cochrane review from 2005 (Alderson and Roberts 2005) states that: "…the largest trial, with about 80% of all randomised participants, found a significant increase in the risk ratio of death with steroids 1.15 (95% CI 1.07–1,24) and a relative risk of death or severe disability of 1,05 (95%; CI 0.99–1.07)".

The risk of gastrointestinal bleeding, hyperglycaemia and infection were also increased. Hyperglycaemia is hazardous in patients with, e.g. cerebral contusions and the importance of keeping blood glucose within normal range has been emphasised in many trials (Jeremitsky et al. 2005; Laird and Miller 2004; Rovlias and Kotsou 2000; Salim et al. 2009; Yag et al. 1989).

So far, the use of corticosteroids has also been directed against the inflammatory response after head injury, but the exact role of inflammatory mediators in brain trauma is not fully elucidated and the use of corticosteroids is not justified on this basis.

Overall, there is no evidence that administration of (high dose) corticosteroids to brain trauma patients has any beneficial effect on survival or long term outcome; actually, Level I evidence states that high-dose corticosteroids to brain trauma patients is directly harmful and raises mortality of any cause without any obvious benefits for the patients.

68.3 Specific Paediatric Concerns

Administration of corticosteroids in paediatric patients with brain trauma should not be initiated.

References

Alderson P, Roberts I (1997) Corticosteroids in acute traumatic brain injury: systematic review of randomised controlled trials. Br Med J 314:1855–1859

Alderson P, Roberts IG (2005) Corticosteroids for acute traumatic brain injury. Cochrane Database Syst Rev (1):CD000196. doi: 10.1002/14651858.CD000196.pub.2

Audibert G, Baumann A et al (2009) Deleterious role of hyperthermia in neurocritical care. Ann Fr Anesth Reanim 28(4):345–351

Dearden NM, Gibson JS et al (1986) Effect of high-dose dexamethasone on outcome from severe head injury. J Neurosurg 64:81–88

Giannotti SL, Weiss MH et al (1984) High dose glucocorticosteroids in the management of severe head injury. Neurosurgery 15:497–501

Ginsbury MD, Busto R (2003) Combating hyperthermia in acute stroke: a significant clinical concern. Stroke 34(1):5–6

Grände PO (2006) The "Lund concept" for the treatment of severe head trauma – physiological principles and clinical applications. Intensive Care Med 32: 1475–1484

Jeremitsky E, Omert LA et al (2005) The impact of hyperglycaemia on patients with severe head injury. J Trauma 58:47–50

Kamano S (2000) Are steroids really ineffective for severely head injured patients? Neurosurg Focus 8(1):Article 7

Laird AM, Miller PR (2004) Relationship of early hyperglycaemia to mortality in trauma patients. J Trauma 56(5):1058–1060

Papadopoulos MC, Saadoun S et al (2004) Molecular mechanisms of brain tumour edema. Neuroscience 129:1011–1020

Poldermann KH (2008) Induced hypothermia and fever control for prevention and treatment of neurological injuries. Lancet 371(9628):1955–1969

Poldermann KH, Herold I (2009) Therapeutic hypothermia and controlled normothermia in the intensive care unit: practical considerations, side effects and cooling methods. Crit Care Med 37:1101–1120

Poungvarin N (2004) Steroids has no role in stroke therapy. Stroke 35:229–230

Rabinstein AA (2006) Treatment of brain edema. Neurologist 12:59–73

Raslan A, Bhardwaj A (2007) Medical management of cerebral edema. Neurosurg Focus 22(5):E12: 1–E12:9

Roberts I, Yates D et al (2004) Effect of intravenous corticosteroids on death within 14 days in 10008 adults with clinically significant head injury (MRS CRASH-trial). Lancet 364:1321–1328

Rovlias A, Kotsou S (2000) The influence of hyperglycaemia on neurological outcome in patients with severe head injury. Neurosurgery 46:335–343

Salim A, Hadjizachoria A et al (2009) Persistent hyperglycaemia in severe traumatic brain injury; an independent predictor of outcome. Am Surg 75(1): 25–29

Sinha S, Bastin ME et al (2004) Effect of dexamethasone on peritumoural oedematous brain: a DT-MRI study. J Neurol Neurosurg Psychiatry 75:1632–1635

Yag B, Ott L et al (1989) Relationship between admission hyperglycaemia and neurologic outcome of severely brain injured patients. Ann Surg 210(4):466–472

Part IX

Early Rehabilitation

Neurorehabilitation in Neurointensive Care

69

Carsten Kock-Jensen and Leanne Enggaard Langhorn

Recommendations

Level I

There are insufficient data to support a Level I recommendation for this topic.

Level II

There are insufficient data to support a Level II recommendation for this topic.

Level III

Observational studies support that physician-driven TBI multidisciplinary rehabilitation programme decrease length of stay (LOS) in acute hospitals.

Prevention of secondary insults due to autonomic dysfunction, upper airway dyscontrol/dysphagia, severe endocrine disturbances and detection and treatment of non-convulsive seizures affects final outcome (tertiary prevention).

Duration of PTA may be used as a prognostic factor to make clinical decisions and to improve and predict outcome during the rehabilitation programme.

C. Kock-Jensen (✉) • L.E. Langhorn
Department of Neurosurgery, Aarhus University Hospital, Noerrebrogade 44, 8000 Aarhus, DK
e-mail: carskock@rm.dk; leanne.langhorn@aarhus.rm.dk

69.1 Overview

During the stay in the neurointensive care unit, it is very important to evaluate patients thoroughly and daily in order to reveal complications to injury and to manage complications, which might threaten the patients' final outcome. Patients must have an overall clinical assessment not only including physical factors but also including functional, behaviour and cognitive problems (risk factor management). It is practical to evaluate the patients' total situation in the frame given by the International Classification of Function (ICF). Special interest must be given to fever and to autonomic dysfunction (see Chap. 65). Seizures, including the non-convulsive type, upper airway control and the need for long-term cuffed tracheotomy tubes as well as severe endocrine disturbances must be given special emphasis.

The duration of post-traumatic amnesia (PTA) might be one of the best prognostic factors to predict the cognitive, neurological and functional outcome in patients with TBI. Furthermore, it is shown that the prognosis and outcome can be improved by using a systematic reality orientation (RO) programme when patients are able to communicate (see below). Therefore, it is recommended to monitor the state of PTA as soon as possible and manage the amnesic patient by using a systematic RO programme in the ICU/acute care. The state and duration of PTA can be monitored by using the Galveston Orientation and Amnesia Test (GOAT) daily.

T. Sundstrøm et al. (eds.), *Management of Severe Traumatic Brain Injury*,
DOI 10.1007/978-3-642-28126-6_69, © Springer-Verlag Berlin Heidelberg 2012

Tips, Tricks, and Pitfalls

- Prevention of secondary insults due to autonomic dysfunction, upper airway dyscontrol/dysphagia, severe endocrine disturbances and detection and treatment of non-convulsive seizures will improve the final outcome (tertiary prevention).
- It is imperative to develop neurointensive care neurohabilitation programmes that are able to encounter adverse reactions to the primary injury (detect and treat secondary and tertiary injury).
- During the recovery phase after end of sedation, patients often present with severe hypertension, tachycardia, spontaneous hyperventilation, fever and profuse sweating and excessive amount of salivation. These symptoms are often misdiagnosed and consequently given the wrong treatment. The patient is returned to sedation, artificially ventilated and given antibiotic treatment. In many cases, these symptoms are due to autonomic dysfunction and they should be treated accordingly.
- Up to 60% of all patients with severe TBI present airway problems, often referred to as dysphagia. Dysphagia with severe risk of aspiration must be ruled out before deflation of tracheostomy tubes. Ruling out the risk for aspiration before deflating cuffs minimises the risk of ventilator associated pneumonias (VAP). Thorough evaluation of the patients' swallowing abilities (which is directly connected to the risk of VAP) can only be done after endoscopic procedure (fiber endoscopic evaluation of swallowing – FEES). Proper management of patients with upper airway dysfunction (dysphagia) should be managed according to the risk for aspiration and pneumonia. New fever episodes affect the already injured brain and finally the outcome after TBI.
- Fever of any course should be treated aggressively, including cooling, to prevent hyperthermia.
- Screening of endocrine disturbances must be done according to the protocol, presented in Chap. 45.
- It is advisable that every neurointensive care unit establishes their own multidisciplinary acute care neurorehabilitation team. In this perspective, it is important that neurosurgeons and neurointensivists do not rely totally on other disciplines (such as occupational therapist and physiotherapist). Responsibility for the overall treatment of TBI patients in neurosurgical and neurointensive care can only founded within the medical profession.
- Up to 70% of patients with TBI will experience PTA. A third of these patients have amnesia for more than 28 days. Monitor patients with PTA daily by using the GOAT. During the PTA period, manage the patient with a systematic RO programme. The RO can be customized to the individual patient and consists of the following items:
  - Ranchos Los Amigos Score (RLAS) 24 h after end of sedation
  - Galveston Orientation Amnesia Test (GOAT) once a day
  - If PTA, place a whiteboard at the patient's bed or close to the patient
  - Orientate the patient constantly to time, place and person
  - Make a day and night schedule including activity and rest
  - Communicate with patient in short terms
  - Avoid confrontations and conflicts
  - Distract the patient from confabulations
  - Involve the relatives in the RO programme

69.2 Background

Traumatic brain injury (TBI) is an acute, sub-acute and a chronic disease. Much is known about the acute management, especially how important it is to correct factors which can add secondary insults to the primary injury: systemic hypoxia and shock, intracranial haematomas and contusions, raised intracranial pressure, cerebral hypoxia and ischemia and a number of adverse reactions influencing body and brain function, exerted by a disturbed homeostasis of the entire body.

The traditional role of the neurointensive/neurosurgery team has been to intervene promptly to correct intracranial pressure, as well as stabilising the total body function in order to improve trauma outcome.

After the battle in the acute stage, in the early hours or days in the intensive care, the pace slackens. It is well known that recovery from severe TBI is gradual, prolonged and incomplete. However, today, more is known about the nature of this process. We know that, under certain circumstances, neurones can repair, regenerate and re-establish functional connections. This neuronal recovery is a delicate process, which is easily disturbed by the same factors that are regarded as secondary insults in the very acute stage. Also, more discrete and often undiagnosed insults of autonomic dysfunction (ADF) leading to poor oxygen transport and loss of nitrogen in the catabolic state may interfere with neuronal recovery, as well as infections. In the sub-acute phase, with the patient still in neurointensive unit, it is therefore mandatory to keep the same surveillance pace as in the early hours following injury.

Today we are facing more survivors from severe TBI, and hopefully all our efforts in improving pre-hospital care, early trauma hospital admission and neurointensive/neurosurgical intervention will minimise the effects of possible secondary insults to the brain.

Many patients do have multiple and wide-ranging impairments of motor function, communication, cognition, behaviour and personality. These form a complex pattern of disability and handicap, which interact to form a clinical kaleidoscope unique to each patient. Some problems are directly related to the primary brain injury; others can be considered consequences of complications, which were not addressed in time.

Brain injury in itself cannot be treated, but complications might be prevented or treated, even after the first few hours and days in the neurointensive care unit (Mac Kay et al. 1992; Turner-Stokes 2008).

PTA is a state of confusion in the early recovery following TBI. On emerging from unconsciousness, the patient's orientation and memory for ongoing events is poor. PTA can last from hours, days, to weeks depending upon the severity of the brain injury. Determination of the duration of PTA is important as an index of severity and is one of the best early predictors of recovery and functional outcome (Teasdale and Jennett 1974; Jennett et al. 1981; Nakase-Richardson et al. 2009). Furthermore, studies have shown that the potential for recovery decreases as duration of PTA increases (Ellenberg et al. 1996; Ponsford et al. 2004; Nakase-Richardson et al. 2009). It is recommended that systematic interventions should be offered as intensively as possible for persons with any documented period of coma or PTA extending more than 30 min (Turner-Stokes 2008). It is suggested that reality orientation (RO) becomes an integrated part of the intervention for patients with difficulties in reality orientation (Spector et al. 2003; Thomas et al. 2003; De Guise et al. 2005). Therefore, initial and follow-up assessment of PTA are essential parts of the rehabilitation programme in acute care (Langhorn 2010).

Survivors after severe TBI constitute a severe health-care problem and a socio-economic burden to the society; in addition, a low quality of life for survivors and their relatives give rise to major family and social problems.

Since 1990, guidelines have been published in Europe (Maas et al. 1997) and USA (Brain Trauma Foundation 1995, 2000, 2007) to guide health-care professionals in trauma management. Many of these guidelines are based on varying degrees of evidence and are used as a template to organise national, regional or local guidance in management of TBI.

In 1995, the Danish National Board of Health published their guidelines for organisation of a neurotrauma system on national basis. It was recommended that cross-sectional neurorehabilitation should be introduced already in the acute phase in the trauma unit and that national specialised centres for early neurorehabilitation of severely brain-injured patients should be organised. It was stressed that early establishment of contact between neurotraumatologists and neurorehabilitation specialists is imperative in this organisation. Since year 2000, there has been a continuous development of two Danish highly specialised centres for acute neurorehabilitation of neurotrauma patients.

In western Denmark, an entire neurorehabilitation hospital, the Hammel Neurorehabilitation Centre, has been established in order to create the possibility of early management for patients still critically ill and on ventilator.

Despite a rapid development of innovative management protocols in neurorehabilitation and an enormous expansion of the care continuum, the scientific foundation for much of commonly accepted practice has unfortunately not kept pace with these developments. Therefore, there is a profound need for systematic development and research programmes in this very delicate field of brain injury management. The process has started in many internationally known neurorehabilitation centres of the world not only focusing directly on neurorehabilitation but – as the case in Hammel Neurorehabilitation Centre – to stimulate research into brain function in the post-acute stage.

Neurosurgeons and neurointensivists should advocate for, and initiate neurointensive care neurorehabilitation programmes, which will, as in the pre-hospital phase and in acute hospital phase, serve to guide clinicians avoid, detect, evaluate and treat complications which may affect the patients' final outcome (tertiary prevention). Each unit should create a multidisciplinary team, including a specialist in neurorehabilitation, to develop local programmes.

It is well known that the neurorehabilitation in Scandinavia is a very non-uniformly established service, and only Denmark has introduced a national programme, which is generally implemented. It must be the role of the caregivers in head injury (TBI) programmes to stimulate and advocate for a process, which can create a full-range trauma system designed to improve quality of survival and minimise burden to families of survivors as well as the burden to society.

69.3 Specific Paediatric Concerns

There are no specific concerns regarding neurorehabilitation in children, except for the fact that younger individuals in general have a better potential for rehabilitation.

References

Brain Trauma Foundation (1995, 2000, 2007) Guidelines for management of severe head injury. Brain Trauma Foundation, New York

De Guise E, Leblanc J, Feyz M, Thomas H, Gosselin N (2005) Effect of an integrated reality orientation programme in acute care on post-traumatic amnesia in patients with traumatic brain injury. Brain Inj 19(4):263–269

Ellenberg JH, Levin HS, Saydjari C (1996) Posttraumatic Amnesia as a predictor of outcome after severe closed head injury. Prospective assessment. Arch Neurol 53(8):782–791

Jennett B, Snoek J, Bond MR, Brooks N (1981) Disability after severe head injury: observations on the use of the Glasgow Outcome Scale. J Neurol Neurosurg Psychiatry 44(4):285–293

Langhorn L (2010) Early rehabilitation of patients with post-traumatic Amnesia in the intensive care unit. Ph.D. dissertation, Faculty of Health Sciences, Aarhus University, Aarhus

Maas AIR, Deardon M, Teasdale GM (1997) EIBC guidelines for management of severe head injury in adults. Acta Neurosur (Wien) 139:286–294

Mac Kay LE et al (1992) Early intervention in severe head injury, long-term benefit of a formalized program. Arch Phys Med Rehabil 73:635–641

Nakase-Richardson R, Sepehri A, Sherer M et al (2009) Classification schema of posttraumatic amnesia duration-based injury severity relative to 1-year outcome: analysis of individuals with moderate and severe traumatic brain injury. Arch Phys Med Rehabil 90(1):17–19

Ponsford J, Willmott C, Rothwell A et al (2004) Use of the Westmead PTA scale to monitor recovery of memory after mild head injury. Brain Inj 18(6):603–614

Spector A, Thorgrimsen L, Woods B et al (2003) Efficacy of an evidence-based cognitive stimulation therapy programme for people with dementia: randomised controlled trial. Br J Psychiatry 183:248–254

Teasdale G, Jennett B (1974) Assessment of coma and impaired consciousness. A practical scale. Lancet 2(7872):81–84

Thomas H, Feyz M, LeBlanc J et al (2003) North Star Project: reality orientation in an acute care setting for patients with traumatic brain injuries. J Head Trauma Rehabil 18(3):292–302

Turner-Stokes L (2008) Evidence for the effectiveness of multi-disciplinary rehabilitation following acquired brain injury: a synthesis of two systematic approaches. J Rehabil Med 40(9):691–701

Part X

Outcome After Severe TBI

Outcome After Severe Traumatic Brain Injury (TBI)

70

Atle Ulvik and Reidar Kvåle

Recommendations

Measuring outcome after therapy is an obvious part of evidence-based medicine. Using standard classification of recommendations may not be appropriate for this topic. To our knowledge, there has not been performed any controlled studies to evaluate whether or not outcome should be measured after traumatic brain injury.

Level I

There is insufficient data to support a Level I recommendation for this topic.

Level II

There is insufficient data to support a Level II recommendation for this topic.

Level III

Survival, quality of life and functional outcomes should be measured after treatment of severe traumatic brain injury.

70.1 Overview

Severe traumatic brain injury is a leading cause of disability and death, especially among young adults. Most TBI deaths occur within the first week, and 30-day mortality is 20–30%. Physical function generally improves quickly and steadily over the first few months, and overall recovery takes place mainly during the first year. Most of the long-term disability from TBI is caused by neurobehavioural problems (cognitive impairment, depression, anxiety and aggression) which constitute an important barrier to reentry to society. The proportion of vegetative patients seems to be stable at 5–10%. Quality of life normally improves during the first year.

Factors predicting poor prognosis are age above 40 years, low Glasgow Coma Score, hypoxia and hypotension, absent pupil reactivity, the presence of major extracranial injury, pre-injury unemployment, pre-injury substance abuse and severe disability at admission to rehabilitation.

A. Ulvik (✉) • R. Kvåle
Department of Anaesthesia and Intensive Care, Haukeland University Hospital, 5021, Bergen, Norway
e-mail: atle.ulvik@helse-bergen.no; reidar.kvale@helse-bergen.no

T. Sundstrøm et al. (eds.), *Management of Severe Traumatic Brain Injury*, DOI 10.1007/978-3-642-28126-6_70, © Springer-Verlag Berlin Heidelberg 2012

Tips, Tricks, and Pitfalls

- Updated population registries are the best tools for follow-up.
- If available, prospectively collected patient data are of great benefit.
- Validated questionnaires and scoring systems should be used.

70.2 Background

Traumatic brain injury is a leading cause of disability and death, especially among young adults (Fleminger and Ponsford 2005). In addition, trauma care is expensive and resources invested must be wisely, ethically and effectively used. Measuring outcomes after TBI is therefore important.

Primary aims of health care are to reduce mortality and morbidity and to maintain or improve functional capacity and quality of life (Black et al. 2001). While a trauma patient is critically ill, the question is whether or not the patient is going to survive. After the acute phase of life-threatening injuries, long-term outcomes become increasingly more important, and the ultimate question is what kind of life the patient can expect to live. For the last decades, there has been more focus on such non-mortality outcomes, especially functional status and quality of life (Ridley 2002).

The length of the follow-up depends on the outcome parameter. Survival should be traced until the survival curves of patients parallel that of a comparative group (Ridley 2001). For non-mortality outcomes, the follow-up should continue until the patients have regained their pre-injury level or until the progress in the rehabilitation process flattens.

The shift of focus towards patients' perspectives implies assessment of outcome beyond the hospital stay. Obviously, long-term outcome after severe TBI depends on the whole health-care system. The rehabilitation period may last for several months or even years. One must therefore be careful in ascribing certain changes in outcome to the performance of only one of the links in the chain of trauma care.

70.2.1 Survival After Traumatic Brain Injury

Survival is clearly defined and easy to measure. Outcome research, however, depends on national databases containing the date of birth and death for the citizens. To limit the number of patients lost to follow-up, the registries need to be updated continuously. A classic trimodal distribution of deaths following trauma has been described (Trunkey 1983):

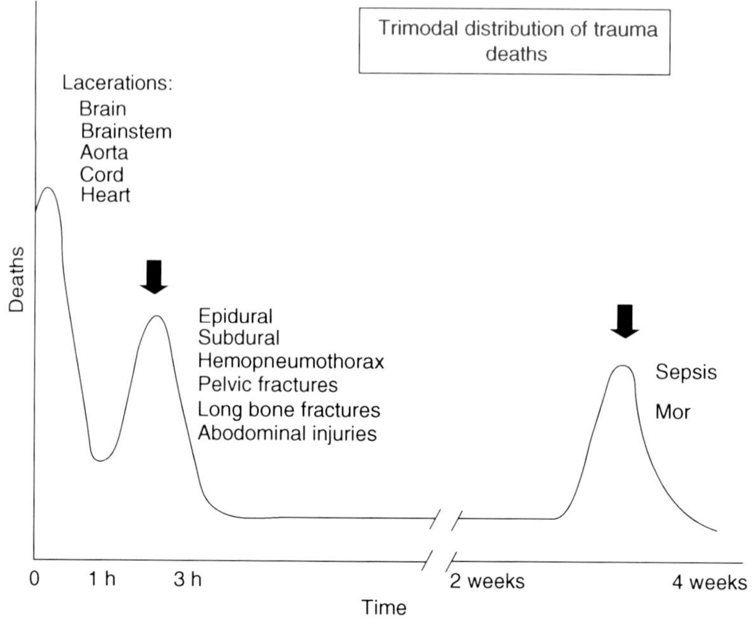

70.2.1.1 Immediate Deaths

Half of trauma deaths occur immediately within seconds to minutes and are due to overwhelming damage to vital structures such as the heart, major vessels, brain and upper spinal cord. In the absence of immediate and aggressive intervention, these deaths are largely unavoidable and can only be limited by preventive measures and legislation.

70.2.1.2 Deaths Occurring from Minutes up to Four Hours After Injury

These deaths account for 30% of trauma deaths and are predominantly a result of major haemorrhage, major chest injuries and traumatic brain injuries. During this period, the so called Golden Hour, a well-organised trauma care system reducing the time interval between injury and definitive treatment, plays an essential role in the improvement of survival after major trauma.

70.2.1.3 Late Deaths Occurring from Days to Weeks After Injury

This third peak, accounting for 20% of trauma deaths, has been attributed to the development of sepsis and multiple organ failure.

Improvements in pre-hospital, resuscitative and operative care of trauma patients have resulted in more patients surviving the initial phases of care and thus requiring intensive care. Critical evaluation of the ICU phase of trauma care has been reported to be the key element in further improvement of outcome after severe trauma (Davis et al. 1991).

Mortality from severe TBI has fallen drastically over the past decades. In the 1970s, a mortality rate of 55% was common. Today, reported 30-day mortality is in the range 20–30% (Ghajar 2000). Most of the deaths occur within the first week after trauma.

70.2.2 Non-mortality Outcomes After Traumatic Brain Injury

Non-mortality outcomes include functional outcome and quality of life.

70.2.2.1 Functional Outcomes

A wide range of sequelae may follow traumatic brain injury, from physical impairment like ataxia or incontinence to neuropsychiatric/neuropsychological problems. Functional outcome describes both physical and mental capability and capacity. The term is frequently and incorrectly used interchangeably with quality of life. Since functional outcome does not include satisfaction or well-being, it can be objectively measured by a researcher. A patient's perception, satisfaction and quality of life may vary independently of functional outcome. Functional outcome can be divided into physical function (impairment and disability), mental function (cognitive and neuropsychological function) and recovery.

Physical Function After TBI

Early post-injury follow-up has traditionally assessed physical disability, which is quite easy to measure and describe. The range of physical sequelae after TBI is, however, wide and includes impairments in motor function, strength, coordination, sensation and cranial nerve function (Wilde et al. 2010). Physical function generally improves quickly and steadily over the first few months following TBI, whereafter a gradual plateauing normally takes place.

Mental Function After TBI

Neuropsychiatric/neuropsychological recovery is a far more complex process, which may not reach baseline even after more than 2 years (Schretlen and Shapiro 2003). Most of the long-term disability from TBI is caused by neurobehavioural problems regarding memory, attention, executive function, behavioural control, mood regulation, anxiety and personality changes. These factors constitute the most important challenge for rehabilitation and interfere with employment, relationships and a normal social life. A review reports prevalence of major depression (25–50%), cognitive impairment (25–70%), anxiety (10–70%) and aggression (30%) following TBI

(Vaishnavi et al. 2009). Another review found that in severe TBI, most of the cognitive recovery takes place within the first 6–18 months after injury, whereafter some improvement may continue at a slower pace (Ruttan et al. 2008). This meta-analysis showed clear cognitive deficits both at approximately 1 and 4.5 years after trauma but found that most of the deficits in attention, executive functions and long-term memory were better explained by primary deficits in working memory. A deficit in speed of processing seems to be a common finding in many studies.

Recovery After TBI

There are numerous outcome measures in TBI research, but the Glasgow Outcome Scale (GOS) is the most commonly used (Wilde et al. 2010). This single-item scale comprises five categories: (1) death, (2) persistent vegetative (minimal responsiveness), (3) severe disability (conscious but disable, dependent for daily support), (4) moderate disability (disable but independent, can work in sheltered settings), and (5) good recovery (resumption of normal life despite minor deficits). A recent study of traumatic brain injury patients with an initial Glasgow Coma Scale ≤ 8 found that at 3 months, almost half of the patients had GOS scores 4 and 5 (favourable outcomes). Other studies have found less favourable outcomes with 46% mortality, 26% persistent vegetative or severely disabled and only 28% having a GOS of 4 and 5 at 6 months (Tasaki et al. 2009).

Several large studies use the GOS at 6 months post injury, since most of the improvements take place during this period. The proportion of vegetative patients seems to be stable at 5–10% (Ghajar 2000).

The Karnofsky Performance Scale (Karnofsky Index) is a generic and useful instrument for measuring functional status, especially the ability to carry out activities of daily living, see Table 70.1 (Schag et al. 1984).

There are two important cut-off points in this scale – score above 50 indicates ability to care for oneself, and score above 70 indicates ability to work and perform normal activities.

Table 70.1 The Karnofsky performance scale

Description	Percentage (%)
Normal; no complaints; no evidence of diseases	100
Abel to carry on normal activity; minor signs and symptoms of diseases	90
Normal activity with effort; some signs and symptoms of diseases	80
Cares for self; unable to carry on normal activity or do work	70
Requires occasional assistance, but is able to care for most personal needs	60
Requires considerable assistance and frequent medical care	50
Disabled; requires special case and assistance	40
Severely disabled; hospitalization indicated although dead not imminent	30
Very risk; hospitalization necessary; requires active support treatment	20
Moribund; fatal processes progressing rapidly	10
Dead	0

70.2.2.2 Quality of Life

Quality of life (QOL) is the subjective experience of life satisfaction and evaluation of life as a whole. Quality of life after TBI should be narrowed to health-related quality of life (HRQOL), which can be defined as the level of well-being and satisfaction associated with an individual's life and how this is affected by disease, accident and treatments (Ridley 2002).

Traumatic brain injury can have serious implications for quality of life, but there are surprisingly few studies published on HRQOL after TBI. Many studies have tried to score quality of life by extrapolating functional status, which is of highly questionable value.

During the acute phase after TBI (<3 months), it can be difficult to assess QOL due to reduced consciousness. In the rehabilitation phase (<1 year) and later, repeated assessment is recommended (Bullinger et al. 2002). Too many different QOL measures have been developed, and for comparison and useful interpretation, only validated measures should be used. The Short Form 36 (SF-36) is a widely used generic measure that has been found to be both reliable and valid for use in many patients groups, including patients with TBI (Findler et al. 2001). The SF-36 is a 36-item questionnaire that assesses eight scales: physical functioning, role limitations due to physical health, body pain, general health, vitality, social functioning, role limitations due to emotional problems and general mental health. A prospective study using the SF-36 found that there is a significant improvement of HRQOL from 6 to 12 months after severe TBI (GCS < 9 for more than 24 h), while there were no major differences between TBI patients with and without polytrauma at 6 or 12 months. This indicates that TBI has a major influence on outcome and QOL after trauma (Lippert-Gruner et al. 2007).

A new trauma-specific international instrument for assessing HRQOL after TBI has been developed, the Quality of Life after Brain Injury (QOLIBRI) (Hawthorne et al. 2011). Validation of the QOLIBRI indicates that this measure is appropriate in TBI studies.

There are some other studies addressing HRQOL after TBI, and they show that TBI has a significant long-term impact on all QOL domains, with lower scores than non-injured controls or normal population reference groups. TBI has a more profound effect on psychosocial domains than on physical domains (Jaracz and Kozubski 2008). Chronic pain is a common complication of TBI with a reported prevalence of up to 58% (Nampiaparampil 2008).

70.2.3 Predictors of Outcome After Traumatic Brain Injury

A predictor gives knowledge in advance about what most likely will happen. Predictors or prognostic factors may constitute a basis for decision making with respect to diagnostic and therapeutic procedures and follow-up. Early identification of patients at risk may improve the outcome after severe TBI through the allocation of expertise, resources and increased attention. Based on risk factors, patients can be stratified into different risk groups. Risk stratification is essential for describing a patient population and is a prerequisite for scientific evaluation of treatment regimens. It is also necessary for comparison of quality of care within and between hospitals and healthcare systems. Identification and evaluation of unexpected non-survivors, i.e. patients who die in spite of low predicted mortality, and unexpected survivors, i.e. patients who survive in spite of high predicted mortality, may improve quality in trauma systems.

In patients with severe TBI the following factors predict poor prognosis, i.e. death or severe disability at 6 months: age above 40 years, low Glasgow Coma Score (linear relation), absent pupil reactivity and the presence of major extracranial injury (Perel et al. 2008). The impact of hypoxia and hypotension is discussed in Chap. 26. Pre-injury unemployment, pre-injury substance abuse and more disability at admission to rehabilitation are found to be important predictors of long-term (more than 1 year) disability (Willemse-van Son et al. 2007).

70.3 Specific Paediatric Concerns

All the uncertainties and doubts regarding pathophysiology, therapy and outcome that apply to TBI in adults are valid also for paediatric TBI. In children, TBI is frequent, but there are little data on prognosis and outcome for these patients (Stocchetti et al. 2010). Based on the concept of greater 'plasticity' in the immature brain, there has been a mistaken optimism concerning outcomes after TBI in children, and a misconception that outcomes in general are superior to those for similar injuries in adults (Forsyth 2010).

Mortality after severe TBI in children is 10–30% (Stocchetti et al. 2010). In a French study reporting a mortality rate of 22%, mortality varied with age and was significantly higher in children <2 years of age (Ducrocq et al. 2006). After 6 months recovery, 39% had a poor outcome defined as GOS ≤ 3, but only 0.8% were in a persistent vegetative state.

References

Black NA, Jenkinson C, Hayes JA, Young D, Vella K, Rowan KM, Daly K, Ridley S (2001) Review of outcome measures used in adult critical care. Crit Care Med 29:2119–2124

Bullinger M, Azouvi P, Brooks N, Basso A, Christensen AL, Gobiet W, Greenwood R, Hutter B, Jennett B, Maas A, Truelle JL, von Wild KR (2002) Quality of life in patients with traumatic brain injury-basic issues, assessment and recommendations. Restor Neurol Neurosci 20:111–124

Davis JW, Hoyt DB, McArdle MS, Mackersie RC, Shackford SR, Eastman AB (1991) The significance of critical care errors in causing preventable death in trauma patients in a trauma system. J Trauma 31:813–818; discussion 818–819

Ducrocq SC, Meyer PG, Orliaguet GA, Blanot S, Laurent-Vannier A, Renier D, Carli PA (2006) Epidemiology and early predictive factors of mortality and outcome in children with traumatic severe brain injury: experience of a French pediatric trauma center. Pediatr Crit Care Med 7:461–467

Findler M, Cantor J, Haddad L, Gordon W, Ashman T (2001) The reliability and validity of the SF-36 health survey questionnaire for use with individuals with traumatic brain injury. Brain Inj 15:715–723

Fleminger S, Ponsford J (2005) Long term outcome after traumatic brain injury. BMJ 331:1419–1420

Forsyth RJ (2010) Back to the future: rehabilitation of children after brain injury. Arch Dis Child 95:554–559

Ghajar J (2000) Traumatic brain injury. Lancet 356: 923–929

Hawthorne G, Kaye AH, Gruen R, Houseman D, Bauer I (2011) Traumatic brain injury and quality of life: initial Australian validation of the QOLIBRI. J Clin Neurosci 18:197–202

Jaracz K, Kozubski W (2008) Quality of life after traumatic brain injury. Neurol Neurochir Pol 42:525–535

Lippert-Gruner M, Maegele M, Haverkamp H, Klug N, Wedekind C (2007) Health-related quality of life during the first year after severe brain trauma with and without polytrauma. Brain Inj 21:451–455

Nampiaparampil DE (2008) Prevalence of chronic pain after traumatic brain injury: a systematic review. JAMA 300:711–719

Perel P, Arango M, Clayton T, Edwards P, Komolafe E, Poccock S, Roberts I, Shakur H, Steyerberg E, Yutthakasemsunt S (2008) Predicting outcome after traumatic brain injury: practical prognostic models based on large cohort of international patients. BMJ 336:425–429

Ridley S (2001) Quality of life and longer term outcomes. In: Sibbald W, Bion JF (eds) Evaluating critical care. Springer, Berlin/Heidelberg/New York/Barcelona/Hong Kong/London/Milan/Paris/Singapore/Tokyo, pp 104–118

Ridley S (2002) Non-mortality outcome measures. In: Ridley S (ed) Outcomes in critical care. Butterworth-Heinemann, Oxford/Auckland/Boston/Johannesburg/Melbourne/New Delhi, pp 120–138

Ruttan L, Martin K, Liu A, Colella B, Green RE (2008) Long-term cognitive outcome in moderate to severe traumatic brain injury: a meta-analysis examining timed and untimed tests at 1 and 4.5 or more years after injury. Arch Phys Med Rehabil 89:S69–S76

Schag CC, Heinrich RL, Ganz PA (1984) Karnofsky performance status revisited: reliability, validity, and guidelines. J Clin Oncol 2:187–193

Schretlen DJ, Shapiro AM (2003) A quantitative review of the effects of traumatic brain injury on cognitive functioning. Int Rev Psychiatry 15:341–349

Stocchetti N, Conte V, Ghisoni L, Canavesi K, Zanaboni C (2010) Traumatic brain injury in pediatric patients. Minerva Anestesiol 76:1052–1059

Tasaki O, Shiozaki T, Hamasaki T, Kajino K, Nakae H, Tanaka H, Shimazu T, Sugimoto H (2009) Prognostic indicators and outcome prediction model for severe traumatic brain injury. J Trauma 66:304–308

Trunkey D (1983) Trauma. Sci Am 249:20–27

Vaishnavi S, Rao V, Fann JR (2009) Neuropsychiatric problems after traumatic brain injury: unraveling the silent epidemic. Psychosomatics 50:198–205

Wilde EA, Whiteneck GG, Bogner J, Bushnik T, Cifu DX, Dikmen S, French L, Giacino JT, Hart T, Malec JF, Millis SR, Novack TA, Sherer M, Tulsky DS, Vanderploeg RD, von Steinbuechel N (2010) Recommendations for the use of common outcome measures in traumatic brain injury research. Arch Phys Med Rehabil 91(1650–1660):e1617

Willemse-van Son AH, Ribbers GM, Verhagen AP, Stam HJ (2007) Prognostic factors of long-term functioning and productivity after traumatic brain injury: a systematic review of prospective cohort studies. Clin Rehabil 21:1024–1037

Subacute MR Imaging: Diffuse Axonal Injury, Brain Stem Lesions and Prognostic Factors

71

Toril Skandsen and Anne Vik

Recommendations

Level I

There is insufficient data to support a Level I recommendation for this topic.

Level II

There is insufficient data to support a Level II recommendation for this topic.

Level III

Patients with severe TBI should preferably be examined with magnetic resonance imaging (MRI) within the first weeks.

Magnetic resonance imaging has shown that brain stem injury is present in almost half of patients with severe TBI surviving the acute phase.

Bilateral brain stem injury has been associated with poor prognosis.

Most patients with severe TBI have diffuse axonal injury (DAI), more often in younger than elderly patients.

71.1 Overview

Computed tomography (CT) is insufficient in the diagnosis of diffuse axonal injury (DAI) and brain stem injury. Such injuries are very common and clinically important in severe traumatic brain injury, especially in the context of high-energy trauma. Magnetic resonance imaging (MRI) is the superior image modality to gain an overview of the traumatic lesions in the brain parenchyma. The neuroanatomic and prognostic information provided by MRI is important during the subacute phase of clinical management and rehabilitation. Thus, MRI should be considered in all patients with severe TBI.

The lesions in diffuse axonal injury are either haemorrhagic or non-haemorrhagic. The haemorrhagic lesions mostly consist of micro-bleeds, detected with a T2*-weighted gradient echo

T. Skandsen (✉)
Department of Neuroscience, Faculty of Medicine, Norwegian University of Science and Technology (NTNU), 7491 Trondheim, Norway

Department of Physical Medicine and Rehabilitation, St. Olavs Hospital, Trondheim University Hospital, Pb 3250, 7006, Sluppen, Trondheim, Norway
e-mail: toril.skandsen@ntnu.no

A. Vik
Department of Neurosurgery, St. Olavs Hospital, Trondheim University Hospital, Trondheim, Norway

Department of Neuroscience, Norwegian University of Science and Technology, Trondheim, Norway
e-mail: anne.vik@ntnu.no

T. Sundstrøm et al. (eds.), *Management of Severe Traumatic Brain Injury*, DOI 10.1007/978-3-642-28126-6_71, © Springer-Verlag Berlin Heidelberg 2012

sequence or susceptibility weighted imaging. The non-haemorrhagic lesions are best visible in T2-weighted imaging, especially fluid-attenuated inversion recovery (FLAIR). Since the non-haemorrhagic lesions attenuate over time, MRI should preferably be performed during the first few weeks post-injury, in order to depict these.

Tips, Tricks, and Pitfalls

- *Important MRI findings and sequences*
  - Most patients with severe TBI have DAI, more often in younger than elderly patients.
  - Commonly, patients have DAI in concert with other lesions, such as hematomas and contusions.
  - Primary brain stem injury is common; mostly these are DAI lesions.
  - Patients with a normal CT scan may have DAI.
  - Patients with a CT scan showing only a few subcortical punctate haemorrhages or modest intraventricular or perimesencephalic subarachnoid haemorrhage may have widespread DAI.
  - Young persons seldom have non-traumatic white matter hyperintensities, and false positive findings are not to be expected.
  - FLAIR: look for high signal in the corpus callosum and rostral part of the brain stem indicating DAI (Fig. 71.1) and non-haemorrhagic cortical contusions in the frontal and temporal lobes. These lesions attenuate with time.
  - T2*-weighted gradient echo or susceptibility weighted imaging: look for dark spots indicating subcortical micro-haemorrhages in the frontal and temporal lobes indicating DAI (Fig. 71.2).
- *Prognosis: information to the family*
  - It is important to know what information has previously been given based on CT findings and the clinical course.
  - MRI often reveals lesions not previously detected by CT, so emphasize that this was to be expected. Especially if MRI was performed during the first weeks, findings may look very extensive due to the depiction of oedema in the tissue.
  - The most serious finding is that of a bilateral brain stem injury, and statistically, this implies a high risk of long-lasting severe disability. In this phase, however, the clinical course is not possible to predict accurately, so stress that also some of these patients eventually have a favourable outcome.
  - Widespread DAI with corpus callosum lesions and/or unilateral brain stem injury often have a favourable outcome, and even a good recovery is possible.
- *Timing and planning*
  - MRI examination in the acute or subacute phase needs to be planned, and communication with the neuroradiologists is essential.
  - If the patient is in the intensive care unit (ICU) and requires continuous monitoring or assisted ventilation, the examination must be planned in cooperation with the staff. Local conditions, such as the number of monitoring ports on the MRI system, distance to the MRI unit and access to anaesthesiology personnel during the examination, can be decisive for timing of the examination.
- *Patient cooperation and MRI quality*
  - The scan protocol takes 30–60 min, and even small patient movements can cause motion artefacts that severely reduce the quality of the scans.

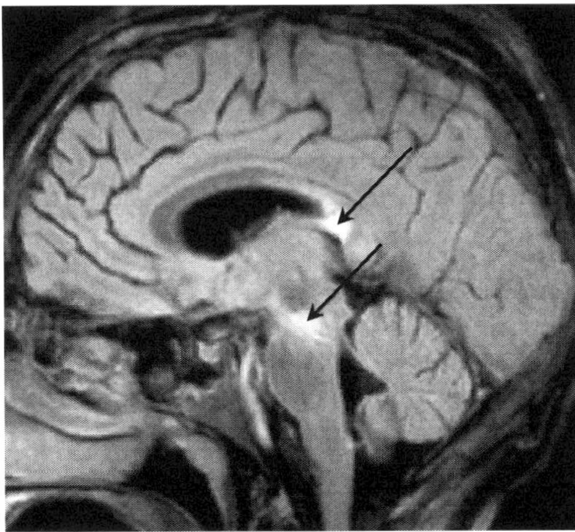

Fig. 71.1 Sagittal FLAIR image. *Arrows* show lesion in the corpus callosum and upper brain stem indicating DAI

- Many patients will enter a phase with confusion and agitation (post-traumatic amnesia) after the sedation has been stopped. One should therefore consider sedation during scanning.
- If the patient is partly cooperative, it is recommended to let a nurse sit close to the patient during scanning in order to repeat the instructions and keep the patient calm.
- To obtain scans of high quality and an assessment by a neuroradiologist experienced with severe traumatic brain injury, it may be beneficial to perform MRI while the patient is still in the trauma centre rather than after transferral to a local hospital.

• *Contraindications and precautions*
  - MRI takes longer time than CT, and MRI findings of lesions not revealed by CT are not decisive for the acute neurosurgical treatment. Thus, MRI should not be performed until the patient's condition is stable regarding intracranial pressure and vital body functions.

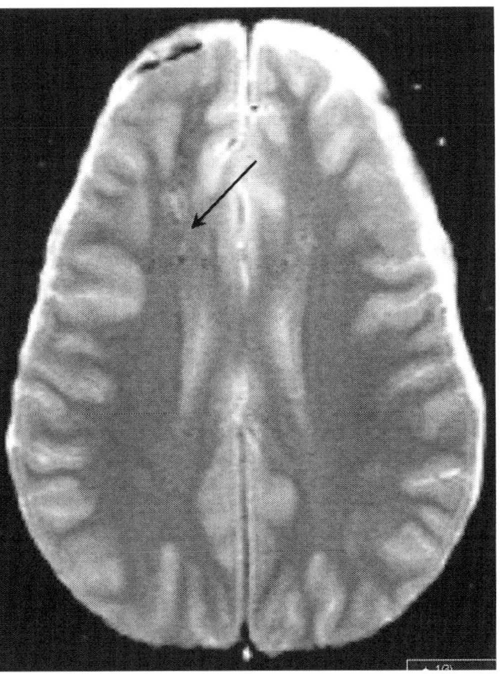

Fig. 71.2 Transversal T2*-weighted gradient echo image. *Arrow* shows micro-haemorrhages in the frontal lobe white matter indicating DAI

- Some external orthopaedic fixations are too magnetic to be in the MRI scanner. Internal orthopaedic fixations as well as material used in craniofacial surgery are usually compatible with MRI.

71.2 Background

71.2.1 Conventional MRI in Patients with Severe TBI

Magnetic resonance imaging is more sensitive than CT in detection of traumatic parenchymal lesions (Gentry et al. 1989) and thus better demonstrates the brain damage. MRI has been recommended if the patient's clinical condition is worse than what should be expected based on the CT scan (Parizel et al. 2005). However, it is not necessarily clear-cut to predict a clinical course from a CT scan which may only show the 'tip of the iceberg'. It should therefore be emphasized that only MRI reliably depicts important traumatic pathoanatomic entities such as diffuse axonal injury or brain stem lesions. These lesions are very common in severe TBI, especially after high-energy trauma. Thus, it has been recommended that patients with moderate-to-severe TBI should preferably be examined with MRI during the first 2 weeks (Hersey et al. 2009).

The common definition of severe TBI is based solely on an initial Glasgow Coma Scale score of 8 or less. This classification is currently debated, and a need for more precise classifications is recognized. New classifications are expected to incorporate also the different pathoanatomic injury types (CT and MRI findings). Recently, as a part of a comprehensive cooperation to agree on common data elements in TBI research, a neuroimaging group published their proposal of state-of-the-art protocols for both CT and MRI (Haacke et al. 2010).

71.2.2 Diffuse Axonal Injury

Diffuse axonal injury increasingly also called 'traumatic axonal injury (TAI)', is an important injury type which has been related to the rotational and deceleration forces associated with high-energy traumas, as traffic accidents, some sports accidents and falls from high heights. It has previously been called 'shearing injury'. The initial mechanical strain and the following cellular events eventually leading to disconnection or recovery of the axons are complex processes and still not fully understood (Andriessen et al. 2010).

In a Norwegian cohort study, DAI was found in 90% of patients under the age of 65 with severe TBI who survived the acute phase. Diffuse axonal injury was often depicted in concert with epidural and subdural haematomas and contusions (Skandsen et al. 2010).

The clinical course of DAI is characterized by initial loss of consciousness which is followed by a period of post-traumatic confusion that can last for weeks (Povlishock and Katz 2005). Patients without large contusions or haematomas, who do not wake up or who exhibit severe agitation and confusion when sedation is stopped, often have a widespread DAI that cannot be diagnosed with CT alone.

The patterns of lesions depicted in the white matter with MRI were found to be identical to what had previously been found in the autopsy and animal studies (Gentry et al. 1988; Adams et al. 1989). Thus, in several MRI studies, a modified grading of DAI has been used: DAI stage 1 (lesions confined to the lobar white matter in the hemispheres), DAI stage 2 (callosal lesions) and DAI stage 3 (in the upper brain stem). The lesions indicating DAI are either haemorrhagic or non-haemorrhagic. The haemorrhagic lesions (micro-bleeds) can be depicted with T2*-weighted gradient echo MRI or a related, more sensitive method, susceptibility weighted imaging (SWI). These are visible for a long time, months or years. The non-haemorrhagic lesions are best visible in T2-weighted images, especially FLAIR. These attenuate during the first weeks and thus may be missed if MRI is performed late.

71.2.3 Prognosis: Diffuse Axonal Injury

Patients with mild and moderate head injury may also have DAI, and therefore DAI per se does not indicate a poor prognosis. DAI in the brain stem (stage 3) has been associated with a poor outcome, defined by Glasgow Outcome Scale Extended 1 scores (death), 2 (vegetative state) or 3 or 4 (two levels of severe disability) (Kampfl et al. 1998a). However, a recent study indicates that in patients with unilateral DAI in the brain stem, outcome was often favourable (Skandsen et al. 2011). The impact of MRI detected DAI in the corpus callosum (stage 2) is less clear since studies have yielded conflicting results (Kampfl et al. 1998b; Pierallini et al. 2000). In a cohort study of patients with moderate and severe TBI, the presence of DAI stage 2 was not a negative prognostic sign in the absence of any BSI (Skandsen et al. 2010).

71.2.4 Brain Stem Injury

Traumatic brain stem injury can be characterized as primary, directly caused by the forces of the trauma, or secondary, resulting from the ischemia associated with herniation of the brain. Primary brain stem lesions comprise DAI, which is the most common, haemorrhage, contusions and lacerations (Blumbergs et al. 2008). Pons and mesencephalon are predilection sites, and the lesions may be unilateral or bilateral. With the increasing use of MRI, it has been shown that brain stem injury is present in almost half of patients with severe TBI surviving the acute phase (Firsching et al. 2001; Skandsen et al. 2011).

Clinical signs of severe brain stem injury in surviving patients are prolonged disorder of consciousness, central motor signs with pareses, spasticity or abnormal posturing and ophthalmoplegia. In the most severely injured patients, periods of autonomic dysfunction (paroxysmal sympathetic hyperactivity) with hypertonia, tachycardia, rigidity and profuse sweating can be observed.

71.2.5 Prognosis: Brain Stem Injury

Bilateral brain stem injury has been associated with poor prognosis (Firsching et al. 2001). In the Norwegian cohort study of 106 patients who survived the acute phase, the patients with a bilateral brain stem injury accounted for most of those who eventually experienced poor outcome. Noteworthy, none were in a vegetative state and only one died (Skandsen et al. 2011). Furthermore, MRI may reveal unilateral brain stem injury, either as more superficial brain stem contusions or DAI lesions. These patients have a better prognosis and often experience only moderate disability or even a good recovery (Shibata et al. 2000; Skandsen et al. 2011).

71.2.6 The MRI Sequences Used in Head Injury

Today, a typical MRI scan protocol in head trauma is performed without contrast at a system with field strength of 1.5 or 3 T and consists of T1- and T2-weighted imaging, a fluid-attenuated inversion recovery (FLAIR) sequence, a T2*-weighted gradient echo sequence or susceptibility weighted imaging (SWI) and diffusion-weighted imaging (DWI).

FLAIR is a T2-weighted sequence where the high T2 signal from the cerebral spinal fluid is suppressed, while the signal from traumatic brain oedema or gliosis remains bright, thus increasing the depictability of tissue injury (Fig. 71.1). In the acute and subacute stage, FLAIR sequences are used for the detection of haemorrhages or oedema in the cortex and the white matter. In the chronic stage, the hyperintensities represent gliotic scarring secondary to the traumatic brain injury (Parizel et al. 2005). High number and large total volume of FLAIR lesions are indications of worse prognosis (Marquez de la Plata et al. 2007; Chastain et al. 2009).

T2*-weighted gradient echo MRI reveals very small haemorrhages associated with DAI, often referred to as 'micro-bleeds'. The technique utilizes the paramagnetic properties of the degradation products of haemoglobin which induce a focal signal loss, a 'blooming effect', and the haemorrhages appear dark on the scan (Fig. 71.2). Even higher sensitivity is found for examinations performed at 3 T (Scheid et al. 2007). Studies have found increased load of micro-bleeds in patients with more severe injury (Tong et al. 2004), but the prognostic value is not yet clear.

Diffusion-weighted imaging is a technique which provides image contrast, resulting from the molecular diffusion of water molecules in the brain tissue (Schaefer 2001). DWI can reliably distinguish between vasogenic oedema (elevated diffusion) and cytotoxic oedema (restricted diffusion). DWI is most useful in the acute phase and could identify white matter lesions not seen on other conventional sequences in a study of TBI patients during the first 48 h (Huisman et al. 2003).

The DWI contains both diffusion and T2 information. These images are compared to the computed apparent diffusion coefficient (ADC) map where the T2 effects have been eliminated while the diffusion effects remain. The areas that appear bright on the DWI scan are dark on the ADC map if they represent abnormal diffusion.

71.2.7 Advanced MR Methods

Several methods require post-processing of MRI data and are therefore less available in clinical diagnostics today. Examples are diffusion tensor imaging (DTI), MR spectroscopy, different methods for measurement of brain volumes and functional magnetic resonance imaging (fMRI). Since DTI is increasingly used in MRI research and is proposed to be a sensitive biomarker of DAI, this method will be briefly described.

In nerve fibres, diffusivity is greater in the direction of the axon (axial), than perpendicular to the fibres; diffusion anisotropy. DTI is based on sampling of diffusion-weighted images for many directions (Le Bihan et al. 2001) and computation of an index of the diffusion anisotropy, e.g. FA (fractional anisotropy) values (Marquez de la Plata et al. 2011). If the microstructure of the axon is damaged (as in TBI), this can result in decreased axial diffusivity and lower FA value.

DTI may depict axonal damage beyond that of conventional MRI (Rutgers et al. 2007). It has also been used longitudinally in patients with very severe injury, and normalization of the DTI indices was larger in the patients who recovered function (Sidaros et al. 2008).

DTI is expected to become more useful in the diagnostic work-up of single patients in the clinic with the development of normative databases of FA values in different brain areas in healthy humans (Haacke et al. 2010).

71.3 Specific Paediatric Concerns

Children with severe TBI are at risk for long-lasting cognitive problems and learning disabilities. It is important for the paediatricians, rehabilitation professionals and neuropsychologists to have a thorough diagnostic of the brain injury. We recommend that MRI is performed in all cases of paediatric TBI. One should consider performing the examination while the child is still under sedation to avoid additional anaesthesia later.

References

Adams JH, Doyle D, Ford I et al (1989) Diffuse axonal injury in head injury: definition, diagnosis and grading. Histopathology 15:49–59

Andriessen TM, Jacobs B, Vos PE (2010) Clinical characteristics and pathophysiological mechanisms of focal and diffuse traumatic brain injury. J Cell Mol Med 14:2381–2392

Blumbergs P, Reilly P, Vink R (2008) Trauma. In: love S, Louis DN, Elison DW (eds) Greenfield's neuropathology. Edward Arnold Ltd., Oxford NY, pp 733–832

Chastain CA, Oyoyo U, Zipperman M et al (2009) Predicting outcomes of traumatic brain injury by imaging modality and injury distribution. J Neurotrauma 26:1183–1196

Firsching R, Woischneck D, Klein S et al (2001) Classification of severe head injury based on magnetic resonance imaging. Acta Neurochir 143:263–271

Gentry LR, Godersky JC, Thompson B (1988) MR imaging of head trauma: review of the distribution and radiopathologic features of traumatic lesions. AJNR Am J Neuroradiol 9:101–110

Gentry LR, Godersky JC, Thompson BH (1989) Traumatic brain stem injury: MR imaging. Radiology 171: 177–187

Haacke EM, Duhaime AC, Gean AD et al (2010) Common data elements in radiologic imaging of traumatic brain injury. J Magn Reson Imaging 32:516–543

Hersey BI, Faro SH, Shah PN et al (2009) Introduction to brain injury imaging. In: Jallo J, Loftus C (eds) Neurotrauma and critical care of the brain. Thieme Medical Publishers Inc., New York, pp 97–141

Huisman TA, Sorensen AG, Hergan K et al (2003) Diffusion-weighted imaging for the evaluation of diffuse axonal injury in closed head injury. J Comput Assist Tomogr 27:5–11

Kampfl A, Franz G, Aichner F et al (1998a) The persistent vegetative state after closed head injury: clinical and magnetic resonance imaging findings in 42 patients. J Neurosurg 88:809–816

Kampfl A, Schmutzhard E, Franz G et al (1998b) Prediction of recovery from post-traumatic vegetative state with cerebral magnetic-resonance imaging. Lancet 351:1763–1767

Le Bihan D, Mangin JF, Poupon C et al (2001) Diffusion tensor imaging: concepts and applications. J Magn Reson Imaging 13:534–546

Marquez de la Plata C, Ardelean A, Koovakkattu D et al (2007) Magnetic resonance imaging of diffuse axonal injury: quantitative assessment of white matter lesion volume. J Neurotrauma 24:591–598

Marquez de la Plata CD, Yang FG, Wang JY et al (2011) Diffusion tensor imaging biomarkers for traumatic axonal injury: analysis of three analytic methods. J Int Neuropsychol Soc 17:24–35

Parizel PM, Van Goethem JW, Ozsarlak O et al (2005) New developments in the neuroradiological diagnosis of craniocerebral trauma. Eur Radiol 15:569–581

Pierallini A, Pantano P, Fantozzi LM et al (2000) Correlation between MRI findings and long-term outcome in patients with severe brain trauma. Neuroradiology 42:860–867

Povlishock JT, Katz DI (2005) Update of neuropathology and neurological recovery after traumatic brain injury. J Head Trauma Rehabil 20:76–94

Rutgers DR, Toulgoat F, Cazejust J et al (2007) White matter abnormalities in mild traumatic brain injury: a diffusion tensor imaging study. AJNR Am J Neuroradiol 29(3):514–519

Schaefer PW (2001) Applications of DWI in clinical neurology. J Neurol Sci 186(Suppl 1):S25–S35

Scheid R, Ott DV, Roth H et al (2007) Comparative magnetic resonance imaging at 1.5 and 3 Tesla for the evaluation of traumatic microbleeds. J Neurotrauma 24:1811–1816

Shibata Y, Matsumura A, Meguro K et al (2000) Differentiation of mechanism and prognosis of traumatic brain stem lesions detected by magnetic resonance imaging in the acute stage. Clin Neurol Neurosurg 102:124–128

Sidaros A, Engberg AW, Sidaros K et al (2008) Diffusion tensor imaging during recovery from severe traumatic brain injury and relation to clinical outcome: a longitudinal study. Brain 131:559–572

Skandsen T, Kvistad KA, Solheim O et al (2010) Prevalence and impact of diffuse axonal injury in patients with moderate and severe head injury: a cohort study of early magnetic resonance imaging findings and 1-year outcome. J Neurosurg 113:556–563

Skandsen T, Kvistad KA, Solheim O et al (2011) Prognostic value of magnetic resonance imaging in moderate and severe head injury: a prospective study of early MRI findings and one-year outcome. J Neurotrauma 28:1–9

Tong KA, Ashwal S, Holshouser BA et al (2004) Diffuse axonal injury in children: clinical correlation with hemorrhagic lesions. Ann Neurol 56:36–50

Part XI

Research in the Neurointensive Care Unit

The Neurointensive Care Unit as a Platform for Advanced Clinical Research

72

Per Enblad, Tim Howells, and Lars Hillered

Recommendations

It is not possible to recommend how the optimal neurointensive care (NIC) platform for advanced clinical research should be organized and equipped according to evidence-based medicine principles. Instead the following advices are given according to the experience from our own and other centres. We believe it is fundamental that the NIC unit is organized in a way that research and development are integrated with routine care. It is also of outmost importance that controlled and standardized conditions are created for the management of the patients. Finally, we believe that information technology systems set up for acquisition and analysis of the large amounts of monitoring data generated will provide unique possibilities for explorative clinical research and that this approach will be beneficial for clinical research and for management and outcome of the patients (Elf et al. 2002).

P. Enblad (✉) • T. Howells • L. Hillered
Department of Neuroscience, Uppsala University Hospital, SE-75185 Uppsala, Sweden
e-mail: per.enblad@neuro.uu.se;
tim.howells@neuro.uu.se; lars.hillered@neuro.uu.se

72.1 Overview

The NIC unit provides an excellent environment for clinical explorative research. Continuous multimodality monitoring of physiological parameters (e.g. arterial blood pressure and temperature) and intracranial parameters (e.g. intracranial pressure, cerebral perfusion pressure, brain tissue oxygenation, neurochemistry and neurophysiology) and computerized collection of high-resolution data makes it possible to obtain a direct insight into human brain injury processes. The use of modern imaging techniques such as magnetic resonance imaging (MRI) and positron emission tomography (PET) are enhancing our understanding of the mechanisms underlying these processes. New monitoring techniques can be validated and critical thresholds defined. The NIC unit also plays an important role in translational research bridging the gap between the laboratory and the patients and in the development of new treatment and management strategies. The Uppsala NIC unit is an important platform in our current network activities: the Uppsala Brain Injury Center (www.neuro.uu.se/ubic), Centre of Excellence Neurotrauma (www.neurotrauma.se/eng), BrainIT Group (www.brainit.org) and Uppsala Berzelii Technology Centre for Neurodiagnostics (www.berzelii.uu.se).

The aims of this chapter are first to describe the cornerstones of the NIC research platform and second to give a few examples of research in which important knowledge was gained by taking advantage of this platform.

T. Sundstrøm et al. (eds.), *Management of Severe Traumatic Brain Injury*,
DOI 10.1007/978-3-642-28126-6_72, © Springer-Verlag Berlin Heidelberg 2012

Tips, Tricks, and Pitfalls

- Establish a research group including various different competences, e.g. neurosurgeons, neurointensivists, research nurses, engineers, programmers and statisticians.
- Involve all members of the staff in the research projects and give them regular feedback.
- Try to make all graduated members of the research group responsible for their own parts of the overall research program to avoid conflicts.
- Try to establish interdisciplinary network activities to enable translation of knowledge between basic science, technological science and the NIC setting.

72.2 Background

72.2.1 Organization of the Neurointensive Care Unit

It is important to create a culture for all members of the NIC staff where research and development are integrated with clinical routine. The goal should be to create a controlled and standardized management environment for the patients resembling the conditions in the laboratory in terms of maintaining clear and consistent standards for patient care. This can be achieved by implementation of standardized management protocol systems similar to the Good Laboratory Practice (GLP) standards. It is also of outmost importance to establish a research group including various different competences, e.g. neurosurgeons, neurointensivists, research nurses, engineers, programmers and statisticians.

72.2.2 Multimodality Monitoring and Computerized Data Acquisition and Analysis Systems

Multimodality monitoring generates enormous amounts of valuable data. It is crucial to set up a computer-based system for collection and acquisition of data. One example is the Odin Monitoring System software (formerly the Edinburgh Browser), which has been developed over several years by the computer scientist Tim Howells in collaboration with clinicians, first in Edinburgh and for the last 10 years in Uppsala. This system can be networked to all beds in the NIC unit for collection, analysis and visualization of demographic data, physiological minute-by-minute monitoring data and treatment data. The software has recently been extended to include functions for high-resolution waveform data analysis, which can be used in autoregulation and compliance studies. Another computer system specially designed for NIC is the ICM+ software developed at the University of Cambridge by Peter Smielewski and Marek Czosnyka. This software is focused on signal acquisition and processing and has been used extensively in autoregulation and compliance studies and also in the management of hydrocephalus patients. The Sensometrics software developed at the National Hospital in Oslo has also been used extensively in brain injury research, based on the analysis of intracranial and systemic pressure signals. A fourth example is the ICU pilot system developed by the former CMA Microdialysis AB in Sweden (M Dialysis AB, Solna, Sweden. www.mdialysis.com) for integration and analysis of microdialysis and other monitoring data.

72.3 Illustrative NIC Research Projects

72.3.1 High-Resolution Waveform Data Analysis for Monitoring of Autoregulation and Compliance

Until recently the dominant school of intensive care management of patients with traumatic brain injury (TBI) held that the most critical factor was maintaining cerebral perfusion pressure (CPP) (Rosner et al. 1995). Other neurosurgical centres have taken a more cautious approach to elevating CPP (CPP-oriented therapy) and have focussed primarily on lowering intracranial pressure (ICP) (ICP-oriented therapy) (Elf et al. 2002; Eker et al. 1998). A study of CPP and ICP management strategies involving our own centre found evidence that some patients responded better to CPP-oriented management and others did better given ICP-oriented treatment (Howells et al. 2005). We also found that pressure autoregulation status was the key to determining the optimal strategy. The most recent Brain Trauma Foundation guidelines have moved in this direction, recommending that CPP management be carefully targeted based in part on pressure autoregulation status (Bratton et al. 2007). Most measures of autoregulation used are based on the response of ICP to changes in systemic blood pressure. The best available measure for continuous assessment of autoregulation status is the pressure reactivity index (PRx) from the Cambridge group, calculated as a moving correlation coefficient between 40 consecutive samples of values for ICP and mean arterial blood pressure averaged for a period of 5 s (Czosnyka et al. 1997). PRx is well validated as a measure of pressure autoregulation, but the investigation of its use in clinical decision making is still in its early stages (Guendling et al. 2006). It is therefore important to refine our understanding of existing measures of autoregulation and to develop new measures, with the goal of clinical application clearly in mind. Modern NIC software systems including functions for high-resolution waveform data analysis provide an excellent tool for such studies.

The monitoring of intracranial compliance in NIC may provide valuable information about intracranial compensatory volume reserve and risk of developing high ICP. Various approaches have been used to estimate intracranial compliance (Marmarou et al. 1975; Robertson et al. 1989; Yau et al. 2002; Czosnyka et al. 2001). There is currently no compliance monitoring method that is widely used in practical clinical care. The most widely studied measures of intracranial compliance are computed from the ICP waveform. One such ICP waveform-based measure of compliance is the RAP index, which has been validated in a number of clinical studies (Castellani et al. 2009; Czosnyka et al. 2007; Kim et al. 2009; Timofeev et al. 2008a, b). The RAP index is calculated as the moving correlation between mean ICP and the ICP pulse amplitude over a time window of about 4 min. The ICP pulse amplitude itself has also been studied and validated as a measure of compliance (Czosnyka et al. 2001; Bentsen et al. 2008; Eide and Sorteberg 2007; Eide et al. 2007, 2011). A third metric that has been proposed is the ascending slope of the ICP pulse waveform (Contant et al. 1995). Compliance-based management of subarachnoid haemorrhage according to the ICP pulse amplitude has recently been the subject of a randomized clinical trial (RCT), which has produced positive preliminary results (Eide et al. 2011). Future NIC studies within this field may foster the development of compliance monitoring into a valuable clinical instrument.

72.3.2 Development of Neurochemical Monitoring Methods from Bench to Bed

Based on cerebral microdialysis (MD) studies in our animal models of stroke and traumatic brain injury (TBI) in the 1980s in collaboration with Ungerstedt et al. (Hillered et al. 1989; Nilsson et al. 1990), we set out to explore the usefulness of MD monitoring in the NIC setting in patients with subarachnoid haemorrhage (SAH) and TBI. Our seminal observations strongly supported a potentially important role for MD as a neurochemical monitoring tool (Persson and Hillered 1992). The MD method has eventually become a widespread tool for neurochemical monitoring and research in neurosurgery and NIC with over 400 publications on the PubMed to date. MD is a unique tool for harvesting of neurochemical signals in the human brain and has together with neuroimaging methods (CT, PET, MRI) provided important new insights into the neurochemistry of acute human brain injury. MD is currently used in the NIC setting mainly for energy metabolic monitoring, monitoring of cellular distress markers, protein biomarker sampling and as an emerging tool in neuropharmacology.

72.3.2.1 Energy Metabolic Monitoring

Low molecular weight cut-off (MWCO) MD in the NIC setting has been chiefly used for monitoring of energy metabolic perturbation (glucose, lactate, pyruvate, lactate/pyruvate ratio [LPR]), excitotoxicity (glutamate), membrane phospholipid

Table 72.1 Typical MD marker pattern of overt cerebral ischaemia

	Glucose	Lactate	Pyruvate	LPR
Ischaemia	↓↓	↑↑	↓↓	↑↑

↓↓ marked decrease, ↑↑ marked increase, *LPR* lactate/pyruvate ratio (For references, see Hillered et al. (2005)

degradation/oxidative stress (glycerol) and urea metabolism, driven by the availability of dedicated point-of-care analytical tools (M Dialysis AB, Solna, Sweden). There are numerous reviews on these topics, with a few of the most recent referred to here (Chefer et al. 2009; Goodman and Robertson 2009; Hillered et al. 2005, 2006; Peerdeman et al. 2003; Ungerstedt and Rostami 2004). The following discussion will focus mainly on TBI.

Ischaemic Energy Metabolic Crisis Following TBI

Based on pioneering work of Graham and colleagues in the 1970s, ischaemia was identified as an important component of severe TBI. This concept was based on autopsy data from patients succumbing to severe TBI (Graham et al. 1978). In the NIC setting, much effort is directed towards minimizing secondary ischaemia owing to intracranial hypertension and low perfusion pressure to prevent progression of the primary brain damage. Studies have been done to validate MD markers of cerebral ischaemia using, e.g. PET. In particular, the LPR has been suggested to be a sensitive and specific marker of ischaemia (Enblad et al. 1996, 2001; Hutchinson et al. 2002). Another advantage of the LPR is that it appears to be a quantitative measure, independent of the extraction efficiency of the MD catheter (Persson and Hillered 1996). A number of validation studies collectively suggest a typical ischaemia pattern of several MD markers as shown in Table 72.1.

Non-ischaemic Energy Metabolic Crisis Following TBI

In recent years, the refinement of modern NIC as well as preventive strategies in Western societies with, e.g. safer cars, the most severe injuries are fewer, and the problem of overt secondary ischaemia has diminished. Instead the complexity of energy metabolic alterations following TBI has been increasingly acknowledged. With the combined use of multimodal monitoring and neuroimaging methods, a new concept of non-ischaemic energy metabolic crisis has emerged (see Hillered and Enblad 2008). Using MD-LPR as a surrogate end point marker, studies by the Houston and UCLA groups revealed that the occurrence of high LPR levels (LPR > 30–40) without hypoxia/ischaemia measured by brain tissue oximetry and PET, respectively, was surprisingly frequent after TBI (Hlatky et al. 2004; Vespa et al. 2005). Apparently, such LPR elevations were often characterized by a pyruvate close to or slightly below the critical level (Table 72.2) but without a marked lactate increment. This phenomenon was tentatively named type 2 LPR elevation (Hillered et al. 2006) to be distinguished from the classical type 1 LPR elevation seen in ischaemia with more pronounced pyruvate reductions in combination with a markedly increased lactate (Table 72.1), reflecting anaerobic glycolysis and a perturbed cellular redox state (see Hillered et al. 2005). The type 2 LPR phenomenon may reflect several possible energy metabolic changes following TBI, including a relative shortage of brain glucose (in spite of normal or high blood glucose), dysfunction of the glycolytic pathway and shunting of glucose to competing pathways such as the pentose phosphate pathway (PPP). In support of this, an increased shunting of glucose to the PPP was recently described after clinical TBI (Dusick et al. 2007). Thus, the emerging picture is that the post-traumatic brain may frequently suffer from a non-ischaemic energy metabolic crisis characterized by an impaired glycolytic activity and/or a relative shortage of brain glucose because of an impaired glucose transport across the BBB and competition for glucose between ATP production and, e.g. the PPP for macromolecular repair and oxidative stress defence, leading to a shortage of glucose and pyruvate, and a type 2 LPR elevation. The potential importance of non-ischaemic energy crisis as a secondary injury mechanism following clinical TBI was suggested by data showing an association between low brain glucose during NIC and poor 6-month clinical

Table 72.2 Tentative critical MD levels in secondary cerebral energy crisis

	Glucose	Lactate	Pyruvate	LPR
Critical level	<1.0 mmol/L	>3.0 mmol/L	<120 μmol/L	>30

Conservatively chosen based on Reinstrup et al. (2000); Schulz et al. (2000); Oddo et al. (2008); Meierhans et al. (2010)

outcome (Vespa et al. 2003). Furthermore, LPR elevations in normal appearing frontal lobe tissue in the NIC setting were related to the extent of frontal lobe atrophy, as measured by volumetric brain MRI at 6-month post-injury (Marcoux et al. 2008). Apparently, in addition to MD-glucose, MD-pyruvate is a biomarker of energy metabolic crisis that deserves increased attention in NIC. Non-ischaemic energy crisis is thought to occur in the NIC setting also in SAH patients (Samuelsson et al. 2007).

Spreading Depolarization (SD) Following Acute Brain Injury

SD is a depolarization wave spreading across the cerebral cortical surface observed in the 1940s following brain injury in experimental animals as a cortical spreading depression (Leao 1947). SD in the form of peri-infarct depolarization is thought to be an important mechanism for the recruitment of penumbral tissue to infarction in experimental stroke (Gill et al. 1992). Because of the difficulty involved in measuring SD, it was not until 2002 that SD was reported to occur in the human brain following acute injury using subdural strip electrodes (Strong et al. 2002). It has now become clear that SD is a common feature of human TBI and neurovascular brain injury. In patients who have undergone craniotomy, SD occurs in 50–60% of TBI and in 70% of SAH patients (Feuerstein et al. 2010). SD is thought to be an important secondary injury mechanism by challenging the energy metabolic capacity of the brain tissue to restore ion homeostasis. By the use of rapid sampling MD in combination with subdural strip electrodes, SDs have been shown to lead to marked, transient reductions of MD-glucose and concomitant increases of MD-lactate, posing a risk of brain glucose depletion when occurring repeatedly, despite an adequate blood supply (Hashemi et al. 2009; Feuerstein et al. 2010). Thus, the SD phenomenon may be an additional important mechanism leading to non-ischaemic energy metabolic crisis following TBI.

Brain Glucose and Insulin Management in the NIC Setting

Experimental studies of decades ago suggested that hyperglycaemia at the onset of cerebral ischaemia aggravates brain damage by producing more pronounced acidosis leading to increased oxidative stress (Siesjö 1981; Li et al. 1999). There is evidence that hyperglycaemia in the acute phase of TBI is associated with poor outcome irrespective of injury severity (Liu-DeRyke et al. 2009). Correcting hyperglycaemia >10 mmol/L was shown to reduce mortality after severe TBI (Jeremitsky et al. 2005), and many neurosurgical centres avoid blood glucose values >10 mmol/L as a routine precaution. A new direction was taken by van den Berghe and colleagues, presenting evidence that keeping blood glucose between 4.4 and 6.1 mmol/L reduced morbidity and mortality in surgical and medical intensive care patients (van den Berghe et al. 2001, 2006). These data created widespread attention even though follow-up studies failed to confirm the positive effects of tight glycemic control in surgical and medical critical care patients (Arabi et al. 2008; Brunkhorst et al. 2008). In the NIC setting, tight glycaemic control (5.0–6.7 mmol/L) produced signs of metabolic distress (reduced MD-glucose and increased MD-LPR and MD-glutamate) without any improvement in 6-month outcome in severe TBI patients (Vespa et al. 2006). Along the same line, Oddo and colleagues showed that tight glycaemic control (4.4–6.7 mmol/L) in NIC patients with severe traumatic and neurovascular brain injury was associated with an increased prevalence of energy metabolic crisis (brain MD-glucose <0.7 mmol/L + MD-LPR >40), associated with a higher mortality rate at discharge (Oddo et al. 2008). Recent data from Meierhans and colleagues studying brain energy metabolic alterations with MD at different blood glucose levels in 20 patients with severe TBI support the notion that MD glucose levels below 1 mmol/L should be avoided and suggest that the optimal blood glucose range may be 6–9 mmol/L in the NIC setting (Meierhans et al. 2010).

In summary, both hyper- and hypoglycaemia are important adverse factors in the NIC setting. It has become increasingly clear that low brain glucose is a common phenomenon during NIC, putting the acutely injured brain at risk for secondary energy metabolic crisis and aggravated brain damage related to the phenomena discussed above. Conversely, blood glucose levels >10 mmol/L should be avoided. The need for controlling brain glucose, particularly to avoid critically low levels frequently observed despite a normal or high blood glucose, has in our view strengthened the indication for brain glucose monitoring with MD in the NIC setting, although a specific treatment algorithm remains to be assessed.

72.3.2.2 Monitoring of Cellular Distress Markers

MD-glutamate and MD-glycerol are widely used biomarkers of cellular distress caused by excitotoxicity and membrane phospholipid degradation/oxidative stress, respectively, in the NIC setting. These biomarkers can be readily analyzed at the bedside with the dedicated MD analyzers available in many neurosurgical centres worldwide. MD-glutamate was recommended as a useful biomarker in NIC monitoring at the Stockholm Consensus Meeting on MD monitoring (Bellander et al. 2004). The importance of MD-glutamate as a biomarker in TBI patients was recently emphasized by the Houston group demonstrating a relationship between MD-glutamate and mortality as well as 6-month functional outcome in a prospective study on 165 severe TBI patients (Chamoun et al. 2010). Although widely used, there is still concern as to the precise interpretation of the biomarker signals. For example, glutamate accumulation in the interstitial fluid (ISF) following brain injury may be derived from several different sources and by different mechanisms making the interpretation problematic (see Hillered et al. 2005). Also glycerol accumulation in the ISF following brain injury may reflect different phenomena, including increased membrane phospholipid degradation, oxidative stress and de novo synthesis from glucose. Recent data using ^{13}C-labelled glucose and MD suggest that de novo synthesis from glucose following experimental TBI only accounts for a few percent of the MD-glycerol signal (Clausen et al. 2011a), leaving membrane phospholipid degradation and oxidative stress as the dominating sources of the MD-glycerol signal.

Oxidative stress following TBI is thought to be closely associated with excitotoxicity, i.e. glutamate-mediated intracellular accumulation of Ca^{2+} leading to, e.g. phospholipase activation, membrane phospholipid degradation and formation of arachidonic acid (see Hillered et al. 2005). Another end product of this phospholipid degradation process is glycerol (Marklund et al. 1997), which has also been implicated as a biomarker of oxidative stress (Lewen and Hillered 1998; Merenda et al. 2008). In an attempt to validate glycerol as a biomarker of oxidative stress, we recently performed a study on MD-8-iso-$PGF_{2\alpha}$, a widely used biomarker of oxidative stress, in six patients with severe TBI (Clausen et al. 2011b). We found significant, strong correlations between MD-8-iso-$PGF_{2\alpha}$ and MD-glycerol and between MD-8-iso-$PGF_{2\alpha}$ and MD-glutamate, supporting the close association between oxidative stress and excitotoxicity also in the human brain following TBI and that the MD-glycerol signal is reflecting oxidative stress to a large degree.

In summary, MD-glutamate and MD-glycerol provide important neurochemical information on excitotoxic and oxidative stress-related secondary injury following acute brain injury in the NIC setting. The combination of MD-8-iso-$PGF_{2\alpha}$ and MD-glycerol may prove useful as biomarkers of oxidative stress pending further validation. These biomarkers may become increasingly useful for proof-of-principle testing before moving to large-scale clinical trials and as surrogate end point markers in neuroprotective drug development.

72.3.2.3 Protein Biomarker Sampling

Biomarkers are currently predicted to play an increasingly important role in future NIC. The introduction of high MWCO (100 kDa or more) MD catheters potentially allowing for studies on the proteomics of acute brain injury has lately been met with considerable enthusiasm. The basic assumption is that sampling of protein biomarkers directly in the injured human brain by MD delivers neurochemical signals with an improved temporal and spatial resolution compared to conventional protein biomarker sampling from vCSF or blood. MD thus offers a unique opportunity for biomarker sampling in the brain potentially avoiding both dilution and chemical degradation of the protein biomarkers. A number of feasibility studies have been published reporting the potential of monitoring various proteins in the NIC setting, including cytokines (Hillman et al. 2005; Helmy et al. 2009, 2010), amyloid β and Tau protein (Brody et al. 2008; Marklund et al. 2009), VEGF and FGF2 (Mellergard et al. 2010) and other proteins (see Dahlin et al. 2010; Maurer 2010). However, several methodological issues have recently emerged, such as potential perfusion fluid loss, low and unstable protein recovery and biofouling, questioning the robustness of high MWCO MD methodology to date (Dahlin et al. 2010). Apparently, protein trafficking across the high MWCO MD membrane is a highly complex process involving a number of aspects potentially affecting the in vivo protein recovery, such as various physical properties of proteins, membrane biofouling and encapsulation (Helmy et al. 2009; Dahlin et al. 2010). When a foreign material is inserted into a living organism, a tissue response will occur, starting with protein adsorption to the material surface followed by the interaction with host cells leading to a phenomenon called biofouling (Anderson et al. 2008). Biofouling has severe implications for MD as it may lead to decreased protein recovery, inflammatory responses and limit the duration of accurate in vivo sampling (Wisniewski et al. 2001). Biofouling of MD catheters following 42-h in vivo dialysis in human brain has been documented by electron microscopy (Helmy et al. 2009). Because of the methodological issues involved with in vivo MD protein sampling, we recently started a collaborative effort with the Uppsala Berzelii Technology Centre for Neurodiagnostics (www.berzelii.uu.se) to improve our understanding of the mechanisms involved with protein trafficking across high MWCO MD membranes. The results from this project thus far point in the direction that surface modification of the high MWCO MD membranes in combination with modification of the perfusate fluid composition may help to improve the robustness of high MWCO MD (Dahlin et al. 2010). This modified technology is currently being tested in a porcine model of acute brain injury (Purins et al. 2011) as a potential step towards a NIC application.

72.3.2.4 Neuropharmacology

Cerebral microdialysis is considered to have a great potential for monitoring of free target drug concentrations and as a tool in clinical drug development in the NIC setting (Helmy et al. 2007). This concept was put forth by Alves et al. (2003) in a study with the glutamate release inhibitor topiramate showing that the initial dose given systemically had to be raised markedly to achieve adequate free drug concentration in NIC patients with severe TBI. Another example is a study by Ederoth et al. (2004) measuring free morphine concentrations in TBI patients. Finally, the topiramate study elegantly showed that MD can be used as a surrogate end point tool in the NIC setting to obtain proof of concept, in this case lowering of interstitial glutamate levels (Alves et al. 2003).

References

Alves OL, Doyle AJ, Clausen T, Gilman C, Bullock R (2003) Evaluation of topiramate neuroprotective effect in severe TBI using microdialysis. Ann N Y Acad Sci 993:25–34

Anderson JM, Rodriguez A, Chang DT (2008) Foreign body reaction to biomaterials. Semin Immunol 20: 86–100

Arabi YM, Dabbagh OC, Tamim HM, Al-Shimemeri AA, Memish ZA, Haddad SH, Syed SJ, Giridhar HR, Rishu AH, Al-Daker MO, Kahoul SH, Britts RJ, Sakkijha MH (2008) Intensive versus conventional insulin therapy: a randomized controlled trial in medical and surgical critically ill patients. Crit Care Med 36: 3190–3197

Bellander BM, Cantais E, Enblad P, Hutchinson P, Nordström CH, Robertson C, Sahuquillo J, Smith M, Stocchetti N, Ungerstedt U, Unterberg A, Olsen NV (2004) Consensus meeting on microdialysis in neurointensive care. Intensive Care Med 30: 2166–2169

Bentsen G, Stubhaug A, Eide PK (2008) Differential effects of osmotherapy on static and pulsatile intracranial pressure. Crit Care Med 36:2414–2419

Bratton SL, Chestnut RM Ghajar J, McConnell Hammond FF, Harris OA, Hartl R, Manley GT, Nemecek A, Newell DW, Rosenthal G, Schouten J, Shutter L, Timmons SD, Ullman JS, Videtta W, Wilberger JE, Wright DW (2007) Guidelines for the management of severe traumatic brain injury. IX. Cerebral perfusion thresholds. J Neurotrauma 24(Suppl 1):S-59–S-64

Brody DL, Magnoni S, Schwetye KE, Spinner ML, Esparza TJ, Stocchetti N, Zipfel GJ, Holtzman DM (2008) Amyloid-beta dynamics correlate with neurological status in the injured human brain. Science 321:1221–1224

Brunkhorst FM, Engel C, Bloos F, Meier-Hellmann A, Ragaller M, Weiler N, Moerer O, Gruendling M, Oppert M, Grond S, Olthoff D, Jaschinski U, John S, Rossaint R, Welte T, Schaefer M, Kern P, Kuhnt E, Kiehntopf M, Hartog C, Natanson C, Loeffler M, Reinhart K (2008) Intensive insulin therapy and pentastarch resuscitation in severe sepsis. N Engl J Med 358:125–139

Castellani G, Zweifel C, Kim DJ, Carrera E, Radolovich DK, Smielewski P, Hutchinson PJ, Pickard JD, Czosnyka M (2009) Plateau waves in head injured patients requiring neurocritical care. Neurocrit Care 11: 143–150

Chamoun R, Suki D, Gopinath SP, Goodman JC, Robertson C (2010) Role of extracellular glutamate measured by cerebral microdialysis in severe traumatic brain injury. J Neurosurg 113:564–570

Chefer VIA, Thompson C, Zapata A, Shippenberg TS (2009) Overview of brain microdialysis. Curr Protoc Neurosci Chapter 7:Unit 7.1

Clausen F, Hillered L, Gustafsson J (2011a) Cerebral glucose metabolism after traumatic brain injury in the rat studied by (13)C-glucose and microdialysis. Acta Neurochir (Wien) 153:653–658

Clausen F, Marklund N, Lewen A, Enblad P, Basu S, Hillered L (2011b) Interstitial F2-isoprostane 8-iso-PGF2α and glycerol as biomarkers of oxidative stress following severe human traumatic brain injury. J Neurotrauma. Sep 13. [Epub ahead of print, PMID: 21639729]

Contant CF, Robertson CS, Crouch J, Gopinath SP, Narayan RK, Grossman RG (1995) Intracranial pressure waveform indices in transient and refractory intracranial hypertension. J Neurosci Methods 57:15–25

Czosnyka M, Smielewski P, Kirkpatrick P, Laing RJ, Menon D, Pickard JD (1997) Continuous assessment of the cerebral vasomotor reactivity in head injury. Neurosurgery 41:11–19

Czosnyka M, Czosnykja ZH, Whitfield PC, Donovan T, Pickard JD (2001) Age dependence of cerebrospinal pressure-volume compensation in patients with hydrocephalus. J Neurosurg 94:482–486

Czosnyka M, Smielewski P, Timofeev I, Lavinio A, Guazzo E, Hutchinson P, Pickard JD (2007) Intracranial pressure: more than a number. Neurosurg Focus 22(5):E10

Dahlin AP, Wetterhall M, Caldwell KD, Larsson A, Bergquist J, Hillered L, Hjort K (2010) Methodological aspects on microdialysis protein sampling and quantification in biological fluids: an in vitro study on human ventricular CSF. Anal Chem 82:4376–4385

Dusick JR, Glenn TC, Lee WN, Vespa PM, Kelly DF, Lee SM, Hovda DA, Martin NA (2007) Increased pentose phosphate pathway flux after clinical traumatic brain injury: a [1,2-(13)C(2)]glucose labelling study in humans. J Cereb Blood Flow Metab 27:1593–1602

Ederoth P, Tunblad K, Bouw R, Lundberg CJ, Ungerstedt U, Nordstrom CH, Hammarlund-Udenaes M (2004) Blood-brain barrier transport of morphine in patients with severe brain trauma. Br J Clin Pharmacol 57(4): 427–435

Eide PK, Sorteberg W (2007) Association among intracranial compliance, intracranial pulse pressure amplitude and intracranial pressure in patients with intracranial bleeds. Neurol Res 29:798–802

Eide PK, Rappaport BI, Gormley WB, Madsen JR (2007) A dynamic nonlinear relationship between the static and pulsatile components of intracranial pressure in patients with subarachnoid hemorrhage. Neurosurg Focus 22(5):E10

Eide PK, Bentsen G, Sorteberg A, Martinsen PB, Stubhaug A, Sorteberg W (2011) Effect of intracranial pressure (ICP) versus ICP wave amplitude guided intensive care management on acute clinical state and 12 months outcome in patients with aneurysmal subarachnoid hemorrhage, a randomized and blinded single-center trial. Neurosurg Focus 30(2):A1

Eker C, Asgeirsson B, Grande PO, Schalen W, Nordstrom CH (1998) Improved outcome after severe head injury with a new therapy based on principles for brain volume regulation and preserved microcirculation. Crit Care Med 26:1881–1886

Elf K, Nilsson P, Enblad P (2002) Treatment results of patients with traumatic brain injury improved by refined neurointensvie care. The Uppsala experience of an organised secondary insult programme. Crit Care Med 30:2129–2134

Enblad P, Valtysson J, Andersson J, Lilja A, Valind S, Antoni G, Långström B, Hillered L, Persson L (1996) Simultaneous intracerebral microdialysis and positron emission tomography performed in the detection of ischemia in patients with subarachnoid hemorrhage. J Cereb Blood Flow Metab 16:637–644

Enblad P, Frykholm P, Valtysson J, Silander HC, Andersson J, Fasth KJ, Watanabe Y, Långström B,

Hillered L, Persson L (2001) Middle cerebral artery occlusion and reperfusion in primates monitored by microdialysis and sequential positron emission tomography. Stroke 32:1574–1580

Feuerstein D, Manning A, Hashemi P, Bhatia R, Fabricius M, Tolias C, Pahl C, Ervine M, Strong AJ, Boutelle MG (2010) Dynamic metabolic response to multiple spreading depolarizations in patients with acute brain injury: an online microdialysis study. J Cereb Blood Flow Metab 30:1343–1355

Gill R, Andine P, Hillered L, Persson L, Hagberg H (1992) The effect of MK-801 on cortical spreading depression in the penumbral zone following focal ischaemia in the rat. J Cereb Blood Flow Metab 12:371–379

Goodman JC, Robertson CS (2009) Microdialysis: is it ready for prime time? Curr Opin Crit Care 15: 110–117

Graham DI, Adams JH, Doyle D (1978) Ischaemic brain damage in fatal non-missile head injuries. J Neurol Sci 39:213–234

Guendling K, Smielewski P, Czosnyka M, Lewis P, Nortje J, Timofeev I, Hutchinson PJ, Pickard JD (2006) Use of ICM+ software for on-line analysis of intracranial and arterial pressures in head-injured patients. Acta Neurochir Suppl 96:108–113, Brain Edema XIII

Hashemi P, Bhatia R, Nakamura H, Dreier JP, Graf R, Strong AJ, Boutelle MG (2009) Persisting depletion of brain glucose following cortical spreading depression, despite apparent hyperaemia: evidence for risk of an adverse effect of Leao's spreading depression. J Cereb Blood Flow Metab 29:166–175

Helmy A, Carpenter KL, Hutchinson PJ (2007) Microdialysis in the human brain and its potential role in the development and clinical assessment of drugs. Curr Med Chem 14:1525–1537

Helmy A, Carpenter KL, Skepper JN, Kirkpatrick PJ, Pickard JD, Hutchinson PJ (2009) Microdialysis of cytokines: methodological considerations, scanning electron microscopy, and determination of relative recovery. J Neurotrauma 26:549–561

Helmy A, Carpenter KL, Menon DK, Pickard JD, Hutchinson PJ (2010) The cytokine response to human traumatic brain injury: temporal profiles and evidence for cerebral parenchymal production. J Cereb Blood Flow Metab 31:658–670

Hillered L, Enblad P (2008) Nonischemic energy metabolic crisis in acute brain injury. Crit Care Med 36:2952–2953

Hillered L, Hallström Å, Segersvärd S, Persson L, Ungerstedt U (1989) Dynamics of extracellular metabolites in the striatum after middle cerebral artery occlusion in the rat monitored by intracerebral microdialysis. J Cereb Blood Flow Metab 9:607–616

Hillered L, Vespa PM, Hovda DA (2005) Translational neurochemical research in acute human brain injury: the current status and potential future for cerebral microdialysis. J Neurotrauma 22:3–41

Hillered L, Persson L, Nilsson P, Ronne-Engstrom E, Enblad P (2006) Continuous monitoring of cerebral metabolism in traumatic brain injury: a focus on cerebral microdialysis. Curr Opin Crit Care 12:112–118

Hillman J, Aneman O, Anderson C, Sjogren F, Saberg C, Mellergard P (2005) A microdialysis technique for routine measurement of macromolecules in the injured human brain. Neurosurgery 56:1264–1268

Hlatky R, Valadka AB, Goodman JC, Contant CF, Robertson CS (2004) Patterns of energy substrates during ischemia measured in the brain by microdialysis. J Neurotrauma 21:894–906

Howells T, Elf K, Jones P, Ronne-Engström E, Piper I, Nilsson P, Andrews P, Enblad P (2005) Pressure reactivity as a guide in the treatment of cerebral perfusion pressure in patients with brain trauma. J Neurosurg 102:311–317

Hutchinson PJ, Gupta AK, Fryer TF, Al-Rawi PG, Chatfield DA, Coles JP, O'Connell MT, Kett-White R, Minhas PS, Aigbirhio FI, Clark JC, Kirkpatrick PJ, Menon DK, Pickard JD (2002) Correlation between cerebral blood flow, substrate delivery, and metabolism in head injury: a combined microdialysis and triple oxygen positron emission tomography study. J Cereb Blood Flow Metab 22:735–745

Jeremitsky E, Omert LA, Dunham CM, Wilberger J, Rodriguez A (2005) The impact of hyperglycemia on patients with severe brain injury. J Trauma 58:47–50

Kim DJM, Czosnyka Z, Keong N, Radolovich D, Smielewski P, Sutcliffe M, Pickard JD, Czosnyka M (2009) Index of cerebrospinal compensatory reserve in hydrocephalus. Neurosurgery 64:494–502

Leao AA (1947) Further observations on the spreading depression of activity in the cerebral cortex. J Neurophysiol 10:409–414

Lewen A, Hillered L (1998) Involvement of reactive oxygen species in membrane phospholipid breakdown and energy perturbation after traumatic brain injury in the rat. J Neurotrauma 15:521–530

Li PA, Liu GJ, He QP, Floyd RA, Siesjo BK (1999) Production of hydroxyl free radical by brain tissues in hyperglycemic rats subjected to transient forebrain ischemia. Free Radic Biol Med 27:1033–1040

Liu-DeRyke X, Collingridge DS, Orme J, Roller D, Zurasky J, Rhoney DH (2009) Clinical impact of early hyperglycemia during acute phase of traumatic brain injury. Neurocrit Care 11:151–157

Marcoux J, McArthur DA, Miller C, Glenn TC, Villablanca P, Martin NA, Hovda DA, Alger JR, Vespa PM (2008) Persistent metabolic crisis as measured by elevated cerebral microdialysis lactate-pyruvate ratio predicts chronic frontal lobe brain atrophy after traumatic brain injury. Crit Care Med 36:2871–2877

Marklund S, Salci K, Lewén A, Hillered L (1997) Glycerol as a marker for post-traumatic membrane phospholipid degradation in rat brain. Neuroreport 8: 1457–1461

Marklund N, Blennow K, Zetterberg H, Ronne-Engstrom E, Enblad P, Hillered L (2009) Monitoring of brain interstitial total tau and beta amyloid proteins by microdialysis in patients with traumatic brain injury. J Neurosurg 110:1227–1237

Marmarou A, Shulman K, La Morgese J (1975) Compartmental analysis of compliance and outflow resistance of the CSF system. J Neurosurg 43: 523–534

Maurer MH (2010) Proteomics of brain extracellular fluid (ECF) and cerebrospinal fluid (CSF). Mass Spectrom Rev 29:17–28

Meierhans R, Bechir M, Ludwig S, Sommerfeld J, Brandi G, Haberthür C, Stocker R, Stover JF (2010) Brain metabolism is significantly impaired at blood glucose below 6 mM and brain glucose below 1 mM in patients with severe traumatic brain injury. Crit Care 14:R13

Mellergard P, Sjogren F, Hillman J (2010) Release of VEGF and FGF in the extracellular space following severe subarachnoidal haemorrhage or traumatic head injury in humans. Br J Neurosurg 24:261–267

Merenda A, Gugliotta M, Holloway R, Levasseur JE, Alessandri B, Sun D, Bullock MR (2008) Validation of brain extracellular glycerol as an indicator of cellular membrane damage due to free radical activity after traumatic brain injury. J Neurotrauma 25:527–537

Nilsson P, Hillered L, Ponten U, Ungerstedt U (1990) Changes in cortical extracellular levels of energy related metabolites and amino acids following concussive brain injury in rats. J Cereb Blood Flow Metab 10:631–637

Oddo M, Schmidt JM, Carrera E, Badjatia N, Connolly ES, Presciutti M, Ostapkovich ND, Levine JM, Le Roux P, Mayer SA (2008) Impact of tight glycemic control on cerebral glucose metabolism after severe brain injury: a microdialysis study. Crit Care Med 36: 3233–3238

Peerdeman SM, van Tulder MW, Vandertop WP (2003) Cerebral microdialysis as a monitoring method in subarachnoid hemorrhage patients, and correlation with clinical events – a systematic review. J Neurol 250:797–805

Persson L, Hillered L (1996) Intracerebral microdialysis. J Neurosurg 85:984–985

Persson L, Hillered L (1992) Chemical monitoring of neurosurgical intensive care patients using intracerebral rnicrodialysis. J Neurosurg 76:72–80

Purins K, Sedigh A, Molnar C, Jansson L, Korsgren O, Lorant T, Tufveson G, Wennberg L, Wiklund L, Lewén A, Enblad P (2011) Standardized experimental brain death model for studies of intracranial dynamics, organ preservation, and organ transplantation in the pig. Crit Care Med 39:512–517

Reinstrup P, Stahl N, Mellergard P, Uski T, Ungerstedt U, Nordstrom CH (2000) Intracerebral microdialysis in clinical practice: baseline values for chemical markers during wakefulness, anesthesia, and neurosurgery. Neurosurgery 47:701–709

Robertson CS, Narayan RK, Contant CF, Grossman RG, Gokaslan ZL, Pahwa R, Caram P, Bray RS, Sherwood A (1989) Clinical experience with a continuous monitor of intracranial compliance. J Neurosurg 71: 673–680

Rosner MJ, Rosner SD, Johnson AH (1995) Cerebral perfusion pressure: management protocol and clinical results. J Neurosurg 83:949–962

Samuelsson C, Hillered L, Zetterling M, Hesselager G, Johansson M, Lewen A, Marklund N, Nilsson P, Salci K, Enblad P, Kumlien E, Ronne-Engstrom E (2007) Cerebral glutamine and glutamate levels in relation to compromised energy metabolism - a microdialysis study in subarachnoid hemorrhage patients. J Cereb Blood Flow Metab 27:1309–1317

Schulz MK, Wang LP, Tange M, Bjerre P (2000) Cerebral microdialysis monitoring: determination of normal and ischemic cerebral metabolisms in patients with aneurysmal subarachnoid hemorrhage. J Neurosurg 93:808–814

Siesjö BK (1981) Cell damage in the brain: a speculative synthesis. J Cereb Blood Flow Metab 1:155–185

Strong AJ, Fabricius M, Boutelle MG, Hibbins SJ, Hopwood SE, Jones R, Parkin MC, Lauritzen M (2002) Spreading and synchronous depressions of cortical activity in acutely injured human brain. Stroke 33:2738–2743

Timofeev I, Czosnyka M, Nortje J, Smielewski P, Kirkpatrick P, Gupta A, Hutchinson P (2008a) Effect of decompressive craniectomy on intracranial pressure and cerebrospinal compensation following traumatic brain injury. J Neurosurg 108:66–73

Timofeev I, Dahyot-Fizelier C, Keong N, Nortje J, Al-Rawi PG, Czosnyka M, Menon DK, Kirkpatrick PJ, Gupta AK, Hutchinson PJ (2008b) Ventriculostomy for control of raised ICP in acute traumatic brain injury. Acta Neurochir Suppl 102:99–104

Ungerstedt U, Rostami E (2004) Microdialysis in neurointensive care. Curr Pharm Des 10:2145–2152

van den Berghe G, Wouters P, Weekers F, Verwaest C, Bruyninckx F, Schetz M, Vlasselaers D, Ferdinande P, Lauwers P, Bouillon R (2001) Intensive insulin therapy in the critically ill patients. N Engl J Med 345:1359–1367

Van den Berghe G, Wilmer A, Hermans G, Meersseman W, Wouters PJ, Milants I, Van Wijngaerden E, Bobbaers H, Bouillon R (2006) Intensive insulin therapy in the medical ICU. N Engl J Med 354:449–461

Vespa PM, McArthur D, Q'Phelan K, Glenn T, Etchepare M, Kelly D, Bergsneider M, Martin NA, Hovda DA (2003) Persistently low extracellular glucose correlates with poor outcome 6 months after human traumatic brain injury despite a lack of increased lactate: a microdialysis study. J Cereb Blood Flow Metab 23:865–877

Vespa P, Bergsneider M, Hattori N, Wu HM, Huang SC, Martin NA, Glenn TC, McArthur DL, Hovda DA (2005) Metabolic crisis without brain ischemia is common after traumatic brain injury: a combined microdialysis and positron emission tomography study. J Cereb Blood Flow Metab 25:763–774

Vespa P, Boonyaputthikul R, McArthur DL, Miller C, Etchepare M, Bergsneider M, Glenn T, Martin N, Hovda D (2006) Intensive insulin therapy reduces microdialysis glucose values without altering glucose utilization or improving the lactate/pyruvate ratio after traumatic brain injury. Crit Care Med 34:850–856

Wisniewski N, Klitzman B, Miller B, Reichert WM (2001) Decreased analyte transport through implanted membranes: differentiation of biofouling from tissue effects. J Biomed Mater Res 57:513–521

Yau Y, Piper I, Contant C, Citerio G, Kiening K, Enblad P, Nilsson P, Ng S, Wasserberg J, Kiefer M, Poon W, Dunn L, Whittle L (2002) Multi-centre assessment of the Spiegelberg compliance monitor: interim results. Acta Neurochir Suppl 81:167–170

Index

T. Sundstrøm et al. (eds.), *Management of Severe Traumatic Brain Injury*,
DOI 10.1007/978-3-642-28126-6, © Springer-Verlag Berlin Heidelberg 2012

Printed by Publishers' Graphics LLC